FAST FACTS
FOR
NURSES

D0645643

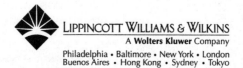

LIPPINCOTT WILLIAMS & WILKINS
A **Wolters Kluwer** Company

Philadelphia • Baltimore • New York • London
Buenos Aires • Hong Kong • Sydney • Tokyo

STAFF

Executive Publisher
Judith A. Schilling McCann, RN, MSN

Editorial Director
H. Nancy Holmes

Clinical Director
Joan M. Robinson, RN, MSN

Senior Art Director
Arlene Putterman

Clinical Project Manager
Mary Perrong, RN, CRNP, MSN, APRN,BC, CPAN

Editor
William Welsh (associate editor)

Clinical Editors
Pamela Kovach, RN, BSN;
Carol Knauff, RN, MSN, CCRN

Copy Editors
Kimberly Bilotta (supervisor),
Tom DeZego, Heather Ditch,
Amy Furman, Dona Hightower,
Carolyn Petersen, Irene Pontarelli,
Pamela Wingrod

Designers
Debra Moloshok (interior design),
Linda Franklin (design project manager),
BJ Crim (cover design)

Digital Composition Services
Diane Paluba (manager), Joyce Rossi Biletz
(senior desktop assistant), Donna S. Morris
(senior desktop assistant)

Manufacturing
Patricia K. Dorshaw (senior manager),
Beth Janae Orr (book production
coordinator)

Editorial Assistants
Megan L. Aldinger, Tara L. Carter-Bell,
Linda K. Ruhf

Librarian
Wani Z. Larsen

Indexer
Ellen S. Brennan

FFN – D N O
05 04   10 9 8 7 6 5 4 3 2

**Library of Congress
Cataloging-in-Publication Data**

Fast facts for nurses.

   p. ; cm.

Includes bibliographical references and index.

   1. Nursing – Handbooks, manuals, etc.

   [DNLM: 1. Nursing Care – methods – Handbooks. WY 49 F251 2003]

I. Lippincott Williams & Wilkins.

   RT51.F37 2003

   610.73 – dc21

ISBN 1-58255-288-6 (alk. paper)   2003013861

CONTENTS

CONTRIBUTORS AND CONSULTANTS

W. Chad Barefoot, MSN, CRNP *Acute Care Nurse Practitioner,* Abington (Pa.) Pulmonary & Critical Care Associates

Nancy P. Blumenthal, MSN, CRNP, CS *Senior Nurse Practitioner, Lung Transplant Program,* University of Pennsylvania Medical Center, Philadelphia

Louise Diehl-Oplinger, RN, MSN, APRN,BC, CLNC, CCRN *Advanced Practice Nurse;* Popkave-Mascarenhas Cardiology; Phillipsburg, N.J.

Diane Dixon, PA-C, MA, MMSc *Assistant Professor,* University of South Alabama, Mobile

Shelba Durston, RN, MSN, CCRN *Adjunct Faculty,* San Joaquin Delta College, Stockton, Calif.; *Staff Nurse,* San Joaquin General Hospital; French Camp, Calif.

M. Susan Emerson, RN, PhD, ANP, BC, CNS *Clinical Assistant Professor and Nurse Practitioner,* University of Missouri — Kansas City

Henry B. Geiter, Jr., RN, CCRN *Adjunct Instructor,* St. Petersburg (Fla.) College; *Critical Care Nurse,* Bayfront Medical Center; *Critical Care Transport,* Sunstar AM

Linda B. Haas, RN, PhC, CDE *Endocrinology Clinical Nurse Specialist,* Veterans Administration Puget South Health Care System, Seattle

René Jackson, RN, BSN, RN *Special Procedures;* Charlotte Regional Medical Center; Punta Gorda, Fla.

Nancy Banfield Johnson, RN, MSN (ANP–inactive), *Nurse Manager,* Kendal at Ithaca (N.Y.)

Kay Luft, MN, CCRN, TNCCP *Assistant Professor;* Saint Luke's College; Kansas City, Mo.

Barbara Maxwell, RNC, MSN *Instructor of Nursing,* State University of New York — Ulster, Stone Ridge

Deanna H. McCarthy, RN, MSN, CCRN *Consultant;* King of Prussia, Pa.

Debi Murphy, MSN, CRNP *Stroke Program Research Coordinator,* Abington (Pa.) Memorial Hospital

Amy C. Shay, RN, MS, CCRN *Staff RN, CT/SICU;* Miami Valley Hospital; Dayton, Ohio

Concha Sitter, MS, APN, CGRN, FNP *GI Nurse Practitioner,* Sterling (Ill.) Rock Falls Clinic

Allison J. Terry, RN, MSN *Staff Development Coordinator;* Beverly Healthcare — Tyson; Montgomery, Ala.

Cynthia Wagner, MS, RNC, CNS *Gerontological Clinical Nurse Specialist;* Doctors Hospital; Columbus, Ohio

Patricia Walters, RN, MSN, APN-C, CCRN *Advanced Practice Nurse — Cardiac Surgery,* Hackensack (N.J.) University Medical Center

Abby Wojahn, RN, BSN *Medical Transcription,* St. Francis Hospital, Milwaukee

FOREWORD

In many ways, this new century represents paradoxes. As health care professionals, we find ourselves in the midst of incredible growth of scientific knowledge, yet have an awareness that we're only in our infancy as far as understanding the complexity of the human body. We're striving for and developing new technology, new equipment, procedures, and tools that tap into our body's secrets. At the same time, we're returning to the earth, herbs, and spirituality. According to the Gallup poll, we are viewed as one of the most respected professionals in the United States, yet we're in the midst of a national shortage in nursing. We're living longer but now have an increasing number of multisystem diseases and co-morbidities.

As a result of this ever-increasing growth, we need to know more, work faster, and do everything in less time. We need to think differently than we did in the last century. We need to multitask, not only procedures but data. We need to acknowledge that the challenges we face will require us to retool ourselves over and over again.

How will you meet the challenges ahead? One of the first ways is to acknowledge that you'll be faced daily with questions that stretch your capacity, techniques that require your senses to be attuned differently, and conflicting data that require a deeper level of analysis. Once you recognize that you must always keep growing, learning, and practicing, you'll prepare yourself with resources to achieve that goal. For those questions you have "in the moment," you'll need to arm yourself with reliable, timely, concise, and condensed information that will inform, alert, and cue you on the spot.

Fast Facts for Nurses is just such a timesaving resource. This remarkable book is jam-packed with illustrations, charts, warnings, and content that's practical and applied. From the basics of lung sounds, to the specialty of managing renal transplant rejection, this book covers it all.

For example, how many of us thought we were well versed in infection control practices? Then SARS came along and woke us up. The speed with which emerging diseases can travel the globe means that we must be able to respond quickly to new health threats. We need sources that will quickly review the difference among droplet, airborne, and contact precautions and the measures we should institute based on patients' symptomatology — not the organism, because we may not know the organism's identity at the start. Infection control is one of many important topics covered just in the Fundamentals chapter alone. This chapter reviews the indications for precautions as well as the recommended barriers and the Centers for Disease Control and Prevention isolation precautions.

Following this are chapters on administering and monitoring drug therapy, including I.V. therapy, anesthesia drugs, blood products. A large part of these chapters involves anticipating, preventing, and managing possible adverse reactions, including drug interactions and latex allergies.

Perhaps best of all, *Fast Facts for Nurses* includes answers to the most frequently asked clinical questions. For example, all nurses know not to crush time-released or enteric-coated medications, but what other drugs shouldn't be crushed? When your patient goes into renal failure, what drugs do you withhold, or alter, or ask to be discontinued? The answers to these questions and so much more are found in the drug therapy chapter.

Another chapter deals solely with older patients and their special needs.

Nine chapters cover the variety of information you need for specific body systems. Each chapter reviews assessment, diagnostic tests, diseases, treatments, procedures and equipment as well as common drugs for the subject body system.

Fast Facts for Nurses is packed with quick-review tables, flow charts, lists, and illustrations that will give you the answers you need — *fast*. A graphic icon, *Alert*, draws your eye right to critical facts, and illustrations make information perfectly clear.

Throughout this book, you'll find "need-to-know" answers for every area of your nursing practice. This handy reference will be worth its weight in gold on your nursing unit and in your pocket. *Fast Facts for Nurses* is a welcome aid to prepare yourself for the 21st century.

Linda Honan Pellico, RN, MSN, CCRN
Lecturer, Yale University School of Nursing

1

FUNDAMENTALS

INFECTION CONTROL PRACTICES

CDC ISOLATION PRECAUTIONS

The Centers for Disease Control and Prevention (CDC) and the Hospital Infection Control Practices Advisory Committee developed the CDC Guideline for Isolation Precautions in Hospitals to help hospitals maintain up-to-date isolation practices.

Standard precautions

The latest (1997) guidelines contain two tiers of precautions. The first—called standard precautions—are to be used when caring for all hospital patients, regardless of their diagnoses or presumed infections. Standard precautions are the primary strategy for preventing nosocomial infection and replace the earlier, universal precautions. Standard precautions refer to protection from:
- blood
- all body fluids, secretions, and excretions except sweat, regardless of whether they contain visible blood
- skin that isn't intact
- mucous membranes.

Transmission-based precautions

The second tier is known as transmission-based precautions. These precautions are instituted when caring for patients with known or suspected highly transmissible infections that necessitate more stringent precautions than those described in the standard precautions. There are three types of transmission-based precautions: airborne precau-

tions, droplet precautions, and contact precautions.

Airborne precautions

Airborne precautions reduce the risk of airborne transmission of infectious agents. Microorganisms carried through the air can be dispersed widely by air currents, making them available for inhalation or deposit on a susceptible host in the same room or a longer distance away from the infected patient. Airborne precautions include special air-handling and ventilation procedures to prevent the spread of infection. They require the use of respiratory protection, such as a mask—in addition to standard precautions—when entering an infected patient's room.

Droplet precautions

Droplet precautions reduce the risk of transmitting infectious agents in large-particle (exceeding 5 micrometers) droplets. Such transmission involves the contact of infectious agents to the conjunctivae or nasal or oral mucous membranes of a susceptible person. Large-particle droplets don't remain in the air

(continued)

CDC ISOLATION PRECAUTIONS *(continued)*

and generally travel short distances of 3' (0.9 m) or less. They require the use of a mask — in addition to standard precautions — to protect the mucous membranes.

Contact precautions

Contact precautions reduce the risk of transmitting infectious agents by direct or indirect contact. Direct-contact transmission can occur through patient care activities that require physical contact. Indirect-contact transmission involves a susceptible host coming in contact with a contaminated object, usually inanimate, in the patient's environment. Contact precautions include the use of gloves, a mask, and a gown — in addition to standard precautions — to avoid contact with the infectious agent. Stringent hand washing is also necessary after removing the protective items.

INDICATIONS FOR AIRBORNE PRECAUTIONS

Disease	Precautionary period
Chickenpox (varicella)	Until lesions are crusted and no new lesions appear
Herpes zoster (disseminated)	Duration of illness
Herpes zoster (localized in immunocompromised patient)	Duration of illness
Measles (rubeola)	Duration of illness
Smallpox (variola major)	Duration of illness, until all scabs fall off
Tuberculosis (TB) — pulmonary or laryngeal, confirmed or suspected	Depends on clinical response; patient must be on effective therapy, be improving clinically (decreased cough and fever and improved findings on chest radiograph), and have three consecutive negative sputum smears collected on different days, or TB must be ruled out.

INDICATIONS FOR DROPLET PRECAUTIONS

Disease	Precautionary period
Adenovirus infection in infants and young children	Duration of illness
Diphtheria (pharyngeal)	Until off antibiotics and two cultures taken at least 24 hours apart are negative
Influenza	Duration of illness
Invasive *Haemophilus influenzae* type B disease, including meningitis, pneumonia, and sepsis	Until 24 hours after initiation of effective therapy
Invasive *Neisseria meningitidis* disease, including meningitis, pneumonia, epiglottiditis, and sepsis	Until 24 hours after initiation of effective therapy
Mumps	For 9 days after onset of swelling
Mycoplasma pneumoniae infection	Duration of illness
Parvovirus B19	Maintain precautions for duration of hospitalization when chronic disease occurs in an immunodeficient patient. For patients with transient aplastic crisis or red-cell crisis, maintain precautions for 7 days.
Pertussis	Until 5 days after initiation of effective therapy
Pneumonic plague	Until 72 hours after initiation of effective therapy
Rubella (German measles)	Until 7 days after onset of rash
Streptococcal pharyngitis, pneumonia, or scarlet fever in infants and young children	Until 24 hours after initiation of effective therapy

INDICATIONS FOR CONTACT PRECAUTIONS

Disease	Precautionary period
Acute viral (acute hemorrhagic) conjunctivitis	Duration of illness
Clostridium difficile enteric infection	Duration of illness
Diphtheria (cutaneous)	Duration of illness
Enteroviral infection, in diapered or incontinent patient	Duration of illness
Escherichia coli disease, in diapered or incontinent patient	Duration of illness
Hepatitis A, in diapered or incontinent patient	Duration of illness
Herpes simplex virus infection (neonatal or mucocutaneous)	Duration of illness
Impetigo	Until 24 hours after initiation of effective therapy
Infection or colonization with multidrug-resistant bacteria	Until off antibiotics and culture is negative
Major abscesses, cellulitis, or pressure ulcer	Until 24 hours after initiation of effective therapy
Parainfluenza virus infection, in diapered or incontinent patients	Duration of illness
Pediculosis (lice)	Until 24 hours after initiation of effective therapy
Respiratory syncytial virus infection, in infants and young children	Duration of illness
Rotavirus infection, in diapered or incontinent patient	Duration of illness
Rubella, congenital syndrome	Precautions during any admission until infant is 1 year old, unless nasopharyngeal and urine cultures negative for virus after age 3 months
Scabies	Until 24 hours after initiation of effective therapy

INDICATIONS FOR CONTACT PRECAUTIONS *(continued)*

Disease	Precautionary period
Shigellosis, in diapered or incontinent patient	Duration of illness
Smallpox	Duration of illness; requires airborne precautions
Staphylococcal furunculosis, in infants and young children	Duration of illness
Viral hemorrhagic infections (Ebola, Lassa, Marburg)	Duration of illness
Zoster (chickenpox, disseminated zoster, or localized zoster in immunodeficient patient)	Until all lesions are crusted; requires airborne precautions

RECOMMENDED BARRIERS TO INFECTION

The list here presents the minimum requirements for using gloves, gowns, masks, and eye protection to avoid coming in contact with and spreading pathogens. In addition to washing your hands thoroughly in all cases, refer to your facility guidelines and use your judgment when assessing the need for barrier protection in specific situations.

Key

Gloves

Gown

Mask

Eyewear

Bathing, for patient with open lesions

if soiling likely

Bedding, changing visibly soiled

if soiling likely

Bleeding or pressure application to control it

if soiling likely

if splattering likely

if splattering likely

(continued)

FUNDAMENTALS

RECOMMENDED BARRIERS TO INFECTION *(continued)*

Blood glucose (capillary) testing

Cardiopulmonary resuscitation

 if splattering likely

 if splattering likely

 if splattering likely

Central venous line insertion and venesection

Chest drainage system change

 if splattering likely

 if splattering likely

 if splattering likely

Chest tube insertion or removal

 if soiling likely

 if splattering likely

 if splattering likely

Cleaning (feces, spilled blood or body substances, or surface contaminated by blood or body fluids)

 if soiling likely

Colonoscopy, flexible sigmoidoscope

Coughing, frequent and forceful by patient; direct contact with secretions

Dialysis, peritoneal (initiating acute treatment, performing an exchange, terminating acute treatment, dismantling tubing from cycler, discarding peritoneal drainage, irrigating peritoneal catheter, changing tubing, or assisting with insertion of acute peritoneal catheter outside sterile field)

 if splattering likely

 if splattering likely

Dressing change for burns

Dressing removal or change for wounds with little or no drainage

RECOMMENDED BARRIERS TO INFECTION *(continued)*

Dressing removal or change for wounds with large amounts of drainage

  if soiling likely

Emptying drainage receptacles, including suction containers, urine receptacles, bedpans, emesis basins

  if soiling likely

  if splattering likely

  if splattering likely

Enema

  if soiling likely

Fecal impaction, removal of

Fecal incontinence, placement of in-dwelling catheter for, and emptying bag of

  if splattering likely

I.V. or intra-arterial line (insertion, removal, tubing change at catheter hub)

Intubation or extubation

  if splattering likely

  if splattering likely

  if splattering likely

Invasive procedures (lumbar puncture, bone marrow aspiration, paracentesis, liver biopsy) outside the sterile field

Irrigation, wound

  if soiling likely

  if splattering likely

  if splattering likely

Nasogastric tube, insertion or irrigation

  if soiling likely

  if splattering likely

(continued)

RECOMMENDED BARRIERS TO INFECTION *(continued)*

Nasogastric tube, insertion or irrigation *(continued)*

 if splattering likely

Ostomy care, irrigation, and teaching

 if soiling likely .

Pelvic examination and Papanicolaou test

Postmortem care

 if soiling likely

Pressure ulcer care

Specimen collection (blood, stool, urine, sputum, wound)

Suctioning, nasotracheal or endo-tracheal

 if soiling likely

 if splattering likely

 if splattering likely

Suctioning, oral or nasal

Tracheostomy suctioning and cannula cleaning

 if soiling likely

 if splattering likely

 if splattering likely

Tracheostomy tube change

 if splattering likely

 if splattering likely

Urine and stool testing

Wound packing

 if soiling likely

REPORTABLE DISEASES AND INFECTIONS

The Centers for Disease Control and Prevention (CDC), the Occupational Safety and Health Administration, the Joint Commission on Accreditation of Healthcare Organizations, and the American Hospital Association all require health care facilities to document and report certain diseases acquired in the community or in hospitals and other health care facilities.

Generally, the health care facility reports diseases to the appropriate local authorities. These authorities notify the state health department, which in turn reports the diseases to the appropriate federal agency or national organization.

The list of diseases that appears below is the CDC's list of nationally notifiable infectious diseases for 2003. Each state also keeps a list of reportable diseases appropriate to its region.

■ Acquired immunodeficiency syndrome (AIDS)
■ Anthrax
■ Botulism (food-borne, infant, other [wound and unspecified])
■ Brucellosis
■ Chancroid
■ *Chlamydia trachomatis*, genital infections
■ Cholera
■ Coccidioidomycosis
■ Cryptosporidiosis
■ Cyclosporiasis
■ Diphtheria
■ Ehrlichiosis (human granulocytic, human monocytic, human [other or unspecified agent])
■ Encephalitis/meningitis: arboviral California serogroup viral, eastern equine, Powassan, St. Louis, western equine, West Nile)
■ Enterohemorrhagic *Escherichia coli* (O157:H7, Shiga toxin positive [serogroup non-O157], Shiga toxin positive [not serogrouped])

■ Giardiasis
■ Gonorrhea
■ *Haemophilus influenzae*, invasive disease
■ Hansen's disease (leprosy)
■ *Hantavirus* pulmonary syndrome
■ Hemolytic uremic syndrome, postdiarrheal
■ Hepatitis, viral, acute (hepatitis A acute, hepatitis B acute, hepatitis B virus perinatal infection, hepatitis C acute)
■ Hepatitis, viral, chronic (chronic hepatitis B, hepatitis C virus infection [past or present])
■ Human immunodeficiency virus (adult ≥ 13 years], pediatric [< 13 years])
■ *Legionella* infections (legionnaires' disease)
■ Listeriosis
■ Lyme disease
■ Malaria
■ Measles
■ Meningococcal disease
■ Mumps
■ Pertussis
■ Plague
■ Poliomyelitis (paralytic)
■ Psittacosis (ornithosis)
■ Q fever
■ Rabies (animal, human)
■ Rocky Mountain spotted fever
■ Rubella (German measles) and congenital syndrome
■ Salmonellosis
■ Severe acute respiratory syndrome
■ Shigellosis
■ Streptococcal disease, invasive, Group A
■ Streptococcal toxic shock syndrome
■ *Streptococcus pneumoniae*, drug-resistant, invasive disease
■ *Streptococcus pneumoniae*, invasive, in children ages < 5 years
■ Syphilis (primary; secondary; latent; early latent; late latent; latent unknown duration; neurosyphilis; late nonneurologic)

(continued)

FUNDAMENTALS

REPORTABLE DISEASES AND INFECTIONS *(continued)*

- Syphilis, congenital (syphilitic still-birth)
- Tetanus
- Toxic shock syndrome
- Trichinosis
- Tuberculosis

- Tularemia
- Typhoid fever
- Varicella (morbidity)
- Varicella (deaths only)
- Yellow fever

HAND HYGIENE AND HAND RUBS

In 2002, the Centers for Disease Control and Prevention (CDC) published its *Guideline for Hand Hygiene in Health Care Settings*. Hand hygiene is a general term that refers to hand washing, antiseptic hand washing, antiseptic hand rubs, and surgical hand antisepsis.

Hand washing

Redefined by the CDC guideline, hand washing refers to washing hands with plain (such as nonantimicrobial) soap and water. Use of an antiseptic agent (such as chlorhexidine, triclosan, or iodophor) to wash hands is an *antiseptic* hand wash. Hand washing is appropriate whenever the hands are soiled or contaminated with infectious material. Surgical personnel preoperatively perform surgical hand antisepsis to eliminate transient bacteria and reduce resident hand flora. Whether it involves a plain or antiseptic agent, hand washing is still the single most effective method to prevent the spread of infection.

Hand rubs

Hand hygiene also includes the use of rubs or hand sanitizers. An antiseptic hand rub involves applying an antiseptic, alcohol-containing product designed to reduce the number of viable microorganisms on the skin to all surfaces of the hands and rubbing until the product has dried (usually within 30 seconds). These products are also referred to as waterless antiseptic agents because no water is required. Alcohol hand rubs usually contain emollients to prevent skin drying and chapping. Hand rubs and sanitizers are appropriate for decontaminating the hands after minimal contamination.

WOUND AND SKIN CARE

STAGING PRESSURE ULCERS

The staging system described here is based on the recommendations of the National Pressure Ulcer Advisory Panel (NPUAP) (Consensus Conference, 1991) and the Agency for Health Care Policy and Research (Clinical Practice Guidelines for Treatment of Pressure Ulcers, 1992). The stage I definition was updated by the NPUAP in 1997.

Stage I

A stage I pressure ulcer is an observable pressure-related alteration of intact skin. The indicators, compared with the adjacent or opposite area on the body, may include changes in one or more of the following factors: skin temperature (warmth or coolness), tissue consistency (firm or boggy feel), or sensation (pain or itching). The ulcer appears as a defined area of persistent redness in lightly pigmented skin; in darker skin, the ulcer may appear with persistent red, blue, or purple hues.

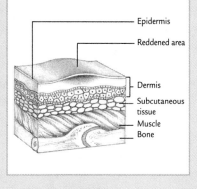

Stage II

A stage II pressure ulcer is characterized by partial-thickness skin loss involving the epidermis or dermis. The ulcer is superficial and appears as an abrasion, blister, or shallow crater.

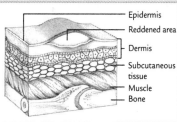

Stage III

A stage III pressure ulcer is characterized by full-thickness skin loss involving damage or necrosis of subcutaneous tissue, which may extend down to, but not through, the underlying fascia. The ulcer appears as a deep crater with or without undermining of adjacent tissue.

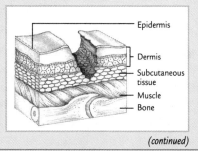

(continued)

FUNDAMENTALS

STAGING PRESSURE ULCERS (continued)

Stage IV

Full-thickness skin loss with extensive destruction, tissue necrosis, or damage to muscle, bone, or support structures (for example, tendon or joint capsule) characterize a stage IV pressure ulcer. Tunneling and sinus tracts may also be associated with stage IV pressure ulcers.

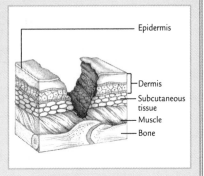

TAILORING WOUND CARE TO WOUND COLOR

With any wound, you can promote healing by keeping the wound moist, clean, and free from debris. For open wounds, using wound color can guide the specific management approach to aid healing.

Wound color	Management technique
Red	■ Cover the wound, keep it moist and clean, and protect it from trauma. ■ Use a transparent dressing (such as Tegaderm or OpSite) over a gauze dressing moistened with normal saline solution, or use a hydrogel, foam, or hydrocolloid dressing to insulate and protect the wound.
Yellow	■ Clean the wound and remove the yellow layer. ■ Cover the wound with a moisture-retentive dressing such as a hydrogel or foam dressing or a moist gauze dressing with or without a debriding enzyme. ■ Consider hydrotherapy with whirlpool or pulsatile lavage.
Black	■ Debride the wound as ordered. Use an enzyme product (such as Accuzyme or Panafil), conservative sharp debridement, or hydrotherapy with whirlpool or pulsatile lavage. ■ For wounds with inadequate blood supply and noninfected heel ulcers, don't debride. Keep them clean and dry.

PRESSURE POINTS: COMMON SITES FOR ULCERS

Ulcers may develop at pressure points, which are shown in these illustrations. To help prevent them, emphasize the importance of frequent repositioning and carefully checking the skin for any changes.

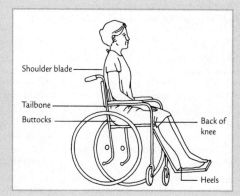

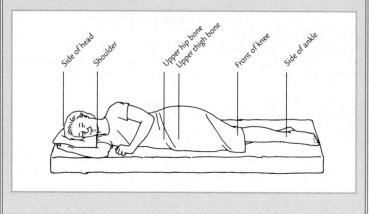

PRESSURE REDUCTION DEVICES

Here are some special pads, mattresses, and beds that help relieve pressure when a patient is confined to one position for long periods.

Gel pads

Gel pads disperse pressure over a wide surface area.

Water mattress or pads

A wave effect provides even distribution of body weight.

Alternating-pressure air mattress

Alternating deflation and inflation of mattress tubes changes areas of pressure.

Foam mattress or pads

Foam areas, which must be at least 3" to 4" (7.6 to 10 cm) thick, cushion skin, minimizing pressure.

Low-air-loss beds

This bed surface consists of inflated air cushions. Each section is adjusted for optimal pressure relief for the patient's body size.

Air-fluidized bed

An air-fluidized bed contains beads that move under an airflow to support the patient, thus reducing shearing force and friction.

Mechanical lifting devices

Lift sheets and other mechanical lifting devices prevent shearing by lifting the patient rather than dragging him across the bed.

Padding

Pillows, towels, and soft blankets can reduce pressure in body hollows.

Foot cradle

A foot cradle lifts the bed linens to relieve pressure over the feet.

PREVENTING SKIN TEARS

As aging occurs, the skin becomes more prone to skin tear injuries. With a little effort and education, you can substantially reduce a patient's risk.

Prevent skin tears by:
- using proper lifting, positioning, transferring, and turning techniques to reduce or eliminate friction or shear
- padding support surfaces where risk is greatest, such as bed rails and limb supports on a wheelchair
- using pillows or cushions to support the patient's arms and legs
- telling the patient to add protection by wearing long-sleeved shirts and long pants, as weather permits
- using nonadhering dressings or those with minimal adherent, such as paper tape, and to use a skin barrier wipe before applying dressings
- removing tape cautiously using the push-pull technique
- using wraps, such as a stockinette or soft gauze, to protect areas of skin where the risk of tearing is high
- telling the patient to avoid sudden or brusque movements that can pull the skin and possibly cause a skin tear
- applying skin lotion twice per day to areas at risk.

WOUND CARE DRESSINGS

Some dressings absorb moisture from a wound bed, whereas others add moisture to it. Use the chart below to quickly determine the category of dressing that's appropriate for your patient.

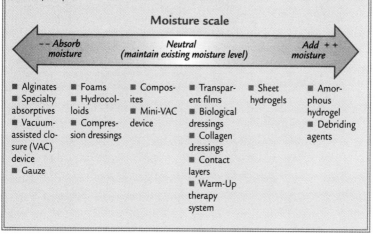

Moisture scale

-- Absorb moisture   *Neutral (maintain existing moisture level)*   Add ++ moisture

■ Alginates ■ Specialty absorptives ■ Vacuum-assisted closure (VAC) device ■ Gauze	■ Foams ■ Hydrocolloids ■ Compression dressings	■ Composites ■ Mini-VAC device	■ Transparent films ■ Biological dressings ■ Collagen dressings ■ Contact layers ■ Warm-Up therapy system	■ Sheet hydrogels	■ Amorphous hydrogel ■ Debriding agents

CHOOSING A WOUND DRESSING

The patient's needs and wound characteristics determine which type of dressing to use on a wound.

Gauze dressings

Made of absorptive cotton or synthetic fabric, gauze dressings are permeable to water, water vapor, and oxygen and may be impregnated with hydrogel or another agent. When uncertain about which dressing to use, you may apply a gauze dressing moistened in saline solution until a wound specialist recommends definitive treatment.

Hydrocolloid dressings

Hydrocolloid dressings are adhesive, moldable wafers made of a carbohydrate-based material and usually have waterproof backings. They're impermeable to oxygen, water, and water vapor, and most have some absorptive properties.

Transparent film dressings

Transparent film dressings are clear, adherent, and nonabsorptive. These polymer-based dressings are permeable to oxygen and water vapor but not to water. Their transparency allows visual inspection. Because they can't absorb drainage, they're used on partial thickness wounds with minimal exudate.

Alginate dressings

Made from seaweed, alginate dressings are nonwoven, absorptive dressings available as soft white sterile pads or ropes. They absorb excessive exudate and may be used on infected wounds. As these dressings absorb exudate, they turn into a gel that keeps the wound bed moist and promotes healing. When exudate is no longer excessive, switch to another type of dressing.

Foam dressings

Foam dressings are spongelike polymer dressings that may be impregnated or coated with other materials. Somewhat absorptive, they may be adherent. These dressings promote moist wound healing and are useful when a nonadherent surface is desired.

Hydrogel dressings

Water-based and nonadherent, hydrogel dressings are polymer-based dressings that have some absorptive properties. They're available as a gel in a tube, as flexible sheets, and as saturated gauze packing strips. They may have a cooling effect, which eases pain, and are used when the wound needs moisture.

CARING FOR A TRAUMATIC WOUND

When treating a patient with a traumatic wound, always begin by assessing the ABCs: airway, breathing, and circulation. Move on to the wound itself only after ABCs are stable. Here are the basic steps to follow in caring for each type of traumatic wound.

Abrasion

■ Flush the area of the abrasion with normal saline solution or wound cleaning solution.

■ Use a sterile 4″ × 4″ gauze pad moistened with normal saline solution to remove dirt or gravel, and gently rub toward the entry point to work contaminants back out the way they entered.

■ If the wound is extremely dirty, you may need to scrub it with a surgical brush. Be as gentle as possible because this is a painful process for your patient.

■ Allow a small wound to dry and form a scab. Cover larger wounds with a non-adherent pad or petroleum gauze and a light dressing. Apply antibacterial ointment if ordered.

Laceration

■ Moisten a sterile 4″ × 4″ gauze pad with normal saline solution or wound cleaning solution. Gently clean the wound, beginning at the center and working out to approximately 2″ (5 cm) beyond the edge of the wound. Whenever the pad becomes soiled, discard it and use a new one. Continue until the wound appears clean.

■ If necessary, irrigate the wound using a 50 ml catheter-tip syringe and normal saline solution.

■ Assist the physician in suturing the wound if necessary; apply sterile strips of porous tape if suturing isn't needed.

■ Apply antibacterial ointment as ordered to prevent infection.

■ Apply a dry sterile dressing over the wound to absorb drainage and help prevent bacterial contamination.

Bite

■ Immediately irrigate the wound with copious amounts of normal saline solution. Don't immerse and soak the wound; this may allow bacteria to float back into the tissue.

■ Clean the wound with sterile 4″ × 4″ gauze pads and an antiseptic solution such as povidone-iodine.

■ Assist with debridement if ordered.

■ Apply a loose dressing. If the bite is on an extremity, elevate it to reduce swelling.

■ Ask the patient about the animal that bit him to determine whether there's a risk of rabies. Administer rabies and tetanus shots as needed.

Penetrating wound

■ If the wound is minor, allow it to bleed for a few minutes before cleaning it. A larger puncture wound may require irrigation.

■ Cover the wound with a dry dressing.

■ If the wound contains an embedded foreign object, such as a shard of glass or metal, stabilize the object until the physician can remove it. When the object is removed and bleeding is under control, clean the wound as you would a laceration.

RECOGNIZING COMMON SKIN LESIONS

Macule

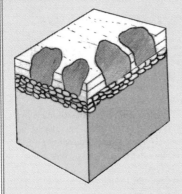

A small (usually less than 1 cm in diameter), flat blemish or discoloration that can be brown, tan, red, or white and has the same texture as surrounding skin

Bulla

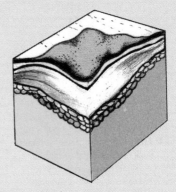

A raised, thin-walled blister greater than 0.5 cm in diameter, containing clear or serous fluid

Vesicle

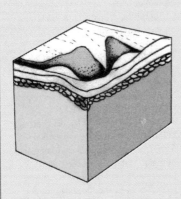

A small (less than 0.5 cm in diameter) thin-walled, raised blister containing clear, serous, purulent, or bloody fluid

Pustule

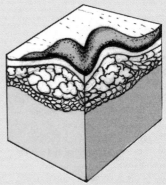

A circumscribed, pus- or lymph-filled elevated lesion that varies in diameter and may be firm or soft, and white or yellow

RECOGNIZING COMMON SKIN LESIONS *(continued)*

Wheal

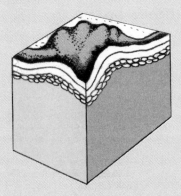

A slightly raised, firm lesion of variable size and shape, surrounded by edema; skin may be red or pale

Nodule

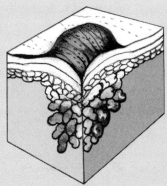

A small, firm, circumscribed, elevated lesion approximately 1 to 2 cm in diameter with possible skin discoloration

Papule

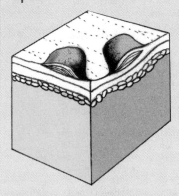

A small, solid, raised lesion less than 1 cm in diameter, with red to purple skin discoloration

Tumor

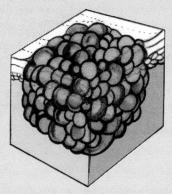

A solid, raised mass usually larger than 2 cm in diameter with possible skin discoloration

NUTRITION

EVALUATING NUTRITIONAL DISORDERS

This chart shows implications for nutritional assessment findings.

Body system or region	Sign or symptom	Implications
General	■ Weakness and fatigue ■ Weight loss	■ Anemia, electrolyte imbalance ■ Decreased calorie intake, increased calorie use, or inadequate nutrient intake or absorption
Skin, hair, and nails	■ Dry, flaky skin ■ Rough, scaly skin with bumps ■ Petechiae or ecchymoses ■ Sore that won't heal ■ Thinning, dry hair ■ Spoon-shaped, brittle, or ridged nails	■ Vitamin A, vitamin B complex, or linoleic acid deficiency ■ Vitamin A deficiency ■ Vitamin C or K deficiency ■ Protein, vitamin C, or zinc deficiency ■ Protein deficiency ■ Iron deficiency
Eyes	■ Night blindness; corneal swelling, softening, or dryness; Bitot's spots ■ Red conjunctiva	■ Vitamin A deficiency ■ Riboflavin deficiency
Throat and mouth	■ Cracks at corner of mouth ■ Magenta tongue ■ Beefy, red tongue ■ Soft, spongy, bleeding gums ■ Swollen neck (goiter)	■ Riboflavin or niacin deficiency ■ Riboflavin deficiency ■ Vitamin B_{12} deficiency ■ Vitamin C deficiency ■ Iodine deficiency
Cardiovascular	■ Edema ■ Tachycardia, hypotension	■ Protein deficiency ■ Fluid volume deficit
GI	■ Ascites	■ Protein deficiency
Musculoskeletal	■ Bone pain and bow leg ■ Muscle wasting	■ Vitamin D or calcium deficiency ■ Protein, carbohydrate, and fat deficiency
Neurologic	■ Altered mental status ■ Paresthesia	■ Dehydration and thiamine or vitamin B_{12} deficiency ■ Vitamin B_{12}, pyridoxine, or thiamine deficiency

HOW TO TAKE
ANTHROPOMETRIC ARM MEASUREMENTS

Follow this procedure when measuring midarm circumference, triceps skin-fold thickness, and midarm muscle circumference.

1. Locate the midpoint on the patient's upper arm using a nonstretching tape measure, and mark the midpoint with a felt-tip pen.

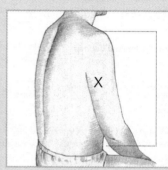

2. Determine the triceps skin-fold thickness by grasping the patient's skin between thumb and forefinger approximately 1 cm above the midpoint. Place the calipers at the midpoint and squeeze the calipers for about 3 seconds. Record the measurement registered on the handle gauge to the nearest 0.5 mm. Take two more readings; then average all three to compensate for possible error.

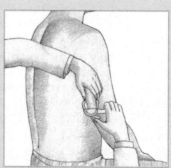

3. From the midpoint, measure the midarm circumference. Calculate midarm muscle circumference by multiplying the triceps skin-fold thickness (in centimeters) by 3.143 and subtracting the result from the midarm circumference.

4. Record all three measurements as percentages of the standard measurements by using the following formula:

$$\frac{\text{actual measurement}}{\text{standard measurement}} \times 100$$

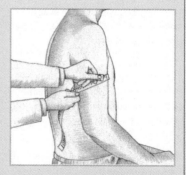

Compare the patient's percentage measurement with the standard. A measurement of less than 90% of the standard indicates caloric deprivation; a measurement of over 90% indicates adequate or more than adequate energy reserves.

(continued)

HOW TO TAKE
ANTHROPOMETRIC ARM MEASUREMENTS *(continued)*

Measurement	Standard	90%
Midarm circumference	*Men:* 29.3 cm *Women:* 28.5 cm	*Men:* 26.4 cm *Women:* 25.7 cm
Triceps skin-fold thickness	*Men:* 12.5 mm *Women:* 16.5 mm	*Men:* 11.3 mm *Women:* 14.9 mm
Midarm muscle circumference	*Men:* 25.3 cm *Women:* 23.2 cm	*Men:* 22.8 cm *Women:* 20.9 cm

Adapted with permission from Blackburn, G., et al. "Nutritional and Metabolic Assessment of the Hospital Patient." *The Journal of Parenteral and Enteral Nutrition* 1(1):11-22, 1977.

TIPS FOR DETECTING NUTRITIONAL PROBLEMS

Nutritional problems may stem from physical conditions, drugs, diet, or lifestyle factors. The list below can help you identify risk factors that make your patient particularly susceptible to nutritional problems.

Physical conditions
■ Chronic illnesses, such as diabetes and neurologic, cardiac, or thyroid problems
■ Family history of diabetes or heart disease
■ Draining wounds or fistulas
■ Weight issues — weight loss of 5% of normal body weight; weight less than 90% of ideal body weight; weight gain or loss of 10 lb or more in last 6 months; obesity; or weight gain of 20% above normal body weight
■ History of GI disturbances
■ Anorexia or bulimia
■ Depression or anxiety
■ Severe trauma
■ Recent chemotherapy or radiation therapy
■ Physical limitations, such as paresis or paralysis
■ Recent major surgery
■ Pregnancy, especially teen or multiple-birth pregnancy

Drugs and diet
■ Fad diets
■ Steroid, diuretic, or antacid use
■ Mouth, tooth, or denture problems
■ Excessive alcohol intake
■ Strict vegetarian diet
■ Liquid diet or nothing by mouth for more than 3 days

Lifestyle factors
■ Lack of support from family or friends
■ Financial problems

MINERAL REQUIREMENTS, DEFICIENCIES, AND TOXICITIES

This table lists the daily requirements of common minerals as well as the signs and symptoms of deficiency and toxicity for each.

Minerals and adult requirements	Signs and symptoms of deficiencies	Signs and symptoms of toxicities
MAJOR MINERALS		
Calcium 1,000 mg (ages 19 to 50) 1,200 mg (> age 50)	■ Arm and leg numbness, brittle fingernails, heart palpitations, insomnia, muscle cramps, osteoporosis	■ Renal calculi, impaired absorption of iron
Chloride 750 mg	■ Disturbance in acid-base balance	■ None
Magnesium *Men:* 400 mg (ages 19 to 39) 420 mg (> age 30) *Women:* 310 mg (ages 19 to 30) 320 mg (> age 30)	■ Confusion, disorientation, nervousness, irritability, rapid pulse, tremors, muscle control loss, neuromuscular dysfunction	■ Cardiac rhythm disturbances, hypotension, respiratory failure
Phosphorus 700 mg	■ Appetite loss, fatigue, irregular breathing, nervous disorders, muscle weakness	■ None
Potassium 2,000 mg	■ Muscular weakness, paralysis, anorexia, confusion, slow irregular heartbeat, weak reflexes	■ Cardiac disturbances, paralysis
Sodium 500 mg	■ Appetite loss, intestinal gas, muscular atrophy, vomiting, weight loss	■ Edema and elevated blood pressure
Sulfur No recommended intake	■ None	■ None
TRACE MINERALS		
Chromium 50 to 200 mcg	■ Glucose intolerance (in diabetic patients)	■ None

(continued)

FUNDAMENTALS

MINERAL REQUIREMENTS, DEFICIENCIES, AND TOXICITIES *(continued)*

Minerals and adult requirements	Signs and symptoms of deficiencies	Signs and symptoms of toxicities
TRACE MINERALS *(continued)*		
Cobalt Unknown	■ Indigestion, diarrhea or constipation, weight loss, fatigue, poor memory	■ None
Copper 1.5 to 3 mg	■ General weakness, impaired respiration, skin sores, bone disease	■ Vomiting, diarrhea
Fluoride *Men:* 3.8 mg *Women:* 3.1 mg	■ Dental caries	■ Mottling and pitting of permanent teeth, increased bone density and calcification
Iodine 150 mcg	■ Cold hands and feet, dry hair, irritability, nervousness, obesity, simple goiter	■ Enlarged thyroid gland
Iron *Men:* 10 mg *Women:* 15 mg (ages 19 to 50) 10 mg (> age 50)	■ Brittle nails, constipation, respiratory problems, tongue soreness or inflammation, anemia, pallor, weakness, cold sensitivity, fatigue	■ Abdominal cramps and pains, nausea, vomiting, hemosiderosis, hemochromatosis
Manganese 2 to 5 mg	■ Ataxia, dizziness, hearing disturbance or loss	■ Severe neuromuscular disturbances
Molybdenum 45 mcg	■ None	■ Headache, dizziness, heartburn, weakness, nausea, vomiting, diarrhea
Selenium 55 mcg	■ None	■ Nausea, vomiting, abdominal pain, hair and nail changes, nerve damage, fatigue
Zinc *Men:* 11 mg *Women:* 8 mg	■ Delayed sexual maturity, fatigue, smell and taste loss, poor appetite, prolonged wound healing, slowed growth, skin disorders	■ Anemia, impaired calcium absorption, fever, muscle pain, dizziness, reproductive failure

VITAMIN REQUIREMENTS, DEFICIENCIES, AND TOXICITIES

This table lists the daily requirements of common vitamins as well as the signs and symptoms of deficiency and toxicity for each.

Vitamins and adult requirements	Signs and symptoms of deficiencies	Signs and symptoms of toxicities
WATER-SOLUBLE VITAMINS		
Vitamin B$_1$ (thiamine) *Men:* 1.2 mg *Women:* 1.1 mg	■ Beriberi (fatigue, muscle weakness, confusion, edema, enlarged heart, heart failure)	■ None
Vitamin B$_2$ (riboflavin) *Men:* 1.3 mg *Women:* 1.1 mg	■ Ariboflavinosis (dermatitis, glossitis, photophobia)	■ None
Vitamin B$_3$ (niacin) *Men:* 16 mg *Women:* 14 mg	■ Pellagra (dermatitis, diarrhea, dementia, death)	■ Flushing, gastric ulcers, low blood pressure, nausea, vomiting, diarrhea, liver damage
Vitamin B$_6$ (pyridoxine) *Men:* 1.3 mg (< age 50) 1.7 mg (> age 50) *Women:* 1.3 mg (< age 50) 1.5 mg (> age 50)	■ Dermatitis, glossitis, seizures, anemia	■ Depression, irritability, headaches, fatigue
Vitamin B$_{12}$ (cobalamin) 2.4 mcg	■ Indigestion, diarrhea or constipation, weight loss, macrocytic anemia, fatigue, poor memory, irritability, paresthesia of hands and feet	■ None
Vitamin C (ascorbic acid) *Men:* 90 mg *Women:* 75 mg	■ Scurvy (bleeding gums, delayed wound healing, hemorrhaging, softening of the bones, easy fractures)	■ Diarrhea, nausea, headaches, fatigue, hot flashes, insomnia

(continued)

VITAMIN REQUIREMENTS, DEFICIENCIES, AND TOXICITIES *(continued)*

Vitamins and adult requirements	Signs and symptoms of deficiencies	Signs and symptoms of toxicities
FAT-SOLUBLE VITAMINS		
Biotin 30 mcg	■ Anorexia, fatigue, depression, dry skin, heart abnormalities	■ None
Folate (folic acid) 400 mcg	■ Diarrhea, macrocytic anemia, confusion, depression, fatigue	■ Masks vitamin B_{12} deficiency
Pantothenic acid 5 mg	■ General failure of all body systems	■ None
FAT-SOLUBLE VITAMINS		
Vitamin A (retinol) *Men:* 1,000 mcg retinol equivalents *Women:* 800 mcg retinol equivalents	■ Night blindness, bone growth cessation, dry skin, decreased saliva, diarrhea	■ Headaches, vomiting, double vision, hair loss, liver damage
Vitamin D (calciferol) 5 mcg (≤ age 50) 10 mcg (ages 51 to 70) 15 mcg (≥ age 70)	■ Rickets (retarded bone growth, bone malformations, decreased serum calcium, abdominal protrusion); osteomalacia (softening of bones, decreased serum calcium, muscle twitching)	■ Renal calculi, kidney damage, muscle and bone weakness, excessive bleeding, headache, excessive thirst
Vitamin E (tocopherol) 15 mg	■ Red blood cell hemolysis, edema, skin lesions	■ None
Vitamin K (menadione) *Men:* 80 mcg *Women:* 65 mcg	■ Hemorrhaging	■ None

FAT: GOOD, BAD, AND WORST

Fats (fatty acids) come in many varieties — some good, some bad, and some really bad. To help your patient plan a heart-healthy diet, make sure you understand the various types.

Good
Monounsaturated fats
Monounsaturated fats are found mainly in canola oil, olive oil, peanut oil, and avocados. These fats are liquid at room temperature.

Polyunsaturated fats
Polyunsaturated fats are found in soybean, sesame, sunflower, and safflower seeds and their oils. They're also the main fats found in seafood. These fats are liquid or soft at room temperature. Specific polyunsaturated fatty acids, such as linoleic acid and alpha-linoleic acid, are called *essential fatty acids* because they're necessary for cell structure and making hormones. Essential fatty acids must be obtained from foods.

Bad
Saturated fats
Saturated fats are found chiefly in animal sources, such as meat, poultry, whole or reduced-fat milk, and butter. Some vegetable oils, such as coconut, palm kernel oil, and palm oil, are saturated. Saturated fats are usually solid at room temperature.

Dietary cholesterol
Dietary cholesterol is found in foods of animal origin, such as meat, pork, poultry, fish, eggs, and full-fat dairy products.

Worst
Trans fatty acids
Trans fatty acids (trans-fats, for short) form when vegetable oils are processed into margarine or shortening. Sources of trans-fats in the diet include snack foods and baked goods made with partially hydrogenated vegetable oil or vegetable shortening. Trans fatty acids also occur naturally in some animal products such as dairy products.

POTASSIUM-RICH FOODS

Fruits
- Avocados
- Bananas
- Cantaloupe
- Grapefruit juice
- Honeydew melon
- Oranges
- Orange juice
- Fresh peaches
- Dried fruit

Beans
- Baked beans
- Black beans
- Black-eyed peas
- Butter beans
- Chickpeas
- Crowder peas
- Great Northern beans
- Kidney beans
- Lentils
- Lima beans
- Navy beans
- Pinto beans
- Split peas

Vegetables
- Broccoli
- Greens
- Spinach
- Tomatoes
- Tomato soup
- Tomato juice

Potatoes
- Baked white potato
- Baked sweet potato
- Potato chips
- French fries

- Instant potato mixes
- Home fries
- Yams

Miscellaneous foods
- Molasses
- Nuts
- Salt substitutes

TIPS TO REDUCE SODIUM INTAKE

Only a small amount of sodium occurs naturally in foods. Most sodium is added to foods during processing. To help your patient cut down on sodium intake, provide the following suggestions.

Read labels
- Read food labels for sodium content.
- Use food products with reduced sodium or no added salt.
- Be aware that soy sauce, broth, and foods that are pickled or cured have high sodium contents.

Cook wisely
- Instead of cooking with salt, use herbs, spices, cooking wines, lemon, lime, or vinegar to enhance food flavors.
- Cook pasta and rice without salt.
- Rinse canned foods, such as tuna, to remove some sodium.

- Avoid adding salt to foods, especially at the table.
- Avoid condiments such as soy and teriyaki sauces and monosodium glutamate (MSG) — or use lower-sodium versions.

Watch your diet
- Eat fresh poultry, fish, and lean meat rather than canned, smoked, or processed versions (which typically contain a lot of sodium).
- Whenever possible, eat fresh foods rather than canned or convenience foods.
- Limit intake of cured foods (such as bacon and ham), foods packed in brine (pickles, olives, and sauerkraut) and condiments (mustard, ketchup, horseradish, and Worcestershire sauce).
- When dining out, ask how food is prepared. Ask that your food be prepared without added salt or MSG.

PAIN MANAGEMENT

PQRST: THE ALPHABET OF PAIN ASSESSMENT

Use the PQRST mnemonic device to obtain more information about the patient's pain. Asking the questions below elicits important details about his pain.

P rovocative or palliative
Ask the patient:
- What provokes or worsens your pain?
- What relieves or causes the pain to subside?

Q uality or quantity
Ask the patient:
- What does the pain feel like? Is it aching, intense, knifelike, burning, or cramping?
- Are you having pain right now? If so, is it more or less severe than usual?
- To what degree does the pain affect your normal activities?
- Do you have other symptoms along with the pain, such as nausea or vomiting?

R egion and radiation
Ask the patient:
- Where is your pain?
- Does the pain radiate to other parts of your body?

S everity
Ask the patient:
- How severe is your pain? How would you rate it on a 0-to-10 scale, with 0 being no pain and 10 being the worst pain imaginable?
- How would you describe the intensity of your pain at its best? At its worst? Right now?

T iming
Ask the patient:
- When did your pain begin?
- At what time of day is your pain best? What time is it worst?
- Is the onset sudden or gradual?
- Is the pain constant or intermittent?

DIFFERENTIATING ACUTE AND CHRONIC PAIN

Acute pain may cause certain physiologic and behavioral changes that you won't observe in a patient with chronic pain.

Type of pain	Physiologic evidence	Behavioral evidence
Acute	■ Increased respirations ■ Increased pulse ■ Increased blood pressure ■ Dilated pupils ■ Diaphoresis	■ Restlessness ■ Distraction ■ Worry ■ Distress
Chronic	■ Normal respirations, pulse, blood pressure, and pupil size ■ No diaphoresis	■ Reduced or absent physical activity ■ Despair, depression ■ Hopelessness

PAIN BEHAVIOR CHECKLIST

A pain behavior is something a patient uses to communicate pain, distress, or suffering. Place a check in the box next to each behavior you observe or infer while talking with your patient.

- ☐ Grimacing
- ☐ Moaning
- ☐ Sighing
- ☐ Clenching teeth
- ☐ Holding or supporting the painful body area
- ☐ Sitting rigidly
- ☐ Frequently shifting posture or position
- ☐ Moving in a guarded or protective manner
- ☐ Moving very slowly
- ☐ Limping

- ☐ Taking medication
- ☐ Using a cane, cervical collar, or other prosthetic device
- ☐ Walking with an abnormal gait
- ☐ Requesting help with walking
- ☐ Stopping frequently while walking
- ☐ Lying down during the day
- ☐ Avoiding physical activity
- ☐ Being irritable
- ☐ Asking such questions as "Why did this happen to me?"
- ☐ Asking to be relieved from tasks or activities

Using the numerical rating scale

A numerical rating scale (NRS) can help the patient quantify his pain. Have him choose a number from 0 (indicating no pain) to 10 (indicating the worst pain imaginable) to reflect his current pain level. He can either circle the number on the scale itself or verbally state the number that best describes his pain.

| **No pain** | 0 | 1 | 2 | 3 | 4 | 5 | 6 | 7 | 8 | 9 | 10 | **Pain as bad as it can be** |

Visual analog scale

To use the visual analog scale, ask the patient to place a mark on the scale to indicate his current level of pain, as shown below

| **No pain** | **Pain as bad as it can be** |

Wong-Baker FACES Pain Rating Scale

A pediatric patient or an adult patient with language difficulties may not be able to express the pain he's feeling. In such instances, use the pain intensity scale below. Ask your patient to choose the face that best represents the severity of his pain on a scale from 0 to 10.

0	2	4	6	8	10
No hurt	Hurts little bit	Hurts little more	Hurts even more	Hurts whole lot	Hurts worst

From Wong, D.L., et al. *Wong's Essentials of Pediatric Nursing*, 6th ed. St. Louis: Mosby, Inc, 2001. Reprinted by permission.

FUNDAMENTALS

SELECTED ANALGESIC COMBINATION PRODUCTS

Many common analgesics are combinations of two or more generic drugs. This table lists components of common nonopioid and opioid analgesics.

Nonopioid analgesics

Trade name	Generic drugs
Anacin, P-A-C Analgesic Tablets	■ Aspirin 400 mg ■ Caffeine 32 mg
Ascriptin, Magnaprin	■ Aspirin 325 mg ■ Magnesium hydroxide 50 mg ■ Aluminum hydroxide 50 mg ■ Calcium carbonate 50 mg
Ascriptin A/D, Magnaprin Arthritis Strength Caplets	■ Aspirin 325 mg ■ Magnesium hydroxide 75 mg ■ Aluminum hydroxide 75 mg ■ Calcium carbonate 75 mg
Aspirin-Free Anacin PM, Extra-Strength Tylenol PM, Sominex Pain Relief	■ Acetaminophen 500 mg ■ Diphenhydramine 25 mg
Cama, Arthritis Pain Reliever	■ Aspirin 500 mg ■ Magnesium oxide 150 mg ■ Aluminum hydroxide 125 mg
Esgic-Plus	■ Acetaminophen 500 mg ■ Caffeine 40 mg ■ Butalbital 50 mg
Excedrin Extra Strength, Excedrin Migraine	■ Aspirin 250 mg ■ Acetaminophen 250 mg ■ Caffeine 65 mg
Excedrin P.M. Caplets	■ Acetaminophen 500 mg ■ Diphenhydramine citrate 38 mg
Fiorinal†, Fiortal†	■ Aspirin 325 mg ■ Caffeine 40 mg ■ Butalbital 50 mg
Sinutab Regular*	■ Acetaminophen 325 mg ■ Chlorpheniramine 2 mg ■ Pseudoephedrine hydrochloride 30 mg
Tecnal*	■ Aspirin 330 mg ■ Caffeine 40 mg ■ Butalbital 50 mg

* Available in Canada only.   † Controlled substance schedule III.

SELECTED ANALGESIC COMBINATION PRODUCTS *(continued)*

Nonopioid analgesics *(continued)*

Trade name	Generic drugs
Vanquish	■ Aspirin 227 mg ■ Acetaminophen 194 mg ■ Caffeine 33 mg ■ Aluminum hydroxide 25 mg ■ Magnesium hydroxide 50 mg

Opioid analgesics

Trade name	Controlled substance schedule	Generic drugs
Aceta with Codeine	III	■ Acetaminophen 300 mg ■ Codeine phosphate 30 mg
Anexsia 7.5/650, Lorcet Plus	III	■ Acetaminophen 650 mg ■ Hydrocodone bitartrate 7.5 mg
Capital with Codeine, Tylenol with Codeine Elixir	V	■ Acetaminophen 120 mg ■ Codeine phosphate 12 mg/5 ml
Darvocet-N 50	IV	■ Acetaminophen 325 mg ■ Propoxyphene napsylate 50 mg
Darvocet-N 100, Propacet 100	IV	■ Acetaminophen 650 mg ■ Propoxyphene napsylate 100 mg
Empirin With Codeine No. 3	III	■ Aspirin 325 mg ■ Codeine phosphate 30 mg
Empirin With Codeine No. 4	III	■ Aspirin 325 mg ■ Codeine phosphate 60 mg
Fioricet With Codeine	III	■ Acetaminophen 325 mg ■ Butalbital 50 mg ■ Caffeine 40 mg ■ Codeine phosphate 30 mg
Fiorinal With Codeine	III	■ Aspirin 325 mg ■ Butalbital 50 mg ■ Caffeine 40 mg ■ Codeine phosphate 30 mg
Lorcet 10/650	III	■ Acetaminophen 650 mg ■ Hydrocodone bitartrate 10 mg

(continued)

FUNDAMENTALS

Selected analgesic combination products *(continued)*

Opioid analgesics *(continued)*

Trade name	Controlled substance schedule	Generic drugs
Lortab 2.5/500	III	■ Acetaminophen 500 mg ■ Hydrocodone bitartrate 2.5 mg
Lortab 5/500	III	■ Acetaminophen 500 mg ■ Hydrocodone bitartrate 5 mg
Lortab 7.5/500	III	■ Acetaminophen 500 mg ■ Hydrocodone bitartrate 7.5 mg
Percocet 5/325	II	■ Acetaminophen 325 mg ■ Oxycodone hydrochloride 5 mg
Percodan-Demi	II	■ Aspirin 325 mg ■ Oxycodone hydrochloride 2.25 mg ■ Oxycodone terephthalate 0.19 mg
Percodan, Roxiprin	II	■ Aspirin 325 mg ■ Oxycodone hydrochloride 4.5 mg ■ Oxycodone terephthalate 0.38 mg
Roxicet	II	■ Acetaminophen 325 mg ■ Oxycodone hydrochloride 5 mg
Roxicet 5/500, Roxilox	II	■ Acetaminophen 500 mg ■ Oxycodone hydrochloride 5 mg
Roxicet Oral Solution	II	■ Acetaminophen 325 mg ■ Oxycodone hydrochloride 5 mg/ 5 ml
Talacen	IV	■ Acetaminophen 650 mg ■ Pentazocine hydrochloride 25 mg
Talwin Compound	IV	■ Aspirin 325 mg ■ Pentazocine hydrochloride 12.5 mg
Tylenol With Codeine No. 2	III	■ Acetaminophen 300 mg ■ Codeine phosphate 15 mg
Tylenol With Codeine No. 3	III	■ Acetaminophen 300 mg ■ Codeine phosphate 30 mg
Tylenol With Codeine No. 4	III	■ Acetaminophen 300 mg ■ Codeine phosphate 60 mg

SELECTED ANALGESIC COMBINATION PRODUCTS *(continued)*

Opioid analgesics *(continued)*

Trade name	Controlled substance schedule	Generic drugs
Tylox	II	■ Acetaminophen 500 mg ■ Oxycodone hydrochloride 5 mg
Vicodin, Zydone	III	■ Acetaminophen 500 mg ■ Hydrocodone bitartrate 5 mg
Vicodin ES	III	■ Acetaminophen 750 mg ■ Hydrocodone bitartrate 7.5 mg

PAIN MANAGEMENT AGENTS

Drug	Indications	Adverse effects
acetaminophen (Acephen, Anacin Aspirin Free, Tylenol)	■ Mild pain ■ Fever	■ Neutropenia, leukopenia, pancytopenia, thrombocytopenia ■ Severe liver damage ■ Hypoglycemia
aspirin (ASA, Ascriptin, Bufferin)	■ Mild pain ■ Fever ■ Transient ischemic attacks and thromboembolic disorders ■ Treatment or reduction of the risk of MI in patients with previous MI or unstable angina ■ Pericarditis following acute MI ■ Prevention of reocclusion in coronary revascularization procedures ■ Stent implantation	■ Tinnitus, hearing loss ■ Nausea, GI distress, occult bleeding, dyspepsia, GI bleeding ■ Acute renal insufficiency ■ Leukopenia, thrombocytopenia, prolonged bleeding time ■ Liver dysfunction, hepatitis ■ Rash ■ Hypersensitivity reactions (anaphylaxis, asthma), Reye's syndrome, angioedema
codeine phosphate; codeine sulfate	■ Mild to moderate pain ■ Nonproductive cough	■ Sedation, clouded sensorium, euphoria, dizziness, light-headedness ■ Hypotension, bradycardia ■ Nausea, vomiting, constipation, dry mouth, ileus ■ Urine retention ■ Respiratory depression ■ Diaphoresis
fentanyl citrate (Sublimaze); Fentanyl Transdermal System (Duragesic-25, Duragesic-50, Duragesic-75, Duragesic-100)	■ Preoperative analgesic ■ Adjunct to general anesthetic; low-dose regimen for minor procedures; moderate-dose regimen for major procedures; high-dose regimen for complicated procedures ■ Postoperative analgesic ■ Management of chronic pain in patients who can't be managed by lesser means ■ Management of breakthrough cancer pain	■ Sedation, somnolence, clouded sensorium, confusion, asthenia ■ Arrhythmias ■ Nausea, vomiting, constipation, dry mouth ■ Urine retention ■ Respiratory depression, apnea

Special considerations

- Use cautiously in patients with history of chronic alcohol abuse because hepatotoxicity has occurred after therapeutic doses. Also use cautiously in patients with hepatic or cardiovascular disease, renal function impairment, or viral infection.
- Know patient's total daily intake of acetaminophen, especially if he's also taking other prescribed drugs containing this component, such as Percocet. Toxicity can occur.
- Monitor the PT and INR values in patients receiving oral anticoagulants and sustained acetaminophen therapy.

- Contraindicated in patients with G6PD deficiency or bleeding disorders such as hemophilia, von Willebrand's disease, or telangiectasia. Also contraindicated in patients with NSAID-induced sensitivity reactions.
- Use cautiously in patients with GI lesions, impaired renal function, hypoprothrombinemia, vitamin K deficiency, thrombotic thrombocytopenic purpura, or hepatic impairment.
- Use cautiously in patients with history of GI disease (especially peptic ulcer disease), increased risk of GI bleeding, or decreased renal function.
- Give 8 oz (237 ml) of water or milk with salicylates to ensure passage into stomach. Have patient sit up for 15 to 30 minutes after taking salicylates to prevent lodging of salicylate in esophagus.
- Monitor vital signs frequently, especially temperature.
- Salicylates may mask the signs and symptoms of acute infection (fever, myalgia, erythema); carefully evaluate patients at risk for infections, such as those with diabetes.
- Monitor CBC, platelets, PT, BUN, serum creatinine, and liver function studies periodically during salicylate therapy to detect abnormalities.
- Assess the patient for signs and symptoms of hemorrhage, such as petechiae, bruising, coffee-ground vomitus, and black, tarry stools.

- Use cautiously in elderly or debilitated patients and in those with impaired renal or hepatic function, head injuries, increased intracranial pressure, increased CSF pressure, hypothyroidism, Addison's disease, acute alcoholism, CNS depression, bronchial asthma, COPD, respiratory depression, or shock.
- Don't mix with other solutions because codeine phosphate is incompatible with many drugs.
- Patients who become physically dependent on drug may experience acute withdrawal syndrome if given a narcotic antagonist.
- The drug may delay gastric emptying, increase biliary tract pressure resulting from contraction of the sphincter of Oddi, and interfere with hepatobiliary imaging studies.

- Use cautiously in elderly or debilitated patients and in those with head injuries, increased CSF pressure, COPD, decreased respiratory reserve, compromised respirations, arrhythmias, or hepatic, renal, or cardiac disease.
- Give an anticholinergic, such as atropine or glycopyrrolate, to minimize possible bradycardic effect of fentanyl.
- Gradually adjust dosage in patients using the transdermal system. Reaching steady state levels of a new dose may take up to 6 days; delay dose adjustment until after at least two applications.
- When reducing opiate therapy or switching to a different analgesic, expect to withdraw the transdermal system gradually. Because the serum level of fentanyl decreases very gradually after removal, give half of the equianalgesic dose of the new analgesic 12 to 18 hours after removal.

(continued)

PAIN MANAGEMENT AGENTS *(continued)*

Drug	Indications	Adverse effects
hydromorphone hydrochloride (Dilaudid)	■ Moderate to severe pain ■ Cough	■ Sedation, somnolence, clouded sensorium, dizziness, euphoria ■ Hypotension, bradycardia ■ Nausea, vomiting, constipation ■ Urine retention ■ Respiratory depression, bronchospasm
ibuprofen (Advil, Motrin, Motrin IB, Nuprin)	■ Arthritis, gout ■ Mild to moderate pain, headache, backache, minor aches associated with the common cold ■ Fever reduction	■ Acute renal failure ■ Neutropenia, pancytopenia, thrombocytopenia, aplastic anemia, leukopenia, agranulocytosis ■ Bronchospasm ■ Stevens-Johnson syndrome
ketorolac tromethamine (Toradol)	■ Short-term management of severe, acute pain ■ Short-term management of moderately severe, acute pain when switching from parenteral to oral administration	■ Drowsiness, sedation, dizziness, headache ■ Arrhythmias ■ Nausea, dyspepsia, GI pain ■ Renal failure ■ Thrombocytopenia
morphine sulfate (Astramorph PF, Avinza, Duramorph, Infumorph, Kadian, MS Contin, MSIR, MS/L, MS/S, OMS Concentrate, Oramorph SR, RMS Uniserts, Roxanol)	■ Severe pain ■ Severe, chronic pain related to cancer ■ Preoperative sedation and adjunct to anesthesia ■ Postoperative analgesia ■ Control of pain caused by acute MI ■ Control of angina pain ■ Adjunctive treatment of acute pulmonary edema	■ Seizures (with large doses), dizziness, nightmares (with long-acting oral forms), light-headedness ■ Hypotension, bradycardia, shock, cardiac arrest ■ Nausea, vomiting, constipation, ileus, dry mouth, biliary tract spasms, anorexia ■ Urine retention ■ Thrombocytopenia ■ Respiratory depression, apnea, respiratory arrest ■ Diaphoresis, edema ■ Physical dependence, decreased libido

Special considerations

■ Contraindicated in patients with intracranial lesions caused by increased intracranial pressure, and whenever ventilator function is depressed, such as in status asthmaticus, COPD, cor pulmonale, emphysema, and kyphoscoliosis.
■ Use cautiously in elderly or debilitated patients and in those with hepatic or renal disease, Addison's disease, hypothyroidism, prostatic hyperplasia, or urethral strictures.
■ For a better analgesic effect, give drug before the patient has intense pain.
■ Give by direct injection over no less than 2 minutes, and monitor the patient constantly. Keep resuscitation equipment available. Respiratory depression and hypotension can occur with I.V. administration.
■ Drug may worsen or mask gallbladder pain. Increased biliary tract pressure resulting from contraction of the sphincter of Oddi may interfere with hepatobiliary imaging studies.

■ Contraindicated in patients who have the syndrome of nasal polyps, angioedema, and bronchospastic reaction to aspirin or other NSAIDs. Contraindicated during the last trimester of pregnancy because it may cause problems with the fetus or complications during delivery.
■ Use cautiously in patients with impaired renal or hepatic function, GI disorders, peptic ulcer disease, cardiac decompensation, hypertension, or coagulation defects. Because chewable tablets contain aspartame, use cautiously in patients with phenylketonuria.
■ Monitor auditory and ophthalmic functions periodically during ibuprofen therapy.
■ Observe the patient for possible fluid retention.
■ Patients older than age 60 may be more susceptible to the toxic effects of ibuprofen, especially adverse GI reactions. Use lowest possible effective dose. The effect of drug on renal prostaglandins may cause fluid retention and edema, a significant drawback for elderly patients, especially those with heart failure.

■ Contraindicated in patients with active peptic ulcer disease, recent GI bleeding or perforation, advanced renal impairment, risk of renal impairment due to volume depletion, suspected or confirmed cerebrovascular bleeding, hemorrhagic diathesis, incomplete hemostasis, or high risk of bleeding.
■ Use cautiously in patients with impaired renal or hepatic function.
■ The combined duration of ketorolac I.M., I.V., or P.O. shouldn't exceed 5 days. Oral use is only for continuation of I.V. or I.M. therapy.

■ Contraindicated in patients with conditions that would preclude administration of opioids by I.V. route (acute bronchial asthma or upper airway obstruction).
■ Use cautiously in elderly or debilitated patients and in those with head injury, increased intracranial pressure, seizures, pulmonary disease, prostatic hyperplasia, hepatic or renal disease, acute abdominal conditions, hypothyroidism, Addison's disease, or urethral strictures.
■ Long-term therapy in patients with advanced renal disease may lead to toxicity as a result of accumulation of the active metabolite.

ELECTROLYTES

INTERPRETING SERUM ELECTROLYTE TEST RESULTS

Use the quick-reference chart below to interpret serum electrolyte test results in adult patients. This chart also lists disorders that can cause imbalances.

Electrolyte	Results	Implications	Common causes
Serum sodium	135 to 145 mEq/L	Normal	
	< 135 mEq/L	Hyponatremia	Syndrome of inappropriate antidiuretic hormone secretion
	> 145 mEq/L	Hypernatremia	Diabetes insipidus
Serum potassium	3.5 to 5 mEq/L	Normal	
	< 3.5 mEq/L	Hypokalemia	Diarrhea
	> 5mEq/L	Hyperkalemia	Burns and renal failure
Total serum calcium	8.5 to 10.5 mg/dl	Normal	
	< 8.5 mg/dl	Hypocalcemia	Acute pancreatitis
	> 10.5 mg/dl	Hypercalcemia	Hyperparathyroidism
Ionized calcium	4.5 to 5.1 mg/dl	Normal	
	< 4.5 mg/dl	Hypocalcemia	Massive transfusion
	> 5.1 mg/dl	Hypercalcemia	Acidosis
Serum phosphates	2.5 to 4.5 mg/dl or 1.8 to 2.6 mEq/L	Normal	
	< 2.5 mg/dl or 1.8 mEq/L	Hypophosphatemia	Diabetic ketoacidosis
	> 4.5 mg/dl or 2.6 mEq/L	Hyperphosphatemia	Renal insufficiency
Serum magnesium	1.5 to 2.5 mEq/L	Normal	
	< 1.5 mEq/L	Hypomagnesemia	Malnutrition
	> 2.5 mEq/L	Hypermagnesemia	Renal failure
Serum chloride	98 to 108 mEq/L	Normal	
	< 98 mEq/L	Hypochloremia	Prolonged vomiting
	> 108 mEq/L	Hyperchloremia	Hypernatremia

ELECTROLYTE IMBALANCES

Signs and symptoms of electrolyte imbalance are often subtle. Blood chemistry tests help diagnose and evaluate electrolyte imbalances.

Electrolyte imbalance	Signs and symptoms	Diagnostic test results
Hyponatremia	■ Muscle twitching and weakness due to osmotic swelling of cells ■ Lethargy, confusion, seizures, and coma due to altered neurotransmission ■ Hypotension and tachycardia due to decreased extracellular circulating volume ■ Nausea, vomiting, and abdominal cramps due to edema affecting receptors in the brain or vomiting center of the brain stem ■ Oliguria or anuria due to renal dysfunction	■ Serum sodium < 135 mEq/L ■ Decreased urine specific gravity ■ Decreased serum osmolality ■ Urine sodium > 100 mEq/24 hours ■ Increased red blood cell count
Hypernatremia	■ Agitation, restlessness, fever, and decreased level of consciousness due to altered cellular metabolism ■ Hypertension, tachycardia, pitting edema, and excessive weight gain due to water shift from intracellular to extracellular fluid ■ Thirst, increased viscosity of saliva, rough tongue due to fluid shift ■ Dyspnea, respiratory arrest, and death from dramatic increase in osmotic pressure	■ Serum sodium > 145 mEq/L ■ Urine sodium < 40 mEq/24 hours ■ High serum osmolality
Hypokalemia	■ Dizziness, hypotension, arrhythmias, electrocardiogram (ECG) changes, and cardiac arrest due to changes in membrane excitability ■ Nausea, vomiting, anorexia, diarrhea, decreased peristalsis, and abdominal distention due to decreased bowel motility ■ Muscle weakness, fatigue, and leg cramps due to decreased neuromuscular excitability	■ Serum potassium < 3.5 mEq/L ■ Coexisting low serum calcium and magnesium levels not responsive to treatment for hypokalemia usually suggest hypomagnesemia ■ Metabolic alkalosis ■ ECG changes include flattened T waves, elevated U waves, depressed ST segment

(continued)

ELECTROLYTE IMBALANCES *(continued)*

Electrolyte imbalance	Signs and symptoms	Diagnostic test results
Hyperkalemia	■ Tachycardia changing to bradycardia, ECG changes, and cardiac arrest due to hypopolarization and alterations in repolarization ■ Nausea, diarrhea, and abdominal cramps due to decreased gastric motility ■ Muscle weakness and flaccid paralysis due to inactivation of membrane sodium channels	■ Serum potassium > 5 mEq/L ■ Metabolic acidosis ■ ECG changes include tented and elevated T waves, widened QRS complex, prolonged PR interval, flattened or absent P waves, depressed ST segment
Hypochloremia	■ Muscle hypertonicity and tetany ■ Shallow, depressed breathing ■ Usually associated with hyponatremia and its characteristic symptoms, such as muscle weakness and twitching	■ Serum chloride < 98 mEq/L ■ Serum pH > 7.45 (supportive value) ■ Serum CO_2 > 32 mEq/L (supportive value)
Hyper-chloremia	■ Deep, rapid breathing ■ Weakness ■ Diminished cognitive ability, possibly leading to coma	■ Serum chloride > 108 mEq/L ■ Serum pH < 7.35, serum CO_2 < 22 mEq/L (supportive values)
Hypocalcemia	■ Anxiety, irritability, twitching around the mouth, laryngospasm, seizures, positive Chvostek's and Trousseau's signs due to enhanced neuromuscular irritability ■ Hypotension and arrhythmias due to decreased calcium influx	■ Serum calcium < 8.5 mg/dl ■ Low platelet count ■ ECG shows lengthened QT interval, prolonged ST segment, arrhythmias ■ Possible changes in serum protein because half of serum calcium is bound to albumin
Hypercalcemia	■ Drowsiness, lethargy, headaches, irritability, confusion, depression, or apathy due to decreased neuromuscular irritability (increased threshold) ■ Weakness and muscle flaccidity due to depressed neuromuscular irritability and release of acetylcholine at the myoneural junction ■ Bone pain and pathological fractures due to calcium loss from bones ■ Heart block due to decreased neuromuscular irritability ■ Anorexia, nausea, vomiting, constipation, and dehydration due to hyperosmolarity ■ Flank pain due to kidney stone formation	■ Serum calcium > 10.5 mg/dl ■ ECG shows signs of heart block and shortened QT interval ■ Azotemia ■ Decreased parathyroid hormone level ■ Sulkowitch urine test shows increased calcium precipitation

ELECTROLYTE IMBALANCES *(continued)*

Electrolyte imbalance	Signs and symptoms	Diagnostic test results
Hypomagne-semia	■ Nearly always coexists with hypokalemia and hypocalcemia ■ Hyperirritability, tetany, leg and foot cramps, positive Chvostek's and Trousseau's signs, confusion, delusions, and seizures due to alteration in neuromuscular transmission ■ Arrhythmias, vasodilation, and hypotension due to enhanced inward sodium current or concurrent effects of calcium and potassium imbalance	■ Serum magnesium < 1.5 mEq/L ■ Coexisting low serum potassium and calcium levels
Hypermagne-semia	■ Hypermagnesemia is uncommon, caused by decreased renal excretion (renal failure) or increased intake of magnesium ■ Diminished reflexes, muscle weakness to flaccid paralysis due to suppression of acetylcholine release at the myoneural junction, blocking neuromuscular transmission and reducing cell excitability ■ Respiratory distress secondary to respiratory muscle paralysis ■ Heart block, bradycardia due to decreased inward sodium current ■ Hypotension due to relaxation of vascular smooth muscle and reduction of vascular resistance by displacing calcium from the vascular wall surface	■ Serum magnesium > 2.5 mEq/L ■ Coexisting elevated potassium and calcium levels
Hypophos-phatemia	■ Muscle weakness, tremor, and paresthesia due to deficiency of adenosine triphosphate ■ Peripheral hypoxia due to 2,3-diphosphoglycerate deficiency	■ Serum phosphate < 2.5 mg/dl ■ Urine phosphate > 1.3 g/24 hours
Hyperphos-phatemia	■ Usually asymptomatic unless leading to hypocalcemia, with tetany and seizures	■ Serum phosphate > 4.5 mg/dl ■ Serum calcium < 9 mg/dl ■ Urine phosphorus < 0.9 g/24 hours

2

I.V. THERAPY AND BLOOD PRODUCTS

I.V. FLUIDS

I.V. solution	Components	Considerations
Dextrose 5% and water (D_5W)	■ 50 g glucose ■ (isotonic — 260 mOsm/L)	■ Rehydration or replace plasma volume ■ Common vehicle for other I.V. medication administration such as potassium ■ Aids in renal excretion of solutes ■ Doesn't replace electrolyte deficits ■ Contraindicated in head injuries—may increase intracranial pressure
Normal saline (0.9% NaCl; 0.9% NS)	■ 154 mEq sodium ■ 154 mEq chloride ■ (isotonic — 308 mOsm/L)	■ Restoration of extracellular fluid volumes ■ Replacement of sodium and chloride deficits ■ Doesn't supply calories ■ Given primarily with blood transfusions and to replace large fluid losses such as in GI fluid loss ■ Contraindicated in heart failure, pulmonary edema, renal impairment, and sodium retention
Lactated Ringer's (LR)	■ 130 mEq sodium ■ 4 mEq potassium ■ 3 mEq calcium ■ 109 mEq chloride ■ 28 mEq lactate ■ (isotonic — 275 mOsm/L)	■ Fluid of choice for acute blood loss replacement ■ Rehydration (similar to electrolyte composition of blood serum or plasma) ■ Hypovolemia ■ Burns ■ Mild metabolic acidosis ■ Sodium depletion ■ Doesn't supply calories ■ Contraindicated in heart failure, renal impairment, head injury, liver disease, alkalosis
0.45 sodium chloride (0.45 NaCl; ½ NS)	■ 77 mEq sodium ■ 77 mEq chloride ■ (hypotonic — 154 mOsm/L)	■ Establishment of renal function ■ Doesn't supply calories ■ Not for replacement therapy

I.V. FLUIDS *(continued)*

I.V. solution	Components	Considerations
Dextrose 5% in 0.45% normal saline (D₅ ½ NS; D₅ 0.45 NaCl	■ 77 mEq sodium ■ 77 mEq chloride ■ 170 calories ■ (hypertonic — 406 mOsm/L)	■ Hypovolemia ■ Maintenance fluid of choice if no electrolyte abnormalities ■ Maintenance of fluid intake
Dextrose 5% in normal saline (D₅NS; D₅0.9% NaCl)	■ 170 calories ■ 154 mEq sodium ■ 154 mEq chloride ■ (hypertonic — 560 mOsm/L)	■ Fluid replacement ■ Sodium, chloride, and calorie replacement ■ Temporary treatment of hypovolemia if plasma expander not available
Dextrose 5% in Lactated Ringer's (D₅LR)	■ 130 mEq sodium ■ 4 mEq potassium ■ 3 mEq chloride ■ 109 mEq chloride ■ 28 mEq lactate ■ 170 calories ■ (hypertonic — 575 mOsm/L)	■ Rehydration (similar to electrolyte composition of blood serum or plasma) ■ Hypovolemia ■ Burns ■ Mild metabolic acidosis ■ Doesn't supply calories ■ Sodium depletion
3% normal saline (3% NS; 3% NaCl)	■ 513 mEq sodium ■ 513 mEq chloride ■ (hypertonic — 810 mOsm/L)	■ Hyponatremia ■ Elimination of intracellular fluid excess
Dextran 40 in normal saline or dextrose 5% in water	■ 170 calories ■ (isotonic — 252 mOsm/L when combined with dextrose 5%; 308 mOsm/L when combined with normal saline)	■ Expansion of plasma volume in early shock when blood products unavailable ■ Improvement of microcirculation ■ Doesn't have electrolyte components

TYPES OF PARENTERAL NUTRITION

Type	Solution components/liter	Special considerations
Standard I.V. therapy	■ Dextrose, water, electrolytes in varying amounts, for example: - dextrose 5% in water (D_5W) = 170 calories/L - $D_{10}W$ = 340 calories/L - normal saline = 0 calories ■ Vitamins as ordered	■ Nutritionally incomplete; doesn't provide sufficient calories to maintain adequate nutritional status
Total parenteral nutrition (TPN) by way of central venous (CV) line	■ $D_{15}W$ to $D_{25}W$ (1 L dextrose 25% = 850 nonprotein calories) ■ Crystalline amino acids 2.5% to 8.5% ■ Electrolytes, vitamins, trace elements, and insulin as ordered ■ Lipid emulsion 10% to 20% (usually infused as a separate solution)	*Basic solution* ■ Nutritionally complete ■ Requires minor surgical procedure for CV line insertion (can be done at bedside by the physician) ■ Highly hypertonic solution ■ May cause metabolic complications (glucose intolerance, electrolyte imbalance, essential fatty acid deficiency) *I.V. lipid emulsion* ■ May not be used effectively in severely stressed patients (especially burn patients) ■ May interfere with immune mechanisms; in patients suffering respiratory compromise, reduces carbon dioxide buildup ■ Given by way of CV line; irritates peripheral vein in long-term use
Protein-sparing therapy	■ Crystalline amino acids in same amounts as TPN ■ Electrolytes, vitamins, minerals, and trace elements as ordered	■ Nutritionally complete ■ Requires little mixing ■ May be started or stopped any time during the hospital stay ■ Other I.V. fluids, medications, and blood by-products may be administered through the same I.V. line ■ Not as likely to cause phlebitis as peripheral parenteral nutrition ■ Adds a major expense; has limited benefits
Total nutrient admixture	■ One day's nutrients are contained in a single, 3-L bag (also called 3:1 solution)	■ See TPN (above) ■ Reduces need to handle bag, cutting risk of contamination

TYPES OF PARENTERAL NUTRITION *(continued)*

Type	Solution components/liter	Special considerations
Total nutrient admixture *(continued)*	■ Combines lipid emulsion with other parenteral solution components	■ Decreases nursing time and reduces need for infusion sets and electronic devices, lowering facility costs, increasing patient mobility, and allowing easier adjustment to home care ■ Has limited use because not all types and amounts of components are compatible ■ Precludes use of certain infusion pumps because they can't accurately deliver large volumes of solution; precludes use of standard I.V. tubing filters because a 0.22-micron filter blocks lipid and albumin molecules
Peripheral parenteral nutrition (PPN)	■ D_5W to $D_{10}W$ ■ Crystalline amino acids 2.5% to 5% ■ Electrolytes, minerals, vitamins, and trace elements as ordered ■ Lipid emulsion 10% or 20% (1 L of dextrose 10% and amino acids 3.5% infused at the same time as 1 L of lipid emulsion = 1,440 nonprotein calories) ■ Heparin or hydrocortisone as ordered	*Basic solution* ■ Nutritionally complete for a short time ■ Can't be used in nutritionally depleted patients ■ Can't be used in volume-restricted patients because PPN requires large fluid volume ■ Doesn't cause weight gain ■ Avoids insertion and care of CV line but requires adequate venous access; site must be changed every 72 hours ■ Delivers less hypertonic solutions than CV line TPN ■ May cause phlebitis and increases risk of metabolic complications ■ Less chance of metabolic complications than with CV line TPN *I.V. lipid emulsion* ■ As effective as dextrose for caloric source ■ Diminishes phlebitis if infused at the same time as basic nutrient solution ■ Irritates vein in long-term use ■ Reduces carbon dioxide buildup when pulmonary compromise is present

CALCULATING DRIP RATES

When calculating the flow rate of I.V. solutions, remember that the number of drops required to deliver 1 ml varies with the type of administration set you're using. To calculate the drip rate, you must know the calibration of the drip rate for each specific manufacturer's product. As a quick guide, refer to the chart below. Use this formula to calculate specific drip rates:

$$\frac{\text{volume of infusion (in ml)}}{\text{time of infusion (in minutes)}} \times \text{drip factor (in drops/ml)} = \text{drops/minute}$$

	Ordered volume	
	500 ml/24 hour or 21 ml/hour	1,000 ml/24 hour or 42 ml/hour
Drops/ml	Drops/minute to infuse	
MACRODRIP		
10	3	7
15	5	11
20	7	14
MICRODRIP		
60	21	42

1,000 ml/20 hour or 50 ml/hour	1,000 ml/10 hour or 100 ml/hour	1,000 ml/8 hour or 125 ml/hour	1,000 ml/6 hour or 166 ml/hour
8	17	21	28
13	25	31	42
17	34	42	56
50	100	125	166

MANAGING I.V. FLOW RATE DEVIATIONS

Problem	Cause	Intervention
Flow rate too slow	■ Venous spasm after insertion	■ Apply warm soaks over site.
	■ Venous obstruction from bending arm	■ Secure with an arm board if necessary.
	■ Pressure change (decreasing fluid in bottle causes solution to run slower because of decreasing pressure)	■ Readjust flow rate.
	■ Elevated blood pressure	■ Readjust flow rate. Use infusion pump or controller to ensure correct flow rate.
	■ Cold solution	■ Allow solution to warm to room temperature before hanging.
	■ Change in solution viscosity from medication added	■ Readjust flow rate.
	■ I.V. container too low or patient's arm or leg too high	■ Hang container higher or remind patient to keep his arm below heart level.
	■ Bevel against vein wall (positional cannulation)	■ Withdraw needle slightly, or place a folded 2″ × 2″ gauze pad over or under catheter hub to change angle.
	■ Excess tubing dangling below insertion site	■ Replace tubing with shorter piece, or tape excess tubing to I.V. pole, below flow clamp. (Make sure tubing isn't kinked.)
	■ Cannula too small	■ Remove cannula in use and insert a larger-bore cannula, or use an infusion pump.
	■ Infiltration or clotted cannula	■ Remove cannula in use and insert a new cannula.
	■ Kinked tubing	■ Check tubing over its entire length and unkink it.
	■ Clogged filter	■ Remove filter and replace with a new one.
	■ Tubing memory (tubing compressed at area clamped)	■ Massage or milk tubing by pinching and wrapping it around a pencil four or five times. Quickly pull pencil out of coiled tubing.
Flow rate too fast	■ Patient or visitor manipulating clamp	■ Instruct patient not to touch clamp. Place tape over it. Administer I.V. solution with infusion pump or controller if necessary.
	■ Tubing disconnected from catheter	■ Wipe distal end of tubing with alcohol, reinsert firmly into catheter hub, and tape at connection site. Consider using tubing with luer-lock connections.
	■ Change in patient position	■ Administer I.V. solution with infusion pump or controller to ensure correct flow rate.
	■ Flow clamp drifting because of patient movement	■ Place tape below clamp.

Risks of peripheral I.V. therapy

Complication and findings	Possible causes	Nursing interventions
LOCAL COMPLICATIONS		
Phlebitis		
■ Tenderness at tip of and proximal to venous access device ■ Redness at tip of cannula and along vein ■ Puffy area over vein ■ Vein hard on palpation ■ Elevated temperature	■ Poor blood flow around venous access device ■ Friction from cannula movement in vein ■ Venous access device left in vein too long ■ Clotting at cannula tip (thrombophlebitis) ■ Drug or solution with high or low pH or high osmolarity	■ Remove venous access device. ■ Apply warm soaks. ■ Notify physician if patient has a fever. ■ Document patient's condition and your interventions. *Prevention* ■ Restart infusion using larger vein for irritating solution, or restart with smaller-gauge device to ensure adequate blood flow. ■ Use filter to reduce risk of phlebitis. ■ Tape device securely to prevent motion.
Infiltration		
■ Swelling at and above I.V. site (may extend along entire limb) ■ Discomfort, burning or pain at site (may be painless) ■ Tight feeling at site ■ Decreased skin temperature around site ■ Blanching at site ■ Continuing fluid infusion even when vein is occluded (although rate may decrease) ■ Absent backflow of blood	■ Venous access device dislodged from vein, or perforated vein	■ Stop infusion. If extravasation is likely, infiltrate the site with an antidote. ■ Apply warm soaks to aid absorption. Elevate limb. ■ Check for pulse and capillary refill periodically to assess circulation. ■ Restart infusion above infiltration site or in another limb. ■ Document patient's condition and your interventions. *Prevention* ■ Check I.V. site frequently. ■ Don't obscure area above site with tape. ■ Teach patient to observe I.V. site and report pain or swelling.

I.V. THERAPY AND BLOOD PRODUCTS

(continued)

RISKS OF PERIPHERAL I.V. THERAPY *(continued)*

Complication and findings	Possible causes	Nursing interventions
LOCAL COMPLICATIONS *(continued)*		
Cannula dislodgment ■ Loose tape ■ Cannula partly backed out of vein ■ Solution infiltrating	■ Loosened tape, or tubing snagged in bed linens, resulting in partial retraction of cannula; pulled out by confused patient	■ If no infiltration occurs, retape without pushing cannula back into vein. If pulled out, apply pressure to I.V. site with sterile dressing. *Prevention* ■ Tape venipuncture device securely on insertion.
Occlusion ■ No increase in flow rate when I.V. container is raised ■ Blood backflow in line ■ Discomfort at insertion site	■ I.V. flow interrupted ■ Heparin lock not flushed ■ Blood backflow in line when patient walks ■ Line clamped too long	■ Use mild flush injection. Don't force it. If unsuccessful, remove I.V. line and insert a new one. *Prevention* ■ Maintain I.V. flow rate. ■ Flush promptly after intermittent piggyback administration. ■ Have patient walk with his arm bent at the elbow to reduce risk of blood backflow.
Vein irritation or pain at I.V. site ■ Pain during infusion ■ Possible blanching if vasospasm occurs ■ Red skin over vein during infusion ■ Rapidly developing signs of phlebitis	■ Solution with high or low pH or high osmolarity, such as 40 mEq/L of potassium chloride, phenytoin, and some antibiotics (vancomycin, erythromycin, and nafcillin)	■ Decrease the flow rate. ■ Try using an electronic flow device to achieve a steady flow. *Prevention* ■ Dilute solutions before administration. For example, give antibiotics in 250-ml solution rather than 100-ml solution. If drug has low pH, ask pharmacist if drug can be buffered with sodium bicarbonate. (Refer to your facility's policy.) ■ If long-term therapy of irritating drug is planned, ask physician to use central I.V. line.

Risks of peripheral I.V. therapy *(continued)*

Complication and findings	Possible causes	Nursing interventions

LOCAL COMPLICATIONS *(continued)*

Complication and findings	Possible causes	Nursing interventions
Hematoma ■ Tenderness at venipuncture site ■ Bruised area around site ■ Inability to advance or flush I.V. line	■ Vein punctured through opposite wall at time of insertion ■ Leakage of blood from needle displacement ■ Inadequate pressure applied when cannula is discontinued	■ Remove venous access device. ■ Apply pressure and warm soaks to affected area. ■ Recheck for bleeding. ■ Document patient's condition and your interventions. *Prevention* ■ Choose a vein that can accommodate the size of venous access device. ■ Release tourniquet as soon as insertion is successful.
Severed cannula ■ Leakage from cannula shaft	■ Cannula inadvertently cut by scissors ■ Reinsertion of needle into cannula	■ If broken part is visible, attempt to retrieve it. If unsuccessful, notify the physician. ■ If portion of cannula enters bloodstream, place tourniquet above I.V. site to prevent progression of broken part. ■ Notify physician and radiology department. ■ Document patient's condition and your interventions. *Prevention* ■ Don't use scissors around I.V. site. ■ Never reinsert needle into cannula. ■ Remove unsuccessfully inserted cannula and needle together.
Venous spasm ■ Pain along vein ■ Flow rate sluggish when clamp completely open ■ Blanched skin over vein	■ Severe vein irritation from irritating drugs or fluids ■ Administration of cold fluids or blood ■ Very rapid flow rate (with fluids at room temperature)	■ Apply warm soaks over vein and surrounding area. ■ Decrease flow rate. *Prevention* ■ Use a blood warmer for blood or packed red blood cells.

(continued)

RISKS OF PERIPHERAL I.V. THERAPY *(continued)*

Complication and findings	Possible causes	Nursing interventions
LOCAL COMPLICATIONS *(continued)*		
Thrombosis ■ Painful, reddened, and swollen vein ■ Sluggish or stopped I.V. flow	■ Injury to endothelial cells of vein wall, allowing platelets to adhere and thrombi to form	■ Remove venous access device; restart infusion in opposite limb if possible. ■ Apply warm soaks. ■ Watch for I.V. therapy–related infection; thrombi provide an excellent environment for bacterial growth. *Prevention* ■ Use proper venipuncture techniques to reduce injury to vein.
Thrombophlebitis ■ Severe discomfort ■ Reddened, swollen, and hardened vein	■ Thrombosis and inflammation	■ Same as for thrombosis. *Prevention* ■ Check site frequently. Remove venous access device at first sign of redness and tenderness.
Nerve, tendon, or ligament damage ■ Extreme pain (similar to electrical shock when nerve is punctured) ■ Numbness and muscle contraction ■ Delayed effects, including paralysis, numbness, and deformity	■ Improper venipuncture technique, resulting in injury to surrounding nerves, tendons, or ligaments ■ Tight taping or improper splinting with arm board	■ Stop procedure. *Prevention* ■ Don't repeatedly penetrate tissues with venous access device. ■ Don't apply excessive pressure when taping; don't encircle limb with tape. ■ Pad arm boards and tape securing arm boards if possible.

Complication and findings	Possible causes	Nursing interventions

SYSTEMIC COMPLICATIONS

Systemic infection (septicemia or bacteremia)

■ Fever, chills, and malaise for no apparent reason ■ Contaminated I.V. site, usually with no visible signs of infection at site	■ Failure to maintain aseptic technique during insertion or site care ■ Severe phlebitis, which can set up ideal conditions for organism growth ■ Poor taping that permits venous access device to move, which can introduce organisms into bloodstream ■ Prolonged indwelling time of device ■ Weak immune system	■ Notify the physician. ■ Administer medications as prescribed. ■ Culture the site and device. ■ Monitor vital signs. *Prevention* ■ Use scrupulous aseptic technique when handling solutions and tubing, inserting venous access device, and discontinuing infusion. ■ Secure all connections. ■ Change I.V. solutions, tubing, and venous access device at recommended times. ■ Use I.V. filters.
Vasovagal reaction ■ Sudden collapse of vein during venipuncture ■ Sudden pallor, sweating, faintness, dizziness, and nausea ■ Decreased blood pressure	■ Vasospasm from anxiety or pain	■ Lower the head of the bed. ■ Have patient take deep breaths. ■ Check vital signs. *Prevention* ■ Prepare patient for therapy to relieve his anxiety. ■ Use local anesthetic to prevent pain.

(continued)

RISKS OF PERIPHERAL I.V. THERAPY *(continued)*

Complication and findings	Possible causes	Nursing interventions
SYSTEMIC COMPLICATIONS *(continued)*		
Allergic reaction ■ Itching ■ Watery eyes and nose ■ Bronchospasm ■ Wheezing ■ Urticarial rash ■ Edema at I.V. site ■ Anaphylactic reaction (flushing, chills, anxiety, itching, palpitations, paresthesia, wheezing, seizures, cardiac arrest) up to 1 hour after exposure	■ Allergens such as medications	■ If reaction occurs, stop infusion immediately. ■ Maintain a patent airway. ■ Notify the physician. ■ Administer antihistamine, steroid, and antipyretic drugs, as prescribed. ■ Give aqueous epinephrine, S.C., as prescribed. Repeat as needed and prescribed. *Prevention* ■ Obtain patient's allergy history. Be aware of cross-allergies. ■ Assist with test dosing and document any new allergies. ■ Monitor patient carefully during first 15 minutes of administration of a new drug.
Circulatory overload ■ Discomfort ■ Neck vein engorgement ■ Respiratory distress ■ Increased blood pressure ■ Crackles ■ Increased difference between fluid intake and output	■ Roller clamp loosened to allow run-on infusion ■ Flow rate too rapid ■ Miscalculation of fluid requirements	■ Raise the head of the bed. ■ Administer oxygen as needed. ■ Notify the physician. ■ Administer medications (probably furosemide) as prescribed. *Prevention* ■ Use pump, controller, or rate minder for elderly or compromised patients. ■ Recheck calculations of fluid requirements. ■ Monitor infusion frequently.

Risks of peripheral I.V. therapy *(continued)*

Complication and findings	Possible causes	Nursing interventions

Systemic complications *(continued)*

Air embolism

Complication and findings	Possible causes	Nursing interventions
■ Respiratory distress ■ Unequal breath sounds ■ Weak pulse ■ Increased central venous pressure ■ Decreased blood pressure ■ Loss of consciousness	■ Solution container empty ■ Solution container empties, and added container pushes air down the line (if line not purged first)	■ Discontinue infusion. ■ Place patient on his left side in Trendelenburg's position to allow air to enter right atrium. ■ Administer oxygen. ■ Notify the physician. ■ Document patient's condition and your interventions. *Prevention* ■ Purge tubing of air completely before starting infusion. ■ Use air-detection device on pump or air-eliminating filter proximal to I.V. site. ■ Secure connections.

I.V. THERAPY AND BLOOD PRODUCTS

GUIDE TO CENTRAL VENOUS CATHETERS

Type	Description	Indications
Groshong catheter	■ Silicone rubber ■ About 35″ (89 cm) long ■ Closed end with pressure-sensitive two-way valve ■ Dacron cuff ■ Single or double lumen ■ Tunneled	■ Long-term central venous (CV) access ■ Patient with heparin allergy

Type	Description	Indications
Short-term single-lumen catheter	■ Polyvinyl chloride (PVC) or polyurethane ■ About 8″ (20 cm) long ■ Lumen gauge varies ■ Percutaneously placed	■ Short-term CV access ■ Emergency access ■ Patient who needs only one lumen

Type	Description	Indications
Short-term multilumen catheter	■ PVC or polyurethane ■ Two, three, or four lumens exiting at ¾″ (2-cm) intervals ■ Lumen gauges vary ■ Percutaneously placed	■ Short-term CV access ■ Patient with limited insertion sites who requires multiple infusions

Advantages and disadvantages	Nursing considerations
Advantages	■ Two surgical sites require dressing after insertion.
■ Less thrombogenic	■ Handle catheter gently.
■ Pressure-sensitive two-way valve eliminates frequent heparin flushes.	■ Check the external portion frequently for kinks and leaks.
■ Dacron cuff anchors catheter and prevents bacterial migration.	
Disadvantages	
■ Requires surgical insertion	■ Repair kit is available.
■ Tears and kinks easily	■ Remember to flush with enough saline solution to clear the catheter, especially after drawing or administering blood.
■ Blunt end makes it difficult to clear substances from its tip.	
Advantages	
■ Easily inserted at bedside	■ Minimize patient movement.
■ Easily removed	■ Assess frequently for signs of infection and clot formation.
■ Stiffness aids central venous pressure (CVP) monitoring.	
Disadvantages	
■ Limited functions	
■ PVC is thrombogenic and irritates inner lumen of vessel.	
■ Should be changed every 3 to 7 days (frequency may depend on facility's CV line infection rate)	
Advantages	
■ Same as single-lumen catheter	■ Know gauge and purpose of each lumen.
■ Allows infusion of multiple (even incompatible) solutions through the same catheter	■ Use the same lumen for the same task.
Disadvantages	
■ Same as single-lumen catheter	

(continued)

GUIDE TO CENTRAL VENOUS CATHETERS (continued)

Type	Description	Indications
Hickman catheter	■ Silicone rubber ■ About 35″ (89 cm) long ■ Open end with clamp ■ Dacron cuff 11¾″ (30 cm) from hub ■ Single lumen or multilumen ■ Tunneled	■ Long-term CV access ■ Home therapy

Broviac catheter	■ Identical to Hickman except smaller inner lumen	■ Long-term CV access ■ Patient with small central vessels (pediatric or geriatric)

Hickman/ Broviac catheter	■ Hickman and Broviac catheters combined ■ Tunneled	■ Long-term CV access ■ Patient who needs multiple infusions

Peripherally inserted central catheter	■ Silicone rubber ■ 20″ (50.8 cm) long ■ Available in 16G, 18G, 20G, and 22G ■ Can be used as midline catheter ■ Percutaneously placed	■ Long-term CV access ■ Patient with poor CV access ■ Patient at risk for fatal complications from CV catheter insertion ■ Patient who needs CV access but is scheduled for or has had head or neck surgery

Advantages and disadvantages	Nursing considerations
Advantages ■ Less thrombogenic ■ Dacron cuff prevents excess motion and migration of bacteria. ■ Clamps eliminate need for Valsalva's maneuver. *Disadvantages* ■ Requires surgical insertion ■ Open end ■ Requires physician for removal ■ Tears and kinks easily	■ Two surgical sites require dressing after insertion. ■ Handle catheter gently. ■ Observe frequently for kinks and tears. ■ Repair kit is available. ■ Clamp catheter with a nonserrated clamp any time it becomes disconnected or opens.
Advantages ■ Smaller lumen *Disadvantages* ■ Small lumen may limit uses. ■ Single lumen	■ Check your facility's policy before drawing blood or administering blood or blood products.
Advantages ■ Double-lumen Hickman catheter allows sampling and administration of blood. ■ Broviac lumen delivers I.V. fluids, including total parenteral nutrition. *Disadvantages* ■ Same as Hickman catheter	■ Know the purpose and function of each lumen. ■ Label lumens to prevent confusion.
Advantages ■ Peripherally inserted ■ Easily inserted at bedside with minimal complications ■ May be inserted by a specially trained nurse in some states *Disadvantages* ■ Catheter may occlude smaller peripheral vessels. ■ May be difficult to keep immobile ■ Long path to CV circulation	■ Check frequently for signs of phlebitis and thrombus formation. ■ Insert catheter above the antecubital fossa. ■ Basilic vein is preferable to cephalic vein. ■ Use arm board, if necessary. ■ Length of catheter may alter CVP measurements.

RISKS OF CENTRAL VENOUS THERAPY

Complication and findings	Possible causes	Nursing interventions
Infection ■ Redness, warmth, tenderness, swelling at insertion or exit site ■ Possible exudate of purulent material ■ Local rash or pustules ■ Fever, chills, malaise ■ Leukocytosis ■ Nausea and vomiting ■ Elevated urine glucose level	■ Failure to maintain aseptic technique during catheter insertion or care ■ Failure to comply with dressing change protocol ■ Wet or soiled dressing remaining on site ■ Immunosuppression ■ Irritated suture line ■ Contaminated catheter or solution ■ Frequent opening of catheter or long-term use of single I.V. access site	■ Monitor temperature frequently. ■ Monitor vital signs closely. ■ Culture the site. ■ Redress aseptically. ■ Possibly use antibiotic ointment locally. ■ Treat systemically with antibiotics or antifungals, depending on culture results and physician order. ■ Catheter may be removed. ■ Draw central and peripheral blood cultures; if the same organism appears in both, then catheter is primary source and should be removed. ■ If cultures don't match but are positive, the catheter may be removed or the infection may be treated through the catheter. ■ If the catheter is removed, culture its tip. ■ Document interventions. *Prevention* ■ Maintain sterile technique. Use sterile gloves, masks, and gowns when appropriate. ■ Observe dressing-change protocols. ■ Teach about restrictions on swimming, bathing, and so on. (With adequate white blood cell count, the physician may allow these activities.) ■ Change wet or soiled dressing immediately. ■ Change dressing more frequently if catheter is located in femoral area or near tracheostomy. Perform tracheostomy care after catheter care. ■ Examine solution for cloudiness and turbidity before infusing; check fluid container for leaks. ■ Monitor urine glucose level in patients receiving total parenteral nutrition (TPN); if greater than 2+, suspect early sepsis. ■ Use a 0.22-micron filter (or a 1.2-micron filter for 3-in-1 TPN solutions). ■ Catheter may be changed frequently. ■ Keep the system closed as much as possible.

Risks of central venous therapy *(continued)*

Complication and findings	Possible causes	Nursing interventions

Pneumothorax, hemothorax, chylothorax, hydrothorax

■ Decreased breath sounds on affected side ■ With hemothorax, decreased hemoglobin level because of blood pooling ■ Abnormal chest X-ray	■ Repeated or long-term use of same vein ■ Preexisting cardiovascular disease ■ Lung puncture by catheter during insertion or exchange over a guidewire ■ Large blood vessel puncture with bleeding inside or outside the lung ■ Lymph node puncture with leakage of lymph fluid ■ Infusion of solution into chest area through infiltrated catheter	■ Notify physician. ■ Remove catheter or assist with removal. ■ Administer oxygen as ordered. ■ Set up and assist with chest tube insertion. ■ Document interventions. *Prevention* ■ Position patient head down with a rolled towel between his scapulae to dilate and expose the internal jugular or subclavian vein as much as possible during catheter insertion. ■ Assess for early signs of fluid infiltration (swelling in the shoulder, neck, chest, and arm). ■ Ensure that the patient is immobilized and prepared for insertion. Active patients may need to be sedated or taken to the operating room.

Air embolism

■ Respiratory distress ■ Unequal breath sounds ■ Weak pulse ■ Increased central venous (CV) pressure ■ Decreased blood pressure ■ Alteration or loss of consciousness	■ Intake of air into the CV system during catheter insertion or tubing changes, or inadvertent opening, cutting, or breaking of catheter	■ Clamp catheter immediately. ■ Turn patient on his left side, head down, so that air can enter the right atrium. Maintain this position for 20 to 30 minutes. ■ Administer oxygen. ■ Notify the physician. ■ Document interventions. *Prevention* ■ Purge all air from tubing before hookup. ■ Teach patient to perform Valsalva's maneuver during catheter insertion and tubing changes. ■ Use air-eliminating filters. ■ Use an infusion device with air detection capability. ■ Use luer-lock tubing, tape the connections, or use locking devices for all connections.

(continued)

I.V. THERAPY AND BLOOD PRODUCTS

RISKS OF CENTRAL VENOUS THERAPY *(continued)*

Complication and findings	Possible causes	Nursing interventions
Thrombosis ■ Edema at puncture site ■ Erythema ■ Ipsilateral swelling of arm, neck, and face ■ Pain along vein ■ Fever, malaise ■ Chest pain ■ Dyspnea ■ Cyanosis	■ Sluggish flow rate ■ Composition of catheter material (polyvinyl chloride catheters are more thrombogenic) ■ Hematopoietic status of patient ■ Preexisting limb edema ■ Infusion of irritating solutions	■ Notify the physician. ■ Possibly remove catheter. ■ Possibly infuse anticoagulant doses of heparin. ■ Verify thrombosis with diagnostic studies. ■ Apply warm, wet compresses locally. ■ Don't use limb on affected side for subsequent venipuncture. ■ Document interventions. *Prevention* ■ Maintain steady flow rate with infusion pump, or flush catheter at regular intervals. ■ Use catheters made of less thrombogenic materials or catheters coated to prevent thrombosis. ■ Dilute irritating solutions. ■ Use a 0.22-micron filter for infusions.

HOW TO AVOID TRANSFUSION ERRORS

Proper identification of the patient and the blood product he's to be given is essential, as is following your facility's policy and taking these precautions:

■ Match the patient's name, medical record number, ABO and Rh status, and blood bank identification numbers with the label on the blood bag.
■ Check the expiration date.
■ Have another nurse verify the information.
■ Sign the blood slip, filling in the required data. The blood slip will prove useful if the patient develops an adverse reaction.
■ Double-check the physician's order to make sure you're transfusing the correct product.
■ Make sure that the blood was typed and crossmatched within the last 48 hours—a Food and Drug Administration requirement for transfusions.

BLOOD COMPATIBILITY

Precise typing and crossmatching of donor and recipient blood can avoid transfusions of incompatible blood, which can be fatal. RBCs are classified as type A, B, or AB, depending on the antigen detected on the cell, or type O, which has no detectable A or B antigens. Similarly, blood plasma has or lacks anti-A or anti-B antibodies.

A person with type O blood is a universal donor. Because his blood lacks A or B antigens, it can be transfused in an emergency in limited amounts to any patient regardless of blood type and with little risk of reaction. A person with AB blood is a universal recipient. Because his blood lacks A and B antibodies, he can receive types A, B, or O blood (given as packed RBCs). This chart shows ABO compatibility at a glance.

Blood group	Antibodies in plasma	Compatible RBCs	Compatible plasma
RECIPIENT			
O	Anti-A and Anti-B	O	O, A, B, AB
A	Anti-B	A, O	A, AB
B	Anti-A	B, O	B, AB
AB	Neither Anti-A nor Anti-B	AB, A, B, O	AB
DONOR			
O	Anti-A and Anti-B	O, A, B, AB	O
A	Anti-B	A, AB	A, O
B	Anti-A	B, AB	B, O
AB	Neither Anti-A nor Anti-B	AB	AB, A, B, O

Transfusing blood and selected components

Blood component	Indications	Crossmatching
Whole blood Complete (pure) blood Volume: 450 or 500 ml	■ To restore blood volume lost from hemorrhaging, trauma, or burns	■ ABO identical: Type A receives A; type B receives B; type AB receives AB; type O receives O ■ Rh match necessary
Packed red blood cells (RBCs) Same RBC mass as whole blood but with 80% of the plasma removed Volume: 250 ml	■ To restore or maintain oxygen-carrying capacity ■ To correct anemia and blood loss that occurs during surgery ■ To increase RBC mass	■ Type A receives A or O ■ Type B receives B or O ■ Type AB receives AB, A, B, or O ■ Type O receives O ■ Rh match necessary
Platelets Platelet sediment from RBCs or plasma Volume: 35 to 50 ml/unit	■ To treat thrombocytopenia caused by decreased platelet production, increased platelet destruction, or massive transfusion of stored blood ■ To treat acute leukemia and marrow aplasia ■ To improve platelet count preoperatively in a patient whose count is 100,000/μl or less	■ ABO compatibility unnecessary but preferable with repeated platelet transfusions ■ Rh match preferred
Fresh frozen plasma (FFP) Uncoagulated plasma separated from RBCs and rich in coagulation factors V, VIII, and IX Volume: 180 to 300 ml	■ To expand plasma volume ■ To treat postoperative hemorrhage or shock ■ To correct an undetermined coagulation factor deficiency ■ To replace a specific factor when that factor alone isn't available ■ To correct factor deficiencies resulting from hepatic disease	■ ABO compatibility unnecessary but preferable with repeated platelet transfusions ■ Rh match preferred
Albumin 5% (buffered saline); albumin 25% (salt poor) A small plasma protein prepared by fractionating pooled plasma Volume: 5% = 12.5 g/250 ml; 25% = 12.5 g/50 ml	■ To replace volume lost because of shock from burns, trauma, surgery, or infections ■ To replace volume and prevent marked hemoconcentration ■ To treat hypoproteinemia (with or without edema)	■ Unnecessary

Nursing considerations

- Use a straight-line or Y-type I.V. set to infuse blood over 2 to 4 hours.
- Avoid giving whole blood when the patient can't tolerate the circulatory volume.
- Reduce the risk of a transfusion reaction by adding a microfilter to the administration set to remove platelets.
- Warm blood if giving a large quantity.

- Use a straight-line or Y-type I.V. set to infuse blood over 2 to 4 hours.
- Bear in mind that packed RBCs provide the same oxygen-carrying capacity as whole blood with less risk of volume overload.
- Give packed RBCs, as ordered, to prevent potassium and ammonia buildup, which may occur in stored plasma.
- Avoid administering packed RBCs for anemic conditions correctable by nutritional or drug therapy.

- Use a component drip administration set to infuse 100 ml over 15 minutes.
- As prescribed, premedicate with antipyretics and antihistamines if the patient's history includes a platelet transfusion reaction.
- Avoid administering platelets when the patient has a fever.
- Prepare to draw blood for a platelet count, as ordered, 1 hour after the platelet transfusion to determine platelet transfusion increments.
- Keep in mind that the physician seldom orders a platelet transfusion for conditions in which platelet destruction is accelerated, such as idiopathic thrombocytopenic purpura and drug-induced thrombocytopenia.

- Use a straight-line I.V. set and administer the infusion rapidly.
- Keep in mind that large-volume transfusions of FFP may require correction for hypocalcemia because citric acid in FFP binds calcium.

- Use a straight-line I.V. set with rate and volume dictated by the patient's condition and response.
- Remember that reactions to albumin (fever, chills, nausea) are rare.
- Avoid mixing albumin with protein hydrolysates and alcohol solutions.
- Consider delivering albumin as a volume expander until the laboratory completes cross-matching for a whole blood transfusion.
- Keep in mind that albumin is contraindicated in severe anemia and administered cautiously in cardiac and pulmonary disease because heart failure may result from circulatory overload.

(continued)

TRANSFUSING BLOOD AND SELECTED COMPONENTS *(continued)*

Blood component	Indications	Crossmatching
Factor VIII (cryoprecipitate) Insoluble portion of plasma recovered from FFP Volume: approximately 30 ml (freeze-dried)	■ To treat a patient with hemophilia A ■ To control bleeding associated with factor VIII deficiency ■ To replace fibrinogen or deficient factor VIII	■ ABO compatibility unnecessary but preferable

GUIDE TO TRANSFUSION REACTIONS

Any patient receiving a transfusion of processed blood products can experience a transfusion reaction. Transfusion reactions typically occur from antigen-antibody reactions; however, they may also occur as a result of bacterial contamination.

Reaction and causes	Signs and symptoms
Allergic ■ Allergen in donor blood ■ Donor blood hypersensitive to certain drugs	■ Anaphylaxis (chills, facial swelling, laryngeal edema, pruritus, urticaria, wheezing), fever, nausea, and vomiting
Bacterial contamination ■ Organisms that can survive cold, such as *Pseudomonas* and *Staphylococcus*	■ Chills, fever, vomiting, abdominal cramping, diarrhea, shock, signs of renal failure
Febrile ■ Bacterial lipopolysaccharides ■ Antileukocyte recipient antibodies directed against donor white blood cells	■ Temperature up to 104° F (40° C), chills, headache, facial flushing, palpitations, cough, chest tightness, increased pulse rate, flank pain
Hemolytic ■ ABO or Rh incompatibility ■ Intradonor incompatibility ■ Improper crossmatching ■ Improperly stored blood	■ Chest pain, dyspnea, facial flushing, fever, chills, shaking, hypotension, flank pain, hemoglobinuria, oliguria, bloody oozing at the infusion site or surgical incision site, burning sensation along vein receiving blood, shock, renal failure
Plasma protein incompatibility ■ Immunoglobulin-A incompatibility	■ Abdominal pain, diarrhea, dyspnea, chills, fever, flushing, hypotension

Nursing considerations

■ Use the administration set supplied by the manufacturer. Administer factor VIII with a filter. Standard dose recommended for treatment of acute bleeding episodes in hemophilia is 15 to 20 U/kg.
■ Half-life of factor VIII (8 to 10 hours) necessitates repeated transfusions at specified intervals to maintain normal levels.

Nursing interventions

■ Administer antihistamines as prescribed.
■ Monitor patient for anaphylactic reaction and administer epinephrine and corticosteroids if indicated.

■ Provide broad-spectrum antibiotics, corticosteroids, or epinephrine as prescribed.
■ Maintain strict blood storage control.
■ Change blood administration set and filter every 4 hours or after every 2 units.
■ Infuse each unit of blood over 2 to 4 hours; stop the infusion if the time span exceeds 4 hours.
■ Maintain sterile technique when administering blood products.

■ Relieve symptoms with an antipyretic, an antihistamine, or meperidine, as prescribed.
■ If the patient requires further transfusions, use frozen RBCs, add a special leukocyte removal filter to the blood line, or premedicate him with acetaminophen, as prescribed, before starting another transfusion.

■ Monitor blood pressure.
■ Manage shock with I.V. fluids, oxygen, epinephrine, a diuretic, and a vasopressor, as prescribed.
■ Obtain posttransfusion-reaction blood samples and urine specimens for analysis.
■ Observe for signs of hemorrhage resulting from disseminated intravascular coagulation.

■ Administer oxygen, fluids, epinephrine, or a corticosteroid as prescribed.

3

DRUG THERAPY AND TABLES

CONVERSION FACTORS

Weight conversion

To convert a patient's weight in pounds to kilograms, divide the number of pounds by 2.2 kg; to convert a patient's weight in kilograms to pounds, multiply the number of kilograms by 2.2 lbs.

Pounds	Kilograms
10	4.5
20	9
30	13.6
40	18.1
50	22.7
60	27.2
70	31.8
80	36.3
90	40.9
100	45.4
110	49.9
120	54.4
130	59
140	63.5
150	68
160	72.6
170	77.1
180	81.6
190	86.2
200	90.8

CONVERSION FACTORS *(continued)*

Temperature conversion

To convert Fahrenheit to Celsius, subtract 32 from the temperature in Fahrenheit and then divide by 1.8; to convert Celsius to Fahrenheit, multiply the temperature in Celsius by 1.8 and then add 32.

$$(F - 32) \div 1.8 = C \text{ degrees}$$
$$(C \times 1.8) + 32 = F \text{ degrees}$$

Fahrenheit degrees (F°)	Celsius degrees (C°)	Fahrenheit degrees (F°)	Celsius degrees (C°)
89.6	32	100.8	38.2
91.4	33	101	38.3
93.2	34	101.2	38.4
94.3	34.6	101.4	38.6
95.0	35	101.8	38.8
95.4	35.2	102	38.9
96.2	35.7	102.2	39
96.8	36	102.6	39.2
97.2	36.2	102.8	39.3
97.6	36.4	103	39.4
98	36.7	103.2	39.6
98.6	37	103.4	39.7
99	37.2	103.6	39.8
99.3	37.4	104	40
99.7	37.6	104.4	40.2
100	37.8	104.6	40.3
100.4	38	104.8	40.4
		105	40.6

(continued)

DRUG THERAPY AND TABLES

CONVERSION FACTORS *(continued)*

Solid equivalents

Milligram (mg)	Gram (g)	Grain (gr)
1,000	1	15
600 (or 650)	0.6	10
500	0.5	7.5
300 (or 325)	0.3	5
200	0.2	3
100	0.1	1.5
60 (or 65)	0.06	1
30	0.03	½
15	0.15	¼

Liquid equivalents

Metric (ml)	Apothecary	Household
—	1 minim = 1 drop (gtt)	—
1	16 minims	—
4	1 dram	—
5	—	1 teaspoon (tsp)
15	4 drams or ½ ounce	1 tablespoon (tbs)
30	8 drams or 1 ounce	1 ounce or 2 tbs
50	—	1 pint
1,000	—	1 quart or 2 pints

DOSAGE CALCULATION FORMULAS AND COMMON CONVERSIONS

Common calculations

Body surface area in $m^2 = \sqrt{\dfrac{\text{height in cm} \times \text{weight in kg}}{3,600}}$

mcg/ml = mg/ml $\times$ 1,000

ml/minute = $\dfrac{\text{ml/hour}}{60}$

gtt/minute = $\dfrac{\text{volume in ml to be infused}}{\text{time in minutes}} \times$ drip factor in gtt/ml

mg/minute = $\dfrac{\text{mg in bag}}{\text{ml in bag}} \times$ flow rate $\div$ 60

mcg/minute = $\dfrac{\text{mg in bag}}{\text{ml in bag}} \div 0.06 \times$ flow rate

mcg/kg/minute = $\dfrac{\text{mcg/ml} \times \text{ml/minute}}{\text{weight in kilograms}}$

DRUG THERAPY
AND TABLES

Common conversions

1 kg = 1,000 g
1 g = 1,000 mg
1 mg = 1,000 mcg

1 oz = 30 g
1 lb = 454 g
2.2 lb = 1 kg

1 L = 1,000 ml
1 ml = 1,000 microliters (µl)
1 tsp = 5 ml
1 tbs = 15 ml
2 tbs = 30 ml
8 oz = 240 ml

1″ = 2.54 cm

BODY SURFACE AREA NOMOGRAM

Height	Body surface area	Weight

Height	Body surface area	Weight
cm 200 — 79 inch	2.80 m²	kg 150 — 330 lb
— 78	2.70	145 — 320
195 — 77	2.60	140 — 310
— 76		135 — 300
190 — 75	2.50	130 — 290
— 74		— 280
185 — 73	2.40	125 — 270
— 72	2.30	120 — 260
180 — 71		115 — 250
— 70	2.20	110 — 240
175 — 69	2.10	105 — 230
— 68		100 — 220
170 — 67	2.00	
— 66	1.95	95 — 210
165 — 65	1.90	90 — 200
— 64	1.85	
160 — 63	1.80	85 — 190
— 62	1.75	80 — 180
155 — 61	1.70	
— 60	1.65	75 — 170
150 — 59	1.60	— 160
— 58	1.55	70 — 150
145 — 57	1.50	
— 56	1.45	65 — 140
140 — 55	1.40	60 — 130
— 54	1.35	
135 — 53	1.30	55 — 120
— 52	1.25	
130 — 51	1.20	50 — 110
— 50	1.15	— 105
125 — 49	1.10	45 — 100
— 48	1.05	— 95
120 — 47	1.00	40 — 90
— 46	0.95	— 85
115 — 45	0.90	— 80
— 44	0.86 m²	35 — 75
110 — 43		— 70
— 42		
105 — 41		kg 30 — 66 lb
— 40		
cm 100 — 39 in		

DISPLACING THE SKIN FOR Z-TRACK INJECTION

By blocking the needle pathway after an injection, the Z-track technique allows I.M. injection while minimizing the risk of subcutaneous irritation and staining from such drugs as iron dextran. The illustrations here show how to perform a Z-track injection.

Before the procedure begins, the skin, subcutaneous fat, and muscle lie in their normal positions.

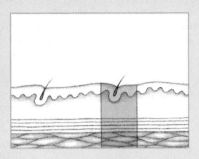

To begin, place your finger on the skin surface and pull the skin and subcutaneous layers out of alignment with the underlying muscle. You should move the skin about ½″ (1 cm).

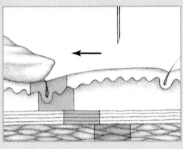

Insert the needle at a 90-degree angle at the site where you initially placed your finger. Inject the drug and withdraw the needle.

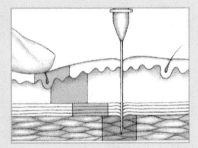

Finally, remove your finger from the skin surface, allowing the layers to return to their normal positions. The needle track (shown by the dotted line) is now broken at the junction of each tissue layer, trapping the drug in the muscle.

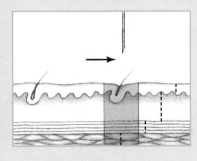

DRUGS THAT SHOULDN'T BE CRUSHED

Many drug forms, such as slow-release, enteric-coated, encapsulated beads, wax-matrix, sublingual, and buccal forms, are made to release their active ingredients over a certain period of time or at preset points after administration. The disruptions caused by crushing these drug forms can dramatically affect the absorption rate and increase the risk of adverse reactions.

Other reasons not to crush these drug forms include such considerations as taste, tissue irritation, and unusual formulation — for example, a capsule within a capsule, a liquid within a capsule, or a multiple-compressed tablet. Avoid crushing the following drugs, listed by brand name, for the reasons noted beside them.

Accutane (irritant)

Aciphex (delayed release)

Adalat CC (sustained release)

Aggrenox (extended release)

Allegra-D (slow release)

Artane Sequels (slow release)

Arthrotec (delayed release)

Asacol (delayed release)

Azulfidine EN-tabs (enteric coated)

Bellergal-S (slow release)

Bisacodyl (enteric coated)

Bontril Slow-Release (slow release)

Breonesin (liquid filled)

Brexin-L.A. (slow release)

Bromfed (slow release)

Bromfed-PD (slow release)

Bromphen (slow release)

Bronkodyl SR (slow release)

Calan SR (slow release)

Carbatrol (extended release)

Carbiset-TR (slow release)

Cardizem CD, SR (slow release)

Ceclor CD (slow release)

Ceftin (taste)

Charcoal Plus DS (enteric coated)

Chloral Hydrate (liquid within a capsule, taste)

Chlor-Trimeton Allergy 8-hour and 12-hour (slow release)

Choledyl SA (slow release)

Chromagen (taste and irritant)

Cipro (taste)

Claritin-D (slow release)

Claritin-D 24-hour (slow release)

Colace (liquid within a capsule, taste)

Colazal (granules within capsules must reach colon intact)

Colestid (protective coating)

Comhist LA (slow release)

Compazine Spansules (slow release)

Concerta (extended release)

Congess SR (sustained release)

Contac 12-hour, Maximum Strength 12-hour (slow release)

Cotazym-S (enteric coated)

Covera-HS (slow release)

Creon (enteric coated)

Cytovene (irritant)

Dallergy (slow release)

Deconamine SR (slow release)

Deconsal, Sprinkle Capsules (slow release)

Demazin Repetabs (sustained release)

Depakene (slow release, mucous membrane irritant)

Drugs that shouldn't be crushed *(continued)*

Depakote (enteric coated)

Desoxyn Gradumets (slow release)

Desyrel (taste)

Dexedrine Spansules (slow release)

Diamox Sequels (slow release)

Dilacor XR (slow release)

Dilatrate-SR (slow release)

Disobrom (slow release)

Ditropan XL (slow release)

Dolobid (irritant)

Donnatal Extentabs (slow release)

Donnazyme (slow release)

Drisdol (liquid filled)

Dristan 12-hour (slow release)

Drixoral (slow release)

Drixoral Plus (slow release)

Drixoral Sinus (slow release)

Drize (slow release)

Dulcolax (enteric coated)

Dura-Vent (slow release)

Dura-Vent A (slow release)

Dura-Vent DA (slow release)

DynaCirc CR (slow release)

Ecotrin (enteric coated)

Ecotrin Maximum Strength (enteric coated)

E.E.S. 400 Filmtab (enteric coated)

Effexor XR (extended release)

E-Mycin (enteric coated)

Endafed (slow release)

Entex LA (slow release)

Entex PSE (slow release)

Equanil (taste)

Eryc (enteric coated)

Ery-Tab (enteric coated)

Erythrocin Stearate (enteric coated)

Erythromycin Base (enteric coated)

Eskalith CR (slow release)

Extendryl JR (slow release)

Extendryl SR (slow release)

Fedahist Gyrocaps, Timecaps (slow release)

Feldene (mucous membrane irritant)

Feocyte (slow release)

Feosol (enteric coated)

Feosol Spansule (slow release)

Feratab (enteric coated)

Fergon (slow release)

Fero-Folic-500 (slow release)

Fero-Grad-500 (slow release)

Ferro-Sequels (slow release)

Feverall Children's Capsules, Sprinkle (taste)

Flomax (slow release)

Fumatinic (slow release)

Geocillin (taste)

Glucotrol XL (slow release)

Gris-PEG (crushing may cause precipitation of larger particles)

Guaifed (slow release)

Guaifed-PD (slow release)

Guaifenex LA (slow release)

Guaifenex PPA 75 (slow release)

Guaifenex PSE (slow release)

Humibid Sprinkle, DM, DM Sprinkle, L.A. (slow release)

Hydergine LC (liquid within a capsule)

Hytakerol (liquid filled)

Iberet (slow release)

Iberet-500 (slow release)

ICAPS Plus (slow release)

(continued)

ICAPS Time Release (slow release)

Ilotycin (enteric coated)

Imdur (slow release)

Inderal LA (slow release)

Inderide LA (slow release)

Indocin SR (slow release)

Ionamin (slow release)

Isoptin SR (slow release)

Isordil Sublingual (sublingual)

Isordil Tembids (slow release)

Isosorbide Dinitrate Sublingual (sublingual)

Isuprel Glossets (sublingual)

Kaon-Cl (slow release)

K-Dur (slow release)

Klor-Con (slow release)

Klotrix (slow release)

K-Tab (slow release)

Levbid (slow release)

Levsinex Timecaps (slow release)

Lithobid (slow release)

Macrobid (slow release)

Mestinon Timespans (slow release)

Methylin ER (extended release)

Micro-K (slow release)

Micro-K Extencaps (slow release)

Motrin (taste)

MS Contin (slow release)

Naprelan (slow release)

Nexium (sustained release)

Nia-Bid (slow release)

Niaspan (slow release)

Nitro-Bid (slow release)

Nitroglyn (slow release)

Nitrong (sublingual)

Nitrostat (sublingual)

Nolamine (slow release)

Norflex (slow release)

Norpace CR (slow release)

Novafed A (slow release)

Oramorph SR (slow release)

Ornade Spansules (slow release)

Oruvail (slow release)

OxyContin (slow release)

Pancrease (enteric coated)

Pancrease MT (enteric coated)

PCE (slow release)

Pentasa (controlled release)

Perdiem (wax coated)

Phazyme (slow release)

Phazyme 95 (slow release)

Phenergan (taste)

Phyllocontin (slow release)

Placidyl (slow release)

Plendil (slow release)

Polaramine Repetabs (slow release)

Prelu-2 (slow release)

Prevacid (delayed release)

Prilosec (slow release)

Pro-Banthine (taste)

Procainamide HCl SR (slow release)

Procan SR (slow release)

Procanbid (slow release)

Procardia (delayed absorption)

Procardia XL (slow release)

Pronestyl-SR (slow release)

Protonix (delayed release)

Proventil Repetabs (slow release)

Prozac (slow release)

Quibron-T/SR (slow release)

DRUGS THAT SHOULDN'T BE CRUSHED *(continued)*

Quinaglute Dura-Tabs (slow release)

Quinidex Extentabs (slow release)

Respaire SR (slow release)

Respbid (slow release)

Ritalin-SR (slow release)

Rondec-TR (slow release)

Roxanol SR (slow release)

Ru-Tuss (slow release)

Ru-Tuss DE, II (slow release)

Sinemet CR (slow release)

Slo-bid Gyrocaps (slow release)

Slo-Niacin (slow release)

Slo-Phyllin GG, Gyrocaps (slow release)

Slow FE (slow release)

Slow-K (slow release)

Slow-Mag (slow release)

Sorbitrate SA (slow release)

Sparine (taste)

Sudafed 12-Hour (slow release)

Sular (slow release)

Sustaire (slow release)

Tamine S.R. (slow release)

Tavist-D (multiple compressed tablet)

Tegretol-XR (extended release)

Teldrin (slow release)

Teldrin Spansules (slow release)

Ten-K (slow release)

Tenuate Dospan (slow release)

Tessalon Perles (slow release)

Theobid Duracaps (slow release)

Theocron (slow release)

Theoclear L.A. (slow release)

Theo-Dur (slow release)

Theolair-SR (slow release)

Theo-Sav (slow release)

Theospan-SR (slow release)

Theo-24 (slow release)

Theovent (slow release)

Theo-X (slow release)

Thorazine Spansules (slow release)

Tiazac (extended release)

Topamax (bitter taste)

Toprol XL (slow release)

T-Phyl (slow release)

Tranxene-SD (slow release)

Trental (slow release)

Triaminic (slow release)

Triaminic TR (slow release)

Triaminic-12 (slow release)

Trilafon Repetabs (slow release)

Trinalin Repetabs (slow release)

Triptone Caplets (slow release)

Tuss-LA (slow release)

Tuss-Ornade Spansules (slow release)

Tylenol Extended Relief (slow relief)

ULR-LA (slow release)

Uniphyl (slow release)

Vantin (taste)

Verelan (slow release)

Volmax (slow release)

Voltaren (enteric coated)

Voltaren-XR (enteric coated)

Wellbutrin SR (sustained release)

Wygesic (taste)

ZORprin (slow release)

Zyban (slow release)

Zymase (enteric coated)

COMPATIBILITY IN A SYRINGE

KEY

Y = compatible for at least 30 minutes

P = provisionally compatible; administer within 15 minutes

P(5) = provisionally compatible; administer within 5 minutes

N = not compatible

* = conflicting data (A blank space indicates no available data.)

	atropine sulfate	butorphanol tartrate	chlorpromazine HCl	cimetidine HCl	codeine phosphate	dexamethasone sodium phosphate	dimenhydrinate	diphenhydramine HCl	droperidol	fentanyl citrate	glycopyrrolate	heparin Na	hydromorphone HCl	hydroxyzine HCl	meperidine HCl	metoclopramide HCl
atropine sulfate	■	Y	P	Y			P	P	P	P	Y	P(5)	Y	P*	P	P
butorphanol tartrate	Y	■	Y	Y			N	Y	Y	Y				Y	Y	Y
chlorpromazine HCl	P	Y	■	N			N	P	P	P	Y	N	Y	P	P	P
cimetidine HCl	Y	Y	N	■			Y	Y	Y	Y	Y	P(5)*	Y	Y	Y	
codeine phosphate					■						Y			Y		
dexamethasone sodium phosphate						■	N*				N		N*			Y
dimenhydrinate	P	N	N				■	P	P	P	N	P(5)	Y	N	P	P
diphenhydramine HCl	P	Y	P	Y		N*	P	■	P	P	Y		Y	P	P	Y
droperidol	P	Y	P	Y			P	P	■	P	Y	N			P	P
fentanyl citrate	P	Y	P	Y			P	P	P	■		P(5)	Y	P	P	P
glycopyrrolate	Y		Y	Y	Y	N	N	Y	Y		■		Y	Y	Y	
heparin Na	P(5)		N	P(5)*			P(5)		N	P(5)		■			N	P(5)*
hydromorphone HCl	Y		Y	Y		N*	Y	Y		Y	Y		■	Y		
hydroxyzine HCl	P*	Y	P	Y	Y		N	P	P	P	Y		Y	■	P	P
meperidine HCl	P	Y	P	Y			P	P	P	P	Y	N		P	■	P
metoclopramide HCl	P	Y	P			Y	P	P	P	P		P(5)*		P	P	■
midazolam HCl	Y	Y	Y	Y			N	Y	Y	Y	Y		Y	Y	Y	Y
morphine sulfate	P	Y	P	Y			P	P	P	P	Y	N*		P	N	N
nalbuphine HCl	Y			Y			Y	Y			Y			Y		
pentazocine lactate	P	Y	P	Y			P	P	P	P	N	N	Y	P	P	P
pentobarbital Na	P	N	N	N			N	N	N	N	N		Y	N	N	
perphenazine	Y	Y	Y	Y			Y	Y	Y	Y				Y	Y	P*
phenobarbital Na												P(5)				
prochlorperazine edisylate	P	Y	P	Y			N	P	P	P	Y		N*	P	P	P
promazine HCl	P		P	Y			N	P	P	P	Y			P	P	P
promethazine HCl	P	Y	P	Y			N	P	P	P	Y	N	Y	P	P	P*
ranitidine HCl	Y		N*			Y	Y	Y			Y	Y	Y	N	Y	Y
scopolamine HBr	P	Y	P	Y			P	P	P	P	Y		Y	P	P	P
sodium bicarbonate												N				N
thiethylperazine maleate		Y												Y		
thiopental Na			N				N	N				N			N	

midazolam HCl	morphine sulfate	nalbuphine HCl	pentazocine lactate	pentobarbital Na	perphenazine	phenobarbital Na	prochlorperazine edisylate	promazine HCl	promethazine HCl	ranitidine HCl	scopolamine HBr	sodium bicarbonate	thiethylperazine maleate	thiopental Na	
Y	P	Y	P	P	Y		P	P	P	Y	P				atropine sulfate
Y	Y		Y	N	Y		Y		Y		Y		Y		butorphanol tartrate
Y	P		P	N	Y		P	P	P	N*	P			N	chlorpromazine HCl
Y	Y	Y	Y	N	Y		Y	Y	Y		Y				cimetidine HCl
															codeine phosphate
										Y					dexamethasone sodium phosphate
N	P		P	N	Y		N	N	N	Y	P			N	dimenhydrinate
Y	P	Y	P	N	Y		P	P	P	Y	P			N	diphenhydramine HCl
Y	P	Y	P	N	Y		P	P	P		P				droperidol
Y	P		P	N	Y		P	P	P	Y	P				fentanyl citrate
Y	Y	Y	N	N			Y	Y	Y	Y	Y	N		N	glycopyrrolate
	N*		N			P(5)		N							heparin Na
Y			Y	Y			N*		Y	Y	Y		Y		hydromorphone HCl
Y	P	Y	P	N	Y		P	P	P	N	P				hydroxyzine HCl
Y	N		P	N	Y		P	P	P	Y	P			N	meperidine HCl
Y	P		P		P*		P	P	P*	Y	P	N			metoclopramide HCl
■	Y	Y		N	N		N	Y	Y	N	Y		Y		midazolam HCl
Y	■	P	P	N*	Y		P*	P	P*	Y	P			N	morphine sulfate
Y	P	■	N	N			Y		N*	Y	Y		Y		nalbuphine HCl
	P	N	■	N	Y		P	P*	P*	Y	P				pentazocine lactate
N	N*	N	N	■	N		N	N	N	N	P	Y		Y	pentobarbital Na
N	Y		Y	N	■		Y		Y	Y	Y		N		perphenazine
						■				N					phenobarbital Na
N	P*	Y	P	N	Y		■	P	P	Y	P			N	prochlorperazine edisylate
Y	P		P*	N			P	■	P		P			N	promazine HCl
Y	P*	N*	P*	N	Y		P	P	■	Y	P			N	promethazine HCl
N	Y	Y	Y	N	Y	N	Y		Y	■	Y		Y		ranitidine HCl
Y	P	Y	P	P	Y		P	P	P	Y	■			Y	scopolamine HBr
				Y								■		N	sodium bicarbonate
Y		Y			N					Y			■		thiethylperazine maleate
	N			Y			N		N		Y	N		■	thiopental Na

DRUG THERAPY AND TABLES

DIALYZABLE DRUGS

The amount of a drug removed by dialysis differs among patients and depends on several factors, including the patient's condition, the drug's properties, length of dialysis and dialysate used, rate of blood flow or dwell time, and purpose of dialysis. This table indicates the effect of hemodialysis on selected drugs.

Drug	Level reduced by hemodialysis	Drug	Level reduced by hemodialysis
Acetaminophen	Yes (may not influence toxicity)	Carbenicillin	Yes
Acyclovir	Yes	Carmustine	No
Allopuril	Yes	Cefaclor	Yes
Alprazolam	No	Cefadroxil	Yes
Amikacin	Yes	Cefazolin	Yes
Amiodarone	No	Cefepime	Yes
Amitriptyline	No	Cefonicid	Yes (only by 20%)
Amoxicillin	Yes	Cefoperazone	Yes
Amoxicillin/ Clavulanate potassium	Yes	Cefotaxime	Yes
		Cefotetan	Yes (only by 20%)
Amphotericin B	No	Cefoxitin	Yes
Ampicillin	Yes	Ceftazidime	Yes
Ampicillin/ Clavulanate potassium	Yes	Ceftizoxime	Yes
		Ceftriaxone	No
Aspirin	Yes	Cefuroxime	Yes
Atenolol	Yes	Cephalexin	Yes
Azathioprine	Yes	Cephradine	Yes
Aztreonam	Yes	Chloral hydrate	Yes
Captopril	Yes	Chlorambucil	No
Carbamazepine	No	Chlordiazepoxide	No

DIALYZABLE DRUGS *(continued)*

Drug	Level reduced by hemodialysis	Drug	Level reduced by hemodialysis
Chloroquine	No	Diphenhydramine	No
Chlorpheniramine	No	Dipyridamole	No
Chlorpromazine	No	Disopyramide	Yes
Chlorthalidone	No	Doxazosin	No
Cimetidine	Yes	Doxepin	No
Ciprofloxacin	Yes (only by 20%)	Doxorubicin	No
Cisplatin	No	Doxycycline	No
Clindamycin	No	Enalapril	Yes
Clofibrate	No	Erythromycin	Yes (only by 20%)
Clonazepam	No	Ethambutol	Yes (only by 20%)
Clonidine	No	Ethosuximide	Yes
Clorazepate	No	Famotidine	No
Cloxacillin	No	Fenoprofen	No
Codeine	No	Flecainide	No
Colchicine	No	Fluconazole	Yes
Cortisone	No	Flucytosine	Yes
Co-trimoxazole	Yes	Fluorouracil	Yes
Cyclophosphamide	Yes	Fluoxetine	No
Diazepam	No	Flurazepam	No
Diclofenac	No	Fosinopril	No
Dicloxacillin	No	Furosemide	No
Digoxin	No	Gabapentin	Yes
Diltiazem	No	Ganciclovir	Yes

(continued)

DIALYZABLE DRUGS *(continued)*

Drug	Level reduced by hemodialysis	Drug	Level reduced by hemodialysis
Gemfibrozil	No	Ketoconazole	No
Gentamicin	Yes	Ketoprofen	Yes
Glipizide	No	Labetalol	No
Glutethimide	Yes	Levofloxacin	No
Glyburide	No	Lidocaine	No
Guanfacine	No	Lithium	Yes
Haloperidol	No	Lomustine	No
Heparin	No	Loracarbef	Yes
Hydralazine	No	Loratadine	No
Hydrochlorothiazide	No	Lorazepam	No
Hydroxyzine	No	Mechlorethamine	No
Ibuprofen	No	Mefenamic acid	No
Imipenem/Cilastatin	Yes	Meperidine	No
Imipramine	No	Mercaptopurine	Yes
Indapamide	No	Methadone	No
Indomethacin	No	Methotrexate	Yes
Insulin	No	Methyldopa	Yes
Irbesartan	No	Methylprednisolone	No
Iron dextran	No	Metoclopramide	No
Isoniazid	Yes	Metolazone	No
Isosorbide	No	Metoprolol	No
Isradipine	No	Metronidazole	Yes
Kanamycin	Yes	Mexiletine	Yes

DIALYZABLE DRUGS *(continued)*

Drug	Level reduced by hemodialysis	Drug	Level reduced by hemodialysis
Miconazole	No	Oxazepam	No
Midazolam	No	Paroxetine	No
Minocycline	No	Penicillin G	Yes
Minoxidil	Yes	Pentamidine	No
Misoprostol	No	Pentazocine	Yes
Morphine	No	Phenobarbital	Yes
Nabumetone	No	Phenylbutazone	No
Nadolol	Yes	Phenytoin	No
Nafcillin	No	Piperacillin	Yes
Naproxen	No	Piroxicam	No
Nelfinavir	Yes	Prazosin	No
Netilmicin	Yes	Prednisone	No
Nifedipine	No	Primidone	Yes
Nimodipine	No	Procainamide	Yes
Nitrofurantoin	Yes	Promethazine	No
Nitroglycerin	No	Propoxyphene	No
Nitroprusside	Yes	Propranolol	No
Nizatidine	No	Protriptyline	No
Nofloxacin	No	Quinidine	Yes
Notriptyline	No	Ramipril	No
Ofloxacin	Yes	Ranitidine	Yes
Olanzapine	No	Rifampin	No
Omeprazole	No	Rofecoxib	No

(continued)

DIALYZABLE DRUGS *(continued)*

Drug	Level reduced by hemodialysis	Drug	Level reduced by hemodialysis
Sertraline	No	Tocainide	Yes
Sotalol	Yes	Tolbutamide	No
Stavudine	Yes	Topirimate	Yes
Streptomycin	Yes	Trazodone	No
Sucralfate	No	Triazolam	No
Sulbactam	Yes	Trimethoprim	Yes
Sulindac	No	Valacyclovir	Yes
Temazepam	No	Valproic acid	No
Theophylline	Yes	Valsartan	No
Ticarcillin	Yes	Vancomycin	No
Timolol	No	Verapamil	No
Tobramycin	Yes	Warfarin	No

DANGEROUS EFFECTS OF DRUG COMBINATIONS

If possible, avoid administering the drug combinations shown below to prevent dangerous drug interactions.

Drug	Interacting drug	Possible effect
Aminoglycosides amikacin gentamicin kanamycin neomycin netilmicin streptomycin tobramycin	Parenteral cephalosporins ■ Ceftazidime ■ Ceftizoxime	Possible enhanced nephrotoxicity
	Loop diuretics ■ Bumetanide ■ Ethacrynic acid ■ Furosemide	Possible enhanced ototoxicity
Amphetamines amphetamine benzphetamine dextroamphetamine methamphetamine	Urine alkalinizers ■ Potassium citrate ■ Sodium acetate ■ Sodium bicarbonate ■ Sodium citrate ■ Sodium lactate ■ Tromethamine	Decreased urinary excretion of amphetamine
Angiotensin-converting enzyme (ACE) inhibitors captopril enalapril lisinopril benazepril fosinopril ramipril quinapril	Indomethacin Nonsteroidal anti-inflammatory drugs (NSAIDs)	Decreased or abolished effectiveness of antihypertensive action of ACE inhibitors
Barbiturate anesthetics methohexital thiopental	Opiate analgesics	Enhanced central nervous system and respiratory depression
Barbiturates amobarbital aprobarbital butabarbital mephobarbital pentobarbital phenobarbital primidone secobarbital	Valproic acid	Increased serum barbiturate levels

(continued)

DANGEROUS EFFECTS OF DRUG COMBINATIONS *(continued)*

Drug	Interacting drug	Possible effect
Beta-adrenergic blockers acebutolol atenolol betaxolol carteolol esmolol levobunolol metoprolol nadolol penbutolol pindolol propranolol timolol	Verapamil	Enhanced pharmacologic effects of both beta-adrenergic blockers and verapamil
Carbamazepine	Erythromycin	Increased risk of carbamazepine toxicity
Carmustine	Cimetidine	Enhanced risk of bone marrow toxicity
Ciprofloxacin	Antacids that contain magnesium or aluminum hydroxide, iron supplements, sucralfate, multivitamins that contain iron or zinc	Decreased plasma levels and effectiveness of ciprofloxacin
Clonidine	Beta-adrenergic blockers	Enhanced rebound hypertension following rapid clonidine withdrawal
Cyclosporine	Carbamazepine, isoniazid, phenobarbital, phenytoin, rifabutin, rifampin	Reduced plasma levels of cyclosporine
Cardiac glycosides	Loop and thiazide diuretics	Increased risk of cardiac arrhythmias due to hypokalemia
	Thiazide-like diuretics	Increased therapeutic or toxic effects
Digoxin	Amiodarone	Decreased renal clearance of digoxin
	Quinidine	Enhanced clearance of digoxin
	Verapamil	Elevated serum digoxin levels
Dopamine	Phenytoin	Hypertension and bradycardia

DANGEROUS EFFECTS OF DRUG COMBINATIONS *(continued)*

Drug	Interacting drug	Possible effect
Epinephrine	Beta-adrenergic blockers	Increased systolic and diastolic pressures; marked decrease in heart rate
Erythromycin	Carbamazepine	Decreased carbamazepine clearance
	Theophylline	Decreased hepatic clearance of theophylline
Ethanol	Disulfiram Furazolidone Metronidazole	Acute alcohol intolerance reaction
Furazolidone	Amine-containing foods Anorexiants	Inhibits monoamine oxidase (MAO), possibly leading to hypertensive crisis
Heparin	Salicylates NSAIDs	Enhanced risk of bleeding
Levodopa	Furazolidone	Enhanced toxic effects of levodopa
Lithium	Thiazide diuretics NSAIDs	Decreased lithium excretion
Meperidine	MAO inhibitors	Cardiovascular instability and increased toxic effects
Methotrexate	Probenecid	Decreased methotrexate elimination
	Salicylates	Increased risk of methotrexate toxicity
MAO inhibitors	Amine-containing foods Anorexiants meperidine	Risk of hypertensive crisis
Nondepolarizing muscle relaxants	Aminoglycosides Inhaled anesthetics	Enhanced neuromuscular blockade
Potassium supplements	Potassium-sparing diuretics	Increased risk of hyperkalemia
Quinidine	Amiodarone	Increased risk of quinidine toxicity
Sympathomimetics	MAO inhibitors	Increased risk of hypertensive crisis

(continued)

DANGEROUS EFFECTS OF DRUG COMBINATIONS *(continued)*

Drug	Interacting drug	Possible effect
Tetracyclines	Antacids containing magnesium, aluminum, or bismuth salts Iron supplements	Decreased plasma levels and effectiveness of tetracyclines
Theophylline	Carbamazepine	Reduced theophylline levels
	Cimetidine	Increased theophylline levels
	Ciprofloxacin	Increased theophylline levels
	Erythromycin	Increased theophylline levels
	Phenobarbital	Reduced theophylline levels
	Rifampin	Reduced theophylline levels
Warfarin	Testosterone	Possible enhanced bleeding caused by increased hypoprothrombinemia
	Barbiturates Carbamazepine	Reduced effectiveness of warfarin
	Amiodarone Cephalosporins (certain ones) Chloral hydrate Cholestyramine Cimetidine Clofibrate Co-trimoxazole Dextrothyroxine Disulfiram	Increased risk of bleeding
	Erythromycin Glucagon Metronidazole Phenylbutazone Quinidine Quinine Salicylates Sulfinpyrazone Thyroid drugs Tricyclic antidepressants	Increased risk of bleeding
	Ethchlorvynol Glutethimide Griseofulvin	Decreased pharmacologic effect
	Rifampin Trazodone	Decreased risk of bleeding
	Methimazole Propylthiouracil	Increased or decreased risk of bleeding

HERB-DRUG INTERACTIONS

Herb	Drug	Possible effects
Aloe	Cardiac glycosides, antiarrhythmics	May lead to hypokalemia, which may potentiate cardiac glycosides and antiarrhythmics
	Thiazide diuretics, licorice, and other potassium-wasting drugs	Increases the effects of potassium wasting with thiazide diuretics, and other potassium-wasting drugs
	Orally administered drugs	Causes potential for decreased absorption of drugs because of more rapid GI transit time
Bilberry	Antiplatelets, anticoagulants	Decreases platelet aggregation
	Insulin, hypoglycemics	May increase serum insulin levels, causing hypoglycemia; increases effect with diabetes drugs
Capsicum	Antiplatelets, anticoagulants	Decreases platelet aggregation and increases fibrinolytic activity, prolonging bleeding time
	Nonsteroidal anti-inflammatory drugs (NSAIDs)	Stimulates GI secretions to help protect against NSAID-induced GI irritation
	ACE inhibitors	May cause cough
	Theophylline	Increases absorption of theophylline, possibly leading to higher serum levels or toxicity
	Monoamine oxidase (MAO) inhibitors	Decreases the effects resulting from the increased catecholamine secretion
	Central nervous system (CNS) depressants, such as opioids, benzodiazepines, barbiturates	Increases sedative effect
	Histamine-2 (H_2) blockers, proton pump inhibitors	Causes potential for decreased effectiveness because of increased acid secretion
Chamomile	Drugs requiring GI absorption	May delay drug absorption
	Anticoagulants	May enhance anticoagulant therapy and prolong bleeding time (if warfarin constituents)
	Iron	May reduce iron absorption because of tannic acid content

(continued)

HERB-DRUG INTERACTIONS *(continued)*

Herb	Drug	Possible effects
Echinacea	Immunosuppressants	May counteract immunosuppressant drugs
	Hepatotoxics	May increase hepatotoxicity with drugs known to elevate liver enzyme levels
	Warfarin	Increases bleeding time withoutan increased International Normalized Ratio (INR)
Evening primrose	Anticonvulsants	Lowers seizure threshold
Feverfew	Antiplatelets, anticoagulants	May decrease platelet aggregation and increase fibrinolytic activity
Garlic	Antiplatelets, anticoagulants	Enhances platelet inhibition, leading to increased anticoagulation
	Insulin, other drugs causing hypoglycemia	May increase serum insulin levels, causing hypoglycemia, an additive effect with antidiabetics
	Antihypertensives	Causes potential for additive hypotension
	Antihyperlipidemics	May have additive lipid-lowering properties
Ginger	Chemotherapy	May reduce nausea associated with chemotherapy
	H_2-blockers, proton pump inhibitors	Causes potential for decreased effectiveness because of increased acid secretion by ginger
	Antiplatelets, anticoagulants	Inhibits platelet aggregation by antagonizing thromboxane synthase and enhancing prostacyclin, leading to prolonged bleeding time
	Calcium channel blockers	May increase calcium uptake by myocardium, leading to altered drug effects
	Antihypertensives	May antagonize antihypertensive effect

HERB-DRUG INTERACTIONS *(continued)*

Herb	Drug	Possible effects
Ginkgo	Antiplatelets, anticoagulants	May enhance platelet inhibition, leading to increased anticoagulation
	Anticonvulsants	May decrease effectiveness of anticonvulsants
	Drugs known to lower seizure threshold	May further reduce seizure threshold
Ginseng	Stimulants	May potentiate stimulant effects
	Warfarin	May antagonize warfarin, resulting in a decreased INR
	Antibiotics	May enhance the effects of some antibiotics (Siberian ginseng)
	Anticoagulants, antiplatelets	Decreases platelet adhesiveness
	Digoxin	May falsely elevate digoxin levels
	MAO inhibitors	Potentiates action of MAO inhibitors
	Hormones, anabolic steroids	May potentiate effects of hormone and anabolic steroid therapies (estrogenic effects of ginseng may cause vaginal bleeding and breast nodules)
	Alcohol	Increases alcohol clearance, possibly by increasing activity of alcohol dehydrogenase
	Furosemide	May decrease diuretic effect of furosemide
	Antipsychotics	May stimulate CNS activity
Goldenseal	Heparin	May counteract anticoagulant effect of heparin
	Diuretics	Increases diuretic effect
	H_2-blockers, proton pump inhibitors	Causes potential for decreased effectiveness because of increased acid secretion by goldenseal
	General anesthetics	May potentiate hypotensive action of general anesthetics
	CNS depressants, such as opioids, barbiturates, benzodiazepines	Increases sedative effect

(continued)

HERB-DRUG INTERACTIONS (continued)

Herb	Drug	Possible effects
Grapeseed	Warfarin	Increases the effects and INR caused by tocopherol content of grapeseed
Green tea	Warfarin	Decreases effectiveness resulting from vitamin content of green tea
Hawthorn berry	Digoxin	Causes additive positive inotropic effect, with potential for digoxin toxicity
Kava	CNS stimulants or depressants	May hinder therapy with CNS stimulants
	Benzodiazepines	May result in comalike states
	Alcohol	Potentiates the depressant effect of alcohol and other CNS depressants
	Levodopa	Decreases the effectiveness of levodopa
Licorice	Digoxin	Causes hypokalemia, which predisposes to digoxin toxicity
	Hormonal contraceptives	Increases fluid retention and potential for increased blood pressure resulting from fluid overload
	Corticosteroids	Causes additive and enhanced effects of the corticosteroids
	Spironolactone	Decreases the effects of spironolactone
Ma huang	MAO inhibitors	Potentiates MAO inhibitors
	CNS stimulants, caffeine, theophylline	Causes CNS stimulation
	Digoxin	Increases the risk of arrhythmias
	Hypoglycemics	Decreases hypoglycemic effect because of hyperglycemia caused by ma huang
Melatonin	CNS depressants (such as opioids, barbiturates, benzodiazepines)	Increases sedative effects

HERB-DRUG INTERACTIONS *(continued)*

Herb	Drug	Possible effects
Milk thistle	Drugs causing diarrhea	Increases bile secretion and often causes loose stools; may increase effect of other drugs commonly causing diarrhea; also causes liver membrane-stabilization and antioxidant effects leading to protection from liver damage from various hepatotoxic drugs such as acetaminophen, phenytoin, ethanol, phenothiazines, butyrophenones
Nettle	Anticonvulsants	May increase sedative adverse effects and risk of seizure
	Narcotics, anxiolytics, hypnotics	May increase sedative adverse effects
	Warfarin	Decreases effectiveness resulting from vitamin K content of aerial parts of nettle
	Iron	May reduce iron absorption because of tannic acid content
Passion flower	CNS depressants (such as opioids, barbiturates, benzodiazepines)	Increases sedative effect
St. John's wort	SSRIs, MAO inhibitors, nefazodone, trazodone	Causes additive effects with SSRIs, MAO inhibitors, and other antidepressants, potentially leading to serotonin syndrome, especially when combined with SSRIs
	Indinavir; HIV protease inhibitors (PIs); nonnucleoside reverse transcriptase inhibitors (NNRTIs)	Induces cytochrome P450 metabolic pathway, which may decrease therapeutic effects of drugs using this pathway for metabolism (use of St. John's wort and PIs or NNRTIs should be avoided because of the potential for subtherapeutic antiretroviral levels and insufficient virologic response that could lead to resistance or class cross-resistance)
	Narcotics, alcohol	Enhances the sedative effect of narcotics and alcohol
	Photosensitizing drugs	Increases photosensitivity
	Sympathomimetic amines (such as pseudoephedrine)	Causes additive effects

(continued)

HERB-DRUG INTERACTIONS *(continued)*

Herb	Drug	Possible effects
St. John's wort *(continued)*	Digoxin	May reduce serum digoxin concentrations, decreasing therapeutic effects
	Reserpine	Antagonizes the effects of reserpine
	Hormonal contraceptives	Increases breakthrough bleeding when taken with hormonal contraceptives; also decreases the contraceptive's effectiveness
	Theophylline	May decrease serum theophylline levels, making the drug less effective
	Anesthetics	May prolong the effect of anesthesia drugs
	Cyclosporine	Decreases cyclosporine levels below therapeutic levels, threatening transplanted organ rejection
	Iron	May reduce iron absorption because of tannic acid content
	Warfarin	Has the potential to alter INR; reduces the effectiveness of anticoagulant, requiring increased dosage of drug
Valerian	Sedative hypnotics, CNS depressants	Enhances the effects of sedative hypnotic drugs
	Alcohol	Increases sedation with alcohol (although debated)
	Iron	May reduce iron absorption because of tannic acid content

4

GERIATRIC PATIENT CARE

PHYSIOLOGIC CHANGES IN AGING

Aging is characterized by the loss of some body cells and reduced metabolism in other cells. These processes cause a decline in body function and changes in body composition. This chart will help you recognize the gradual changes in body function that normally accompany aging so you can adjust your assessment techniques accordingly.

Body system	Age-related changes
Nutrition	■ Protein, vitamin, and mineral requirements usually unchanged ■ Energy requirements possibly decreased by about 200 calories per day because of diminished activity ■ Loss of calcium and nitrogen (in patients who aren't ambulatory) ■ Diminished absorption of calcium and vitamins B_1 and B_2 due to reduced pepsin and hydrochloric acid secretion ■ Decreased salivary flow and decreased sense of taste (may reduce appetite) ■ Diminished intestinal motility and peristalsis of the large intestine ■ Brittle teeth due to thinning of tooth enamel ■ Decreased biting force ■ Diminished gag reflex ■ Limited mobility (may affect ability to obtain or prepare food)
Skin	■ Facial lines resulting from subcutaneous fat loss, dermal thinning, decreasing collagen and elastin, and 50% decline in cell replacement ■ Delayed wound healing due to decreased rate of cell replacement ■ Decreased skin elasticity (may seem almost transparent) ■ Brown spots on skin due to localized melanocyte proliferation ■ Dry mucous membranes and decreased sweat gland output (as the number of active sweat glands declines) ■ Difficulty regulating body temperature because of decrease in size, number, and function of sweat glands and loss of subcutaneous fat
Hair	■ Decreased pigment, causing gray or white hair ■ Thinning as the number of melanocytes declines ■ Pubic hair loss resulting from hormonal changes ■ Facial hair increase in postmenopausal women and decrease in men

PHYSIOLOGIC CHANGES IN AGING *(continued)*

Body system	Age-related changes
Eyes and vision	■ Baggy and wrinkled eyelids due to decreased elasticity, with eyes sitting deeper in sockets ■ Thinner and yellow conjunctivae; possible pingueculae (fat pads) ■ Decreased tear production due to loss of fatty tissue in lacrimal apparatus ■ Corneal flattening and loss of luster ■ Fading or irregular pigmentation of iris ■ Smaller pupil, requiring three times more light to see clearly; diminished night vision and depth perception ■ Scleral thickening and rigidity; yellowing due to fat deposits ■ Vitreous degeneration, revealing opacities and floating debris ■ Lens enlargement; loss of transparency and elasticity, decreasing accommodation ■ Impaired color vision due to deterioration of retinal cones ■ Decreased reabsorption of intraocular fluid, predisposing to glaucoma
Ears and hearing	■ Atrophy of the organ of Corti and the auditory nerve (sensory presbycusis) ■ Inability to distinguish high-pitched consonants ■ Degenerative structural changes in the entire auditory system
Respiratory system	■ Nose enlargement from continued cartilage growth ■ General atrophy of tonsils ■ Tracheal deviation due to changes in the aging spine ■ Increased anteroposterior chest diameter as a result of altered calcium metabolism and calcification of costal cartilage ■ Lung rigidity; decreased number and size of alveoli ■ Kyphosis ■ Respiratory muscle degeneration or atrophy ■ Declining diffusing capacity ■ Decreased inspiratory and expiratory muscle strength; diminished vital capacity ■ Lung tissue degeneration, causing decrease in lungs' elastic recoil capability and increase in residual capacity ■ Poor ventilation of the basal areas (from closing of some airways), resulting in decreased surface area for gas exchange and reduced partial pressure of oxygen ■ Oxygen saturation decreased by 5% ■ 30% reduction in respiratory fluids, heightening risk of pulmonary infection and mucus plugs ■ Lower tolerance for oxygen debt

PHYSIOLOGIC CHANGES IN AGING *(continued)*

Body system	Age-related changes
Cardiovascular system	■ Slightly smaller heart size ■ Loss of cardiac contractile strength and efficiency ■ 30% to 35% diminished cardiac output by age 70 ■ Heart valve thickening, causing incomplete closure (systolic murmur) ■ 25% increase in left ventricular wall thickness between ages 30 and 80 ■ Fibrous tissue infiltration of the sinoatrial node and internodal atrial tracts, causing atrial fibrillation and flutter ■ Vein dilation and stretching ■ 35% decrease in coronary artery blood flow between ages 20 and 60 ■ Increased aortic rigidity, causing increased systolic blood pressure disproportionate to diastolic, resulting in widened pulse pressure ■ Electrocardiogram changes: increased PR, QRS complex, and QT interval; decreased amplitude of QRS complex; shift of QRS axis to the left ■ Heart rate takes longer to return to normal after exercise ■ Decreased strength and elasticity of blood vessels, contributing to arterial and venous insufficiency ■ Decreased ability to respond to physical and emotional stress
GI system	■ Diminished mucosal elasticity ■ Reduced GI secretions, affecting digestion and absorption ■ Decreased motility, bowel wall and anal sphincter tone, and abdominal wall strength ■ Liver changes: decreases in weight, regenerative capacity, and blood flow ■ Decline in hepatic enzymes involved in oxidation and reduction, causing less efficient metabolism of drugs and detoxification of substances
Renal system	■ Decline in glomerular filtration rate ■ 53% decrease in renal blood flow secondary to reduced cardiac output and atherosclerotic changes ■ Decrease in size and number of functioning nephrons ■ Reduction in bladder size and capacity ■ Weakening of bladder muscles, causing incomplete emptying and chronic urine retention ■ Diminished kidney size ■ Impaired clearance of drugs ■ Decreased ability to respond to variations in sodium intake

(continued)

PHYSIOLOGIC CHANGES IN AGING *(continued)*

Body system	Age-related changes
Male reproductive system	■ Reduced testosterone production, resulting in decreased libido as well as atrophy and softening of testes ■ 48% to 69% decrease in sperm production between ages 60 and 80 ■ Prostate gland enlargement, with decreasing secretions ■ Decreased volume and viscosity of seminal fluid ■ Slower and weaker physiologic reaction during intercourse, with lengthened refractory period
Female reproductive system	■ Declining estrogen and progesterone levels (about age 50) cause: – cessation of ovulation; atrophy, thickening, and decreased size of ovaries – loss of pubic hair and flattening of labia majora – shrinking of vulval tissue, constricted introitus, and loss of tissue elasticity – vaginal atrophy; thin and dry mucus lining; more alkaline pH of vaginal environment – shrinking uterus – cervical atrophy, failure to produce mucus for lubrication, thinner endometrium and myometrium – pendulous breasts; atrophy of glandular, supporting, and fatty tissue – nipple flattening and decreased size – more pronounced inframammary ridges.
Neurologic system	■ Degenerative changes in neurons of central and peripheral nervous system ■ Slower nerve transmission ■ Decrease in number of brain cells by about 1% per year after age 50 ■ Hypothalamus less effective at regulating body temperature ■ 20% neuron loss in cerebral cortex ■ Slower corneal reflex ■ Increased pain threshold ■ Decrease in stage III and IV of sleep, causing frequent awakenings; rapid eye movement sleep also decreased
Immune system	■ Decline beginning at sexual maturity and continuing with age ■ Loss of ability to distinguish between self and nonself ■ Loss of ability to recognize and destroy mutant cells, increasing incidence of cancer ■ Decreased antibody response, resulting in greater susceptibility to infection ■ Tonsillar atrophy and lymphadenopathy ■ Lymph node and spleen size slightly decreased ■ Some active blood-forming marrow replaced by fatty bone marrow, resulting in inability to increase erythrocyte production as readily as before in response to such stimuli as hormones, anoxia, hemorrhage, and hemolysis ■ Diminished vitamin B_{12} absorption, resulting in reduced erythrocyte mass and decreased hemoglobin level and hematocrit

Physiologic changes in aging *(continued)*

Body system	Age-related changes
Musculoskeletal system	■ Increased adipose tissue ■ Diminished lean body mass and bone mineral contents ■ Decreased height from exaggerated spinal curvature and narrowing intervertebral spaces ■ Decreased collagen formation and muscle mass ■ Increased viscosity of synovial fluid, more fibrotic synovial membranes
Endocrine system	■ Decreased ability to tolerate stress ■ Blood glucose concentration increases and remains elevated longer than in a younger adult ■ Diminished levels of estrogen and increasing levels of follicle-stimulating hormone during menopause, causing coronary thrombosis and osteoporosis ■ Reduced progesterone production ■ 50% decline in serum aldosterone levels ■ 25% decrease in cortisol secretion rate

COMPARING DELIRIUM AND DEMENTIA

The following characteristics can help distinguish delirium from dementia.

Characteristics	Delirium	Dementia
Onset	Acute	Insidious
Duration	Days to weeks	Permanent
Associated conditions	Systemic illness commonly present	No systemic conditions necessary
Attention span	Poor	Typically unaffected until late stages
Arousal level	Fluctuates from lethargic to agitation	Normal until later stages
Orientation to person, place, and time	Variably impaired for person and place, almost always for time	Variably impaired for person and place, almost always for time
Cognition	Disorganized thoughts; hallucinations and delusions common	Hallucinations, illusions, and delusions common
Speech and language	Dysarthric, slow, often inappropriate and incoherent	Aphasia common in middle and late stages
Memory	Temporarily impaired	Loss of recent memory; remote memory impaired in later stages
Treatment	Protect the patient and treat the causes	Protect the patient and treat the behaviors

Adapted with permission from Ignatavicius, D. "Resolving the Delirium Dilemma," *Nursing99* 20(10):41-46, October 1999.

PREVENTING ADVERSE DRUG REACTIONS IN OLDER PATIENTS

A drug's action in the body and its interaction with body tissues (pharmacodynamics) change significantly in older people. In the chart below, you'll find the information you need to help prevent adverse drug reactions in your elderly patients.

Pharmacology	Indications	Special considerations
Adrenergics, direct- and indirect-acting ■ Exert excitatory actions on the heart, glands, and vascular smooth muscle and peripheral inhibitory actions on smooth muscles of the bronchial tree	■ Hypotension ■ Cardiac stimulation ■ Bronchodilation ■ Shock	■ An elderly patient may be more sensitive to therapeutic and adverse effects of some adrenergics and may require lower doses.
Adrenocorticoids, systemic ■ Stimulate enzyme synthesis needed to decrease the inflammatory response	■ Inflammation ■ Immunosuppression ■ Adrenal insufficiency ■ Rheumatic and collagen diseases ■ Acute spinal cord injury	■ These drugs may aggravate hyperglycemia, delay wound healing, or contribute to edema, insomnia, or osteoporosis in an elderly patient. ■ Decreased metabolic rate and elimination may cause increased plasma levels and increase the risk of adverse effects. Monitor the elderly patient carefully.
Alpha-adrenergic blockers ■ Block the effects of peripheral neurohormonal transmitters (norepinephrine, epinephrine) on adrenergic receptors in various effector systems	■ Peripheral vascular disorders ■ Hypertension ■ Benign prostatic hyperplasia	■ Hypotensive effects may be more pronounced in an elderly patient. ■ These drugs should be administered at bedtime to reduce potential for dizziness or light-headedness.
Aminoglycosides ■ Inhibit bacterial protein synthesis	■ Infection caused by susceptible organisms	■ The elderly patient may have decreased renal function and thus be at greater risk for nephrotoxicity, ototoxicity, and superinfection (common).

(continued)

PREVENTING ADVERSE DRUG REACTIONS IN OLDER PATIENTS *(continued)*

Pharmacology	Indications	Special considerations
Angiotensin-converting enzyme (ACE) inhibitors ■ Prevent the conversion of angiotensin I to angiotensin II ■ Decrease vasoconstriction and adrenocortical secretion of aldosterone	■ Hypertension ■ Heart failure	■ Diuretic therapy should be discontinued before ACE inhibitors are started to reduce the risk of hypotension. ■ An elderly patient may need lower doses because of impaired drug clearance.
Anticholinergics ■ Exert antagonistic action on acetylcholine and other cholinergic agonists within the parasympathetic nervous system	■ Hypersecretory conditions ■ GI tract disorders ■ Sinus bradycardia ■ Dystonia and parkinsonism ■ Perioperative use ■ Motion sickness	■ These drugs should be used cautiously in an elderly adult, who may be more sensitive to the effects of these drugs; a lower dosage may be indicated.
Antihistamines ■ Prevent access and subsequent activity of histamine	■ Allergy ■ Pruritus ■ Vertigo ■ Nausea and vomiting ■ Sedation ■ Cough suppression ■ Dyskinesia	■ An elderly patient is usually more sensitive to the adverse effects of antihistamines; he's especially likely to experience a greater degree of dizziness, sedation, hypotension, and urine retention.
Barbiturates ■ Decrease presynaptic and postsynaptic excitability, producing central nervous system (CNS) depression	■ Seizure disorders ■ Sedation (including preanesthesia) ■ Hypnosis	■ An elderly patient and a patient receiving subhypnotic doses may experience hyperactivity, excitement, or hyperanalgesia. Use with caution.
Benzodiazepines ■ Act selectively on polysynaptic neuronal pathways throughout the CNS; synthetically produced sedative-hypnotic	■ Seizure disorders ■ Anxiety, tension, insomnia ■ Surgical adjuncts for conscious sedation or amnesia ■ Skeletal muscle spasm, tremor	■ These drugs should be used cautiously in an elderly patient, who is sensitive to the drugs' CNS effects; parenteral administration is more likely to cause apnea, hypotension, bradycardia, and cardiac arrest.

PREVENTING ADVERSE DRUG REACTIONS
IN OLDER PATIENTS *(continued)*

Pharmacology	Indications	Special considerations
Beta-adrenergic blockers ■ Compete with beta agonists for available beta-receptor sites; individual agents differ in their ability to affect beta receptors	■ Hypertension ■ Angina ■ Arrhythmias ■ Glaucoma ■ Myocardial infarction ■ Migraine prophylaxis	■ Increased bioavailability or delayed metabolism in the elderly patient may require a lower dosage; an elderly patient may also experience enhanced adverse effects.
Calcium channel blockers ■ Inhibit calcium influx across the slow channels of myocardial and vascular smooth muscle cells, causing dilation of coronary arteries, peripheral arteries, and arterioles and slowing cardiac conduction	■ Angina ■ Arrhythmias ■ Hypertension	■ These drugs should be used cautiously in an elderly patient because the half-life of calcium channel blockers may be increased as a result of decreased clearance.
Cardiac glycosides ■ Directly increase myocardial contractile force and velocity, atrioventricular node refractory period, and total peripheral resistance ■ Indirectly depress sinoatrial node and prolong conduction to the atrioventricular node	■ Heart failure ■ Arrhythmias ■ Paroxysmal atrial tachycardia or atrioventricular junctional rhythm ■ Myocardial infarction (MI) ■ Cardiogenic shock ■ Angina	■ These drugs should be used cautiously in an elderly patient with renal or hepatic dysfunction or with electrolyte imbalance that may predispose him to toxicity.
Cephalosporins ■ Inhibit bacterial cell wall synthesis, causing rapid cell lysis	■ Infection caused by susceptible organisms	■ Because the elderly patient commonly has impaired renal function, he may require a lower dosage. ■ An older adult is more susceptible to superinfection and coagulopathies.
Coumarin derivatives ■ Interfere with the hepatic synthesis of vitamin K-dependent clotting factors II, VII, IX, and X, decreasing the blood's coagulation potential	■ Treatment for or prevention of thrombosis or embolism	■ An older adult has an increased risk of hemorrhage because of altered hemostatic mechanisms or age-related hepatic and renal deterioration.

(continued)

PREVENTING ADVERSE DRUG REACTIONS IN OLDER PATIENTS *(continued)*

Pharmacology	Indications	Special considerations
Diuretics, loop ■ Inhibit sodium and chloride reabsorption in the ascending loop of Henle and increase excretion of potassium, sodium, chloride, and water	■ Edema ■ Hypertension	■ An elderly or debilitated patient is more susceptible to drug-induced diuresis and can quickly develop dehydration, hypovolemia, hypokalemia, and hyponatremia, which may cause circulatory collapse.
Diuretics, potassium-sparing ■ Act directly on the distal renal tubules, inhibiting sodium reabsorption and potassium excretion	■ Edema ■ Hypertension ■ Diagnosis of primary hyperaldosteronism	■ An older patient may need a smaller dosage because of his susceptibility to drug-induced diuresis and hyperkalemia.
Diuretics, thiazide and thiazide-like ■ Interfere with sodium transport, thereby increasing renal excretion of sodium, chloride, water, potassium, and calcium	■ Edema ■ Hypertension ■ Diabetes insipidus	■ Age-related changes in cardiovascular and renal function make the elderly patient more susceptible to excessive diuresis, which may lead to dehydration, hypovolemia, hyponatremia, hypomagnesemia, and hypokalemia.
Estrogens ■ Promote development and maintenance of the female reproductive system and secondary sexual characteristics; inhibition of the release of pituitary gonadotropins	■ Moderate to severe vasomotor symptoms of menopause ■ Atrophic vaginitis ■ Carcinoma of the breast and prostate ■ Prophylaxis of postmenopausal osteoporosis	■ A postmenopausal woman on long-term estrogen therapy has an increased risk of developing endometrial cancer.
Histamine-2 receptor antagonists ■ Inhibit histamine's action at histamine-2 receptors in gastric parietal cells, reducing gastric acid output and concentration, regardless of the stimulatory agent or basal conditions	■ Duodenal ulcer ■ Gastric ulcer ■ Hypersecretory states ■ Reflux esophagitis ■ Stress ulcer prophylaxis	■ These drugs should be used cautiously in an elderly patient because of his increased risk of developing adverse reactions, particularly those affecting the CNS.

PREVENTING ADVERSE DRUG REACTIONS
IN OLDER PATIENTS *(continued)*

Pharmacology	Indications	Special considerations
Insulin ■ Increases glucose transport across muscle and fat-cell membranes to reduce blood glucose levels ■ Promotes conversion of glucose to glycogen ■ Stimulates amino acid uptake and conversion to protein in muscle cells ■ Inhibits protein degradation ■ Stimulates triglyceride formation and lipoprotein lipase activity; inhibits free fatty acid release from adipose tissue	■ Diabetic ketoacidosis ■ Diabetes mellitus ■ Diabetes mellitus inadequately controlled by diet and oral antidiabetic agents ■ Hyperkalemia	■ Insulin is available in many forms that differ in onset, peak, and duration of action; the physician will specify the individual dosage and form. ■ Blood glucose measurement is an important guide to dosage and management. ■ The elderly patient's diet and his ability to recognize hypoglycemia are important. ■ A source of diabetic teaching should be provided, especially for the elderly patient, who may need follow-up home care.
Iron supplements, oral ■ Are needed in adequate amounts for erythropoiesis and efficient oxygen transport; essential component of hemoglobin	■ Iron deficiency anemia	■ Iron-induced constipation is common among elderly patients; stress proper diet to minimize constipation. ■ An elderly patient may also need higher doses because of reduced gastric secretions and because achlorhydria may lower his capacity for iron absorption.
Nitrates ■ Relax smooth muscle; generally used for vascular effects (vasodilatation)	■ Angina pectoris ■ Acute MI	■ Severe hypotension and cardiovascular collapse may occur if nitrates are combined with alcohol. ■ Transient dizziness, syncope, or other signs of cerebral ischemia may occur; instruct the elderly patient to take nitrates while sitting.

(continued)

Preventing adverse drug reactions in older patients *(continued)*

Pharmacology	Indications	Special considerations
Nonsteroidal anti-inflammatory drugs (NSAIDs) ■ Interfere with prostaglandins involved with pain; anti-inflammatory action that contributes to analgesic effect	■ Pain ■ Inflammation ■ Fever	■ A patient over age 60 may be more susceptible to the toxic effects of NSAIDs because of decreased renal function; these drugs' effects on renal prostaglandins may cause fluid retention and edema, a drawback for a patient with heart failure.
Opioid agonists ■ Act at specific opiate receptor-binding sites in the CNS and other tissues; alteration of pain perception without affecting other sensory functions	■ Analgesia ■ Pulmonary edema ■ Preoperative sedation ■ Anesthesia ■ Cough suppression ■ Diarrhea	■ Lower doses are usually indicated for elderly patients, who tend to be more sensitive to the therapeutic and adverse effects of these drugs.
Opioid agonist-antagonists ■ Act, in theory, on different opiate receptors in the CNS to a greater or lesser degree, thus yielding slightly different effects	■ Pain	■ Lower doses may be indicated in patients with renal or hepatic dysfunction to prevent drug accumulation.
Opioid antagonists ■ Act differently, depending on whether an opioid agonist has been administered previously, the actions of that opioid, and the extent of physical dependence on it	■ Opioid-induced respiratory depression ■ Adjunct in treating opiate addiction	■ These drugs are contraindicated for narcotic addicts, in whom they may produce an acute abstinence syndrome.
Penicillins ■ Inhibit bacterial cell-wall synthesis, causing rapid cell lysis; most effective against fast-growing susceptible organisms	■ Infection caused by susceptible organisms	■ An elderly patient (and others with low resistance from immunosuppressants or radiation therapy) should be taught the signs and symptoms of bacterial and fungal superinfection.

PREVENTING ADVERSE DRUG REACTIONS IN OLDER PATIENTS *(continued)*

Pharmacology	Indications	Special considerations
Phenothiazine ■ Believed to function as dopamine antagonists, blocking postsynaptic dopamine receptors in various parts of the CNS; antiemetic effects resulting from blockage of the chemoreceptor trigger zones	■ Psychosis ■ Nausea and vomiting ■ Anxiety ■ Severe behavior problems ■ Tetanus ■ Porphyria ■ Intractable hiccups ■ Neurogenic pain ■ Allergies and pruritus	■ An older adult needs a lower dosage because he's more sensitive to these drugs' therapeutic and adverse effects, especially cardiac toxicity, tardive dyskinesia, and other extrapyramidal effects. ■ Dosage should be titrated to patient response.
Salicylates ■ Decrease formation of prostaglandins involved in pain and inflammation	■ Pain ■ Inflammation ■ Fever	■ A patient over age 60 with impaired renal function may be more susceptible to these drugs' toxic effects. ■ The effect of salicylates on renal prostaglandins may cause fluid retention and edema, a significant disadvantage for a patient with heart failure.
Serotonin-reuptake inhibitors ■ Inhibit reuptake of serotonin; have little or no effect on other neurotransmitters	■ Major depression ■ Obsessive compulsive disorder ■ Bulimia nervosa	■ These drugs should be used cautiously in a patient with hepatic impairment.
Sulfonamides ■ Inhibit folic acid biosynthesis needed for cell growth	■ Bacterial and parasitic infections ■ Inflammation	■ These drugs should be used cautiously in an elderly patient, who is more susceptible to bacterial and fungal superinfection, folate deficiency anemia, and renal and hematologic effects because of diminished renal function.

GERIATRIC PATIENT CARE

(continued)

PREVENTING ADVERSE DRUG REACTIONS
IN OLDER PATIENTS *(continued)*

Pharmacology	Indications	Special considerations
Tetracyclines ■ Inhibit bacterial protein synthesis	■ Bacterial, protozoal, rickettsial, and fungal infections ■ Sclerosing agent	■ Some elderly patients have decreased esophageal motility; administer tetracyclines with caution and monitor for local irritation from slowly passing oral forms.
Thrombolytic enzymes ■ Convert plasminogen to plasmin for promotion of clot lysis	■ Thrombosis, thromboembolism	■ Patients age 75 and older are at greater risk for cerebral hemorrhage because they're more apt to have pre-existing cerebrovascular disease.
Thyroid hormones ■ Have catabolic and anabolic effects ■ Influence normal metabolism, growth and development, and every organ system; vital to normal CNS function	■ Hypothyroidism ■ Nontoxic goiter ■ Thyrotoxicosis ■ Diagnostic use	■ In a patient over age 60, the initial hormone replacement dose should be 25% less than the recommended dose.
Thyroid hormone antagonists ■ Inhibit iodine oxidation in the thyroid gland through a block of iodine's ability to combine with tyrosine to form thyroxine	■ Hyperthyroidism ■ Preparation for thyroidectomy ■ Thyrotoxic crisis ■ Thyroid carcinoma	■ Serum thyroid-stimulating hormone should be monitored as a sensitive indicator of thyroid hormone levels. Dosage adjustment may be required.
Tricyclic antidepressants ■ Inhibit neurotransmitter reuptake, resulting in increased concentration and enhanced activity of neurotransmitters in the synaptic cleft	■ Depression ■ Obsessive compulsive disorder ■ Enuresis ■ Severe, chronic pain	■ Lower doses are indicated in an elderly patient because he's more sensitive to both the therapeutic and adverse effects of tricyclic antidepressants.

ADVERSE REACTIONS MISINTERPRETED AS AGE-RELATED CHANGES

Some conditions result from aging, others from drug therapy; however, some can result from aging and drug therapy. This chart indicates drug classes and their associated adverse reactions.

Adverse reactions

Drug classifications	Agitation	Anxiety	Arrhythmias	Ataxia	Changes in appetite	Confusion	Constipation	Depression	Difficulty breathing	Disorientation	Dizziness	Drowsiness	Edema	Fatigue	Hypotension	Insomnia	Memory loss	Muscle weakness	Restlessness	Sexual dysfunction	Tremors	Urinary dysfunction	Visual changes
Alpha1-adrenergic blockers		•					•	•			•	•	•	•	•	•				•		•	•
Angiotensin-converting enzyme inhibitors					•	•	•				•			•	•	•				•			•
Antianginals	•	•	•			•					•			•	•	•			•	•		•	•
Antiarrhythmics			•				•		•		•			•	•	•							
Anticholinergetics	•	•				•	•	•		•	•	•		•		•			•	•	•		•	•
Anticonvulsants	•		•	•	•	•	•	•	•		•	•	•	•	•	•					•		•
Antidepressants, tricyclic	•	•	•	•	•	•	•	•		•	•	•		•	•	•			•	•	•	•	•
Antidiabetics, oral											•			•									
Antihistimines					•	•	•			•	•	•		•						•		•	•
Antilipemics							•				•			•		•		•		•		•	•
Antiparkinsonians	•	•		•	•	•	•	•		•	•	•		•	•	•		•		•	•	•	•
Antipsychotics	•	•	•	•	•	•	•	•	•		•	•		•	•	•			•	•	•	•	•
Barbiturates	•	•	•			•			•	•			•		•	•		•					
Benzodiazepines	•			•		•	•	•	•	•	•	•		•		•	•	•		•		•	•
Beta-adrenergic blockers		•	•					•	•		•			•	•	•		•		•	•	•	•
Calcium channel blockers		•	•				•		•		•		•	•	•	•				•		•	•
Corticosteroids	•					•		•						•	•		•		•				•
Diuretics						•					•			•	•		•					•	
Nonsteroidal anti-inflammatory drugs		•				•	•	•			•	•	•	•		•		•					•
Opioids	•	•				•	•	•	•	•	•	•		•	•	•	•		•	•		•	•
Skeletal muscle relaxants	•	•		•		•		•			•	•		•	•	•					•		
Thyroid hormones			•		•											•					•		

5

ANESTHESIA DRUGS AND LATEX ALLERGY

REVIEWING COMMON GENERAL ANESTHETICS

Drug	Indications	Advantages
INHALATION AGENTS		
Nitrous oxide	■ Maintains anesthesia ■ May provide an adjunct for inducing general anesthesia	■ Has little effect on heart rate, myocardial contractility, respiration, blood pressure, liver, kidneys, or metabolism in absence of hypoxia ■ Produces excellent analgesia ■ Allows for rapid induction and recovery ■ Doesn't increase capillary bleeding ■ Doesn't sensitize myocardium to epinephrine
Halothane Fluothane	■ Maintains general anesthesia	■ Is easy to administer ■ Allows for rapid, smooth induction and recovery ■ Has a relatively pleasant odor and is nonirritating ■ Depresses salivary and bronchial secretions ■ Causes bronchodilation ■ Easily suppresses pharyngeal and laryngeal reflexes
Enflurane Ethrane	■ Maintains anesthesia ■ Occasionally used to induce anesthesia	■ Allows for rapid induction and recovery ■ Is nonirritating and eliminates secretions ■ Causes bronchodilation ■ Provides good muscle relaxation ■ Allows cardiac rhythm to remain stable
Isoflurane Forane	■ Maintains general anesthesia ■ Occasionally used to induce general anesthesia	■ Allows for rapid induction and recovery ■ Causes bronchodilation ■ Provides excellent muscle relaxation ■ Allows for extremely stable cardiac rhythm

Disadvantages	Nursing interventions
■ May cause hypoxia with excessive amounts ■ Doesn't relax muscles (procedures requiring muscular relaxation require addition of a neuromuscular blocker) ■ Soluble gas has ability to diffuse into air-containing cavities such as chest or bowel	■ Monitor for signs of hypoxia. (Must always be given with oxygen to prevent hypoxia.)
■ May cause myocardial depression, leading to arrhythmias ■ Sensitizes heart to action of catecholamine ■ May cause circulatory or respiratory depression, depending on the dose ■ Has no analgesic property	■ Watch for arrhythmias, hypotension, respiratory depression. ■ Monitor for a fall in body temperature; the patient may shiver after prolonged use. Shivering increases oxygen consumption.
■ Causes myocardial depression ■ Lowers seizure threshold ■ Increases hypotension as depth of anesthesia increases ■ May cause shivering during recovery ■ May cause circulatory or respiratory depression, depending on the dose ■ May increase intracranial pressure (ICP)	■ Monitor for decreased heart and respiratory rates and hypotension. ■ Watch for shivering, which increases oxygen consumption.
■ May cause circulatory or respiratory depression, depending on the dose ■ Potentiates the action of nondepolarizing muscular relaxants ■ May cause the patient to shiver ■ Tends to lower blood pressure as depth of anesthesia increases; pulse remains somewhat elevated	■ Watch for respiratory depression and hypotension. ■ Watch for shivering, which increases oxygen consumption.

(continued)

REVIEWING COMMON GENERAL ANESTHETICS *(continued)*

Drug	Indications	Advantages
INHALATION AGENTS *(continued)*		
Desflurane Suprane	■ Induces and maintains general anesthesia	■ Can use decreased doses for neuromuscular blockers ■ Increased doses for maintenance anesthesia may produce dose-dependent hypotension
Sevoflurane Ultane	■ Induces and maintains general anesthesia for adults and children	■ Nonpungent odor ■ No respiratory irritability ■ Suitable for use with mask induction
I.V. BARBITURATES		
Thiopental sodium Pentothal	■ Used primarily to induce general anesthesia	■ Promotes rapid, smooth, and pleasant induction and quick recovery ■ Infrequently causes complications ■ Doesn't sensitize autonomic tissues of heart to catecholamines
I.V. BENZODIAZEPINES		
Diazepam Valium	■ Induces general anesthesia ■ Provides amnesia during balanced anesthesia	■ Minimally affects the cardiovascular system ■ Acts as a potent anticonvulsant ■ Produces amnesia
Midazolam hydro-chloride Versed	■ Induces general anesthesia ■ Provides amnesia during balanced anesthesia	■ Minimally affects the cardiovascular system ■ Acts as a potent anticonvulsant ■ Produces amnesia
Ketamine hydro-chloride Ketalar	■ Produces a dissociative state of consciousness; induces anesthesia when a barbiturate is contraindicated; sole anesthetic for short diagnostic and surgical procedures not requiring skeletal muscle relaxation	■ Produces rapid anesthesia and profound analgesia ■ Doesn't irritate veins or tissues ■ Maintains a patent airway without endotracheal intubation because it suppresses laryngeal and pharyngeal reflexes

Disadvantages	Nursing interventions
■ May increase heart rate ■ Respiratory irritant is more likely in adults during induction of anesthesia via mask ■ Not recommended for induction of general anesthesia in infants or children because of high incidence of laryngospasm or other respiratory adverse effects (after anesthesia is induced and tracheal intubation is achieved, it can be used for maintenance anesthesia) ■ Not indicated for patients with coronary artery disease or in those who will be adversely affected by increases in heart rate	■ Monitor the patient's vital signs, especially heart rate and blood pressure. ■ Watch for shivering, which increases oxygen consumption.
■ Dose-related cardiac depressant	■ Monitor the patient's vital signs. ■ Watch for shivering, which increases oxygen consumption.
■ Is associated with airway obstruction, respiratory depression, and laryngospasm, possibly leading to hypoxia ■ Doesn't provide muscle relaxation and produces little analgesia ■ May cause cardiovascular depression, especially in hypovolemic or debilitated patients	■ Watch for signs and symptoms of hypoxia, airway obstruction, and cardiovascular and respiratory depression.
■ May cause irritation when injected into a peripheral vein ■ Has a long elimination half-life	■ Monitor the patient's vital signs, respiratory rate, and volume.
■ Can cause respiratory depression	■ Monitor the patient's vital signs, especially respiratory rate, and volume.
■ May cause unpleasant dreams, hallucinations, and delirium during recovery ■ Increases heart rate, blood pressure, and intraocular pressure ■ Preserves muscle tone, leading to poor relaxation during surgery	■ Protect the patient from visual, tactile, and auditory stimuli during recovery. ■ Monitor the patient's vital signs.

(continued)

REVIEWING COMMON GENERAL ANESTHETICS *(continued)*

Drug	Indications	Advantages
I.V. NONBARBITURATES		
Propofol Diprivan	■ Used for induction and mainte- nance of anesthesia; is particularly useful for short procedures and outpatient surgery	■ Allows for quick, smooth induction ■ Permits rapid awakening and recovery ■ Causes less vomiting
I.V. TRANQUILIZERS		
Droperidol Inapsine	■ Used preoperatively and during induction and maintenance of anesthesia as an adjunct to general or regional anesthesia	■ Allows for rapid, smooth induction and recovery ■ Produces sleepiness and mental de- tachment for several hours
NARCOTICS		
Fentanyl citrate Sublimaze	■ Used preoperatively for minor and major surgery, urologic proce- dures, and gastroscopy; also used as an adjunct to regional anesthe- sia and for inducing and maintain- ing general anesthesia	■ Promotes rapid, smooth induction and recovery ■ Doesn't cause histamine release ■ Minimally affects cardiovascular sys- tem ■ Can be reversed by a narcotic antago- nist (naloxone)

Disadvantages	Nursing interventions
■ Can cause hypotension ■ Can cause pain if injected into small veins ■ May cause clonic or myoclonic movements upon emergence ■ May interact with benzodiazepines, increasing propofol's effects ■ Doesn't cause profound analgesia	■ Monitor the patient for hypotension. ■ Prepare for rapid emergence.
■ May cause hypotension because it's a peripheral vasodilator ■ Contraindicated in patients with known or suspected prolonged QT interval	■ Monitor the patient for increased pulse rate hypotension and prolonged QT interval
■ May cause respiratory depression, euphoria, bradycardia, bronchoconstriction, nausea, vomiting, and miosis ■ May cause skeletal-muscle and chest-wall rigidity	■ Observe the patient for respiratory depression. ■ Watch for nausea and vomiting. If vomiting occurs, position the patient to prevent aspiration. ■ Monitor blood pressure. ■ Decrease postoperative narcotics to one-third to one-fourth the usual dose.

REVIEWING COMMON NEUROMUSCULAR BLOCKERS

Drug	Adverse effects	Special considerations
NONDEPOLARIZING NEUROMUSCULAR BLOCKERS		
Atracurium besylate Tracrium	■ Slight hypertension in some patients	■ Acts for 20 to 30 minutes ■ May cause slight histamine release ■ Doesn't accumulate with repeated doses ■ Is useful for patients with underlying hepatic, renal, and cardiac disease
Gallamine triethiodide Flaxedil	■ Tachycardia and hypertension ■ Allergic reaction in patients sensitive to iodine	■ Acts for 15 to 35 minutes ■ May cause tachycardia after doses of 0.5 mg/kg; avoid using in cardiac disease ■ Doesn't cause bronchospasm ■ Accumulates; don't administer to patients with impaired renal function
Pancuronium bromide	■ Tachycardia ■ Transient skin rashes and a burning sensation at the injection site	■ Acts for 35 to 45 minutes ■ Is five times more potent than curare ■ Doesn't cause ganglion blockage, so it doesn't usually lead to hypotension ■ Has a vagolytic action that increases heart rate
Tubocurarine chloride Tubarine	■ Hypotension ■ Bronchospasm	■ Acts for 25 to 90 minutes with single large dose or multiple single doses; may last 24 hours in some patients ■ Causes histamine release; in higher doses, causes sympathetic ganglion blockade ■ May have prolonged action in elderly or debilitated patients and in those with renal or liver disease
Vecuronium bromide Norcuron	■ Minimal and transient cardiovascular effects ■ Skeletal muscle weakness or paralysis; respiratory insufficiency; respiratory paralysis; prolonged, dose-related apnea	■ Acts for 25 to 40 minutes ■ Probably metabolized mostly in the liver ■ Has a short duration of action and causes fewer cardiovascular effects than other nondepolarizing neuromuscular blockers

REVIEWING COMMON NEUROMUSCULAR BLOCKERS *(continued)*

Drug	Adverse effects	Special considerations
DEPOLARIZING NEUROMUSCULAR BLOCKERS		
Succinylcholine chloride Anectine	■ Respiratory depression ■ Bradycardia ■ Excessive salivation ■ Hypotension ■ Arrhythmias ■ Tachycardia ■ Hypertension ■ Increased intraocular and intragastric pressure ■ Fasciculations ■ Muscle pain ■ Malignant hyperthermia	■ Acts for 5 to 10 minutes ■ Is metabolized mostly in plasma by pseudocholinesterase; therefore, it's contraindicated in patients with a deficiency of plasma cholinesterase due to a genetic variant defect, liver disease, uremia, or malnutrition ■ Is used cautiously in patients with glaucoma or penetrating wounds of the eye; those undergoing eye surgery; or those with burns, severe trauma, spinal cord injuries, muscular dystrophy, or cardiovascular, hepatic, pulmonary, metabolic, or renal disorders; may cause sudden hyperkalemia and consequent cardiac arrest ■ Can cause pregnant patients who also receive magnesium sulfate to experience increased neuromuscular blockade because of decreased pseudocholinesterase levels

LATEX ALLERGY SCREENING QUESTIONNAIRE

To determine whether your patient has a latex sensitivity or allergy, ask the following screening questions:

Allergies

■ Do you have a history of hay fever, asthma, eczema, allergies, or rashes? If so, what type of reaction do you have?

■ Have you experienced an allergic reaction, local sensitivity, or itching following exposure to any latex products, such as balloons or condoms?

■ Do you have shortness of breath or wheezing after blowing up balloons or after a dental visit? Do you have itching in or around your mouth after eating a banana?

■ If you experience shortness of breath or wheezing when blowing up latex balloons, describe your reaction.

■ Are you allergic to any foods, especially bananas, avocados, kiwi, or chestnuts? If so, describe your reaction.

Occupation

■ What's your occupation?

■ Are you exposed to latex in your occupation?

■ Do you experience a reaction to latex products at work? If so, describe your reaction.

■ If you've had a rash develop on your hands after wearing latex gloves, how long after putting on the gloves did it take for the rash to develop?

■ What did the rash look like?

Personal history

■ Do you have any congenital abnormalities? If yes, explain.

■ Have you ever had itching, swelling, hives, cough, shortness of breath, or other allergic symptoms during or after using condoms, diaphragms, or following a vaginal or rectal examination?

Surgical history

■ Have you had any previous surgical procedures? Did you experience associated complications? If so, describe them.

■ Have you had previous dental procedures? Did complications result? If so, describe them.

■ Do you have spina bifida or any urinary tract problem that requires surgery or catheterization?

CREATING A LATEX-SAFE ENVIRONMENT

■ Ask all patients about latex sensitivity. Use a screening questionnaire to determine whether your patient has latex sensitivity.

■ Include information about latex allergy on the patient's identification bracelet. Make sure the information is also noted on the front of the patient's chart and in the facility's database.

■ Post a LATEX ALLERGY sign in the patient's room and on the patient's door.

■ Implement and disseminate latex allergy protocols and lists of nonlatex substitutes that can be used to care for the patient.

■ Remove all latex-containing products that may come in contact with the patient.

■ Use tubing made of polyvinyl chloride.

■ Check adhesives and tapes, including electrocardiogram electrodes and dressing supplies, for latex content.

■ Have a special latex-free crash cart available at all times during the patient's hospitalization.

■ Notify central supply and pharmacy that the patient has a latex allergy so that latex contact is eliminated from drugs and other materials prepared for the patient.

■ Notify dietary staff of relevant food allergies and instruct them to avoid handling the patient's food with powdered latex gloves.

Choosing the right glove

Health care workers may develop allergic reactions as a result of their exposure to latex gloves and other products containing natural rubber latex. Patients may also have latex sensitivity. Take the following steps to protect yourself and your patient from allergic reactions to natural rubber latex:

■ Use nonlatex (for example, vinyl or synthetic) gloves for activities that aren't likely to involve contact with infectious materials (food preparation, routine cleaning, and so forth).

■ Use appropriate barrier protection when handling infectious materials. If you choose latex gloves, select the powder-free gloves with reduced protein content.

■ After wearing and removing gloves, wash your hands with soap and dry them thoroughly.

■ When wearing latex gloves, don't use oil-based hand creams or lotions (which can cause gloves to deteriorate) unless they've been shown to maintain glove-barrier protection.

■ Refer to the material safety data sheet provided by OSHA for the appropriate glove to wear when handling chemicals.

■ Learn procedures for preventing latex allergy, and learn to recognize the following symptoms of latex allergy: skin rashes, hives, flushing, itching, asthma, shock, and nasal, eye, or sinus symptoms.

■ If you have (or suspect you have) a latex sensitivity, use nonlatex gloves, avoid contact with latex gloves and other latex-containing products, and consult a physician experienced in treating latex allergy.

For latex allergy

If you have a latex allergy, consider the following precautions:

■ Avoid contact with latex gloves and other products containing latex. Check package labels prior to use to see if any item contains latex.

■ Avoid areas where you might inhale the powder from latex gloves worn by other workers.

■ Tell your employers and your health care providers (physicians, nurses, dentists, and others).

■ Wear a medical identification bracelet.

■ Follow your physician's instructions for dealing with allergic reactions to latex.

ANESTHESIA INDUCTION AND LATEX ALLERGY

Latex allergy can cause signs and symptoms in both conscious and anesthetized patients.

Causes of intraoperative reaction	Signs and symptoms in a conscious patient	Signs and symptoms in an anesthetized patient
■ Latex contact with mucous membrane ■ Latex contact with intraperitoneal serosal lining ■ Inhalation of airborne latex particles during anesthesia ■ Injection of antibiotics and anesthetic agents through latex ports	■ Abdominal cramping ■ Anxiety ■ Bronchoconstriction ■ Diarrhea ■ Feeling of faintness ■ Generalized pruritus ■ Itchy eyes ■ Nausea ■ Shortness of breath ■ Swelling of soft tissue (hands, face, tongue) ■ Vomiting ■ Wheezing	■ Bronchospasm ■ Cardiopulmonary arrest ■ Facial edema ■ Flushing ■ Hypotension ■ Laryngeal edema ■ Tachycardia ■ Urticaria ■ Wheezing

MANAGING A LATEX ALLERGY REACTION

If you determine that your patient is having an allergic reaction to a latex product, act immediately. Make sure you perform emergency interventions using latex-free equipment. If the latex product that caused the reaction is known, remove it and perform the following measures:

■ If the allergic reaction develops during medication administration or a procedure, stop it immediately.
■ Assess airway, breathing, and circulation.
■ Administer 100% oxygen and monitor oxygen saturation.
■ Start an I.V. with lactated Ringer's solution or normal saline solution.
■ Administer epinephrine according to the patient's symptoms.
■ Administer famotidine by I.V. route as ordered.
■ If bronchospasm is evident, treat it with nebulized albuterol.

■ Secondary treatment for latex allergy reaction is aimed at treating the swelling and tissue reaction to the latex as well as breaking the chain of events associated with the allergic reaction. It includes:
  - diphenhydramine I.V.
  - methylprednisolone I.V.
■ Document the event and the exact cause (if known). If latex particles have entered the I.V. line, insert a new I.V. line with a new catheter, new tubing, and new infusion attachments as soon as possible.

6

CARDIOVASCULAR CARE

CARDIOVASCULAR SYSTEM: NORMAL FINDINGS

Inspection
■ No pulsations are visible, except at the point of maximal impulse (PMI).
■ No lifts (heaves) or retractions are detectable in the four valve areas of the chest wall.

Palpation
■ No vibrations or thrills are detectable.
■ No lifts, or heaves, are detectable.
■ No pulsations are detectable, except at the PMI and epigastric area. At the PMI, a localized (less than ½″ (1.3 cm) diameter area) tapping pulse may be felt at the start of systole. In the epigastric area, pulsation from the abdominal aorta may be palpable.

Auscultation
■ A first heart sound (S_1); the lub sound is best heard with the diaphragm of the stethoscope over the mitral area when the patient is in a left lateral position. It sounds longer, lower, and louder there than a second heart sound (S_2). S_1 splitting may be audible in the tricuspid area.

■ An S_2 sound: The dub sound is best heard with the diaphragm of the stethoscope in the aortic area while the patient sits and leans over. It sounds shorter, sharper, higher, and louder there than an S_1. Normal S_2 splitting may be audible in the pulmonic area on inspiration.
■ A third heart sound (S_3) in children and slender, young adults with no cardiovascular disease is normal. It usually disappears when adults reach ages 25 to 35. In an older adult, it may signify heart failure. S_3 is heard best with the bell of the stethoscope over the mitral area with the patient in a supine position and exhaling. It sounds short, dull, soft, and low.
■ Murmurs may be functional in children and young adults, but are abnormal in older adults. Innocent murmurs are soft, short, and vary with respirations and patient position. They occur in early systole and are best heard in pulmonic or mitral areas with the patient in a supine position.

DETERMINING PULSE AMPLITUDE

To record your patient's pulse amplitude, use this standard scale:

0: Pulse isn't palpable.

+1: Pulse is thready, weak, difficult to find, may fade in and out, and disappears easily with pressure.

+2: Pulse is constant but not strong; light pressure must be applied or pulse will disappear.

+3: Pulse considered normal. It's easily palpable and doesn't disappear with pressure.

+4: Pulse is strong, bounding, and doesn't disappear with pressure.

EVALUATING JUGULAR VEIN DISTENTION

First, position the supine patient so that you can visualize jugular vein pulsations reflected from the right atrium. Elevate the head of the bed 45 to 90 degrees. (In the normal patient, veins distend only when the patient lies flat.) Next, locate the angle of Louis (sternal notch) — the reference point for measuring venous pressure. To do so, palpate the clavicles where they join the sternum (the suprasternal notch). Place your first two fingers on the suprasternal notch. Then, without lifting them from the skin, slide them down the sternum until you feel a bony protuberance — this is the angle of Louis.

Find the internal jugular vein (which indicates venous pressure more reliably than the external jugular vein). Shine a flashlight across the patient's neck to create shadows that highlight his venous pulse. Be sure to distinguish jugular venous pulsations from carotid arterial pulsations. One way to do this is to palpate the vessel: Arterial pulsations continue, whereas venous pulsations disappear with light finger pressure. Also, venous pulsations increase or decrease with changes in body position, but arterial pulsations remain constant.

Next, locate the highest point along the vein where you can see pulsations. Using a centimeter ruler, measure the distance between that high point and the sternal notch. Record this finding as well as the angle at which the patient was lying. A finding greater than 3 or 4 cm above the sternal notch with the head of the bed at a 45-degree angle indicates jugular vein distention.

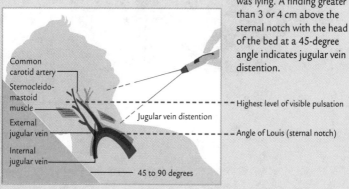

Common carotid artery

Sternocleidomastoid muscle

External jugular vein

Internal jugular vein

Jugular vein distention

Highest level of visible pulsation

Angle of Louis (sternal notch)

45 to 90 degrees

IDENTIFYING CARDIOVASCULAR LANDMARKS

These views show where to find critical landmarks used in cardiovascular assessment.

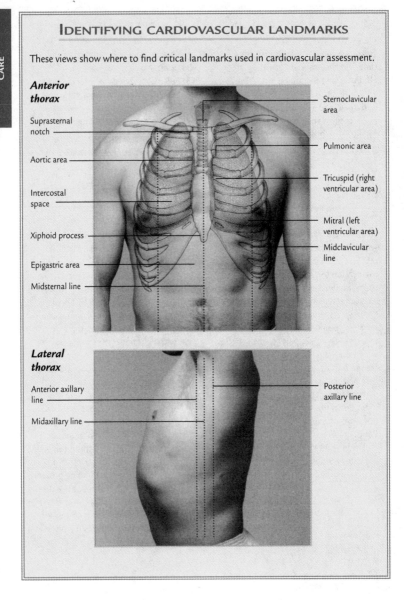

Anterior thorax

Suprasternal notch

Aortic area

Intercostal space

Xiphoid process

Epigastric area

Midsternal line

Sternoclavicular area

Pulmonic area

Tricuspid (right ventricular area)

Mitral (left ventricular area)

Midclavicular line

Lateral thorax

Anterior axillary line

Midaxillary line

Posterior axillary line

POSITIONING THE PATIENT FOR CARDIAC AUSCULTATION

During auscultation, you'll typically stand to the right of the patient, who's in a supine position. The patient may lie flat or at a comfortable elevation.

If heart sounds seem faint or undetectable, try repositioning the patient. Alternate positioning may enhance heart sounds or make them seem louder by bringing the heart closer to the surface of the chest. Common alternate positions include a seated, forward-leaning position and left-lateral decubitus position.

Forward-leaning position

This position is best for hearing high-pitched sounds related to semilunar valve problems such as aortic and pulmonic valve murmurs. To auscultate these sounds, help the patient to the forward-leaning position, and place the diaphragm of the stethoscope over the aortic and pulmonic areas in the right and left second intercostal space.

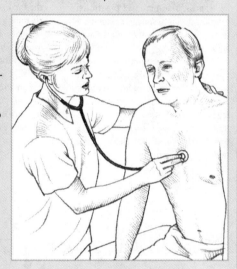

Left-lateral decubitus position

This position is best for hearing low-pitched sounds related to atrioventricular valve problems, such as mitral valve murmurs and extra heart sounds. To auscultate these sounds, help the patient to the left-lateral decubitus position, and place the bell of the stethoscope over the apical area. If these positions don't enhance heart sounds, try auscultating with the patient standing or squatting.

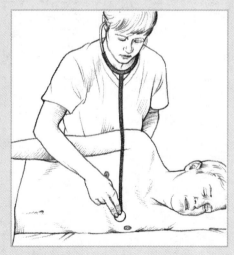

HEART SOUND ABNORMALITIES

Auscultation sites

When auscultating for heart sounds, place the stethoscope over four different sites. Follow the same auscultation sequence during every cardiovascular assessment.

■ Place the stethoscope in the aortic area, the second intercostal space along the right sternal border, as shown. In the aortic area, blood moves from the left ventricle during systole, crossing the aortic valve and flowing through the aortic arch.

■ Move to the pulmonary area, located in the second intercostal space at the left sternal border. In the pulmonary area, blood ejected from the right ventricle during systole crosses the pulmonic valve and flows through the main pulmonary artery.

■ In the third auscultation site, assess the tricuspid area, which lies in the fifth inter-costal space along the left sternal border. In the tricuspid area, sounds reflect blood movement from the right atrium across the tricuspid valve, filling the right ventricle during diastole.

■ Finally, listen in the mitral area, located in the fifth intercostal space near the midclavicular line. (If the patient's heart is enlarged, the mitral area may be closer to the anterior axillary line.) In the mitral (apical) area, sounds represent blood flow across the mitral valve and left ventricular filling during diastole.

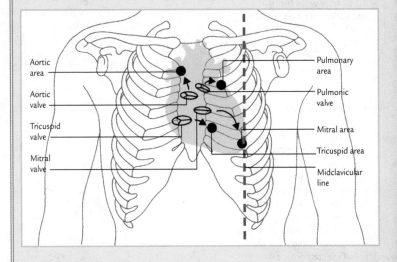

Implications of abnormal heart sounds

Upon detecting an abnormal heart sound, you must accurately identify the sound as well as its location and timing in the cardiac cycle. This information will help you identify the possible cause of the sound. The chart below lists abnormal heart sounds with their possible causes.

Abnormal heart sound	Timing	Possible causes
Accentuated S_1	Beginning of systole	Mitral stenosis; fever
Diminished S_1	Beginning of systole	Mitral insufficiency; severe mitral regurgitation with calcified immobile valve; heart block
Accentuated S_2	End of systole	Pulmonary or systemic hypertension
Diminished or inaudible S_2	End of systole	Aortic or pulmonic stenosis
Persistent S_2 split	End of systole	Delayed closure of the pulmonic valve, usually from overfilling of the right ventricle, causing prolonged systolic ejection time
Reversed or paradoxical S_2 split that appears on expiration and disappears on inspiration	End of systole	Delayed ventricular stimulation; left bundle-branch block or prolonged left ventricular ejection time
S_3 (ventricular gallop)	Early diastole	Normal in children and young adults; overdistention of ventricles in rapid-filling segment of diastole; mitral insufficiency or ventricular failure
S_4 (atrial gallop or presystolic extra sound)	Late diastole	Forceful atrial contraction from resistance to ventricular filling late in diastole; left ventricular hypertrophy; pulmonic stenosis; hypertension; coronary artery disease; and aortic stenosis
Pericardial friction rub (grating or leathery sound at left of sternal border; usually muffled, high-pitched, and transient)	Throughout systole and diastole	Pericardial inflammation
Click	Early systole or midsystole	Aortic stenosis; aortic dilation; hypertension; chordae tendineae damage of the mitral valve
Opening snap	Early diastole	Mitral or tricuspid valve abnormalities
Summation gallop	Diastole	Tachycardia

WHERE EXTRA HEART SOUNDS OCCUR IN THE CARDIAC CYCLE

To understand where extra heart sounds fall in relation to systole, diastole, and normal heart sounds, compare the illustrations of normal and extra heart sounds.

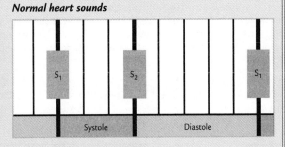

Normal heart sounds

Extra heart sounds

GRADING MURMURS

Use the system outlined below to describe the intensity of a murmur. When recording your findings, use Roman numerals as part of a fraction, always with VI as the denominator. For instance, a grade III murmur would be recorded as "grade III/VI."

- Grade I is a barely audible murmur.
- Grade II is audible but quiet and soft.
- Grade III is moderately loud, without a thrust or thrill.
- Grade IV is loud, with a thrill.

- Grade V is very loud, with a thrust or a thrill.
- Grade VI is loud enough to be heard before the stethoscope comes into contact with the chest.

CHARACTERIZING MURMURS

Identify a heart murmur by first listening closely to determine its timing in the cardiac cycle. Then determine its other characteristics one at a time, including its quality, pitch, location, and radiation. Use the chart below to identify the underlying condition.

Quality	Pitch	Location	Radiation	Condition
MIDSYSTOLIC (SYSTOLIC EJECTION)				
Harsh, rough	Medium to high	Pulmonary	Toward left shoulder and neck, possibly along left sternal border	Pulmonic stenosis
Harsh, rough	Medium to high	Aortic and suprasternal notch	Toward carotid arteries or apex	Aortic stenosis
HOLOSYSTOLIC (PANSYSTOLIC)				
Harsh	High	Tricuspid	Precordium	Ventricular septal defect
Blowing	High	Mitral, lower left sternal border	Toward left axilla	Mitral insufficiency
Blowing	High	Tricuspid	Toward apex	Tricuspid insufficiency
EARLY DIASTOLIC				
Blowing	High	Mid-left sternal edge (not aortic area)	Toward sternum	Aortic insufficiency
Blowing	High	Pulmonary	Toward sternum	Pulmonic insufficiency
MID- TO LATE DIASTOLIC				
Rumbling	Low	Apex	Usually none	Mitral stenosis
Rumbling	Low	Tricuspid, lower right sternal border	Usually none	Tricuspid stenosis

CARDIOVASCULAR SYSTEM:
INTERPRETING YOUR FINDINGS

Your assessment will reveal a group of findings that may lead you to suspect a particular disorder. The chart below shows some common groups of findings for signs and symptoms of the cardiovascular system, along with their probable causes.

Sign or symptom and findings	Probable cause
CHEST PAIN	
■ A feeling of tightness or pressure in the chest described as pain or a sensation of indigestion or expansion ■ Pain that may radiate to the neck, jaw, and arms; classically to the inner aspect of the left arm ■ Pain begins gradually, reaches a maximum, then slowly subsides ■ Pain is provoked by exertion, emotional stress, or a heavy meal ■ Pain typically lasts 2 to 10 minutes (usually no more than 20 minutes) ■ Dyspnea ■ Nausea and vomiting ■ Tachycardia ■ Dizziness ■ Diaphoresis	Angina
■ A crushing substernal pain, unrelieved by rest or nitroglycerin ■ Pain that may radiate to the left arm, jaw, neck, or shoulder blades ■ Pain that lasts from 15 minutes to hours ■ Pallor ■ Clammy skin ■ Dyspnea ■ Diaphoresis ■ Feeling of impending doom	Myocardial infarction
■ Sharp, severe pain aggravated by inspiration, coughing, or pressure ■ Shallow, splinted breaths ■ Dyspnea ■ Cough ■ Local tenderness and edema	Rib fracture
FATIGUE	
■ Fatigue following mild activity ■ Pallor ■ Tachycardia ■ Dyspnea	Anemia

CARDIOVASCULAR SYSTEM:
INTERPRETING YOUR FINDINGS *(continued)*

Sign or symptom and findings	Probable cause
FATIGUE *(continued)*	
■ Persistent fatigue unrelated to exertion ■ Headache ■ Anorexia ■ Constipation ■ Sexual dysfunction ■ Loss of concentration ■ Irritability	Depression
■ Progressive fatigue ■ Cardiac murmur ■ Exertional dyspnea ■ Cough ■ Hemoptysis	Valvular heart disease
PALPITATIONS	
■ Paroxysmal palpitations ■ Diaphoresis ■ Facial flushing ■ Trembling ■ Impending sense of doom ■ Hyperventilation ■ Dizziness	Acute anxiety attack
■ Paroxysmal or sustained palpitations ■ Dizziness ■ Weakness ■ Fatigue ■ Irregular, rapid, or slow pulse rate ■ Decreased blood pressure ■ Confusion ■ Diaphoresis	Cardiac arrhythmias
■ Sustained palpitations ■ Fatigue ■ Irritability ■ Hunger ■ Cold sweats ■ Tremors ■ Anxiety	Hypoglycemia

(continued)

CARDIOVASCULAR SYSTEM:
INTERPRETING YOUR FINDINGS (continued)

Sign or symptom and findings	Probable cause
PERIPHERAL EDEMA	
■ Headache ■ Bilateral leg edema with pitting ankle edema ■ Weight gain despite anorexia ■ Nausea ■ Chest tightness ■ Hypotension ■ Pallor ■ Palpitations ■ Inspiratory crackles	Heart failure
■ Bilateral arm edema accompanied by facial and neck edema ■ Edematous areas marked by dilated veins ■ Headache ■ Vertigo ■ Visual disturbances	Superior vena cava syndrome
■ Moderate to severe, unilateral or bilateral leg edema ■ Darkened skin ■ Stasis ulcers around the ankle	Venous insufficiency

CHARACTERIZING CHEST PAIN

Pericarditis	Angina	Myocardial infarction
ONSET AND DURATION		
Sudden onset, continuous pain lasting for days, residual soreness	Gradual or sudden onset, pain usually lasting less than 15 minutes and not more than 30 minutes (average: 3 minutes)	Sudden onset, pain lasting 30 minutes to 2 hours, residual soreness for 1 to 3 days
LOCATION AND RADIATION		
Substernal pain to left of midline, radiation to back or subclavicular area	Substernal or anterior chest pain or pressure; not sharply localized; radiation to back, neck, arms, jaws, also upper abdomen or fingers	Substernal, midline, or anterior chest pain, radiation to jaws, neck, back, shoulders, and one or both arms
QUALITY AND INTENSITY		
Mild ache to severe pain, deep or superficial, "stabbing" and "knifelike"	Mild to moderate pressure; deep sensation; varied pattern of attacks; "tightness," "squeezing," or "crushing"	Persistent, severe pressure; deep sensation; "crushing," "squeezing," "heavy," or "oppressive"; sudden death
SIGNS AND SYMPTOMS		
Pericardial friction rub; increased pain with movement, inspiration, laughing, coughing; increased pain with sitting or leaning forward (sitting up pulls the heart away from the diaphragm)	Dyspnea, diaphoresis, nausea, desire to void, belching, or apprehension	Nausea, vomiting, apprehension, dyspnea, diaphoresis, increased or decreased blood pressure; gallop heart sound; "sensation of impending doom"; chest pressure may fluctuate initially and then become persistent
PRECIPITATING FACTORS		
Myocardial infarction or upper respiratory tract infection; no relation to effort; cardiac surgery, cardiac tumor, or penetrating chest wound	Exertion, stress, eating, cold or hot and humid weather	Physical exertion or emotional stress; may also occur when person is at rest

FACTORS THAT AFFECT PRELOAD AND AFTERLOAD

Preload

Preload refers to the passive stretching force exerted on the ventricular muscle at the end of diastole by the amount of blood in the chamber. According to Starling's law, the more cardiac muscles are stretched, the more forcefully they contract in systole.

Factors that increase preload

■ Increased blood volume returning to the heart
■ Control of fluid loss with replacement therapy such as I.V. or transfusion therapy; fluid overload
■ Decreased ventricular compliance
■ Mitral stenosis or insufficiency
■ Venous congestion, such as with cardiac tamponade and heart failure
■ Poor contractility of the right ventricle, such as from infarction or pericarditis
■ Conditions associated with high pulmonary vascular resistance, such as pulmonary edema or chronic obstructive pulmonary disease

Factors that decrease preload

■ Fluid losses, such as with hemorrhage, excessive diaphoresis, vomiting, or diarrhea
■ Third-space shifting
■ Diuresis
■ Fluid and sodium restriction
■ Extreme vasodilation

■ Medications, such as loop diuretics, nitrates, and cardiac glycosides

Afterload

Afterload refers to the pressure the ventricular muscles must generate to overcome the higher pressure in the aorta. Normally, end-diastolic pressure in the left ventricle is 5 to 10 mm Hg; in the aorta, however, it's 70 to 80 mm Hg. This difference means that the ventricle must develop enough pressure to force open the aortic valve.

Factors that increase afterload

■ Peripheral vasoconstriction
■ Decreased stroke volume
■ Hypovolemia
■ Hypothermia
■ Hypertension
■ Cardiogenic shock
■ Cardiac tamponade
■ Massive pulmonary embolism
■ Vasopressor agents, such as epinephrine, norepinephrine, and dopamine

Factors that decrease afterload

■ Peripheral vasodilation
■ Increased stroke volume
■ Medications, such as angiotensin-converting enzyme inhibitors (captopril [Capoten] and enalapril [Vasotec]), hydralazine (Apresoline), and sodium nitroprusside (Nitropress)
■ Early septic shock

DIAGNOSTIC TESTS

CARDIAC BLOOD POOL IMAGING

Overview

- A noninvasive evaluation of regional and global ventricular performance after I.V. injection of human serum albumin, or red blood cells (RBCs), tagged with the isotope technetium 99m pertechnetate
- First-pass imaging: scintillation camera records the radioactivity emitted by the isotope in its initial pass through the left ventricle, allowing calculation of the ejection fraction
- Gated cardiac blood pool imaging: performed after first-pass imaging or as a separate test; commonly uses signals from an electrocardiogram to trigger the scintillation camera
- Two-frame gated imaging: the camera records left ventricular end-systole and end-diastole for 500 to 1,000 cardiac cycles, allowing assessment of left ventricular contractility
- Multiple-gated acquisition (MUGA) scanning: the camera records 14 to 64 points of a single cardiac cycle; used to evaluate regional wall motion and determine indices of cardiac function
- Stress MUGA test: MUGA scanning done at rest and after exercise to detect changes in ejection fraction and cardiac output
- Nitro MUGA test: the camera records points in the cardiac cycle after sublingual administration of nitroglycerin; used to assess the drug's effect on ventricular function
- Blood pool imaging: involves less risk than left ventriculography in assessing cardiac function

PURPOSE

- To evaluate left ventricular function
- To detect and evaluate left ventricular aneurysms
- To detect and evaluate myocardial wall-motion abnormalities (areas of akinesia or dyskinesia)
- To detect and evaluate intracardiac shunting

PATIENT PREPARATION

- Make sure the patient has signed an appropriate consent form.
- Note and report all allergies.
- Restriction of food and fluids isn't necessary.
- Warn the patient that the needle puncture may cause transient discomfort, but that the imaging procedure is painless.

Teaching points

Be sure to cover:
- the purpose of the study and how it's done
- who will perform the test and where
- that the study takes about 1½ hours
- that the tracer used for the study poses no radiation hazard, and rarely produces adverse effects.

POSTPROCEDURE CARE

- No specific postprocedure care is required.

PRECAUTIONS

- Cardiac blood pool imaging is contraindicated during pregnancy.

COMPLICATIONS

- Adverse reaction to tracer (rare)

Interpretation

NORMAL FINDINGS

- The left ventricle contracts symmetrically.
- The isotope appears evenly distributed.
- The ejection fraction is 55% to 65%.

ABNORMAL RESULTS

- Globally reduced ejection fractions suggest possible cardiomyopathy.
- Prolongation of the radioisotope's activity may indicate a left-to-right shunt.
- Early arrival of radioisotope activity in the left ventricle or aorta may signify a right-to-left shunt.
- Segmental abnormalities of ventricular wall motion suggest possible coronary artery disease or myocarditis.
- Ejection fraction less than 35% to 40% suggests left ventricular systolic dysfunction.

CARDIAC CATHETERIZATION

Overview

- Involves passage of a catheter into the right, left, or both sides of the heart
- Used to measure pressures in chambers of the heart; records films of the ventricles (contrast ventriculography) and arteries (coronary arteriography)
- Left-sided heart catheterization: used to assess patency of the coronary arteries and function of left ventricle
- Right-sided heart catheterization: used to assess pulmonary artery pressures

PURPOSE

- To evaluate valvular insufficiency or stenosis, septal defects, congenital anomalies, myocardial function, myocardial blood supply, and cardiac wall motion
- To aid in diagnosing left ventricular enlargement, aortic root enlargement, ventricular aneurysms, and intracardiac shunts

PATIENT PREPARATION

- Make sure the patient has signed an appropriate consent form.
- Note and report all allergies.
- Discontinue anticoagulant therapy to reduce complications of bleeding.
- Restrict food and fluids for at least 6 hours before the test.
- Explain that if a mild sedative is given the patient remains conscious.
- Warn the patient that a transient hot, flushing sensation or nausea may occur.
- Stress the need to cough or breathe deeply.

Teaching points

Be sure to cover:

- the test's purpose and how it's done
- that the test will take 1 to 2 hours.

POSTPROCEDURE CARE

- Reinforce the dressing as needed.
- Enforce bed rest for 8 hours.
- If the femoral route was used for catheter insertion, keep the leg straight at the hip for 6 to 8 hours.
- If the antecubital fossa route was used, keep the arm straight at the elbow for at least 3 hours.
- Resume medications and administer analgesics as ordered.
- Encourage fluid intake.

Monitoring

- Vital signs
- Intake and output

- Cardiac rhythm
- Neurologic and respiratory status
- Peripheral vascular status distal to the puncture site
- Catheter insertion site and dressings
- Signs and symptoms of infection
- Complications

PRECAUTIONS

- Notify the physician of hypersensitivity to shellfish, iodine, or contrast media.
- Contraindications to right- and left-heart catheterization include uncorrected coagulopathy, poor renal function, and debilitation.
- Contraindications to right-heart catheterization include left bundle-branch block, unless a temporary pacemaker is inserted to counteract possible ventricular asystole.
- The brachial artery causes a higher incidence of complications.
- Prophylactic antibiotics prevent infective endocarditis in a patient with valvular heart disease.

COMPLICATIONS

- With left-or right-sided catheterization: myocardial infarction, arrhythmias, cardiac tamponade, infection, hypovolemia, pulmonary edema, hematoma, blood loss, adverse reaction to contrast media, and vasovagal response
- With left-sided catheterization: arterial thrombus or embolism, and stroke
- With right-sided catheterization: thrombophlebitis and pulmonary embolism

Interpretation

NORMAL FINDINGS

- There are no abnormalities of heart valves, chamber size, pressures, configuration, wall motion or thickness, and blood flow.
- Coronary arteries have a smooth and regular outline.

ABNORMAL RESULTS

- Coronary artery narrowing greater than 70% suggests significant coronary artery disease.
- Narrowing of the left main coronary artery and occlusion or narrowing high in the left anterior descending artery suggests the need for revascularization surgery.
- Impaired wall motion suggests myocardial incompetence.
- A pressure gradient, or difference in pressures above and below a heart valve indicates valvular heart disease.
- Retrograde flow of the contrast medium across a valve during systole indicates valvular incompetence.

CARDIAC MAGNETIC RESONANCE IMAGING

Overview

- Magnetic resonance imaging (MRI): Noninvasive procedure that enables visualization of cross-sectional images of bone and delineation of fluid-filled soft tissue in great detail; produces images of organs and vessels in motion
- Most commonly relies on the magnetic properties of hydrogen, the most abundant and magnetically sensitive of the body's atoms
- Cardiac MRI: Involves placing the patient in a magnetic field, obtaining cross-sectional images of the heart and related structures in multiple planes, and recording them for permanent record
- Magnetic fields and radiofrequency (RF) energy used for MRI are imper-

ceptible to the patient; no harmful effects have been documented
- Optimal magnetic fields and RF waves for each type of tissue under investigation

PURPOSE

- To identify anatomic sequelae related to myocardial infarction, such as formation of ventricular aneurysm and mural thrombus
- To detect and evaluate cardiomyopathy
- To detect and evaluate pericardial disease
- To identify paracardiac or intracardiac masses
- To detect and evaluate congenital heart disease, such as atrial or ventricular septal defects and malposition of the great vessels
- To identify vascular disease such as thoracic aortic aneurysm and dissection
- To assess the structure of the pulmonary vasculature

PATIENT PREPARATION

- Make sure the patient has signed an appropriate consent form.
- Note and report all allergies.
- Restriction of food and fluids isn't necessary.
- Have the patient remove all metal objects.
- Make sure the patient doesn't have a pacemaker or surgically implanted joints, pins, clips, valves, or pumps containing metal that could be attracted to the strong MRI magnet.
- Ask if the patient has ever worked with metals or has any metal in his eyes.
- Explain that MRI is painless, but discomfort may be associated with remaining still inside a small space throughout the test.

- The patient may be given earplugs because the scanner makes clicking, whirring, and thumping noises as it moves.
- Provide reassurance that the patient will be able to communicate with the technician at all times, and the procedure will be stopped if he feels claustrophobic.
- Administer a sedative if ordered, especially for a claustrophobic patient.

Teaching points

Be sure to cover:
- the purpose of the study and how it's done
- who will perform the test and where
- that the test takes up to 90 minutes.

POSTPROCEDURE CARE

- No specific postprocedure care is usually required unless the patient required sedation.

Monitoring

Monitor the sedated patient's hemodynamic, cardiac, respiratory, and mental status until the effects of the sedative have worn off.

PRECAUTIONS

- If claustrophobia is an issue, the patient may need sedation, or may not be able to tolerate the procedure.
- Monitor cardiac patients for signs of ischemia secondary to anxiety.
- No metal can enter the testing area because the MRI works through a powerful magnetic field.
- MRI can't be performed on patients with pacemakers, intracranial aneurysm clips, or other ferrous metal implants.
- Ventilators, I.V. infusion pumps, and other metallic or computer-based equipment cannot be used in the MRI area.

■ Unstable patients need an I.V. access without metal components, and all equipment must be MRI-compatible.

■ Excessive patient movement can blur images.

■ If necessary, monitor the patient's oxygen saturation, cardiac rhythm, and respiratory status during the test.

■ A member of the anesthesia department may be needed to monitor a heavily sedated patient.

■ A nurse or radiology technician should maintain verbal contact with a conscious patient.

COMPLICATIONS

■ Panic attacks related to claustrophobia

■ Adverse reactions to sedation

Interpretation

NORMAL FINDINGS

■ No cardiovascular anatomic and structural abnormalities are present.

ABNORMAL RESULTS

■ Cardiovascular anatomic or structural abnormalities may suggest:

– cardiomyopathy and pericardial disease

– atrial or ventricular septal defects

– congenital defects

– paracardiac or intracardiac masses

– pericardiac or vascular disease.

CARDIAC POSITRON EMISSION TOMOGRAPHY

Overview

■ Combines elements of both computed tomography scanning and conventional radionuclide imaging

■ Works by measuring emissions of particles of injected radioisotopes, called positrons, and converting them to tomographic images

■ Unlike conventional radionuclide imaging, uses radioisotopes of biologically important elements, oxygen, nitrogen, carbon, and fluorine

■ Positron emitters: can be chemically tagged to biologically active molecules, such as carbon monoxide, neurotransmitters, hormones, and metabolites (particularly glucose), allowing study of their uptake and distribution in tissue

■ Radiation is 25% of that received by computed tomography scan

■ Costly because of short half-lives of the radioisotopes, which must be produced at an on-site cyclotron and attached quickly to the desired tracer molecules

■ Also known as PET scanning

PURPOSE

■ To detect coronary artery disease

■ To evaluate myocardial metabolism

■ To distinguish viable from infarcted cardiac tissue, especially during early stages of myocardial infarction

PATIENT PREPARATION

■ Make sure the patient has signed an appropriate consent form.

■ Note and report all allergies.

■ Provide reassurance that the test is painless, other than possible minor discomfort if an I.V. access is inserted.

■ Fasting after midnight the night before the test may be required.

■ Abstinence from caffeinated beverages, alcohol, and tobacco products may be required for 24 hours before the test.

■ Stress the importance of remaining still during the study.

Teaching points

Be sure to cover:
- the purpose of the study and how it's done
- who will perform the test and where
- that the test takes 1 to 1½ hours.

POSTPROCEDURE CARE

- Instruct the patient to move slowly immediately after the procedure to avoid postural hypotension.
- Encourage increased oral fluid intake to help flush the radioisotope from the bladder.

PRECAUTIONS

- Carefully screen female patients of childbearing age because the radioisotope may be harmful to a fetus.
- Failure of the patient to maintain proper positioning can prevent accurate imaging.

COMPLICATIONS

- Postural hypotension

Interpretation

NORMAL FINDINGS

- No areas of ischemic tissue are present.
- If the patient receives two tracers, the flow and distribution should match, indicating normal tissue.

ABNORMAL RESULTS

- Reduced blood flow, with increased glucose use, indicates ischemia.
- Reduced blood flow, with decreased glucose use, indicates necrotic, scarred tissue.

DOPPLER ULTRASONOGRAPHY

Overview

- A noninvasive test to evaluate blood flow in the major veins and arteries of the arms and legs and in the extracranial cerebrovascular system
- Handheld transducer directs high-frequency sound waves to artery or vein; transducer amplifies the sound waves to permit direct listening and graphic recording of blood flow
- Measurement of systolic pressure helps to detect the presence, location, and extent of peripheral arterial occlusive disease
- Accuracy rate: 95% in detecting arteriovenous disease that impairs at least 50% of blood flow

PURPOSE

- To aid the diagnosis of:
- Venous insufficiency
- Superficial and deep vein thromboses
- Peripheral artery disease and arterial occlusion
- To monitor patients who have had arterial reconstruction and bypass grafts
- To detect abnormalities of carotid artery blood
- To evaluate possible arterial trauma

PATIENT PREPARATION

- Make sure the patient has signed an appropriate consent form.
- Note and report all allergies.

Teaching points

Be sure to cover:
- the purpose of the study and how it's done
- who will perform the test and where
- that the test takes about 20 minutes

- that the test doesn't involve risk or discomfort.

POSTPROCEDURE CARE
- Remove the conductive jelly from the patient's skin.

PRECAUTIONS
- The Doppler probe shouldn't be placed over an open or draining lesion.
- It may fail to detect mild arteriosclerotic plaques and smaller thrombi.

COMPLICATIONS
- Possible bradyarrhythmias when probe is placed in carotid sinus region

Interpretation

NORMAL FINDINGS
- Arterial waveforms of the arms and legs are multiphasic, with a prominent systolic component and one or more diastolic sounds.
- Proximal thigh pressure is normally 20 to 30 mm Hg greater than arm pressure.
- Arm pressure readings should remain unchanged despite postural changes.
- Venous blood flow velocity is normally phasic with respiration, with a lower pitch than arterial flow.
- Distal compression, or release of proximal limb compression, increases blood flow velocity.
- In the legs, abdominal compression eliminates respiratory variations but release increases blood flow.
- Valsalva's maneuver interrupts venous flow velocity.
- In cerebrovascular testing, a strong velocity signal is present.
- In the common carotid artery, blood flow velocity increases during diastole.

- Periorbital arterial flow is normally anterograde out of the orbit.

ABNORMAL RESULTS
- Diminished blood flow velocity signal suggests arterial stenosis or occlusion.
- Absent velocity signals suggest complete occlusion and lack of collateral circulation.
- An abnormal ankle-brachial index (ABI) is directly proportional to the degree of circulatory impairment:
  – ABI > 0.9: normal
  – ABI 0.5 to 0.9: claudication
  – ABI < 0.5: resting ischemic pain
  – ABI < 0.2: gangrenous extremity.
- Venous blood flow velocity unchanged by respirations, not increased with compression or Valsalva's maneuver, or absent, indicates venous thrombosis.
- Reversed flow velocity signal may indicate chronic venous insufficiency and varicose veins.
- Ability to identify Doppler signals during cerebrovascular examination implies total arterial occlusion.

ECHOCARDIOGRAPHY

Overview

- Noninvasive test to examine the size, shape, and motion of cardiac structures
- Transducer directs ultra-high-frequency sound waves toward cardiac structures, which reflect these waves; the transducer picks up the echoes, converts them to electrical impulses, and relays them to an echocardiography machine for display
- In M-mode (motion mode): a single, pencil-like ultrasound beam strikes the heart and produces a vertical view;

useful for recording the motion and dimensions of intracardiac structures
- In two-dimensional echocardiography: a cross-sectional view of cardiac structures is used for recording lateral motion and spatial relationship between structures

PURPOSE
- To diagnose and evaluate valvular abnormalities
- To measure and evaluate the size of the heart's chambers and valves
- To aid the diagnosis of cardiomyopathies and atrial tumors
- To evaluate cardiac function or wall motion after myocardial infarction
- To detect pericardial effusion or mural thrombi

PATIENT PREPARATION
- Restriction of food and fluids isn't necessary.
- Explain that the patient may be asked to breathe in and out slowly, and to hold his breath while changes in heart function are recorded.
- Stress the need to remain still during the test because movement may distort results.

Teaching points
Be sure to cover:
- the purpose of the study and how it's done
- who will perform the test and where
- that the test takes 15 to 30 minutes.

POSTPROCEDURE CARE
- Remove the conductive gel from the patient's skin.

PRECAUTIONS
- None known

Interpretation

NORMAL FINDINGS
Mitral valve
- Anterior and posterior mitral valve leaflets separate in early diastole and attain maximum excursion rapidly, then move toward each other during ventricular diastole; after atrial contraction, they come together and remain so during ventricular systole.

Aortic valve
- Aortic valve cusps move anteriorly during systole and posteriorly during diastole.

Tricuspid valve
- Motion of the tricuspid valve resembles that of the mitral valve.

Pulmonic valve
- The pulmonic valve moves posteriorly during atrial systole and during ventricular systole. During right ventricular ejection, the cusp moves anteriorly, attaining its most anterior position during diastole.

Ventricular cavities
- The left ventricular cavity normally appears as an echo-free space between the interventricular septum and the posterior left ventricular wall.
- The right ventricular cavity normally appears as an echo-free space between the anterior chest wall and the interventricular septum.

ABNORMAL RESULTS
- In mitral stenosis, the valve narrows abnormally because of the leaflets' thickening and disordered motion; during diastole both mitral valve leaflets move anteriorly instead of posteriorly.

■ In mitral valve prolapse, one or both leaflets balloon into the left atrium during systole.

■ In aortic insufficiency, leaflet fluttering of the aortic valve during diastole occurs.

■ In stenosis, the aortic valve thickens and thus generates more echoes.

■ In bacterial endocarditis, valve motion is disrupted and fuzzy echoes usually appear on or near the valve.

■ A large chamber size may indicate cardiomyopathy, valvular disorders, or heart failure.

■ A small chamber may indicate restrictive pericarditis.

■ Hypertrophic cardiomyopathy can be identified by systolic anterior motion of the mitral valve and asymmetrical septal hypertrophy.

■ Myocardial ischemia or infarction may cause absent or paradoxical motion in ventricular walls.

■ Pericardial effusion is suggested when fluid accumulates in the pericardial space, causing an abnormal echo-free space to appear. In large effusions, pressure exerted by excess fluid can restrict pericardial motion.

ELECTRO-CARDIOGRAPHY

Overview

■ Graphically records the electrical current generated by the heart and measured by electrodes connected to an amplifier and strip chart recorder

■ Standard resting ECG: measures the electrical potential from 12 different leads: the standard limb leads (I, II, III), the augmented limb leads (aV_F, aV_L, and aV_R), and the precordial, or chest, leads (V_1 through V_6) (see *Limb lead placement,* pages 146 and 147; *Precordial lead placement,* page 148; *Right precordial lead placement* and *Posterior lead electrode placement,* page 149; and *Quadrant method for axis determination,* page 152)

■ Also known as ECG

PURPOSE

■ To identify conduction abnormalities, cardiac arrhythmias, myocardial ischemia or infarction (MI)

■ To monitor recovery from MI

■ To document pacemaker performance

PATIENT PREPARATION

■ Explain the need to lie still, relax, and breathe normally during the procedure.

■ Note current cardiac drug therapy on the test request form as well as any other pertinent clinical information, such as chest pain or pacemaker.

Teaching points

Be sure to cover:

■ test's purpose and how it's done

■ who will perform the test and where

■ that the test is painless and takes 5 to 10 minutes.

POSTPROCEDURE CARE

■ Disconnect the equipment, remove the electrodes, and remove the gel with a moist cloth towel.

■ Electrode patches are left in place if the patient is having recurrent chest pain or if serial ECGs are ordered.

PRECAUTIONS

■ All recording and other nearby electrical equipment should be properly grounded.

■ Ensure that electrodes are firmly attached.

COMPLICATIONS

■ Skin sensitivity to electrodes

LIMB LEAD PLACEMENT

Proper lead placement is critical for the accurate recording of cardiac rhythms. The diagrams here show electrode placement for the six limb leads. RA indicates right arm; LA, left arm; RL, right leg; and LL, left leg. The plus sign (+) indicates the positive pole, the minus sign (-) indicates the negative pole, and G indicates the ground. Below each diagram is a sample ECG recording for that lead.

Lead I
Lead I connects the right arm (negative pole) with the left arm (positive pole).

Lead II
Lead II connects the right arm (negative pole) with the left leg (positive pole).

Lead III
Lead III connects the left arm (negative pole) with the left leg (positive pole).

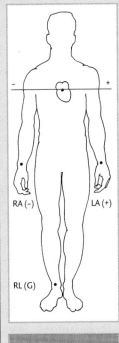

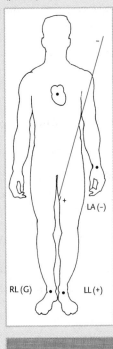

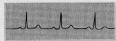

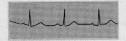

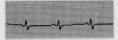

Interpretation

NORMAL FINDINGS
Common, basic findings include:
■ ECG tracings normally consist of P wave, QRS complex, and T wave. (See *Reviewing ECG waveform components,*

pages 150 and 151 and *ECG grid,* page 151.)
■ The normal cardiac rate is 60 to 100 beats/minute.
■ The cardiac rhythm should be normal sinus rhythm.

Lead aV_R

Lead aV$_R$ connects the right arm (positive pole) with the heart (negative pole).

Lead aV_L

Lead aV$_L$ connects the left arm (positive pole) with the heart (negative pole).

Lead aV_F

Lead aV$_F$ connects the left leg (positive pole) with the heart (negative pole).

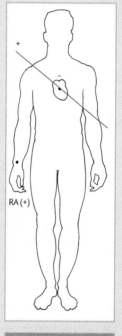

RA (+)

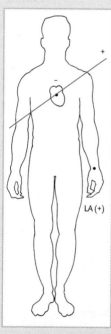

LA (+)

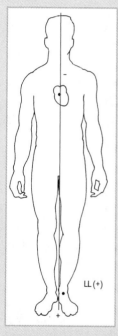

LL (+)

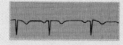

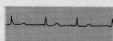

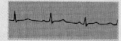

- The P wave precedes each QRS complex.
- The PR interval has a duration of 0.12 to 0.20 second.
- The QRS complex has a duration of 0.06 to 0.10 second.

- The ST segment is usually not more than 0.1 mV.
- The T wave is usually rounded and smooth and is usually positive in leads I, II, and V$_3$ to V$_6$.

PRECORDIAL LEAD PLACEMENT

To record the 12-lead electrocardiogram, place electrodes on the patient's arms and legs (with the ground lead on the patient's right leg). The three standard limb leads (I, I, and III) and the three augmented leads (aV$_R$, aV$_L$, and aV$_F$) are recorded using these electrodes.

To record the precordial chest leads, place the electrodes as follows:

- V$_1$ — fourth intercostal space (ICS), right sternal border
- V$_2$ — fourth ICS, left sternal border
- V$_3$ — midway between V$_2$ and V$_4$
- V$_4$ — fifth ICS, left midclavicular line
- V$_5$ — fifth ICS, left anterior axillary line
- V$_6$ — fifth ICS, left midaxillary line.

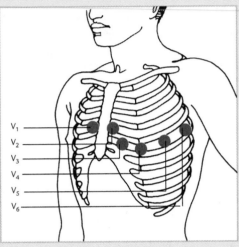

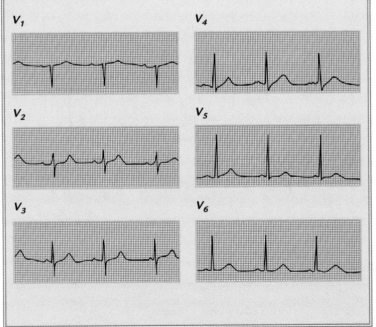

RIGHT PRECORDIAL LEAD PLACEMENT

The standard 12-lead electrocardiogram (ECG) evaluates only the left ventricle. The six right precordial leads provide specific information about right ventricular function. With this type of ECG, the six leads are placed on the right side of the chest in a mirror image of the standard precordial lead placement.

V_1R: fourth intercostal space (ICS), left sternal border
V_2R: fourth ICS, right sternal border
V_3R: halfway between V_2R and V_4R
V_4R: fifth ICS, right midclavicular line
V_5R: fifth ICS, right anterior axillary line
V_6R: fifth ICS, right midaxillary line

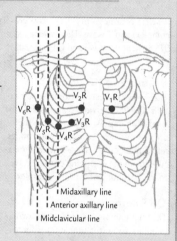

POSTERIOR LEAD ELECTRODE PLACEMENT

Evidence-based research has proven that a 12-lead electrocardiogram (ECG) has limited sensitivity in detecting posterior myocardial infarction. Because of the heart's posterior surface, changes associated with myocardial damage aren't apparent on a standard 12-lead ECG. These studies have shown that the addition of posterior leads V_7, V_8, and V_9 to the 12-lead ECG increases the sensitivity and specificity of identifying posterior wall infarction and may provide clues to posterior wall infarction so that appropriate treatment can begin.

To ensure an accurate ECG reading, make sure the posterior electrodes V_7, V_8, and V_9 are placed at the same level horizontally as the V_6 lead at the fifth intercostal space. Place lead V_7 at the posterior axillary line, lead V_9 at the paraspinal line, and lead V_8 halfway between leads V_7 and V_9.

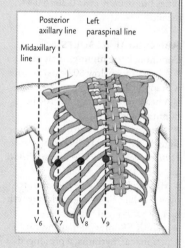

REVIEWING ECG WAVEFORM COMPONENTS

An electrocardiogram (ECG) waveform has three basic components: the P wave, QRS complex, and T wave. These elements can be further divided into the PR interval, J point, ST segment, U wave, and QT interval.

P wave and PR interval

The P wave represents atrial depolarization. The PR interval represents the time it takes an impulse to travel from the atria through the atrioventricular nodes and bundle of His. The PR interval measures from the beginning of the P wave to the beginning of the QRS complex.

QRS complex

The QRS complex represents ventricular depolarization (the time it takes for the impulse to travel through the bundle branches to the Purkinje fibers).

The Q wave appears as the first negative deflection in the QRS complex; the R wave, as the first positive deflection. The S wave appears as the second negative deflection or the first negative deflection after the R wave.

J point and ST segment

Marking the end of the QRS complex, the J point also indicates the beginning

---

■ The duration of the QT interval varies but usually lasts 0.36 to 0.44 second.

ABNORMAL RESULTS

Common, basic findings include:
■ A heart rate below 60 beats/minute is bradycardia.
■ A heart rate greater than 100 beats/ minute is tachycardia.
■ Abnormalities in cardiac rhythm suggest arrhythmias. (See *Recognizing LBBB,* page 153, and *Recognizing RBBB,* page 154.)
■ Missing P waves may indicate atrioventricular (AV) block, atrial arrhythmia, or junctional rhythm.
■ A short PR interval may indicate a junctional arrhythmia; a prolonged PR interval may indicate AV block.
■ A prolonged QRS complex may indicate intraventricular conduction defects; missing QRS complexes may indicate AV block or ventricular asystole.

■ ST-segment elevation of 0.2 mV or more above baseline may indicate myocardial injury; ST-segment depression may indicate myocardial ischemia or injury. (See *Vessels that supply the heart,* page 155; *Locating myocardial damage,* page 156; and *Reciprocal changes in MI,* page 157.)
■ T-wave inversion in leads I, II, and V_3 to V_6 may indicate myocardial ischemia; peaked T waves may indicate hyperkalemia or myocardial ischemia; variations in T-wave amplitude may indicate electrolyte imbalances.
■ A prolonged QT interval may suggest life-threatening ventricular arrhythmias.

of the ST segment. The ST segment represents part of ventricular repolarization.

T wave and U wave
Usually following the same deflection pattern as the P wave, the T wave represents ventricular repolarization. The U wave follows the T wave, but isn't always seen.

QT interval
The QT interval represents ventricular depolarization and repolarization. It extends from the beginning of the QRS complex to the end of the T wave.

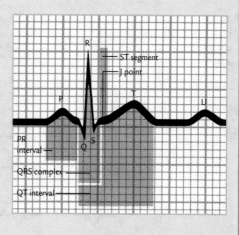

ECG GRID

This electrocardiogram (ECG) grid shows the horizontal and vertical axes and their respective measurement values.

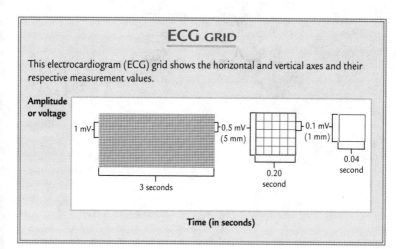

QUADRANT METHOD FOR AXIS DETERMINATION

This chart will help you quickly determine the direction of a patient's electrical axis. Observe the deflections of the QRS complexes in leads I and aV$_F$. Then check the chart to determine whether the patient's axis is normal or has a left, right, or extreme axis deviation.

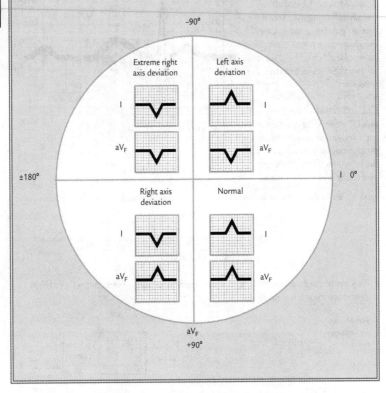

RECOGNIZING LBBB

This 12-lead electrocardiogram shows characteristic changes of a left bundle-branch block (LBBB). All leads have prolonged QRS complexes. In lead V_1, note the QS wave pattern. In lead V_6, you'll see the slurred R wave and T-wave inversion. The elevated ST segments and upright T waves in leads V_1 to V_4 are also common in LBBB.

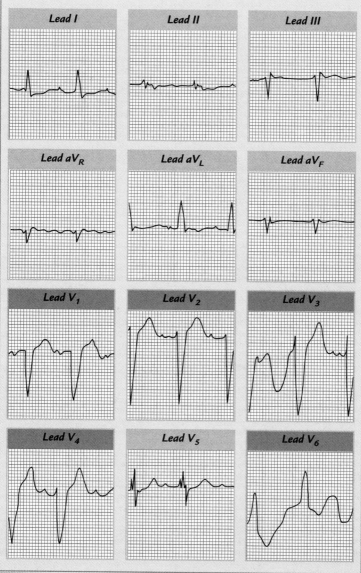

RECOGNIZING RBBB

This 12-lead electrocardiogram shows the characteristic changes of right bundle-branch block (RBBB). In lead V_1, note the rsR' pattern and T-wave inversion. In lead V_6, see the widened S wave and the upright T wave. Also note the prolonged QRS complexes.

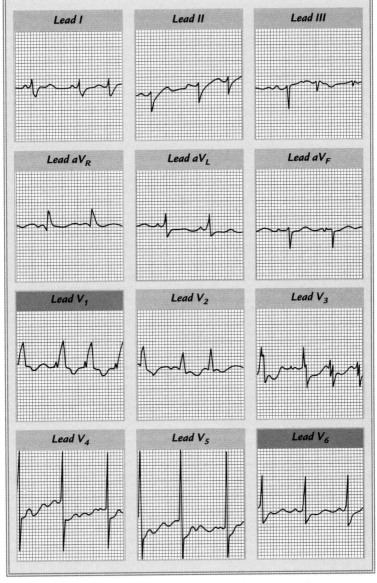

VESSELS THAT SUPPLY THE HEART

The coronary circulation involves the arterial system of blood vessels that supply oxygenated blood to the heart and the venous system that removes oxygen-depleted blood from it.

Anterior view

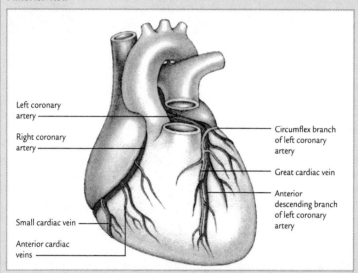

Left coronary artery

Right coronary artery

Circumflex branch of left coronary artery

Great cardiac vein

Anterior descending branch of left coronary artery

Small cardiac vein

Anterior cardiac veins

Posterior view

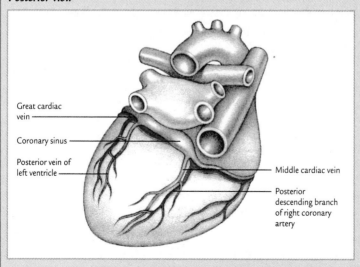

Great cardiac vein

Coronary sinus

Posterior vein of left ventricle

Middle cardiac vein

Posterior descending branch of right coronary artery

LOCATING MYOCARDIAL DAMAGE

After you've noted characteristic lead changes in an acute myocardial infarction, use this chart to identify the areas of damage. Match the lead changes in the second column with the affected wall in the first column and the artery involved in the third column. The fourth column shows reciprocal lead changes.

Wall affected	Leads	Artery involved	Reciprocal changes
Inferior (diaphragmatic)	II, III, aV_F	Right coronary artery	1, aV_L and, possibly, V_4
Lateral	I, aV_L, V_5, V_6	Circumflex artery, branch of left coronary artery	V_1, V_2
Anterior	V_2 to V_4	Left coronary artery, left anterior descending (LAD) artery	II, III, aV_F
Posterior	V_1, V_2, V_7, V_8, V_9	Right coronary artery, circumflex artery	R wave greater than S wave in V_1 and V_2; depressed ST segments; elevated T wave
Anterolateral	I, aV_L, V_4 to V_6	LAD artery, circumflex artery	II, III, aV_F
Anteroseptal	V_1 to V_4	LAD artery	None
Right ventricular	V_4R, V_5R, V_6R	Right coronary artery	None

RECIPROCAL CHANGES IN MI

Ischemia, injury, and infarction (the three I's of myocardial infarction [MI]) produce characteristic electrocardiogram (ECG) changes. The changes shown by leads that reflect electrical activity in damaged areas are shown to the right of the illustration below.

Reciprocal leads, those opposite the damaged area, show opposing ECG changes, as shown to the left of the illustration.

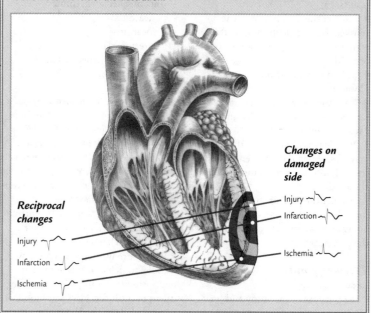

Changes on damaged side

Injury

Infarction

Ischemia

Reciprocal changes

Injury

Infarction

Ischemia

ELECTRO-CARDIOGRAPHY, EXERCISE

Overview

- Monitors patient's electrocardiogram (ECG) and blood pressure while the patient walks on a treadmill or pedals a stationary bicycle; response to a constant or increasing workload is observed
- Used to evaluate the heart during physical stress
- Commonly known as an exercise stress test

PURPOSE

- To diagnose the cause of chest pain
- To determine functional capacity of the heart
- To screen for asymptomatic coronary artery disease
- To help set limitations for an exercise program
- To identify cardiac arrhythmias that develop during physical exercise
- To evaluate effectiveness of antiarrhythmic or antianginal therapy
- To evaluate myocardial perfusion

PATIENT PREPARATION

- Make sure the patient has signed an appropriate consent form.
- Note and report all allergies.
- Check the patient's history for a recent physical examination (within 1 week) and for baseline 12-lead ECG results.
- Instruct the patient not to eat, smoke, or drink alcoholic or caffeine-containing beverages before the test as ordered.
- Continue medications unless the physician directs otherwise.
- Warn the patient that he may feel fatigued, slightly breathless, and sweaty during the test.
- Provide reassurance that the test may be stopped if the patient experiences significant symptoms such as chest pain.
- Instruct the patient to wear comfortable socks and shoes and loose, lightweight shorts or slacks during the procedure.

Teaching points

Be sure to cover:
- the purpose of the study and how it's done
- who will perform the test and where
- that the test takes approximately 30 minutes.

POSTPROCEDURE CARE

- Assist the patient to a chair and continue monitoring heart rate and blood pressure for 10 to 15 minutes or until the ECG returns to baseline.
- Remove the electrodes and clean the application sites.
- Resume a normal diet and activities as ordered.

Monitoring

- Vital signs
- ECG
- Heart sounds
- Anginal symptoms

PRECAUTIONS

- The procedure may be contraindicated in a patient with:
 – ventricular or dissecting aortic aneurysm
 – uncontrolled arrhythmias
 – pericarditis
 – myocarditis
 – severe anemia
 – uncontrolled hypertension
 – unstable angina
 – heart failure.

⚡ *Stop the test immediately if the ECG shows significant arrhythmias or increase in ectopy, if systolic blood pressure falls below resting level, if the heart rate falls 10 beats/minute or more below resting level, or if the patient becomes exhausted or experiences severe symptoms such as chest pain.*

- Conditions that cause left ventricular hypertrophy may interfere with testing for ischemia.
- The test may be stopped for new bundle-branch block, ST-segment depression exceeding 1.5 mm, or frequent or multifocal PVCs; if blood pressure fails to rise above resting level; if systolic pressure exceeds 220 mm Hg; or if the patient experiences angina.
- The test may also be stopped if the examiner suspects that persistent ST-segment elevation may indicate myocardial injury.

COMPLICATIONS

- Cardiac arrhythmias
- Myocardial ischemia or infarction

Interpretation

NORMAL FINDINGS

- The heart rate increases in direct proportion to the workload and metabolic oxygen demand.

■ Systolic blood pressure increases as workload increases.

■ The patient attains the endurance levels appropriate for his age and the exercise protocol.

ABNORMAL RESULTS

■ T-wave inversion or ST-segment depression may signify ischemia.

■ Significant coronary artery disease may be indicated by:
– exercise-induced hypotension
– ST-segment depression of 2 mm or more
– downsloping ST segments
– ST-segment elevation may indicate myocardial injury.

ELECTRO-CARDIOGRAPHY, SIGNAL-AVERAGED

Overview

■ The amplification, averaging, and filtering of an electrocardiogram signal recorded on the body surface

■ Used to detect high-frequency, low-amplitude cardiac electrical signals in the last part of the QRS complex and in the ST segment

PURPOSE

■ To detect late potentials

■ To evaluate risk of life-threatening arrhythmias

PATIENT PREPARATION

■ Make sure the patient has signed an appropriate consent form.

■ Note and report all allergies.

■ Record the use of antiarrhythmics on the patient's chart.

■ Tell the patient that electrodes will be attached to his arms, legs, and chest and that the procedure is painless.

■ Instruct the patient to lie still and breathe normally during the procedure.

■ There's no need to restrict food and fluids before the test.

Teaching points

Be sure to cover:

■ the purpose of the study and how it's done

■ who will perform it and where

■ that the test takes about 30 minutes.

POSTPROCEDURE CARE

■ Wash conductive gel from the skin.

PRECAUTIONS

■ Electrical equipment should be properly grounded to prevent electrical interference.

■ Antiarrhythmics may interfere with the accuracy of test results.

■ Poor tissue-electrode contact produces artifact.

COMPLICATIONS

■ Possible skin sensitivity to the electrodes

Interpretation

NORMAL FINDINGS

■ QRS complexes lack low potentials.

ABNORMAL RESULTS

■ Late potentials after the QRS complex indicate a risk for ventricular arrhythmias.

ELECTROPHYSIOLOGY STUDIES

Overview

■ Permits measurement of discrete conduction intervals

- Records electrical conduction during the slow withdrawal of an electrode catheter from the right ventricle through the bundle of His to the sinoatrial node
- Also known as EPS or bundle of His electrography

PURPOSE
- To diagnose arrhythmias and conduction anomalies
- To determine the need for an implanted pacemaker, internal cardioverter-defibrillator, and cardioactive drugs
- To locate the site of a bundle-branch block, especially in asymptomatic patients with conduction disturbances
- To determine the presence and location of accessory conducting pathways

PATIENT PREPARATION
- Make sure the patient has signed an appropriate consent form.
- Note and report all allergies.
- Instruct the patient to restrict food and fluids for at least 6 hours before the test.
- Provide reassurance that the patient will remain conscious during the test. Instruct him to report any discomfort or pain.

Teaching points
Be sure to cover:
- the purpose of the study and how it's done
- who will perform the test and where
- that the test takes 1 to 3 hours.

POSTPROCEDURE CARE
- Monitor the patient's vital signs, as ordered.
- Enforce bed rest, as ordered.
- If bleeding occurs, apply pressure and inform the physician at once.

- Resume a normal diet, as ordered.
- Obtain a 12-lead resting electrocardiogram (ECG).

Monitoring
- Vital signs
- Insertion site
- Bleeding
- Signs and symptoms of infection
- Cardiac arrhythmias
- Anginal symptoms
- Signs and symptoms of embolism
- ECG changes

PRECAUTIONS
- The procedure is contraindicated in a patient with:
  - severe uncorrected coagulopathy
  - recent thrombophlebitis
  - acute pulmonary embolism.

Emergency resuscitation equipment should be immediately available in case of arrhythmias during the test.

COMPLICATIONS
- Arrhythmias
- Pulmonary emboli
- Thromboemboli
- Hemorrhage
- Infection

Interpretation

NORMAL FINDINGS
- The HV interval (conduction time from the bundle of His to the Purkinje fibers) is 35 to 55 msec.
- The AH interval (conduction time from the atrioventricular node to the bundle of His) is 45 to 150 msec.
- The PA (intra-atrial) interval is 20 to 40 msec.

ABNORMAL RESULTS
- A prolonged HV interval suggests possible acute or chronic disease.

■ AH interval delays suggest atrial pacing, chronic conduction system disease, carotid sinus pressure, recent myocardial infarction, and use of certain drugs.

■ PA interval delays suggest possible acquired, surgically induced, or congenital atrial disease and atrial pacing.

HOLTER MONITORING

Overview

■ Continuous recording of heart activity as the patient follows his normal routine, usually for 24 hours

■ Patient-activated monitor: worn for 5 to 7 days, allows patient to manually initiate recording of heart activity when symptoms are experienced

■ Also known as ambulatory electrocardiography (ECG) or dynamic monitoring

PURPOSE

■ To detect cardiac arrhythmias

■ To evaluate chest pain

■ To evaluate effectiveness of antiarrhythmic drug therapy

■ To monitor pacemaker function

■ To correlate symptoms and palpitations with actual cardiac events and patient activities

■ To detect sporadic arrhythmias missed by an exercise or resting ECG

PATIENT PREPARATION

■ Make sure the patient has signed an appropriate consent form.

■ Note and report all allergies.

■ Provide bathing instructions because some equipment must not get wet.

■ Instruct the patient to avoid magnets, metal detectors, high-voltage areas, and electric blankets.

Teaching points

Be sure to cover:

■ the purpose of the study and how it's done

■ routine activities during the monitoring period

■ the importance of logging activities as well as emotional upsets, physical symptoms, and ingestion of medication in a diary

■ how to mark the tape at the onset of symptoms if applicable

■ how to check the recorder to make sure it's working properly.

POSTPROCEDURE CARE

■ Remove all chest electrodes.

■ Clean the electrode sites.

PRECAUTIONS

■ Avoid placing electrodes over large muscles masses, such as the pectorals, to limit artifact.

COMPLICATIONS

■ Skin sensitivity to the electrodes

Interpretation

NORMAL FINDINGS

■ The ECG shows no significant arrhythmias or ST-segment changes.

■ Changes in heart rate occur during various activities.

ABNORMAL RESULTS

■ Abnormalities in cardiac rate or rhythm suggest possible serious arrhythmias, which may be symptomatic or asymptomatic.

■ ST-T wave changes may coincide with patient symptoms or increased patient activity, and suggest possible myocardial ischemia.

MYOCARDIAL PERFUSION IMAGING, RADIOPHARMACEUTICAL

Overview

■ Alternative method of assessing coronary arteries for patients who can't tolerate exercise stress tests
■ A drug (adenosine, dobutamine, or dipyridamole) is used to chemically stress the patient; this simulates the effects of exercise by increasing blood flow in the coronary arteries or by increasing heart rate and contractility
■ Radiopharmaceutical is injected and resting and stress images are obtained and compared to evaluate coronary perfusion
■ Also known as chemical stress test imaging

PURPOSE

■ To assess the presence and degree of coronary artery disease
■ To evaluate patient's response after therapeutic procedures (such as bypass surgery and coronary angioplasty)

PATIENT PREPARATION

■ Make sure the patient has signed an appropriate consent form.
■ Note and report all allergies.
■ Confirm that the patient isn't pregnant.
■ Weigh the patient to determine the appropriate drug dosage.
■ Withhold nitrates 6 hours before testing as ordered.
■ Fasting for 3 to 4 hours is required before the test; the patient may have water.
■ A cardiologist, nurse, electrocardiogram (ECG) technician, and nuclear medicine technologist are usually present during the test.

■ Warn the patient that he may experience flushing, shortness of breath, dizziness, headache, chest pain, increased heart rate, or palpitations during the infusion, depending on the drug used.
■ Provide reassurance that emergency equipment will be available if needed.

Adenosine or dipyridamole administration

■ Withhold all theophylline medications for 24 to 36 hours before the examination as ordered.
■ Instruct the patient to avoid all caffeine-containing products for 12 hours before testing.

Dobutamine administration

■ Withhold beta-adrenergic blockers for 48 hours before the test as ordered.
■ Administer medications, such as antihypertensives, as ordered.

Teaching points

Be sure to cover:
■ the purpose of the study and how it's done
■ who will perform the test and where
■ that the study takes 1 to 2 hours, and the time can be longer depending on the type of nuclear medicine equipment
■ that signs and symptoms generally stop as soon as the infusion ends.

POSTPROCEDURE CARE

■ Regular diet and activity are resumed as ordered.

Monitoring

■ Vital signs
■ ECG
■ Cardiac rhythm
■ Respiratory status
■ Anginal symptoms
■ Heart sounds
■ Breath sounds

PRECAUTIONS

■ Keep resuscitation equipment readily available.

■ Screen for bronchospastic lung disease or asthma (adenosine and dipyridamole are contraindicated).

■ Screen for the presence of a pacemaker; dobutamine may be contraindicated.

■ Reversal agents that should be readily available include:

– I.V. aminophylline for adenosine and dipyridamole

– I.V. beta-adrenergic blocker for dobutamine.

■ Contraindications include:

– myocardial infarction within 10 days of testing

– acute myocarditis and pericarditis

– unstable angina

– arrhythmias

– hypertension or hypotension

– severe aortic or mitral stenosis

– hyperthyroidism.

COMPLICATIONS

■ Serious arrhythmias

■ Myocardial ischemia or infarction

Interpretation

NORMAL FINDINGS

■ No perfusion defects are found on imaging.

■ No ischemic changes are found on ECG.

ABNORMAL RESULTS

■ Cold spots, indicating areas of decreased uptake, may suggest:

– coronary artery disease (most common)

– myocardial fibrosis

– attenuation caused by soft tissue (breast and diaphragm)

– coronary spasm.

PERICARDIOCENTESIS

Overview

■ Needle aspiration and analysis of pericardial fluid

■ Useful as an emergency measure to treat cardiac tamponade

PURPOSE

■ To identify the cause of pericardial effusion

■ To determine appropriate therapy

■ To treat cardiac tamponade

PATIENT PREPARATION

■ Make sure the patient has signed an appropriate consent form, if the clinical situation persists.

■ Note and report all allergies.

■ Restriction of food or fluids before the test usually isn't necessary.

■ Explain the need to use a local anesthetic.

■ Advise that the patient will feel pressure when the needle is inserted into the pericardial sac.

■ Explain the need to insert an I.V. line before the procedure.

■ Administer I.V. sedation as ordered.

■ Explain the need to monitor vital signs and heart rhythm throughout the procedure.

Teaching points

Be sure to cover:

■ the purpose of the study and how it's done

■ who will perform the test and where

■ that the test takes 10 to 20 minutes.

POSTPROCEDURE CARE
Monitoring

■ Vital signs

■ Cardiac rhythm

■ Serial electrocardiograms

■ Serial echocardiograms

- Bleeding
- Infection
- Insertion site
- Respiratory status
- Heart sounds
- Neck veins

Be alert for respiratory or cardiac distress. Watch especially for signs of cardiac tamponade, including muffled and distant heart sounds, distended jugular veins, paradoxical pulse, and shock. Cardiac tamponade may result from rapid reaccumulation of pericardial fluid or puncture of a coronary vessel, causing bleeding into the pericardial sac.

COMPLICATIONS
- Bleeding
- Infection
- Cardiac arrhythmias
- Coronary artery laceration
- Myocardial perforation
- Respiratory distress
- Cardiac tamponade

Interpretation

NORMAL FINDINGS
- The pericardium normally contains 10 to 30 ml of sterile fluid.
- The fluid is clear and straw-colored, without evidence of pathogens, blood, or malignant cells.
- White blood cell (WBC) count in the fluid is usually less than 1,000/μl.
- Glucose concentration should approximate the glucose levels in whole blood.

ABNORMAL RESULTS
- Effusions suggest various possible disorders, including:
  - pericarditis
  - neoplasms
  - acute myocardial infarction
  - tuberculosis
  - rheumatoid disease
  - systemic lupus erythematosus.
- The presence of most exudates, containing large amounts of protein, suggests inflammation.
- An elevated WBC count or neutrophil fraction suggests possible inflammatory conditions such as bacterial pericarditis.
- A high lymphocyte fraction suggests possible fungal or tuberculous pericarditis.
- Turbid or milky effusions may result from the accumulation of lymph or pus in the pericardial sac or from tuberculosis or rheumatoid disease.
- Bloody pericardial fluid suggests hemopericardium, hemorrhagic pericarditis, or traumatic tap.
- A glucose concentration less than that of whole blood suggests possible cancer, inflammation, or infection.

TECHNETIUM-99M PYROPHOSPHATE SCANNING

Overview

- Used to detect and determine extent of recent myocardial infarction (MI)
- I.V. tracer isotope (^{99m}Tc pyrophosphate) accumulates in damaged myocardial tissue (possibly by combining with calcium in the damaged myocardial cells), where it forms a hot spot on a scan made with a scintillation camera
- Useful when serum cardiac enzyme tests are unreliable or when patients have equivocal electrocardiograms such as in left bundle-branch block
- Also known as hot spot myocardial imaging and infarct avid imaging

PURPOSE
- To confirm recent MI

■ To define size and location of recent MI
■ To assess prognosis after acute MI

PATIENT PREPARATION
■ Make sure the patient has signed an appropriate consent form.
■ Note and report all allergies.
■ Restriction of food and fluids isn't necessary.
■ Provide reassurance that only transient discomfort will be felt during isotope injection; the scan itself is painless.
■ Stress the need to remain quiet and motionless during scanning.

Teaching points
Be sure to cover:
■ the purpose of the study and how it's done
■ who will perform the 30- to 60-minute test and where
■ that radiation exposure is minimal.

POSTPROCEDURE CARE
■ No specific posttest care is necessary.

COMPLICATIONS
■ None known

Interpretation

NORMAL FINDINGS
■ No isotope is found in the myocardium.

ABNORMAL RESULTS
■ Isotope is taken up by the sternum and ribs, and their activity is compared with the heart's; 2+, 3+, and 4+ activity (equal to or greater than bone) suggests a positive myocardial scan.
■ Areas of isotope accumulation, or hot spots, suggest damaged myocardium.

THALLIUM IMAGING

Overview

■ Used to evaluate blood flow after I.V. injection of the radioisotope thallium-201 or Cardiolite
■ Cardiolite: shown to have a better energy spectrum for imaging; requires living myocardial cells for uptake and allows for imaging the myocardial blood flow both before and after reperfusion
■ Thallium: concentrates in healthy myocardial tissue but not in necrotic or ischemic tissue; taken up rapidly in areas of the heart with normal blood supply and intact cells; fails to be taken up by areas with poor blood flow and ischemic cells, which appear as cold spots on a scan
■ May be performed in a resting state or after stress
■ Rest imaging: can disclose acute myocardial infarction (MI) within the first few hours of symptoms, but doesn't distinguish old from new infarct
■ Stress imaging: performed after exercise stress testing or after pharmacologic stress testing; used to assess known or suspected coronary artery disease (CAD)
■ Also known as cardiac nuclear imaging, cold spot myocardial imaging, or myocardial perfusion scan

PURPOSE
■ To assess myocardial perfusion
■ To demonstrate location and extent of MI
■ To diagnose CAD (stress imaging)
■ To evaluate coronary artery patency following surgical revascularization
■ To evaluate effectiveness of antianginal therapy or percutaneous revascu-

larization interventions (stress imaging)

PATIENT PREPARATION
■ Make sure the patient has signed an appropriate consent form.
■ Note and report all allergies.

Stress imaging
■ Instruct the patient to wear comfortable walking shoes during the treadmill exercise.
■ Restriction of alcohol, tobacco, and nonprescription medications is necessary for 24 hours before the test.
■ Fasting is necessary after midnight the night before the test.
■ Tell the patient to report fatigue, pain, shortness of breath, or other anginal symptoms immediately.

Teaching points
Be sure to cover:
■ the purpose of the study and how it's done
■ who will perform the test and where
■ that the initial test takes 45 to 90 minutes; additional scans may be required
■ that radiation exposure is minimal.

POSTPROCEDURE CARE
■ If further scanning is required, have the patient rest, and restrict foods and beverages other than water.

Monitoring
■ Vital signs
■ Cardiac arrhythmias
■ Anginal symptoms
■ Electrocardiograms (ECGs)

PRECAUTIONS
■ The results may be normal if the patient has narrowed coronary arteries but adequate collateral circulation.

■ Thallium imaging is contraindicated in:
– pregnancy
– impaired neuromuscular function
– acute MI
– myocarditis
– critical aortic stenosis
– acute infection
– unstable metabolic conditions (such as diabetes)
– digoxin toxicity
– recent pulmonary infarction.

Stress imaging is stopped immediately if the patient develops chest pain, dyspnea, fatigue, syncope, hypotension, ischemic ECG changes, significant arrhythmias, or other critical signs or symptoms (confusion, staggering, or pale, clammy skin).

COMPLICATIONS
■ Cardiac arrhythmias
■ Myocardial ischemia
■ MI
■ Respiratory distress
■ Cardiac arrest
■ Hypotension or hypertension

Interpretation

NORMAL FINDINGS
■ There's normal distribution of the isotope throughout the left ventricle without defects (cold spots).
■ After coronary artery bypass surgery, improved regional perfusion suggests patency of the graft.
■ Improved perfusion after nonsurgical revascularization interventions suggests increased coronary flow.

ABNORMAL RESULTS
■ Persistent defects suggest MI.
■ Transient defects (those that disappear after a 3- to 6-hour rest) suggest myocardial ischemia caused by CAD.

TRANSESOPHAGEAL ECHOCARDIOGRAPHY

Overview

- Combines ultrasonography with endoscopy to provide a better view of the heart's structures
- Involves small transducer attached to the end of a gastroscope and inserted into the esophagus, allowing images to be taken from the posterior aspect of the heart
- Causes less tissue penetration and interference from chest wall structures and produces high-quality images of the thoracic aorta, except for the superior ascending aorta, which is shadowed by the trachea

PURPOSE

- To visualize and evaluate many disorders:
- – Thoracic and aortic disorders, such as dissection and aneurysm
- – Valvular disease (especially of the mitral valve)
- – Endocarditis
- – Congenital heart disease
- – Intracardiac thrombi
- – Cardiac tumors
- – Cardiac tamponade
- – Ventricular dysfunction

PATIENT PREPARATION

- Make sure the patient has signed an appropriate consent form.
- Note and report all allergies.
- Review the patient's medical history and report possible contraindications to the test, such as esophageal obstruction or varices, GI bleeding, previous mediastinal radiation therapy, or severe cervical arthritis.
- Note and report loose teeth.
- Fasting is required for 6 hours before the procedure.
- Instruct the patient to remove dentures or oral prostheses.
- Explain the use of a topical anesthetic throat spray.
- Warn about possible gagging when the tube is inserted.
- Explain the need for I.V. sedation and continuous monitoring during the study.

Teaching points

Be sure to cover:
- the purpose of the study and how it's done
- who will perform the test and when
- that the study takes about 2 hours including preparation and recovery.

POSTPROCEDURE CARE

- Ensure patient safety and patent airway until the sedative wears off.
- Withhold food and water until his gag reflex returns.
- If the procedure is done on an outpatient basis, advise the patient to have someone drive him home.

Monitoring

- Level of consciousness
- Vital signs
- Respiratory status
- Cardiac arrhythmias
- Bleeding
- Gag reflex

PRECAUTIONS

- Keep resuscitation equipment immediately available.
- Keep suction equipment immediately available to avoid aspiration if vomiting occurs.
- Observe closely for a vasovagal response, which may occur with gagging.
- Use pulse oximetry to detect hypoxia.
- If bleeding occurs, stop the procedure immediately.

■ Laryngospasm, arrhythmias, or bleeding increases the risk of complications. If any of these occurs, postpone the test.
■ Possible contraindications include esophageal obstruction or varices, GI bleeding, previous mediastinal radiation therapy, or severe cervical arthritis.

COMPLICATIONS
■ Laryngospasm
■ Cardiac arrhythmias
■ Bleeding
■ Adverse reaction to sedation

Interpretation

NORMAL FINDINGS
■ The heart is without structural abnormalities.
■ No vegetations or thrombus is visible.
■ No tumors are visible.

ABNORMAL RESULTS
■ Structural thoracic and aortic abnormalities suggest possible endocarditis, congenital heart disease, intracardiac thrombi, or tumors.
■ Congenital defects suggest possible patent ductus arteriosus.

ULTRASONOGRAPHY OF THE ABDOMINAL AORTA

Overview

■ Transducer directs high-frequency sound waves into the abdomen over a wide area from the xiphoid process to the umbilical region; sound waves echoing to transducer from tissue of different densities are transmitted as electrical impulses and displayed on a monitor to reveal internal organs, the vertebral column and, most important, the size and course of the abdominal aorta and other major vessels
■ Used to confirm a suspected aortic aneurysm and method of choice for determining its diameter; performed to detect expansion of a known aneurysm because the risk of rupture is highest when aneurysmal diameter is 7 cm or greater
■ Used every 6 months to monitor changes in patient's status

PURPOSE
■ To detect and measure a suspected abdominal aortic aneurysm
■ To monitor expansion of a known abdominal aortic aneurysm

PATIENT PREPARATION
■ Make sure the patient has signed an appropriate consent form.
■ Note and report all allergies.
■ Administer simethicone to reduce bowel gas if ordered.
■ Fasting is required for 12 hours before the test to minimize bowel gas and motility.
■ Inform the patient that he will feel slight pressure during the study.
■ Instruct the patient to remain still during scanning and to hold his breath when requested.

Teaching points
Be sure to cover:
■ the purpose of the study and how it's done
■ who will perform the test and where
■ that the test takes 30 to 45 minutes.

POSTPROCEDURE CARE
■ Remove residual gel from the skin.
■ Resume the patient's usual diet and medications as ordered.

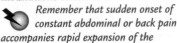 *Remember that sudden onset of constant abdominal or back pain accompanies rapid expansion of the*

aneurysm; sudden, excruciating pain with weakness, sweating, tachycardia, and hypotension signals rupture.

PRECAUTIONS
■ No precautions are necessary.

COMPLICATIONS
■ None known

Interpretation

NORMAL FINDINGS
■ In adults, the abdominal aorta tapers from about 2.5 to 1.5 cm in diameter along its length from the diaphragm to the bifurcation.
■ The abdominal aorta descends through the retroperitoneal space, anterior to the vertebral column and slightly left of the midline.
■ Four of the abdominal aorta's major branches are usually well visualized: the celiac trunk, the renal arteries, the superior mesenteric artery, and the common iliac arteries.

ABNORMAL RESULTS
■ Luminal diameter of the abdominal aorta greater than 4 cm indicates an aneurysm.
■ Luminal diameter of the abdominal aorta greater than 7 cm indicates an aneurysm with a high risk of rupture.

VENOGRAPHY OF THE LOWER LIMB

Overview

■ Radiographic examination of veins in the lower extremity
■ Commonly used to assess the condition of the deep leg veins after injection of a contrast medium
■ Not used for routine screening because it exposes the patient to relatively high doses of radiation and can cause complications, such as phlebitis, local tissue damage and, occasionally, deep vein thrombosis (DVT)
■ Used in patients whose duplex ultrasound findings are equivocal
■ Also known as ascending contrast phlebography

PURPOSE
■ To confirm diagnosis of DVT
■ To distinguish clot formation from venous obstruction (such as a large tumor of the pelvis impinging on the venous system)
■ To evaluate congenital venous abnormalities
■ To assess deep vein valvular competence (especially helpful in identifying underlying causes of leg edema)
■ To locate a suitable vein for arterial bypass grafting
■ To evaluate chronic venous disease

PATIENT PREPARATION
■ Make sure the patient has signed an appropriate consent form.
■ Note and report all allergies.
■ Check the patient's history for and report hypersensitivity to iodine, iodine-containing foods, or contrast media.
■ Reassure the patient that contrast media complications are rare, but tell him to report nausea, severe burning or itching, constriction in the throat or chest, or dyspnea at once.
■ Discontinue anticoagulant therapy as ordered.
■ Administer sedation as ordered.
■ Instruct the patient to restrict food and drink only clear liquids for 4 hours before the test.
■ Warn the patient that he might experience a burning sensation in the leg when the contrast medium is injected and some discomfort during the procedure.

Teaching points

Be sure to cover:
- the purpose of the study and how it's done
- who will perform the test and where
- that the test takes 30 to 45 minutes.

POSTPROCEDURE CARE

- Administer analgesics as ordered.
- Resume the patient's usual diet and medications as ordered.
- Encourage oral fluid intake as ordered.
- If DVT is documented, initiate therapy (heparin infusion, bed rest, leg elevation or support) as ordered.

Monitoring

- Vital signs
- Intake and output
- Injection site
- Bleeding
- Infection
- Hematoma
- Erythema
- Renal function
- Hydration

PRECAUTIONS

- Improper needle placement in a superficial vein, weight bearing or muscle contraction, or use of tourniquets can produce artifacts of poor filling.
- Errors in diagnosis are commonly the result of incomplete filling of vessels.
- Fluoroscopy is essential for establishing that the contrast medium has reached the vessels being filmed and that opacification is adequate.

Because of the high volume of contrast used, especially if bilateral venography is necessary, monitor renal function and hydration status very carefully.

Because most allergic reactions to the contrast medium occur within 30 minutes of injection, carefully observe the patient for signs and symptoms of anaphylaxis, such as flushing, urticaria, and laryngeal stridor.

Complications

- Adverse reactions to contrast media or medications
- Thrombophlebitis
- Local tissue damage
- Renal insufficiency or failure

Small extravasations of contrast media (less than 10 ml) don't usually pose a problem. However, tissue necrosis and ulceration may occur, especially with larger extravasations and in patients with arterial insufficiency.

Interpretation

NORMAL FINDINGS

- Test shows steady opacification of the superficial and deep vasculature with no filling defects.

ABNORMAL RESULTS

- Consistent filling defects, abrupt termination of a column of contrast material, unfilled major deep veins, or diversion of flow (through collaterals, for example) suggests DVT.

DISEASES

ANEURYSM, ABDOMINAL AORTIC

Overview

DESCRIPTION
■ Abnormal dilation in the arterial wall
■ Generally occurs in the aorta between the renal arteries and iliac branches
■ Can be fusiform (spindle-shaped), saccular (pouchlike), or dissecting (see *Types of aortic aneurysms,* page 172)

PATHOPHYSIOLOGY
■ Focal weakness in the tunica media layer of the aorta
■ Due to degenerative changes, which allows the tunica intima and tunica adventitia layers to stretch outward
■ Blood pressure within the aorta that progressively weakens vessel walls and enlarges aneurysm

CAUSES
■ Arteriosclerosis or atherosclerosis (95%)
■ Trauma
■ Syphilis; other infections

COMPLICATIONS
■ Hemorrhage
■ Shock
■ Dissection

Assessment

HISTORY
■ Asymptomatic until the aneurysm enlarges and compresses surrounding tissue
■ Syncope when aneurysm ruptures
■ When clot forms and bleeding stops, he may again be asymptomatic or have abdominal pain because of bleeding into the peritoneum

PHYSICAL FINDINGS
Intact aneurysm
■ Gnawing, generalized, steady abdominal pain
■ Lower back pain unaffected by movement
■ Gastric or abdominal fullness
■ Sudden onset of severe abdominal pain or lumbar pain with radiation to flank and groin

Ruptured aneurysm
■ Into the peritoneal cavity, severe, persistent abdominal and back pain
■ Into the duodenum, GI bleeding with massive hematemesis and melena
■ May note a pulsating mass in the periumbilical area: don't palpate
■ Mottled skin; poor distal perfusion
■ Decreased level of consciousness
■ Diaphoresis
■ Hypotension
■ Tachycardia
■ Oliguria
■ Distended abdomen
■ Ecchymosis or hematoma in the abdominal, flank, or groin area
■ Paraplegia if aneurysm rupture reduces blood flow to the spine
■ Systolic bruit over the aorta
■ Tenderness over affected area
■ Absent peripheral pulses distally

TEST RESULTS
Imaging
■ Abdominal ultrasonography or echocardiography can determine the size, shape, and location of the aneurysm.

TYPES OF AORTIC ANEURYSMS

Saccular aneurysm	Fusiform aneurysm	Dissecting aneurysm	False aneurysm

| Unilateral pouch-like bulge with a narrow neck | A spindle-shaped bulge encompassing the entire diameter of the vessel | A hemorrhagic separation of the medial layers of the vessel wall, which create a false lumen | A pulsating hematoma resulting from trauma and commonly mistaken for an abdominal aneurysm |

■ Anteroposterior and lateral abdominal X-rays can detect aortic calcification, which outlines the mass, at least 75% of the time.
■ Computed tomography scan can visualize aneurysm's effect on nearby organs.
■ Aortography shows condition of vessels proximal and distal to the aneurysm and extent of aneurysm; aneurysm diameter may be underestimated because it shows only the flow channel and not the surrounding clot.

Treatment

GENERAL
■ If the aneurysm is small and asymptomatic, surgery may be delayed
■ Careful control of hypertension
■ Fluid and blood replacement

DIET
■ Weight reduction, if appropriate
■ Low-fat

ACTIVITY
■ No restrictions unless surgery

MEDICATION
■ Beta-adrenergic blockers
■ Antihypertensives
■ Analgesics
■ Antibiotics

SURGERY
■ Resection of large aneurysms or those that produce symptoms
■ Bypass procedures for poor perfusion distal to aneurysm

MONITORING
■ Cardiac rhythm and hemodynamics

■ Vital signs, intake and hourly output, neurologic status, and arterial blood gas levels
■ Respirations and breath sounds at least every hour
■ Daily weight
■ Fluid status
■ Nasogastric intubation for patency, amount, and type of drainage
■ Monitor for signs and symptoms of renal failure
■ Abdominal dressings
■ Wound site for infection

ANEURYSM, THORACIC AORTIC

Overview

DESCRIPTION
■ Abnormal widening of the ascending, transverse, or descending part of the aorta
■ May be saccular (outpouching), fusiform (spindle-shaped), or dissecting

PATHOPHYSIOLOGY
■ Circumferential or transverse tear of the aortic wall intima, usually within the medial layer
■ Occurs in about 60% of patients, is usually an emergency, and has a poor prognosis

CAUSES
■ Atherosclerosis
■ Blunt chest trauma
■ Bacterial infections, usually at an atherosclerotic plaque
■ Coarctation of the aorta
■ Syphilis infection
■ Rheumatic vasculitis

RISK FACTORS
■ Cigarette smoking
■ Hypertension

COMPLICATIONS
■ Cardiac tamponade
■ Dissection

Assessment

HISTORY
■ Without signs and symptoms until aneurysm expands and begins to dissect
■ Sudden pain and possibly syncope

PHYSICAL FINDINGS
■ Pallor, diaphoresis, dyspnea, cyanosis, leg weakness, or transient paralysis
■ Abrupt onset of intermittent neurologic deficits
■ Abrupt loss of radial and femoral pulses and right and left carotid pulses
■ Increasing area of flatness over the heart, suggesting cardiac tamponade and hemopericardium

In dissecting ascending aneurysm
■ Pain with a boring, tearing, or ripping sensation in the thorax or the right anterior chest; may extend to the neck, shoulders, lower back, and abdomen
■ Pain most intense at onset
■ Murmur of aortic insufficiency, a diastolic murmur
■ Pericardial friction rub (if hemopericardium present)
■ Blood pressure may be normal or significantly elevated, with a large difference in systolic blood pressure between the right and left arms

In dissecting descending aneurysm
■ Sharp, tearing pain located between the shoulder blades that usually radiates to the chest

- Carotid and radial pulses present and equal bilaterally
- Systolic blood pressure is equal
- May detect bilateral crackles and rhonchi if pulmonary edema is present

In dissecting transverse aneurysm
- Sharp, boring, and tearing pain that radiates to the shoulders
- Hoarseness, dyspnea, throat pain, dysphagia, and a dry cough

TEST RESULTS
Laboratory
- Normal or decreased hemoglobin levels from blood loss caused by a leaking aneurysm

Imaging
- Posteroanterior and oblique chest X-rays show widening of the aorta and mediastinum.
- Aortography shows lumen of the aneurysm and its size and location.
- Magnetic resonance imaging and computed tomography scan help confirm and locate the presence of aortic dissection.

Diagnostic procedures
- Electrocardiography helps rule out the presence of myocardial infarction.
- Echocardiography may help identify dissecting aneurysm of the aortic root.
- Transesophageal echocardiography can be used to measure the aneurysm in the ascending and descending aorta.

Treatment

GENERAL
- I.V. fluids and whole blood transfusions, if needed

DIET
- Weight reduction, if appropriate
- Low-fat

ACTIVITY
- No restrictions unless surgery

MEDICATION
- Beta-adrenergic blockers
- Antihypertensives
- Negative inotropic agents
- Analgesics
- Antibiotics

SURGERY
- Surgical resection with a Dacron or Teflon graft replacement

MONITORING
- Vital signs and hemodynamics
- Chest tube drainage
- Heart and lung sounds
- Ordered laboratory tests
- Distal pulses
- Level of consciousness and pain
- Signs of infection
- I.V. therapy and intake and output

After surgical repair, monitor for signs that resemble those of the initial dissecting aneurysm, suggesting a tear at the graft site.

AORTIC INSUFFICIENCY

Overview

DESCRIPTION
- Blood flows back into the left ventricle, causing excess fluid volume
- Also called aortic regurgitation

PATHOPHYSIOLOGY
- Blood flows back into the left ventricle during diastole, causing increased left ventricular diastolic pressure

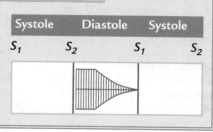

IDENTIFYING THE MURMUR OF AORTIC INSUFFICIENCY

A high-pitched, blowing decrescendo murmur that radiates from the aortic valve area to the left sternal border characterizes aortic insufficiency.

■ Results in volume overload, dilation and, eventually, hypertrophy of the left ventricle
■ Excess fluid volume also eventually results in increased left atrial pressure and increased pulmonary vascular pressure

CAUSES
■ Rheumatic fever
■ Primary disease of the aortic valve leaflets, the wall or the aortic root, or both
■ Hypertension
■ Infective endocarditis
■ Trauma
■ Idiopathic valve calcification
■ Aortic dissection
■ Aortic aneurysm
■ Connective tissue diseases

COMPLICATIONS
■ Left-sided heart failure
■ Pulmonary edema
■ Myocardial ischemia

Assessment

HISTORY
■ Exertional dyspnea, orthopnea, paroxysmal nocturnal dyspnea
■ Sensation of a forceful heartbeat, especially in supine position
■ Angina, especially nocturnal

■ Fatigue
■ Palpitations, head pounding
■ Symptoms of heart failure, in late stages

PHYSICAL FINDINGS
■ Corrigan's pulse
■ Bisferious pulse
■ Water-hammer pulse
■ Pulsating nail beds and Quincke's sign
■ Wide pulse pressure
■ Diffuse, hyperdynamic apical impulse, displaced laterally and inferiorly
■ Systolic thrill at base or suprasternal notch
■ S_3 gallop with increased left ventricular (LV) end-diastolic pressure
■ High frequency, blowing early-peaking, diastolic decrescendo murmur best heard with the patient sitting leaning forward and in deep fixed expiration (see *Identifying the murmur of aortic insufficiency*)
■ Austin Flint murmur
■ Head bobbing with each heartbeat
■ Tachycardia, peripheral vasoconstriction, and pulmonary edema if severe aortic insufficiency

TEST RESULTS
Imaging
■ Chest X-rays may show LV enlargement and pulmonary vein congestion.

■ Echocardiography may show LV enlargement, increased motion of the septum and posterior wall, thickening of valve cusps, prolapse of the valve, flail leaflet, vegetations, or dilation of the aortic root.

Diagnostic procedures
■ Electrocardiography shows sinus tachycardia, left axis deviation, LV hypertrophy, and left atrial hypertrophy in severe disease.
■ Cardiac catheterization shows presence and degree of aortic insufficiency, LV dilation and function, and coexisting coronary artery disease.

Treatment

GENERAL
■ Periodic noninvasive monitoring of aortic insufficiency and LV function with echocardiogram
■ Medical control of hypertension

DIET
■ Low-sodium

ACTIVITY
■ Planned periodic rest periods to avoid fatigue

MEDICATION
■ Cardiac glycosides
■ Diuretics
■ Vasodilators
■ Antihypertensives
■ Antiarrhythmics
■ Infective endocarditis prophylaxis
Avoid using beta-adrenergic blockers due to negative inotropic effects.

SURGERY
■ Valve replacement

MONITORING
■ Signs and symptoms of heart failure

■ Pulmonary edema
■ Adverse reactions to drug therapy
■ Complications

After surgery
■ Vital signs and cardiac rhythm
■ Heart tones
■ Chest tube drainage
■ Neurologic status
■ Arterial blood gas levels
■ Intake and output; daily weights
■ Blood chemistry studies, prothrombin time, and International Normalized Ratio values
■ Chest X-ray results
■ Pulmonary artery catheter pressures

AORTIC STENOSIS

Overview

DESCRIPTION
■ Narrowing of the aortic valve
■ Classified as either acquired or rheumatic

PATHOPHYSIOLOGY
■ Stenosis of the aortic valve results in impedance to forward blood flow.
■ The left ventricle requires greater pressure to open the aortic valve.
■ Added workload increases myocardial oxygen demands.
■ Diminished cardiac output reduces coronary artery blood flow.
■ Left ventricular (LV) hypertrophy and failure result.

CAUSES
■ Idiopathic fibrosis and calcification
■ Congenital aortic bicuspid valve
■ Rheumatic fever
■ Atherosclerosis

RISK FACTORS
■ Diabetes mellitus
■ Hypercholesterolemia

IDENTIFYING THE MURMUR OF AORTIC STENOSIS

A low-pitched, harsh crescendo-decrescendo murmur that radiates from the aortic valve area to the carotid artery characterizes aortic stenosis.

Systole	Diastole	Systole	
S_1	S_2	S_1	S_2

COMPLICATIONS
- Left-sided heart failure
- Right-sided heart failure
- Infective endocarditis
- Cardiac arrhythmias, especially atrial fibrillation
- Sudden death

Assessment

HISTORY
- May be asymptomatic
- Dyspnea on exertion
- Angina
- Exertional syncope
- Fatigue
- Palpitations
- Paroxysmal nocturnal dyspnea

PHYSICAL FINDINGS
- Small, sustained arterial pulses that rise slowly
- Distinct lag between carotid artery pulse and apical pulse
- Orthopnea
- Prominent jugular vein *a* waves
- Peripheral edema
- Diminished carotid pulses with delayed upstroke
- Apex of the heart may be displaced inferiorly and laterally
- Suprasternal thrill

An early systolic ejection murmur may be present in children and adolescents who have noncalcified valves. The murmur is low-pitched, rough, and rasping and is loudest at the base in the second intercostal space.
- Split S_2 develops as stenosis becomes more severe
- Prominent S_4
- Harsh, rasping, mid-to late-peaking systolic murmur that's best heard at the base and commonly radiates to carotids and apex (see *Identifying the murmur of aortic stenosis*)

TEST RESULTS
Imaging
- Chest X-ray shows valvular calcification, LV enlargement, pulmonary vein congestion and, in later stages, left atrial, pulmonary artery, right atrial, and right ventricular enlargement.
- Echocardiography shows decreased valve area, increased gradient, and increased LV wall thickness.

Diagnostic procedures
- Cardiac catheterization shows increased pressure gradient across the aortic valve, increased LV pressures, and presence of coronary artery disease.

Other
- Electrocardiography may show LV hypertrophy, atrial fibrillation, or other arrhythmia.

Treatment

GENERAL
- Periodic noninvasive evaluation of the severity of valve narrowing
- Lifelong treatment and management of congenital aortic stenosis

DIET
- Low-sodium
- Low-fat, low-cholesterol

ACTIVITY
- Planned rest periods

MEDICATION
- Cardiac glycosides
- Antibiotic infective endocarditis prophylaxis

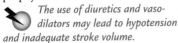

The use of diuretics and vasodilators may lead to hypotension and inadequate stroke volume.

SURGERY
- In adults, valve replacement after they become symptomatic with hemodynamic evidence of severe obstruction
- Percutaneous balloon aortic valvuloplasty
- In children without calcified valves, simple commissurotomy under direct visualization
- Ross procedure may be performed in patients younger than age 5

MONITORING
- Vital signs
- Intake and output
- Signs and symptoms of heart failure
- Signs and symptoms of progressive aortic stenosis
- Daily weight
- Arrhythmias
- Respiratory status

If the patient has surgery
- Signs and symptoms of thrombus formation
- Hemodynamics
- Arterial blood gas results
- Blood chemistry results
- Chest X-ray results

ARTERIAL OCCLUSIVE DISEASE

Overview

DESCRIPTION
- An obstruction or narrowing of the lumen of the aorta and its major branches
- May affect arteries including the carotid, vertebral, innominate, subclavian, femoral, iliac, renal, mesenteric, and celiac arteries (see *Types of arterial occlusive disease*)
- Prognosis depends on location of the occlusion and the development of collateral circulation that counteracts reduced blood flow

PATHOPHYSIOLOGY
- Narrowing leads to interrupted blood flow, usually to the legs and feet
- During times of increased activity or exercise, blood flow to surrounding muscles is unable to meet the metabolic demand
- Results in pain in affected areas

CAUSES
- Atherosclerosis
- Immune arteritis
- Embolism
- Thrombosis
- Thromboangiitis obliterans
- Raynaud's disease
- Fibromuscular disease
- Atheromatous debris (plaques)
- Indwelling arterial catheter
- Direct blunt or penetrating trauma

TYPES OF ARTERIAL OCCLUSIVE DISEASE

Site of occlusion	Signs and symptoms
Carotid arterial system ■ Internal carotids ■ External carotids	Neurologic dysfunction; transient ischemic attacks (TIAs) due to reduced cerebral circulation produce unilateral sensory or motor dysfunction (transient monocular blindness, hemiparesis), possible aphasia or dysarthria, confusion, decreased mentation, and headache. These recurrent clinical features usually last 5 to 10 minutes, but may persist up to 24 hours and may herald a stroke. Absent or decreased pulsation with an auscultatory bruit over the affected vessels.
Vertebrobasilar system ■ Vertebral arteries ■ Basilar arteries	Neurologic dysfunction: TIAs of brain stem and cerebellum produce binocular visual disturbances, vertigo, dysarthria, and "drop attacks" (falling down without loss of consciousness). Less common than carotid TIAs.
Innominate ■ Brachiocephalic artery	Neurologic dysfunction: signs and symptoms of vertebrobasilar occlusion. Indications of ischemia (claudication) of right arm; possible bruit over right side of neck.
Subclavian artery	Subclavian steal syndrome (characterized by blood backflow from the brain through the vertebral artery on the same side as the occlusion, into the subclavian artery distal to the occlusion); clinical effects of vertebrobasilar occlusion and exercise-induced arm claudication. Possible gangrene, usually limited to the digits.
Mesenteric artery ■ Superior (most commonly affected) ■ Celiac axis ■ Inferior	Bowel ischemia, infarct necrosis, and gangrene; sudden, acute abdominal pain; nausea and vomiting; diarrhea; leukocytosis; and shock due to massive intraluminal fluid and plasma loss.
Aortic bifurcation (saddle block occlusion, a medical emergency associated with cardiac embolization)	Sensory and motor deficits (muscle weakness, numbness, paresthesia, paralysis) and signs of ischemia (sudden pain; cold, pale legs with decreased or absent peripheral pulses) in both legs.
Iliac artery (Leriche's syndrome)	Intermittent claudication of lower back, buttocks, and thighs, relieved by rest; absent or reduced femoral or distal pulses; possible bruit over femoral arteries; impotence in males.
Femoral and popliteal artery (associated with aneurysm formation)	Intermittent claudication of the calves on exertion; ischemic pain in feet; pretrophic pain (heralds necrosis and ulceration); leg pallor and coolness; blanching of feet on elevation; gangrene; no palpable pulses in ankles and feet.

RISK FACTORS
- Smoking
- Hypertension
- Dyslipidemia
- Diabetes mellitus
- Advanced age

COMPLICATIONS
- Severe ischemia
- Skin ulceration
- Gangrene
- Limb loss

Assessment

HISTORY
- One or more risk factors
- Family history of vascular disease
- Intermittent claudication
- Rest pain
- Poor-healing wounds or ulcers
- Impotence
- Dizziness or near syncope
- Transient ischemic attack symptoms

PHYSICAL FINDINGS
- Trophic changes of involved limb
- Diminished or absent limb pulses
- Presence of ischemic ulcers
- Pallor with elevation of extremity
- Pallor, dependent rubor
- Arterial bruit
- Hypertension
- Pain
- Pulselessness distal to the occlusion
- Paralysis and paresthesia occurring in the affected extremity
- Poikilothermy

TEST RESULTS
Imaging
- Arteriography shows type, location, and degree of obstruction, and the establishment of collateral circulation.
- Ultrasonography and plethysmography show decreased blood flow distal to the occlusion.
- Doppler ultrasonography shows a relatively low-pitched sound and a monophasic waveform.
- Electroencephalography and computed tomography scan may show the presence of brain lesions.

Other
- Segmental limb pressures and pulse volume measurements show the location and extent of the occlusion.
- Ophthalmodynamometry shows the degree of obstruction in the internal carotid artery.
- Electrocardiogram may show presence of cardiovascular disease.

Treatment

GENERAL
- Elimination of smoking
- Hypertension, diabetes, and dyslipidemia control
- Foot and leg care
- Weight control

DIET
- Low-fat

ACTIVITY
- Regular walking program

MEDICATION
- Antiplatelets
- Lipid-lowering agents
- Hypoglycemic agents
- Antihypertensives
- Thrombolytics
- Anticoagulation

SURGERY
- Embolectomy
- Endarterectomy
- Atherectomy
- Laser angioplasty
- Endovascular stent placement
- Percutaneous transluminal angioplasty

NORMAL SINUS RHYTHM

Normal sinus rhythm, shown below, represents normal impulse conduction through the heart.

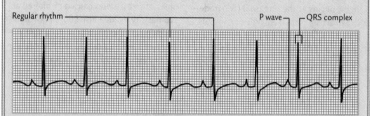

Regular rhythm — P wave — QRS complex

Lead II
Atrial rhythm: regular
Ventricular rhythm: regular
Atrial rate: 60 to 100 beats/minute (80 beats/minute shown)
Ventricular rate: 60 to 100 beats/minute (80 beats/minute shown)
P wave: normally shaped (All P waves have a similar size and shape; a P wave precedes each QRS complex.)
PR interval: within normal limits (0.12 to 0.20 second) and constant (0.20-second duration shown)

QRS complex: within normal limits (0.06 to 0.10 second) (All QRS complexes have the same configuration. The duration shown here is 0.12 second.)
T wave: normally shaped; upright and rounded (Each QRS complex is followed by a T wave.)
QT interval: within normal limits (0.36 to 0.44 second) and constant (0.44-second duration shown)

- Laser surgery
- Patch grafting
- Bypass graft
- Lumbar sympathectomy
- Amputation
- Bowel resection

MONITORING
- Signs and symptoms of fluid and electrolyte imbalance and renal failure
- Signs and symptoms of stroke
- Vital signs
- Intake and output
- Distal pulses
- Neurologic status
- Bowel sounds

CARDIAC ARRHYTHMIAS

To recognize an arrhythmia, you first must recognize normal sinus rhythm. (See *Normal sinus rhythm*.) Normal sinus rhythm records an impulse that starts in the sinus node and progresses to the ventricles through the normal conduction pathway. (See *Comparing normal and abnormal conduction,* pages 182 and 183.) Alterations in this pathway may lead to cardiac arrhythmias. (See *Types of cardiac arrhythmias,* pages 182 to 191.) Prompt identifica-
(Text continues on page 190.)

COMPARING NORMAL AND ABNORMAL CONDUCTION

Normal cardiac conduction

The heart's conduction system, shown at right, begins at the sinoatrial (SA) node — the heart's pacemaker. When an impulse leaves the SA node, it travels through the atria along Bachmann's bundle and the internodal pathways to the atrioventricular (AV) node, and then down the bundle of His, along the bundle branches and, finally, down the Purkinje fibers to the ventricles.

Abnormal cardiac conduction

Altered automaticity, reentry, or conduction disturbances may cause cardiac arrhythmias.

Altered automaticity

Altered automaticity is the result of partial depolarization, which may increase the intrinsic rate of the SA node or lateral pacemakers, or may induce ectopic pacemakers to reach threshold and depolarize.

Automaticity may be altered by drugs, such as epinephrine, atropine, and digoxin, and such conditions as acidosis, alkalosis, hypoxia, myocardial infarction (MI), hypokalemia, and hypocalcemia. Examples of arrhythmias caused by altered automaticity include atrial fibrillation and flutter; supraventricular tachycardia; premature atrial, junctional, and ventricular complexes; ventricular tachycardia and fibrillation; and accelerated idioventricular and junctional rhythms.

Reentry

Ischemia or a deformity causes an abnormal circuit to develop within conductive fibers. Although current flow is blocked in one direction within the circuit, the descending impulse can travel in the other direction. By the time the impulse completes the circuit, the previously depolarized tissue within the circuit is no longer refractory to stimulation, allowing reentry of the impulse and repetition of this cycle.

Conditions that increase the likelihood of reentry include hyperkalemia, myocardial ischemia, and the use of certain antiarrhythmic drugs. Reentry may be responsible for such arrhythmias as parox-

TYPES OF CARDIAC ARRHYTHMIAS

This chart reviews many common cardiac arrhythmias and outlines their features, causes, and treatments.

Arrhythmia and features

Sinus tachycardia

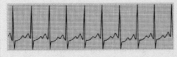

- Atrial and ventricular rhythms regular
- Rate > 100 beats/minute; rarely, > 160 beats/minute
- Normal P wave preceding each QRS complex

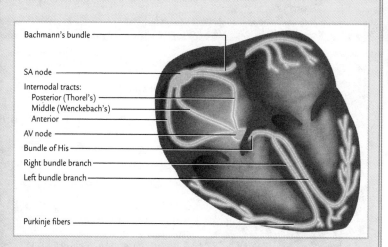

ysmal supraventricular tachycardia; premature atrial, junctional, and ventricular complexes; and ventricular tachycardia.

An alternative reentry mechanism depends on the presence of a congenital accessory pathway linking the atria and the ventricles outside the AV junction; for example, Wolff-Parkinson-White syndrome.

Conduction disturbances

Conduction disturbances occur when impulses are conducted too quickly or too slowly. Possible causes include trauma, drug toxicity, myocardial ischemia, MI, and electrolyte abnormalities. The AV blocks occur as a result of conduction disturbances.

Causes

■ Normal physiologic response to fever, exercise, anxiety, pain, dehydration; may also accompany shock, left ventricular failure, cardiac tamponade, hyperthyroidism, anemia, hypovolemia, pulmonary embolism, and anterior wall myocardial infarction (MI)
■ May also occur with atropine, epinephrine, isoproterenol, quinidine, caffeine, alcohol, cocaine, amphetamine, and nicotine use

Treatment

■ Correction of underlying cause
■ Beta-adrenergic blockers or calcium channel blockers

(continued)

CARDIOVASCULAR
CARE

Arrhythmia and features

Sinus bradycardia

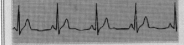

- Atrial and ventricular rhythms regular
- Rate < 60 beats/minute
- Normal P waves preceding each QRS complex

Paroxysmal supraventricular tachycardia

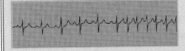

- Atrial and ventricular rhythms regular
- Heart rate > 160 beats/minute; rarely exceeds 250 beats/minute
- P waves regular but aberrant; difficult to differentiate from preceding T wave
- P wave preceding each QRS complex
- Sudden onset and termination of arrhythmia

Atrial flutter

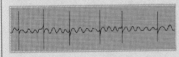

- Atrial rhythm regular; rate 250 to 400 beats/minute
- Ventricular rate variable, depending on degree of AV block (usually 60 to 100 beats/minute)
- No P waves, atrial activity appears as flutter waves (F waves); sawtooth configuration common in lead II
- QRS complexes uniform in shape, but usually irregular in rate

Causes	Treatment

- Normal, in well-conditioned heart, as in an athlete
- Increased intracranial pressure; increased vagal tone due to straining during defecation, vomiting, intubation, or mechanical ventilation; sick sinus syndrome; hypothyroidism; and inferior wall MI
- May also occur with anticholinesterase, beta-adrenergic blocker, digoxin, and morphine use

- Correction of underlying cause
- For low cardiac output, dizziness, weakness, altered level of consciousness, or low blood pressure; advanced cardiac life support (ACLS) protocol for administration of atropine
- Temporary or permanent pacemaker
- Dopamine or epinephrine infusion

- Intrinsic abnormality of atrioventricular (AV) conduction system
- Physical or psychological stress, hypoxia, hypokalemia, cardiomyopathy, congenital heart disease, MI, valvular disease, Wolff-Parkinson-White syndrome, cor pulmonale, hyperthyroidism, and systemic hypertension
- Digoxin toxicity; use of caffeine, marijuana, or central nervous system stimulants

- If patient is unstable, immediate cardioversion
- If patient is stable, vagal stimulation: Valsalva's maneuver, carotid sinus massage, and adenosine
- If cardiac function is preserved, treatment priority; calcium channel blocker, beta-adrenergic blocker, digoxin, and cardioversion; then consider procainamide or amiodarone, if each preceding treatment is ineffective in rhythm conversion
- If the ejection fraction is less than 40% or if the patient is in heart failure, treatment order: digoxin, amiodarone, then diltiazem

---

- Heart failure, tricuspid or mitral valve disease, pulmonary embolism, cor pulmonale, inferior wall MI, and pericarditis
- Digoxin toxicity

- If patient is unstable with a ventricular rate > 150 beats/minute, immediate cardioversion
- If patient is stable, follow ACLS protocol for cardioversion and drug therapy, which may include calcium channel blockers, beta-adrenergic blockers, amiodarone, or digoxin
- Anticoagulation therapy may also be necessary
- Radio-frequency ablation to control rhythm

(continued)

TYPES OF CARDIAC ARRHYTHMIAS *(continued)*

Arrhythmia and features

Atrial fibrillation

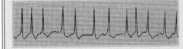

- Atrial rhythm grossly irregular; rate > 400 beats/minute
- Ventricular rhythm grossly irregular
- QRS complexes of uniform configuration and duration
- PR interval indiscernible
- No P waves, atrial activity appears as erratic, irregular, baseline fibrillatory waves (f waves)

Junctional rhythm

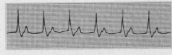

- Atrial and ventricular rhythms regular; atrial rate 40 to 60 beats/minute; ventricular rate usually 40 to 60 beats/minute (60 to 100 beats/minute is accelerated junctional rhythm)
- P waves preceding, hidden within (absent), or after QRS complex; usually inverted if visible
- PR interval (when present) < 0.12 second
- QRS complex configuration and duration normal, except in aberrant conduction

First-degree AV block

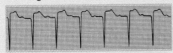

- Atrial and ventricular rhythms regular
- PR interval > 0.20 second
- P wave precedes QRS complex
- QRS complex normal

Second-degree AV block
Mobitz I (Wenckebach)

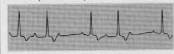

- Atrial rhythm regular
- Ventricular rhythm irregular
- Atrial rate exceeds ventricular rate
- PR interval progressively longer with each cycle until QRS complex disappears (dropped beat); PR interval shorter after dropped beat

Causes	Treatment
■ Heart failure, chronic obstructive pulmonary disease, thyrotoxicosis, constrictive pericarditis, ischemic heart disease, sepsis, pulmonary embolus, rheumatic heart disease, hypertension, mitral stenosis, atrial irritation, or complication of coronary bypass or valve replacement surgery ■ Nifedipine and digoxin use	■ If patient is unstable with a ventricular rate > 150 beats/minute, immediate cardioversion ■ If patient is stable, follow ACLS protocol and drug therapy, which may include calcium channel blockers, beta-adrenergic blockers, amiodarone, or digoxin ■ Anticoagulation therapy may also be necessary ■ In a patient with refractory atrial fibrillation uncontrolled by drugs, radio-frequency catheter ablation
■ Inferior wall MI or ischemia, hypoxia, vagal stimulation, and sick sinus syndrome ■ Acute rheumatic fever ■ Valve surgery ■ Digoxin toxicity	■ Correction of underlying cause ■ Atropine for symptomatic slow rate ■ Pacemaker insertion if patient doesn't respond to drugs ■ Discontinuation of digoxin if appropriate
■ May be seen in healthy persons ■ Inferior wall MI or ischemia, hypothyroidism, hypokalemia, and hyperkalemia ■ Digoxin toxicity; use of quinidine, procainamide, beta-adrenergic blockers, calcium channel blockers, or amiodarone	■ Correction of underlying cause ■ Possibly atropine if severe symptomatic bradycardia develops ■ Cautious use of digoxin, calcium channel blockers, and beta-adrenergic blockers
■ Inferior wall MI, cardiac surgery, acute rheumatic fever, and vagal stimulation ■ Digoxin toxicity; use of propranolol, quinidine, or procainamide	■ Treatment of underlying cause ■ Atropine or temporary pacemaker for symptomatic bradycardia ■ Discontinuation of digoxin if appropriate

(continued)

TYPES OF CARDIAC ARRHYTHMIAS *(continued)*

Arrhythmia and features

Mobitz II

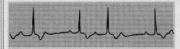

- Atrial rhythm regular
- Ventricular rhythm regular or irregular, with varying degree of block
- P-R interval constant for conducted beats
- P waves normal size and configuration, but some P waves aren't followed by a QRS complex

Third-degree AV block
(complete heart block)

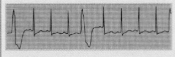

- Atrial rhythm regular
- Ventricular rhythm regular and rate slower than atrial rate
- No relation between P waves and QRS complexes
- No constant PR interval
- QRS duration normal (junctional pacemaker) or wide and bizarre (ventricular pacemaker)

Premature ventricular contraction (PVC)

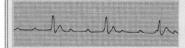

- Atrial rhythm regular
- Ventricular rhythm irregular
- QRS complex premature, usually followed by a complete compensatory pause
- QRS complex wide and distorted, usually > 0.12 second
- Premature QRS complexes occurring alone, in pairs, or in threes, alternating with normal beats; focus from one or more sites
- Ominous when clustered, multifocal, with R wave on T pattern

Causes	Treatment
■ Severe coronary artery disease, anterior wall MI, and acute myocarditis ■ Digoxin toxicity	■ Temporary or permanent pacemaker ■ Atropine, dopamine, or epinephrine for symptomatic bradycardia ■ Discontinuation of digoxin, if appropriate
■ Inferior or anterior wall MI, congenital abnormality, rheumatic fever, hypoxia, postoperative complication of mitral valve replacement, postprocedure complication of radiofrequency ablation in or near AV nodal tissue, Lev's disease (fibrosis and calcification that spreads from cardiac structures to the conductive tissue), and Lenègre's disease (conductive tissue fibrosis) ■ Digoxin toxicity	■ Temporary or permanent pacemaker ■ Atropine, dopamine, or epinephrine for symptomatic bradycardia
■ Heart failure; old or acute MI, ischemia, or contusion; myocardial irritation by ventricular catheter or a pacemaker; hypercapnia; hypokalemia; hypocalcemia and hypomagnesemia ■ Drug toxicity (digoxin, aminophylline, tricyclic antidepressants, beta-adrenergic blockers, isoproterenol, or dopamine) ■ Caffeine, tobacco, or alcohol use ■ Psychological stress, anxiety, pain, or exercise	■ If warranted, procainamide, amiodarone, or lidocaine I.V. ■ Treatment of underlying cause ■ Discontinuation of drug causing toxicity ■ Potassium chloride I.V. if PVC induced by hypokalemia ■ Magnesium sulfate I.V. if PVC induced by hypomagnesemia

(continued)

TYPES OF CARDIAC ARRHYTHMIAS *(continued)*

Arrhythmia and features

Ventricular tachycardia

- Ventricular rate 100 to 220 beats/minute, rhythm usually regular
- QRS complexes wide, bizarre, and independent of P waves
- P waves not discernible
- May start and stop suddenly

Ventricular fibrillation

- Ventricular rhythm and rate chaotic and rapid
- QRS complexes wide and irregular; no visible P waves

Asystole

- No atrial or ventricular rate or rhythm
- No discernible P waves, QRS complexes, or T waves

tion and treatment of arrhythmias is especially important with ventricular fibrillation and pulseless ventricular tachycardia. (See *Ventricular fibrillation and pulseless ventricular tachycardia algorithm,* page 192.)

Causes	Treatment
■ Myocardial ischemia, MI, or aneurysm; coronary artery disease; rheumatic heart disease; mitral valve prolapse; heart failure; cardiomyopathy; ventricular catheters; hypokalemia; hypercalcemia; hypomagnesemia; and pulmonary embolism ■ Digoxin, procainamide, epinephrine, or quinidine toxicity ■ Anxiety	■ With pulse: If hemodynamically stable with monomorphic QRS complexes, administration of procainamide, sotalol, amiodarone, or lidocaine (follow ACLS protocol); if drug is unsuccessful, cardioversion ■ If polymorphic QRS complexes and normal QT interval, administer beta-adrenergic blockers, lidocaine, amiodarone, procainamide, or sotalol (follow ACLS protocol); if drug is unsuccessful, cardioversion ■ If polymorphic QRS and QT interval is prolonged, magnesium I.V., then overdrive pacing if rhythm persists; may also administer isoproterenol, phenytoin, or lidocaine ■ Pulseless: Initiate CPR; follow ACLS protocol for defibrillation, endotracheal (ET) intubation, and administration of epinephrine or vasopressin, followed by amiodarone or lidocaine and, if ineffective, magnesium sulfate or procainamide ■ Implanted cardioverter-defibrillator if recurrent ventricular tachycardia
■ Myocardial ischemia, MI, untreated ventricular tachycardia, R-on-T phenomenon, hypokalemia, hyperkalemia, hypercalcemia, hypoxemia, alkalosis, electric shock, and hypothermia ■ Digoxin, epinephrine, or quinidine toxicity	■ CPR; follow ACLS protocol for defibrillation, ET intubation, and administration of epinephrine or vasopressin, amiodarone, or lidocaine and, if ineffective, magnesium sulfate or procainamide ■ Implanted cardioverter-defibrillator if at risk for recurrent ventricular fibrillation
■ Myocardial ischemia, MI, aortic valve disease, heart failure, hypoxia, hypokalemia, severe acidosis, electric shock, ventricular arrhythmia, AV block, pulmonary embolism, heart rupture, cardiac tamponade, hyperkalemia, and electromechanical dissociation ■ Cocaine overdose	■ Continue CPR; follow ACLS protocol for ET intubation, transcutaneous pacing, and administration of epinephrine and atropine

VENTRICULAR FIBRILLATION AND PULSELESS VENTRICULAR TACHYCARDIA ALGORITHM

Ventricular fibrillation (VF) and pulseless ventricular tachycardia (VT) require aggressive, systematic treatment. Follow the algorithm below for patients with these arrhythmias.

Primary ABCD survey

Focus: Basic cardiopulmonary resuscitation and defibrillation.

- Check responsiveness.
- Activate emergency response system.
- Call for defibrillator.
- **A** Airway: Open the airway.
- **B** Breathing: Provide positive-pressure ventilations.
- **C** Circulation: Give chest compressions.
- **D** Defibrillation: Assess for VF or pulseless VT and defibrillate up to three times (200 joules, 200 to 300 joules, 360 joules, or equivalent biphasic), if necessary.

Rhythm after first three cardioversions?

↓

Persistent or recurrent VF or VT

Secondary ABCD survey

Focus: More advanced assessments and treatments

- **A** Airway: Insert airway device as soon as possible.
- **B** Breathing: Confirm airway device placement by examination plus confirmation device.
- **B** Breathing: Secure airway device; purpose-made tube holders preferred.
- **B** Breathing: Confirm effective oxygenation and ventilation.
- **C** Circulation: Establish I.V. access.
- **C** Circulation: Identify rhythm and monitor.
- **C** Circulation: Administer drugs appropriate for rhythm and condition.
- **D** Differential diagnosis: Search for and treat identified reversible causes.

- Epinephrine I.V. push; repeat every 3 to 5 minutes
  or
- Vasopressin I.V.; single dose, one time only

Resume attempts to defibrillate.

1 × 360 joules (or equivalent biphasic) within 30 to 60 seconds

↓

Consider antiarrhythmics.

- Amiodarone (class IIb intervention)
- Lidocaine (indeterminate)
- Magnesium (IIb if hypomagnesemic state)
- Procainamide (IIb for intermittent or recurrent VF or VT)
- Consider buffers.

↓

Resume attempts to defibrillate.

CARDIAC TAMPONADE

Overview

DESCRIPTION
- Rapid increase in intrapericardial pressure
- Impaired diastolic filling of the heart

PATHOPHYSIOLOGY
- Progressive accumulation of fluid in the pericardial sac causes compression of the heart chambers.
- Compression of the heart chambers obstructs blood flow into the ventricles and reduces the amount of blood pumped out with each contraction.
- With each contraction more fluid accumulates, decreasing cardiac output.

CAUSES
- May be idiopathic
- Effusion in cancer, bacterial infections, tuberculosis and, rarely, acute rheumatic fever
- Trauma
- Hemorrhage from nontraumatic cause
- Viral, postirradiation, or idiopathic pericarditis
- Acute myocardial infarction
- Chronic renal failure
- Drug reaction
- Connective tissue disorders
- Cardiac catheterization
- Cardiac surgery

COMPLICATIONS
- Cardiogenic shock
- Death

Assessment

HISTORY
- Presence of one or more causes

- Dyspnea
- Shortness of breath
- Chest pain

PHYSICAL FINDINGS
- Vary with volume of fluid and speed of fluid accumulation
- Diaphoresis
- Anxiety and restlessness
- Pallor or cyanosis
- Jugular vein distention
- Edema
- Rapid, weak pulses
- Hepatomegaly
- Decreased arterial blood pressure
- Increased central venous pressure
- Pulsus paradoxus
- Narrow pulse pressure
- Muffled heart sounds

TEST RESULTS
Imaging
- Chest X-rays show slightly widened mediastinum and enlargement of the cardiac silhouette.

Diagnostic procedures
- Electrocardiography may show low voltage complexes in the precordial leads.
- Hemodynamic monitoring shows equalization of mean right atrial, right ventricular diastolic, pulmonary capillary wedge pressure, and left ventricular diastolic pressures.
- Echocardiography may show an echo-free space, indicating fluid accumulation in the pericardial sac.

Treatment

GENERAL
- Pericardiocentesis may be necessary

DIET
- As tolerated

ACTIVITY
- Bed rest

MEDICATION
- Intravascular volume expansion
- Inotropic agents
- Oxygen

SURGERY
- Pericardiocentesis
- Pericardial window
- Subxiphoid pericardiotomy
- Complete pericardectomy
- Thoracotomy

MONITORING
- Vital signs
- Intake and output
- Signs and symptoms of increasing tamponade
- Arrhythmias
- Hemodynamics
- Arterial blood gas levels
- Heart and breath sounds
- Complications

CARDIOMYOPATHY, DILATED

Overview

DESCRIPTION
- Disease of the heart muscle fibers
- Also called congestive cardiomyopathy

PATHOPHYSIOLOGY
- Extensively damaged myocardial muscle fibers reduce contractility of left ventricle.
- As systolic function declines, cardiac output falls.
- The sympathetic nervous system is stimulated to increase heart rate and contractility.
- When compensatory mechanisms can no longer maintain cardiac output, the heart begins to fail.

CAUSES
- Viral or bacterial infections
- Hypertension
- Peripartum syndrome related to toxemia
- Ischemic heart disease
- Valvular disease
- Drug hypersensitivity
- Chemotherapy
- Cardiotoxic effects of drugs or alcohol

COMPLICATIONS
- Intractable heart failure
- Arrhythmias
- Emboli

Assessment

HISTORY
- Possible history of a disorder that can cause cardiomyopathy
- Gradual onset of shortness of breath, orthopnea, dyspnea on exertion, paroxysmal nocturnal dyspnea, fatigue, dry cough at night, palpitations, and vague chest pain

PHYSICAL FINDINGS
- Peripheral edema
- Jugular vein distention
- Ascites
- Peripheral cyanosis
- Tachycardia even at rest and pulsus alternans in late stages
- Hepatomegaly and splenomegaly
- Narrow pulse pressure
- Irregular rhythms, diffuse apical impulses, pansystolic murmur
- S_3 and S_4 gallop rhythms
- Pulmonary crackles
- Dilated cardiomyopathy may need to be differentiated from other types of cardiomyopathy

TEST RESULTS
Imaging
- Angiography results are used to rule out ischemic heart disease.
- Chest X-rays demonstrate moderate to marked cardiomegaly and possible pulmonary edema.
- Echocardiography may reveal ventricular thrombi, global hypokinesis, and the degrees of left ventricular dilation and dysfunction.
- Gallium scans may be used to identify patients with dilated cardiomyopathy and myocarditis.

Diagnostic procedures
- Cardiac catheterization can show left ventricular dilation and dysfunction, elevated left ventricular and, commonly, right ventricular filling pressures, and diminished cardiac output.
- Transvenous endomyocardial biopsy may be useful in some patients to determine the underlying disorder.
- Electrocardiography is used to rule out ischemic heart disease.

Treatment

GENERAL
- With cardiomyopathy caused by alcoholism, ingestion of alcohol must be stopped.

 A woman of childbearing age with dilated cardiomyopathy should avoid pregnancy.

DIET
- Low-sodium diet supplemented by vitamin therapy

ACTIVITY
- Rest

MEDICATION
- Cardiac glycosides
- Diuretics
- Angiotensin-converting enzyme inhibitors
- Oxygen
- Anticoagulants
- Vasodilators
- Antiarrhythmics
- Beta-adrenergic blockers

SURGERY
- Heart transplantation
- Possible cardiomyoplasty

MONITORING
- Vital signs
- Hemodynamics
- Intake and output
- Daily weights
- Signs and symptoms of progressive heart failure

CARDIOMYOPATHY, HYPERTROPHIC

Overview

DESCRIPTION
- Primary disease of cardiac muscle
- Also known as idiopathic hypertrophic subaortic stenosis, hypertrophic obstructive cardiomyopathy, and muscular aortic stenosis

PATHOPHYSIOLOGY
- The hypertrophied ventricle becomes stiff, noncompliant, and unable to relax during ventricular filling.
- Ventricular filling time is reduced as compensation to tachycardia.
- Reduced ventricular filling leads to low cardiac output.

CAUSES
- Transmission by autosomal dominant trait (about 50% of all cases)
- Associated with hypertension

COMPLICATIONS
- Pulmonary hypertension
- Heart failure
- Ventricular arrhythmias

Assessment

HISTORY
- Generally, no visible clinical features until disease is well advanced
- Atrial dilation and, sometimes, atrial fibrillation abruptly reduce blood flow to left ventricle
- Possible family history of hypertrophic cardiomyopathy
- Orthopnea and dyspnea on exertion
- Anginal pain
- Fatigue
- Syncope, even at rest

PHYSICAL FINDINGS
- Rapidly rising carotid arterial pulse possible
- Pulsus biferiens
- Double or triple apical impulse, possibly displaced laterally
- Bibasilar crackles if heart failure is present
- Harsh systolic murmur heard after S_1 at the apex near the left sternal border
- S_4 also possibly audible

TEST RESULTS
Imaging
- Chest X-rays may show a mild to moderate increase in heart size.
- Thallium scan usually reveals myocardial perfusion defects.

Diagnostic procedures
- Echocardiography shows left ventricular hypertrophy and a thick, asymmetrical intraventricular septum in obstructive hypertrophic cardiomyopathy, whereas hypertrophy affects various ventricular areas in nonobstructive hypertrophic cardiomyopathy.

- Cardiac catheterization reveals elevated left ventricular end-diastolic pressure and, possibly, mitral insufficiency.
- Electrocardiography usually shows left ventricular hypertrophy, ST-segment and T-wave abnormalities, Q waves in leads II, III, aV_F, and V_4 to V_6 (due to hypertrophy, not infarction), left anterior hemiblock, left axis deviation, and ventricular and atrial arrhythmias.

Treatment

GENERAL
- Cardioversion for atrial fibrillation

DIET
- Low-fat, low-salt
- Fluid restriction
- Avoidance of alcohol

ACTIVITY
- Limitations vary
- Bed rest may be necessary

MEDICATION
- Beta-adrenergic blockers
- Calcium channel blockers
- Amiodarone may be used, unless atrioventricular block exists
- Antibiotic prophylaxis

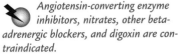 *Angiotensin-converting enzyme inhibitors, nitrates, other beta-adrenergic blockers, and digoxin are contraindicated.*

SURGERY
- Ventricular myotomy alone or combined with mitral valve replacement
- Heart transplantation

MONITORING
- Vital signs
- Hemodynamics
- Intake and output

CORONARY ARTERY DISEASE

Overview

DESCRIPTION
- Results from narrowing of coronary arteries over time due to atherosclerosis
- Primary effect: loss of oxygen and nutrients to myocardial tissue because of diminished coronary blood flow

PATHOPHYSIOLOGY
- Fatty, fibrous plaques narrow the coronary artery lumina, reducing the blood volume that flows through them, leading to myocardial ischemia.
- As atherosclerosis progresses, luminal narrowing is accompanied by vascular changes that impair the ability of the diseased vessel to dilate. This can lead to tissue injury or necrosis.
- Oxygen deprivation forces the myocardium to shift from aerobic to anaerobic metabolism, leading to accumulation of lactic acid and reduction of cellular pH.
- The combination of hypoxia, reduced energy availability, and acidosis rapidly impairs left ventricular function.
- The strength of contractions in the affected myocardial region is reduced as the fibers shorten inadequately, resulting in less force and velocity.
- Wall motion is abnormal in the ischemic area, resulting in less blood being ejected from the heart with each contraction.

CAUSES
- Atherosclerosis
- Dissecting aneurysm
- Infectious vasculitis
- Syphilis
- Congenital defects
- Coronary artery spasm

COMPLICATIONS
- Arrhythmias
- Myocardial infarction (MI)
- Heart failure

Assessment

HISTORY
- Angina that may radiate to the left arm, neck, jaw, or shoulder blade
- Commonly occurs after physical exertion but may also follow emotional excitement, exposure to cold, or a large meal
- May develop during sleep; symptoms wake the patient
- Nausea
- Vomiting
- Fainting
- Sweating
- Stable angina (predictable and relieved by rest or nitrates)
- Unstable angina (increases in frequency and duration and is more easily induced and generally indicates extensive or worsening disease and, left untreated, may progress to MI)
- Crescendo angina (an effort-induced pain that occurs with increasing frequency and with decreasing provocation)
- Prinzmetal's or variant angina pectoris (severe non-effort-produced pain occurs at rest without provocation)

PHYSICAL FINDINGS
- Cool extremities
- Xanthoma
- Arteriovenous nicking of the eye
- Obesity
- Hypertension
- Decreased or absent peripheral pulses

TEST RESULTS
Imaging
- Myocardial perfusion imaging with thallium 201 during treadmill exercise

shows ischemic areas of the myocardium, visualized as "cold spots."

■ Pharmacologic myocardial perfusion imaging in arteries with stenosis shows decrease in blood flow proportional to the percentage of occlusion.

■ Multiple-gated acquisition scanning demonstrates cardiac wall motion and reflects injury to cardiac tissue.

DIAGNOSTIC PROCEDURES

■ Electrocardiography may be normal between anginal episodes. During angina, it may show ischemic changes.

■ Exercise testing may be performed to detect ST-segment changes during exercise, indicating ischemia, and to determine a safe exercise prescription.

■ Coronary angiography reveals the location and degree of coronary artery stenosis or obstruction, collateral circulation, and the condition of the artery beyond the narrowing.

■ Stress echocardiography may show abnormal wall motion.

Treatment

GENERAL

■ Stress reduction techniques essential, especially if known stressors precipitate pain

■ Lifestyle modifications, such as smoking cessation and maintaining ideal body weight

DIET

■ Low-fat
■ Low-sodium

ACTIVITY

■ Restrictions possible
■ Regular exercise

MEDICATION

■ Nitrates
■ Beta-adrenergic blockers
■ Calcium channel blockers
■ Antiplatelets
■ Antilipemics
■ Antihypertensives
■ Estrogen replacement therapy

SURGERY

■ Coronary artery bypass graft
■ "Keyhole" or minimally invasive surgery
■ Angioplasty
■ Endovascular stent placement
■ Laser angioplasty
■ Atherectomy

MONITORING

■ Vital signs
■ Intake and output
■ Anginal episodes
■ Abnormal bleeding and distal pulses following intervention procedures
■ Breath sounds
■ Chest tube drainage, after surgery
■ Cardiac rate and rhythm

Not all patients experience angina in the same way.

■ Some patients, particularly women, may not experience chest discomfort. Their symptoms may be primarily dyspnea and fatigue.

■ This presentation, called anginal equivalent, may also be found in Black and Hispanic patients.

■ Patients with diabetes may develop central neuropathies and therefore not experience chest pain. Signs of sympathetic stimulation may be their primary angina symptom.

ENDOCARDITIS

Overview

DESCRIPTION

■ Infection of the endocardium, heart valves, or cardiac prosthesis

PATHOPHYSIOLOGY

■ Fibrin and platelets cluster on valve tissue and engulf circulating bacteria or fungi.

■ This produces vegetation, which in turn may cover the valve surfaces, causing deformities and destruction of valvular tissue and may extend to the chordae tendineae, causing them to rupture, leading to valvular insufficiency.

■ Vegetative growth on the heart valves, endocardial lining of a heart chamber, or the endothelium of a blood vessel may embolize to the spleen, kidneys, central nervous system, and lungs.

CAUSES

■ Cardiac valvular disease
■ I.V. drug use
■ Rheumatic heart disease
■ Prosthetic heart valves
■ Congenital heart disease
■ Mitral valve prolapse
■ Degenerative heart disease
■ Calcific aortic stenosis (in elderly patients)
■ Asymmetrical septal hypertrophy
■ Marfan syndrome
■ Syphilitic aortic valve
■ Long-term hemodialysis

COMPLICATIONS

■ Left-sided heart failure
■ Valve stenosis or regurgitation
■ Myocardial erosion
■ Embolic debris lodged in the small vasculature of the visceral tissue

Assessment

HISTORY

■ Patient may report predisposing condition and complain of nonspecific symptoms, such as weakness, fatigue, weight loss, anorexia, arthralgia, night sweats, and intermittent fever that may recur for weeks

PHYSICAL FINDINGS

■ Petechiae on the skin (especially common on the upper anterior trunk) and on the buccal, pharyngeal, or conjunctival mucosa
■ Splinter hemorrhages under the nails
■ Clubbing of the fingers in patients with long-standing disease
■ Heart murmur in all patients except those with early acute endocarditis and I.V. drug users with tricuspid valve infection
■ Osler's nodes
■ Roth's spots
■ Janeway lesions
■ A murmur that changes suddenly or a new murmur that develops in the presence of fever — a classic physical sign
■ Splenomegaly in long-standing disease
■ Dyspnea, tachycardia, and bibasilar crackles possible with left-sided heart failure
■ Splenic infarction causing pain in the upper left quadrant, radiating to the left shoulder, and abdominal rigidity
■ Renal infarction causing hematuria, pyuria, flank pain, and decreased urine output
■ Cerebral infarction causing hemiparesis, aphasia, and other neurologic deficits
■ Pulmonary infarction causing cough, pleuritic pain, pleural friction rub, dyspnea, and hemoptysis
■ Peripheral vascular occlusion causing numbness and tingling in arm, leg, finger, or toe or signs of impending peripheral gangrene

TEST RESULTS
Laboratory
■ Three or more blood cultures during a 24- to 48-hour period identifying the causative organism (in up to 90% of patients)
■ White blood cell count and differential normal or elevated
■ Complete blood count and anemia panel showing normocytic, normochromic anemia in subacute infective endocarditis
■ Erythrocyte sedimentation rate and serum creatinine levels elevated
■ Serum rheumatoid factor positive in about one-half of all patients with endocarditis after the disease is present for 6 weeks
■ Urinalysis showing proteinuria and microscopic hematuria

Imaging
■ Echocardiography may identify valvular damage in up to 80% of patients with native valve disease.

Diagnostic procedures
■ An electrocardiogram reading may show atrial fibrillation and other arrhythmias that accompany valvular disease.

Treatment

GENERAL
■ Prompt therapy that continues for several weeks
■ Selection of anti-infective drug based on type of infecting organism and sensitivity studies
■ If blood cultures negative (10% to 20% of subacute cases), possible I.V. antibiotic therapy (usually for 4 to 6 weeks) against probable infecting organism

DIET
■ Sufficient fluid intake
■ No restrictions

ACTIVITY
■ Bed rest

MEDICATION
■ Aspirin
■ Antibiotics

SURGERY
■ With severe valvular damage, especially aortic insufficiency or infection of a cardiac prosthesis, possible corrective surgery if refractory heart failure develops or if an infected prosthetic valve must be replaced

MONITORING
Watch for signs of embolization, a common occurrence during the first 3 months of treatment. Tell the patient to watch for and report these signs.
■ Renal status
■ Frequent cardiovascular status assessment
■ Arterial blood gas evaluation as needed

HEART FAILURE

Overview

DESCRIPTION
■ The myocardium can't pump effectively enough to meet the body's metabolic needs (see *Classifying heart failure*)
■ Usually occurs in a damaged left ventricle, but it may happen in right ventricle primarily, or secondary to left-sided heart failure

PATHOPHYSIOLOGY
Left-sided heart failure
■ Pumping ability of the left ventricle fails and cardiac output falls.
■ Blood backs up into the left atrium and lungs, causing pulmonary congestion.

Right-sided heart failure
■ Ineffective contractile function of the right ventricle leads to blood backing up into the right atrium and the peripheral circulation, which results in peripheral edema and engorgement of the kidneys and other organs.

CAUSES
■ Mitral stenosis secondary to rheumatic heart disease, constrictive pericarditis, or atrial fibrillation
■ Mitral or aortic insufficiency
■ Arrhythmias
■ Pregnancy
■ Thyrotoxicosis
■ Pulmonary embolism
■ Infections
■ Anemia
■ Emotional stress
■ Increased salt or water intake

COMPLICATIONS
■ Pulmonary edema
■ Organ failure, especially the brain and kidneys
■ Myocardial infarction

Assessment

HISTORY
■ A disorder or condition that can precipitate heart failure
■ Dyspnea or paroxysmal nocturnal dyspnea
■ Peripheral edema
■ Fatigue
■ Weakness
■ Insomnia
■ Anorexia
■ Nausea
■ Sense of abdominal fullness (particularly in right-sided heart failure)

PHYSICAL FINDINGS
■ Cough that produces pink, frothy sputum
■ Cyanosis of the lips and nail beds

CLASSIFYING HEART FAILURE

The New York Heart Association classification is a universal gauge of heart failure severity based on physical limitations.

Class I: Minimal
■ No limitations
■ Ordinary physical activity doesn't cause undue fatigue, dyspnea, palpitations, or angina

Class II: Mild
■ Slightly limited physical activity
■ Comfortable at rest
■ Ordinary physical activity results in fatigue, palpitations, dyspnea, or angina

Class III: Moderate
■ Markedly limited physical activity
■ Comfortable at rest
■ Less than ordinary activity produces symptoms

Class IV: Severe
■ Unable to perform physical activity without discomfort
■ Angina or symptoms of cardiac insufficiency may develop at rest

---

■ Pale, cool, clammy skin
■ Diaphoresis
■ Jugular vein distention
■ Ascites
■ Tachycardia
■ Pulsus alternans
■ Hepatomegaly and, possibly, splenomegaly
■ Decreased pulse pressure
■ S_3 and S_4 heart sounds
■ Moist, bibasilar crackles, rhonchi, and expiratory wheezing

VAD: HELP FOR THE FAILING HEART

The ventricular assist device (VAD) functions somewhat like an artificial heart. The major difference is that the VAD assists the heart, whereas the artificial heart replaces it. The VAD is designed to aid one or both ventricles. The pumping chambers themselves aren't usually implanted in the patient.

The permanent VAD is implanted in the patient's chest cavity. Although it usually provides only temporary support, in November 2002, the Food and Drug Administration approved the use of a left ventricular assist device as a permanent implant for terminally ill patients with end-stage heart failure who aren't eligible for a heart transplant. The device receives power through the skin by a belt of electrical transformer coils (worn externally as a portable battery pack). It can also operate off an implanted, rechargeable battery for up to 1 hour at a time.

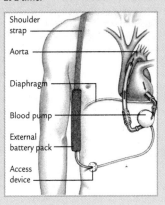

Labels: Shoulder strap, Aorta, Diaphragm, Blood pump, External battery pack, Access device

TEST RESULTS
Imaging
■ Chest X-rays show increased pulmonary vascular markings, interstitial edema, or pleural effusion and cardiomegaly.

Diagnostic procedures
■ Electrocardiography reflects heart strain or enlargement or ischemia. It may also reveal atrial enlargement, tachycardia, and extrasystole.
■ Pulmonary artery pressure monitoring typically shows elevated pulmonary artery and pulmonary artery wedge pressures, left ventricular end-diastolic pressure in left-sided heart failure, and elevated right atrial or central venous pressure in right-sided heart failure.

Treatment

GENERAL
■ Antiembolism stockings

DIET
■ Sodium restriction
■ Fluid restriction
■ Calorie restriction, if indicated
■ Low-fat, if indicated

ACTIVITY
■ Walking program
■ Activity as tolerated

MEDICATION
■ Diuretics
■ Oxygen
■ Inotropic drugs
■ Vasodilators
■ Angiotensin-converting enzyme inhibitors
■ Angiotensin II receptor antagonists
■ Cardiac glycosides
■ Diuretics
■ Potassium supplements
■ Beta-adrenergic blockers

SURGERY

- For valvular dysfunction with recurrent acute heart failure, surgical replacement
- Heart transplantation
- Ventricular assist device (see *VAD: Help for the failing heart*)

MONITORING

- Daily weight for peripheral edema and other signs and symptoms of fluid overload
- Intake and output
- Vital signs and mental status
- Abnormal heart and breath sounds

Auscultate for abnormal heart and breath sounds and report changes immediately.

- Blood urea nitrogen and serum creatinine, potassium, sodium, chloride, and magnesium levels

HYPERTENSION

Overview

DESCRIPTION

- Intermittent or sustained elevation of diastolic or systolic blood pressure (see *Classifying blood pressure readings,* page 204)
- Usually begins as benign disease, slowly progressing to accelerated or malignant state
- Two major types: essential (also called primary or idiopathic) hypertension and secondary hypertension, which results from renal disease or another identifiable cause
- Malignant hypertension, a medical emergency, is severe, fulminant form commonly arising from both types

PATHOPHYSIOLOGY
Several theories

- Changes in arteriolar bed, causing increased peripheral vascular resistance
- Abnormally increased tone in the sympathetic nervous system that originates in the vasomotor system centers, causing increased peripheral vascular resistance
- Increased blood volume resulting from renal or hormonal dysfunction
- An increase in arteriolar thickening caused by genetic factors, leading to increased peripheral vascular resistance
- Abnormal renin release, resulting in the formation of angiotensin II, which constricts the arterioles and increases blood volume

CAUSES

- Essential hypertension: unknown
- Secondary hypertension: may be cause by chronic kidney disease, renovascular disease, primary aldosteronism, pheochromocytoma, coarctation of the aorta, or sleep apnea.

RISK FACTORS

- Family history
- Black race in United States
- Stress
- Obesity
- Diabetes mellitus
- Diet high in sodium or saturated fat
- Use of tobacco or hormonal contraceptives
- Excess alcohol intake
- Sedentary lifestyle
- Aging

COMPLICATIONS

- Stroke
- Cardiac disease
- Renal failure
- Blindness

(See *What happens in hypertensive crisis,* page 205.)

CLASSIFYING BLOOD PRESSURE READINGS

In 2003, the National Institutes of Health issued the Seventh Report of the Joint National Committee on Prevention, Detection, Evaluation, and Treatment of High Blood Pressure (The JNC 7 Report). Updates since the JNC6 report include a new category, prehypertension, and the combining of stages 2 and 3 hypertension. Categories now are normal, prehypertension, and stages 1 and 2 hypertension.

The revised categories are based on the average of two or more readings taken on separate visits after an initial screening. They apply to adults age 18 and older. (If the systolic and diastolic pressures fall into different categories, use the higher of the two pressures to classify the reading. For example, a reading of 160/92 mm Hg should be classified as stage 2.)

Normal blood pressure with respect to cardiovascular risk is a systolic reading below 120 mm Hg and a diastolic reading below 80 mm Hg. Patients with prehypertension are at increased risk for developing hypertension and should follow health-promoting lifestyle modifications to prevent cardiovascular disease.

In addition to classifying stages of hypertension based on average blood pressure readings, clinicians should also take note of target organ disease and additional risk factors, such as a patient with diabetes, left ventricular hypertrophy, and chronic renal disease. This additional information is important to obtain a true picture of the patient's cardiovascular health.

Category	Systolic		Diastolic
Normal	< 120 mm Hg	and	< 80 mm Hg
Prehypertension	120 to 139 mm Hg	or	80 to 89 mm Hg
Hypertension Stage 1	140 to 159 mm Hg	or	90 to 99 mm Hg
Stage 2	≥160 mm Hg	or	≥ 100 mm Hg

Assessment

HISTORY

■ In many cases, no symptoms, and disorder revealed incidentally during evaluation for another disorder or during a routine blood pressure screening program

■ Symptoms that reflect the effect of hypertension on the organ systems

■ Awakening with a headache in the occipital region, which subsides spontaneously after a few hours

■ Dizziness, fatigue, and confusion

■ Palpitations, chest pain, dyspnea

■ Epistaxis

■ Hematuria

■ Blurred vision

WHAT HAPPENS IN HYPERTENSIVE CRISIS

Hypertensive crisis is a severe increase in arterial blood pressure caused by a disturbance in one or more of the regulating mechanisms. If untreated, hypertensive crisis may result in renal, cardiac, or cerebral complications and, possibly, death.

Causes of hypertensive crisis

- Abnormal renal function
- Hypertensive encephalopathy
- Intracerebral hemorrhage
- Withdrawal of antihypertensive drugs (abrupt)

- Myocardial ischemia
- Eclampsia
- Pheochromocytoma
- Monoamine oxidase inhibitor interactions

↓

Prolonged hypertension

↓

Inflammation and necrosis of arterioles

↓

Narrowing of blood vessels

↓

Restriction of blood flow to major organs

↓

Organ damage

↓   ↓   ↓

Renal
- Decreased renal perfusion
- Progressive deterioration of nephrons
- Decreased ability to concentrate urine
- Increased serum creatinine and blood urea nitrogen
- Increased renal tubule permeability with protein leakage into tubules
- Renal insufficiency
- Uremia
- Renal failure

Cardiac
- Decreased cardiac perfusion
- Coronary artery disease
- Angina or myocardial infarction
- Increased cardiac workload
- Left ventricular hypertrophy
- Heart failure

Cerebral
- Decreased cerebral perfusion
- Increased stress on vessel wall
- Arterial spasm
- Ischemia
- Transient ischemic attacks
- Weakening of vessel intima
- Aneurysm formation
- Intracranial hemorrhage

PHYSICAL FINDINGS

■ Elevated blood pressure on at least two consecutive occasions after initial screenings
■ Bruits over the abdominal aorta and femoral arteries or the carotids
■ Peripheral edema in late stages
■ Hemorrhages, exudates, and papilledema of the eye in late stages if hypertensive retinopathy present
■ Pulsating abdominal mass, suggesting an abdominal aneurysm

TEST RESULTS
Laboratory

■ Urinalysis possibly showing protein, red blood cells, or white blood cells, suggesting renal disease, or glucose, suggesting diabetes mellitus
■ Serum potassium levels less than 3.5 mEq/L possibly indicating adrenal dysfunction (primary hyperaldosteronism)
■ Blood urea nitrogen levels normal or elevated to more than 20 mg/dl and serum creatinine levels normal or elevated to more than 1.5 mg/dl, suggesting renal disease

Imaging

■ Excretory urography may reveal renal atrophy, indicating chronic renal disease; one kidney more than ⅝″ (1.6 cm) shorter than the other suggests unilateral renal disease.
■ Chest X-rays may demonstrate cardiomegaly.
■ Renal arteriography may show renal artery stenosis.

Diagnostic procedures

■ Electrocardiography may show left ventricular hypertrophy or ischemia.
■ An oral captopril challenge may be done to test for renovascular hypertension.

■ Ophthalmoscopy reveals arteriovenous nicking and, in hypertensive encephalopathy, edema.

Treatment

GENERAL

■ Lifestyle modification, such as weight control, limiting alcohol, regular exercise, and smoking cessation
■ For a patient with secondary hypertension, correction of the underlying cause and control of hypertensive effects

DIET

■ Low-saturated fat and sodium
■ Adequate calcium, magnesium, and potassium

ACTIVITY

■ Regular exercise program

MEDICATION

■ Diuretics
■ Beta-adrenergic blockers
■ Calcium channel blockers
■ Angiotensin-converting enzyme inhibitors
■ Alpha-receptor antagonists
■ Vasodilators
■ Angiotensin II receptor antagonists

MONITORING

■ Vital signs, especially blood pressure
■ Signs and symptoms of target end-organ damage
■ Complications
■ Response to treatment
■ Risk factor modification
■ Adverse effects of antihypertensive agents

MITRAL STENOSIS

Overview

DESCRIPTION
■ Narrowing of the mitral valve orifice, which is normally 3 to 6 cm
■ Mild mitral stenosis (also called MS): valve orifice of 2 cm
■ Severe MS: valve orifice of 1 cm

PATHOPHYSIOLOGY
■ Valve leaflets become diffusely thickened by fibrosis and calcification.
■ The mitral commissures and the chordae tendineae fuse and shorten, the valvular cusps become rigid, and the valve's apex becomes narrowed.
■ This obstructs blood flow from the left atrium to the left ventricle.
■ Left atrial volume and pressure increase and the atrial chamber dilates.
■ Increased resistance to blood flow causes pulmonary hypertension, right ventricular hypertrophy and, eventually, right-sided heart failure and reduced cardiac output.

CAUSES
■ Rheumatic fever
■ Congenital anomalies
■ Atrial myxoma
■ Endocarditis
■ Adverse effects of fenfluramine and phentermine (Fen-phen) diet drug combination (Fen-phen was removed from the market in 1997.)

COMPLICATIONS
■ Cardiac arrhythmias, especially atrial fibrillation
■ Thromboembolism

Assessment

HISTORY
Mild mitral stenosis
■ Asymptomatic

Moderate to severe mitral stenosis
■ Gradual decline in exercise tolerance
■ Dyspnea on exertion; shortness of breath
■ Paroxysmal nocturnal dyspnea
■ Orthopnea
■ Weakness
■ Fatigue
■ Palpitations
■ Cough

PHYSICAL FINDINGS
■ Hemoptysis
■ Peripheral and facial cyanosis
■ Malar rash
■ Jugular vein distention
■ Ascites
■ Peripheral edema
■ Hepatomegaly
■ A loud S_1 or opening snap
■ A diastolic murmur at the apex (see *Identifying the murmur of mitral stenosis,* page 208)
■ Crackles over lung fields
■ Right ventricular lift
■ Resting tachycardia; irregularly irregular heart rhythm

TEST RESULTS
Imaging
■ Chest X-rays show left atrial and ventricular enlargement (in severe mitral stenosis), straightening of the left border of the cardiac silhouette, enlarged pulmonary arteries, dilation of the upper lobe pulmonary veins, and mitral valve calcification.
■ Echocardiography discloses thickened mitral valve leaflets and left atrial enlargement.

IDENTIFYING THE MURMUR OF MITRAL STENOSIS

A low, rumbling crescendo-decrescendo murmur in the mitral valve area characterizes mitral stenosis.

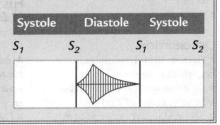

Systole	Diastole	Systole	
S_1	S_2	S_1	S_2

Diagnostic procedures
■ Cardiac catheterization shows a diastolic pressure gradient across the valve, elevated pulmonary artery wedge pressure (greater than 15 mm Hg), and pulmonary artery pressure in the left atrium with severe pulmonary hypertension.
■ Electrocardiography reveals left atrial enlargement, right ventricular hypertrophy, right axis deviation, and (in 40% to 50% of cases) atrial fibrillation.

Treatment

GENERAL
■ Synchronized electrical cardioversion to correct atrial fibrillation

DIET
■ Sodium-restricted

ACTIVITY
■ As tolerated

MEDICATION
■ Digoxin
■ Diuretics
■ Oxygen
■ Beta-adrenergic blockers
■ Calcium channel blockers
■ Anticoagulants
■ Infective endocarditis antibiotic prophylaxis
■ Nitrates

SURGERY
■ Commissurotomy or valve replacement
■ Percutaneous balloon valvuloplasty

MONITORING
■ Vital signs and hemodynamics
■ Intake and output
■ Signs and symptoms of heart failure and pulmonary edema
■ Signs and symptoms of thromboembolism
■ Adverse drug reactions
■ Cardiac arrhythmias
■ Postoperatively: hypotension, arrhythmias, and thrombus formation

MITRAL VALVE PROLAPSE

Overview

DESCRIPTION
■ Portion of the mitral valve (MV) prolapses into the left atrium during ventricular contraction (systole)

PATHOPHYSIOLOGY
■ Myxomatous degeneration of MV leaflets with redundant tissue leads to prolapse of the MV into the left atrium during systole.

■ In some patients, this results in leakage of blood into the left atrium from the left ventricle.

CAUSES
■ Connective tissue disorders, such as systemic lupus erythematosus and Marfan syndrome
■ Congenital heart disease
■ Acquired heart disease, such as coronary artery disease and rheumatic heart disease

COMPLICATIONS
■ Arrhythmias
■ Infective endocarditis
■ Mitral insufficiency from chordal rupture

Assessment

HISTORY
■ Usually asymptomatic
■ Possible fatigue, syncope, palpitations, chest pain, or dyspnea on exertion

PHYSICAL FINDINGS
■ Orthostatic hypotension
■ Mid-to-late systolic click and late systolic murmur

TEST RESULTS
Imaging
■ Echocardiography may reveal mitral valve prolapse with or without mitral insufficiency.

Diagnostic procedures
■ Electrocardiography (ECG) is usually normal but may reveal atrial or ventricular arrhythmia.
■ Signal-averaged ECG may show ventricular and supraventricular arrhythmias.
■ Holter monitor worn for 24 hours may show an arrhythmia.

Treatment

GENERAL
■ Usually requires no treatment; regular monitoring necessary

DIET
■ Decreased caffeine intake
■ Fluid intake to maintain hydration

ACTIVITY
■ No restrictions

MEDICATION
■ Antibiotic prophylaxis
■ Beta-adrenergic blockers
■ Anticoagulants
■ Antiarrhythmics

MONITORING
■ Vital signs
■ Blood pressure while lying, sitting, and standing
■ Heart sounds
■ Signs and symptoms of mitral insufficiency
■ Serial echocardiograms
■ ECG for arrhythmias

MYOCARDIAL INFARCTION

Overview

DESCRIPTION
■ Reduced blood flow through one or more coronary arteries causing myocardial ischemia and necrosis
■ Infarction site depends on the vessels involved
■ Also called MI and heart attack; it's part of a broader category of disease known as acute coronary syndromes that includes Q-wave MI, non-Q-wave MI, and unstable angina.

PATHOPHYSIOLOGY

■ One or more coronary arteries becomes occluded. The degree and duration of blockage determines the type of infarct that occurs. Damage to the innermost layer of the heart muscle results in a non-Q-wave MI. When damage extends through all myocardial layers, a Q-wave MI results.

■ If coronary occlusion causes prolonged ischemia, lasting longer than 30 to 45 minutes, irreversible myocardial cell damage and muscle death occur.

■ Every MI has a central area of necrosis surrounded by an area of hypoxic injury. This injured tissue is potentially viable and may be salvaged if circulation is restored, or it may progress to necrosis.

CAUSES

■ Atherosclerosis
■ Thrombosis
■ Platelet aggregation
■ Coronary artery stenosis or spasm

RISK FACTORS

■ Increased age
■ Diabetes mellitus
■ Elevated serum triglyceride, low-density lipoprotein, and cholesterol levels, and decreased serum high-density lipoprotein levels
■ Excessive intake of saturated fats, carbohydrates, or salt
■ Hypertension
■ Obesity
■ Positive family history of coronary artery disease (CAD)
■ Sedentary lifestyle
■ Smoking
■ Stress or type A personality
■ Use of drugs, such as amphetamines or cocaine

COMPLICATIONS

■ Arrhythmias
■ Cardiogenic shock
■ Heart failure causing pulmonary edema
■ Pericarditis
■ Rupture of the atrial or ventricular septum, ventricular wall
■ Ventricular aneurysm
■ Cerebral or pulmonary emboli
■ Extensions of the original infarction
■ Mitral insufficiency

Assessment

HISTORY

■ Possible CAD with increasing anginal frequency, severity, or duration
■ Cardinal symptom of MI: persistent, crushing substernal pain possibly radiating to the left arm, jaw, neck, and shoulder blades, and possibly persisting for 12 or more hours
■ In elderly patient or one with diabetes, pain possibly absent; in others, pain possibly mild and confused with indigestion
■ Women may experience atypical symptoms, such as vague chest pain, a lack of chest pain, nausea, fatigue, or heartburn.
■ A feeling of impending doom, fatigue, nausea, vomiting, and shortness of breath
■ Sudden death (may be the first and only indication of MI)

PHYSICAL FINDINGS

■ Extreme anxiety and restlessness
■ Dyspnea
■ Diaphoresis
■ Tachycardia
■ Hypertension
■ Bradycardia and hypotension, in inferior MI
■ An S_4, an S_3, and paradoxical splitting of S_2 with ventricular dysfunction
■ Systolic murmur of mitral insufficiency
■ Pericardial friction rub with transmural MI or pericarditis

- Low-grade fever possibly developing during the next few days

TEST RESULTS
Laboratory

- Elevated serum creatine kinase (CK) level, especially the CK-MB isoenzyme, the cardiac muscle fraction of CK (see *Release of cardiac enzymes and proteins,* page 212)
- Elevated serum lactate dehydrogenase (LD) level; higher LD_1 isoenzyme (found in cardiac tissue) than LD_2 (in serum)
- Elevated white blood cell count usually appearing on the second day and lasting 1 week
- Detection of myoglobin (the hemoprotein found in cardiac and skeletal muscle) that's released with muscle damage as soon as 2 hours after MI
- Elevated troponin I, a structural protein found in cardiac muscle, only in cardiac muscle damage; more specific than the CK-MB level (Troponin levels increase within 4 to 6 hours of myocardial injury and may remain elevated for 5 to 11 days.)

Imaging

- Nuclear medicine scans, using I.V. technetium 99m pertechnetate, can identify acutely damaged muscle by picking up accumulations of radioactive nucleotide, which appears as a "hot spot" on the film. Myocardial perfusion imaging with thallium 201 reveals a "cold spot" in most patients during the first few hours after a Q-wave MI.
- Echocardiography shows ventricular wall dyskinesia with a Q-wave MI and helps to evaluate the ejection fraction.

Diagnostic procedures

- Serial 12-lead electrocardiography (ECG) readings may be normal or inconclusive during the first few hours after an MI. Characteristic abnormalities include serial ST-segment depression in non-Q-wave MI and ST-segment elevation and Q waves, representing scarring and necrosis in Q-wave MI.
- Pulmonary artery catheterization may be performed to detect left- or right-sided heart failure and to monitor response to treatment.

Treatment

GENERAL

- To relieve chest pain, stabilize heart rhythm, and reduce cardiac workload
- For arrhythmias, a pacemaker, or electrical cardioversion
- I.V. thrombolytic therapy started within 3 hours of the onset of symptoms
- Intra-aortic balloon pump for cardiogenic shock

DIET

- Low-fat, low-cholesterol
- Calorie restriction if indicated

ACTIVITY

- Bed rest with bedside commode
- Gradual increase in activity as tolerated

MEDICATION

- Aspirin
- Antiarrhythmics
- Antianginals
- Calcium channel blockers
- Heparin I.V.
- Morphine I.V.
- Inotropic drugs
- Beta-adrenergic blockers
- Angiotensin-converting enzyme inhibitors
- Stool softeners
- Oxygen

RELEASE OF CARDIAC ENZYMES AND PROTEINS

Because they're released by damaged tissue, serum proteins and isoenzymes (catalytic proteins that vary in concentration in specific organs) can help identify the compromised organ and assess the extent of damage. After acute myocardial infarction, cardiac enzymes and proteins rise and fall in a characteristic pattern, as shown in the graph below.

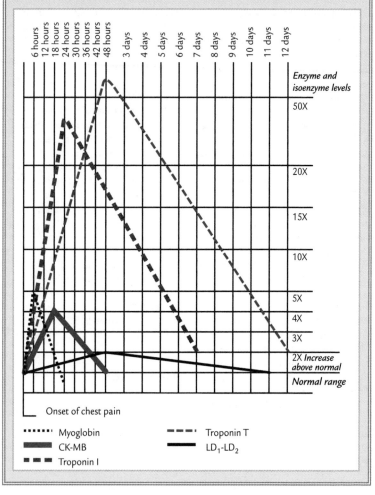

SURGERY

- Surgical revascularization
- Percutaneous revascularization

MONITORING

- Serial ECGs
- Vital signs and heart and breath sounds

> Watch for crackles, cough, tachypnea, and edema, which may indicate impending left-sided heart failure.

- Daily weight; intake and output
- Cardiac enzyme levels; coagulation studies
- Cardiac rhythm for reperfusion arrhythmias (treat according to facility protocol)

PERICARDITIS

Overview

DESCRIPTION
- Inflammation of the pericardium—the fibroserous sac that envelops, supports, and protects the heart
- Occurs in acute and chronic forms
- Acute form: can be fibrinous or effusive; characterized by serous, purulent, or hemorrhagic exudate
- Chronic form (called constrictive pericarditis): characterized by dense fibrous pericardial thickening

PATHOPHYSIOLOGY
- Pericardial tissue is damaged by bacteria or another substance that releases chemical mediators of inflammation into surrounding tissue.
- Friction occurs as the inflamed layers rub against each other.
- Chemical mediators dilate blood vessels and increase vessel permeability.
- Vessel walls leak fluids and proteins, causing extracellular edema.

CAUSES
- Bacterial, fungal, or viral infection (in infectious pericarditis)
- Neoplasms (primary or metastatic)
- High-dose chest radiation
- Uremia

- Hypersensitivity or autoimmune disease
- Drugs, such as hydralazine or procainamide
- Idiopathic factors
- Myocardial infarction (MI)
- Chest trauma
- Aortic aneurysm with pericardial leakage
- Myxedema with cholesterol deposits in pericardium

COMPLICATIONS
- Pericardial effusion
- Cardiac tamponade

Assessment

HISTORY
- Predisposing factor
- Sharp, sudden pain, usually starting over the sternum and radiating to the neck, shoulders, back, and arms
- Pleuritic pain, increasing with deep inspiration and decreasing when the patient sits up and leans forward
- Dyspnea
- Chest pain (may mimic MI pain)

PHYSICAL FINDINGS
- Pericardial friction rub
- Diminished apical impulse
- Fluid retention, ascites, hepatomegaly (resembling those of chronic right-sided heart failure)
- With pericardial effusion: tachycardia
- With cardiac tamponade: pallor, clammy skin, hypotension, pulsus paradoxus, jugular vein distention, and dyspnea

TEST RESULTS
Laboratory
- Elevated white blood cell count (especially in infectious pericarditis)
- Elevated erythrocyte sedimentation rate

■ Slightly elevated serum creatine kinase-MB levels (with associated myocarditis)
■ Pericardial fluid culture; may identify a causative organism in bacterial or fungal pericarditis
■ Elevated blood urea nitrogen in uremia
■ Elevated antistreptolysin-O titers; may indicate rheumatic fever
■ Positive reaction in purified protein derivative skin test; indicates tuberculosis

Imaging
■ Echocardiography showing an echo-free space between the ventricular wall and the pericardium indicates pericardial effusion.

Diagnostic procedures
■ Electrocardiography shows initial ST-segment elevation across the precordium.

Treatment

GENERAL
■ Management of rheumatic fever, uremia, tuberculosis, or other underlying disorder

DIET
■ Restrictions, based on underlying disorder

ACTIVITY
■ Bed rest as long as fever and pain persist

MEDICATION
■ Nonsteroidal anti-inflammatory drugs
■ Corticosteroids
■ Antibiotics

SURGERY
■ Surgical drainage

■ Pericardiocentesis
■ Partial pericardectomy (for recurrent pericarditis)
■ Total pericardectomy (for constrictive pericarditis)

MONITORING
■ Vital signs
■ Heart rhythm
■ Heart sounds
■ Hemodynamic values

SHOCK, CARDIOGENIC

Overview

DESCRIPTION
■ A condition of diminished cardiac output that severely impairs tissue perfusion
■ Sometimes called pump failure

PATHOPHYSIOLOGY
■ Left ventricular dysfunction initiates a series of compensatory mechanisms that attempt to increase cardiac output.
■ As cardiac output decreases, aortic and carotid baroreceptors activate sympathetic nervous responses.
■ Responses increase heart rate, left ventricular filling pressure, and peripheral resistance to flow to enhance venous return to the heart.
■ This action initially stabilizes the patient but later causes deterioration with increasing oxygen demands on the already compromised myocardium.
■ These events consist of a cycle of low cardiac output, sympathetic compensation, myocardial ischemia, and even lower cardiac output.

CAUSES
■ Myocardial infarction (or MI; most common)

- Myocardial ischemia
- Papillary muscle dysfunction
- End-stage cardiomyopathy
- Myocarditis
- Acute mitral or aortic insufficiency
- Ventricular septal defect
- Ventricular aneurysm

COMPLICATIONS
- Multisystem organ failure
- Death

Assessment

HISTORY
- Disorder, such as MI or cardiomyopathy, that severely decreases left ventricular function
- Anginal pain

PHYSICAL FINDINGS
- Urine output less than 20 ml/hour
- Pale, cold, and clammy skin
- Decreased sensorium
- Rapid, shallow respirations
- Rapid, thready pulse
- Mean arterial pressure of less than 60 mm Hg in adults
- Gallop rhythm, faint heart sounds and, possibly, a holosystolic murmur

TEST RESULTS
Laboratory
- Serum enzyme measurements showing elevated levels of creatine kinase (CK), lactate dehydrogenase (LD), aspartate aminotransferase, and alanine aminotransferase, pointing to MI or ischemia and suggesting heart failure or shock; CK and LD isoenzyme levels possibly confirming acute MI

Imaging
- Cardiac catheterization and echocardiography reveal other conditions that can lead to pump dysfunction and failure, such as cardiac tamponade, papillary muscle infarct or rupture, ventricular septal rupture, pulmonary emboli, venous pooling (associated with venodilators and continuous intermittent positive-pressure breathing), and hypovolemia.

Diagnostic procedures
- Pulmonary artery pressure monitoring reveals increased pulmonary artery pressure and pulmonary artery wedge pressure, reflecting an increase in left ventricular end-diastolic pressure (preload) and heightened resistance to left ventricular emptying (afterload) caused by ineffective pumping and increased peripheral vascular resistance.
- Invasive arterial pressure monitoring shows systolic arterial pressure less than 80 mm Hg caused by impaired ventricular ejection.
- Arterial blood gas (ABG) analysis may show metabolic and respiratory acidosis and hypoxia.
- Electrocardiography demonstrates possible evidence of acute MI, ischemia, or ventricular aneurysm.

Treatment

GENERAL
- Intra-aortic balloon pump

DIET
- Possible parenteral nutrition or tube feedings

ACTIVITY
- Bed rest

MEDICATION
- Vasopressors
- Inotropics
- Vasoconstrictors
- Analgesics; sedatives
- Osmotic diuretics
- Vasodilators
- Oxygen

SURGERY
- Possible ventricular assist device
- Possible heart transplant

MONITORING
- ABG levels (acid-base balance)
- Complete blood count and electrolyte levels
- Vital signs and peripheral pulses
- Cardiac rate and rhythm continuously
- Hemodynamics
- Hourly urine output with an indwelling urinary catheter
- Heart sounds and breath sounds
- Level of consciousness

SHOCK, HYPOVOLEMIC

Overview

DESCRIPTION
- Reduced intravascular blood volume causes circulatory dysfunction and inadequate tissue perfusion
- Potentially life-threatening

PATHOPHYSIOLOGY
- When fluid is lost from the intravascular space, venous return to the heart is reduced.
- This decreases ventricular filling, which leads to a drop in stroke volume.
- Cardiac output falls, causing reduced perfusion to tissues and organs.
- Tissue anoxia prompts a shift in cellular metabolism from aerobic to anaerobic pathways.
- This produces an accumulation of lactic acid, resulting in metabolic acidosis.

CAUSES
- Acute blood loss (about one-fifth of total volume)
- Intestinal obstruction

- Burns
- Peritonitis
- Acute pancreatitis
- Ascites
- Dehydration from excessive perspiration, severe diarrhea or protracted vomiting, diabetes insipidus, diuresis, and inadequate fluid intake

COMPLICATIONS
- Acute respiratory distress syndrome
- Acute tubular necrosis and renal failure
- Disseminated intravascular coagulation
- Multisystem organ dysfunction syndrome

HISTORY
- Disorders or conditions that reduce blood volume, such as GI hemorrhage, trauma, and severe diarrhea and vomiting
- Patient with cardiac disease: possible anginal pain because of decreased myocardial perfusion and oxygenation

PHYSICAL FINDINGS
- Pale, cool, and clammy skin
- Decreased sensorium
- Rapid, shallow respirations
- Urine output usually less than 20 ml/hour
- Rapid, thready pulse
- Mean arterial pressure less than 60 mm Hg in adults (with chronic hypotension, mean pressure may fall below 50 mm Hg before signs of shock)
- Orthostatic vital signs and tilt test results consistent with hypovolemic shock (see *Checking for early hypovolemic shock*)

TEST RESULTS
Laboratory
- Low hematocrit and decreased hemoglobin levels and red blood cell and platelet counts
- Elevated serum potassium, sodium, lactate dehydrogenase, creatinine, and blood urea nitrogen levels
- Increased urine specific gravity (greater than 1.020) and urine osmolality
- Decreased pH and partial pressure of oxygen in arterial blood and increased partial pressure of carbon dioxide in arterial blood
- Aspiration of gastric contents through a nasogastric tube identifying internal bleeding
- Positive occult blood tests
- Coagulation studies showing coagulopathy from disseminated intravascular coagulation

Imaging
- X-rays (chest or abdominal) help to identify internal bleeding sites.

Diagnostic procedures
- Gastroscopy helps to identify internal bleeding sites.
- Invasive hemodynamic monitoring shows reduced central venous pressure, right atrial pressure, pulmonary artery pressure, pulmonary artery wedge pressure, and cardiac output.

Treatment

GENERAL
- In severe cases, an intra-aortic balloon pump, ventricular assist device, or pneumatic antishock garment
- Oxygen administration
- Bleeding control by direct application of pressure and related measures

---

CHECKING FOR EARLY HYPOVOLEMIC SHOCK

Orthostatic vital signs and tilt test results can help in assessing for the possibility of impending hypovolemic shock.

Orthostatic vital signs
Measure the patient's blood pressure and pulse rate while he's lying in a supine position, sitting, and standing. Wait at least 1 minute between each position change. A systolic blood pressure decrease of 10 mm Hg or more between positions or a pulse rate increase of 10 beats/minute or more is a sign of volume depletion and impending hypovolemic shock.

Tilt test
With the patient lying in a supine position, raise his legs above heart level. If his blood pressure increases significantly, the test is positive, indicating volume depletion and impending hypovolemic shock.

DIET
- Possible parenteral nutrition or tube feedings

ACTIVITY
- Bed rest

MEDICATION
- Prompt and vigorous blood and fluid replacement
- Positive inotropes
- Possible diuretics

SURGERY
- Possibly, to correct underlying problem

MONITORING

- Vital signs and peripheral pulses
- Cardiac rhythm continuously
- Coagulation studies for signs of impending coagulopathy
- Complete blood count and electrolyte measurements
- Arterial blood gas levels
- Intake and output
- Hemodynamics

SHOCK, SEPTIC

Overview

DESCRIPTION

- Low systemic vascular resistance and an elevated cardiac output
- Probably a response to infections that release microbes or an immune mediator

PATHOPHYSIOLOGY

- Initially, the body's defenses activate chemical mediators in response to the invading organisms.
- The release of these mediators results in low systemic vascular resistance and increased cardiac output.
- Blood flow is unevenly distributed in the microcirculation, and plasma leaking from capillaries causes functional hypovolemia.
- Eventually, cardiac output decreases, and poor tissue perfusion and hypotension cause multisystem dysfunction syndrome and death.

CAUSES

- Any pathogenic organism
- Gram-negative bacteria, such as *Escherichia coli, Klebsiella pneumoniae, Serratia, Enterobacter,* and *Pseudomonas,* most common causes (up to 70% of cases)

COMPLICATIONS

- Disseminated intravascular coagulation
- Renal failure
- Heart failure
- GI ulcers
- Abnormal liver function

Assessment

HISTORY

- Possible disorder or treatment that can cause immunosuppression
- Possibly, previous invasive tests or treatments, surgery, or trauma
- Possible fever and chills (although 20% of patients possibly hypothermic)

PHYSICAL FINDINGS
Hyperdynamic or warm phase

- Peripheral vasodilation
- Skin possibly pink and flushed or warm and dry
- Altered level of consciousness (LOC) reflected in agitation, anxiety, irritability, and shortened attention span
- Respirations rapid and shallow
- Urine output below normal
- Rapid, full, bounding pulse
- Blood pressure normal or slightly elevated

Hypodynamic or cold phase

- Peripheral vasoconstriction and inadequate tissue perfusion
- Pale skin and possible cyanosis
- Decreased LOC; possible obtundation and coma
- Respirations possibly rapid and shallow
- Urine output possibly less than 25 ml/hour or absent
- Rapid pulse that's weak, thready
- Irregular pulse if arrhythmias are present
- Cold and clammy skin
- Hypotension

- Crackles or rhonchi if pulmonary congestion present

TEST RESULTS
Laboratory
- Positive blood cultures for the causative organism
- Complete blood count showing the presence or absence of anemia and leukopenia, severe or absent neutropenia, and usually the presence of thrombocytopenia
- Increased blood urea nitrogen and creatinine levels and decreased creatinine clearance
- Abnormal prothrombin time and partial thromboplastin time
- Elevated serum lactate dehydrogenase levels with metabolic acidosis
- Urine studies showing increased specific gravity (more than 1.020) and osmolality and decreased sodium
- Arterial blood gas (ABG) analysis demonstrating elevated blood pH and partial pressure of arterial oxygen and decreased partial pressure of arterial carbon dioxide with respiratory alkalosis in early stages

Diagnostic procedures
- Invasive hemodynamic monitoring shows:
  - increased cardiac output and decreased systemic vascular resistance in warm phase
  - decreased cardiac output and increased systemic vascular resistance in cold phase.

Treatment

GENERAL
- Removal of I.V., intra-arterial, or urinary drainage catheters whenever possible
- In patients who are immunosuppressed because of drug therapy, drugs discontinued or reduced if possible
- Mechanical ventilation if respiratory failure occurs

DIET
- Possible parenteral nutrition or tube feedings

ACTIVITY
- Bed rest

MEDICATION
- Antimicrobials
- Granulocyte transfusions
- Colloid or crystalloid infusions
- Oxygen
- Diuretics
- Vasopressors

MONITORING
- ABG levels
- Hourly intake and urine output
- Vital signs and peripheral pulses
- Hemodynamics
- Cardiac rhythm continuously
- Heart and breath sounds

THROMBOPHLEBITIS

Overview

DESCRIPTION
- An acute condition characterized by inflammation and thrombus formation
- May occur in deep or superficial veins
- Typically occurs at the valve cusps because venous stasis encourages accumulation and adherence of platelet and fibrin

PATHOPHYSIOLOGY
- Alteration in epithelial lining causes platelet aggregation and fibrin entrap-

ment of red blood cells, white blood cells, and additional platelets.
■ The thrombus initiates a chemical inflammatory process in the vessel epithelium that leads to fibrosis, which may occlude the vessel lumen or embolize.

CAUSES
■ May be idiopathic
■ Prolonged bed rest
■ Trauma
■ Surgery
■ Pregnancy and childbirth
■ Hormonal contraceptives such as estrogens
■ Neoplasms
■ Fracture of the spine, pelvis, femur, or tibia
■ Venous stasis
■ Venulitis

COMPLICATIONS
■ Pulmonary embolism
■ Chronic venous insufficiency

Assessment

HISTORY
■ Asymptomatic in up to 50% of patients with deep vein thrombophlebitis
■ Possible tenderness, aching, or severe pain in the affected leg or arm; fever, chills, and malaise

PHYSICAL FINDINGS
■ Redness, swelling, and tenderness of the affected leg or arm
■ Possible positive Homans' sign
■ Positive cuff sign
■ Possible warm feeling in affected leg or arm
■ Lymphadenitis in case of extensive vein involvement

TEST RESULTS
Diagnostic procedures
■ Doppler ultrasonography shows reduced blood flow to a specific area and any obstruction to venous flow, particularly in iliofemoral deep vein thrombophlebitis.
■ Plethysmography shows decreased circulation distal to the affected area; it's more sensitive than ultrasonography in detecting deep vein thrombophlebitis.
■ Phlebography is usually used to confirm the diagnosis and shows filling defects and diverted blood flow.

Treatment

GENERAL
■ Application of warm, moist compresses to the affected area
■ Antiembolism stockings

DIET
■ No restrictions

ACTIVITY
■ Bed rest, with elevation of the affected extremity

MEDICATION
■ Anticoagulants
■ Thrombolytics
■ Analgesics

SURGERY
■ Simple ligation to vein plication, or clipping
■ Embolectomy
■ Caval interruption with transvenous placement of a vena cava filter

MONITORING
■ Signs and symptoms of bleeding
■ Vital signs
■ Partial thromboplastin time for patient on heparin therapy

- Prothrombin time for patient on warfarin
- Signs and symptoms of heparin-induced thrombocytopenia
- Signs and symptoms of pulmonary embolism
- Response to treatment

TREATMENTS

ANGIOPLASTY, PERCUTANEOUS TRANSLUMINAL CORONARY

Overview

- Nonsurgical alternative to coronary artery bypass surgery; commonly called PTCA
- Uses a tiny balloon catheter to dilate a coronary artery narrowed by atherosclerotic plaque (see *Relieving occlusions with angioplasty,* page 222)
- Less expensive than coronary artery bypass surgery, with shorter length of stay
- Most likely to be performed on a patient who has had disabling angina for less than 1 year
- May require that patient be pre-screened for eligibility for coronary artery bypass surgery, which may be done if PTCA fails

INDICATIONS
- Documented myocardial ischemia
- Proximal lesion in a single coronary artery
- Multivessel disease
- Acute myocardial infarction (MI)
- Totally occluded coronary arteries
- Postthrombolytic therapy with high-grade stenosis
- Previous coronary artery bypass surgery
- High risk for complications associated with coronary artery bypass surgery
- Stenosis that narrows the arterial lumen by 70% or greater

COMPLICATIONS
- Arterial dissection
- Coronary artery rupture
- Cardiac tamponade
- Myocardial ischemia
- MI
- Abrupt reclosure of the affected artery (occurs within a few hours of PTCA)
- Restenosis (occurs 3 to 6 months later)
- Coronary artery spasm
- Arrhythmias
- Bleeding
- Hematoma
- Thromboembolism
- Adverse reactions to contrast medium

Nursing interventions

PRETREATMENT CARE
- Explain the treatment and preparation to the patient and his family.
- Make sure the patient has signed an appropriate consent form.
- Tell the patient that contrast medium injection may cause a flushing sensation or transient nausea.
- Check for and report a history of allergies or adverse reactions to shellfish, iodine, or contrast medium.

RELIEVING OCCLUSIONS WITH ANGIOPLASTY

For a patient with an occluded coronary artery, percutaneous transluminal coronary angioplasty can open the artery without opening the chest — an important advantage over bypass surgery.

First, coronary angioplasty must confirm the presence and location of the arterial occlusion. Then, a guide catheter is threaded through the patient's femoral artery into the coronary artery under fluoroscopic guidance.

When angiography shows the guide catheter positioned at the occlusion site (top illustration), a smaller double-lumen balloon catheter is carefully inserted through the guide catheter and the balloon is directed through the occlusion (below, left). A marked pressure gradient is obvious.

The balloon is alternately inflated and deflated until an angiogram verifies successful arterial dilation (below, right) and that the pressure gradient has decreased.

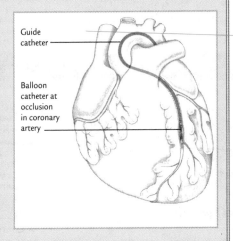

Guide catheter

Balloon catheter at occlusion in coronary artery

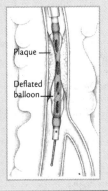

Plaque

Deflated balloon

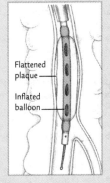

Flattened plaque

Inflated balloon

■ Restrict food and fluid intake for at least 6 hours before the procedure.
■ Obtain results of coagulation studies, complete blood count, serum electrolyte studies, blood area nitrogen, and blood typing and crossmatching as ordered.
■ Locate and mark bilateral distal pulses.
■ Administer a sedative as ordered.

Monitoring
■ Vital signs

■ Color, temperature, and sensation of extremities

POSTTREATMENT CARE
■ Administer anticoagulants and I.V. nitroglycerin as ordered.
■ Administer I.V. fluids as ordered.
■ Keep the affected extremity straight as ordered.
■ Elevate the head of the bed no more than 15 degrees as ordered.
■ If an expanding ecchymosis appears, mark the area, and obtain he-

moglobin and hematocrit samples as ordered.
■ Report bleeding sites to the physician, and apply direct pressure to them.
■ After sheath removal, apply direct pressure to the insertion site until hemostasis occurs.
■ Apply a pressure dressing as ordered.

MONITORING
■ Vital signs
■ Intake and output
■ Heart rate and rhythm
■ Electrocardiogram
■ Invasive arterial pressures
■ Peripheral pulses
■ Neurovascular status of extremities
■ Hematoma formation, ecchymosis, or bleeding at the catheter insertion site
■ Chest pain or other angina symptoms
■ Signs and symptoms of infection
■ Fluid overload
■ Abrupt arterial reclosure

PATIENT TEACHING
Be sure to cover:
■ medications and possible adverse reactions
■ puncture site care
■ activity restrictions if applicable
■ follow-up care and testing
■ signs and symptoms of bleeding, infection, and restenosis
■ complications
■ when to notify the physician.

CORONARY ARTERY BYPASS GRAFTING

Overview

■ Grafting of a blood vessel segment from another part of the body to create an alternate circulatory route that bypasses an occluded area of a coronary artery, thus restoring normal blood flow to the myocardium
■ Usually the saphenous vein or internal mammary artery is used for grafting
■ Can relieve anginal pain and improve cardiac function, and may enhance the quality of life
■ Commonly called CABG
■ Sometimes involves a minimally invasive surgical procedure

INDICATIONS
■ Medically uncontrolled angina that adversely affects the quality of life
■ Left main coronary artery disease (CAD)
■ Severe proximal left anterior descending coronary artery stenosis
■ Three-vessel CAD with proximal stenoses or left ventricular dysfunction
■ Three-vessel CAD with normal left ventricular function at rest, but with inducible ischemia and poor exercise capacity

COMPLICATIONS
■ Cardiac arrhythmias
■ Hypertension or hypotension
■ Cardiac tamponade
■ Thromboembolism
■ Hemorrhage
■ Postpericardiotomy syndrome
■ Myocardial infarction
■ Stroke
■ Postoperative depression or emotional instability
■ Pulmonary embolism
■ Decreased renal function
■ Infection
■ Graft rupture or closure

Nursing interventions

PRETREATMENT CARE
■ Explain the treatment and preparation to the patient and his family.

■ Make sure the patient has signed an appropriate consent form.
■ Explain what to expect during the immediate postoperative period including:
- endotracheal tube and mechanical ventilator
- cardiac monitor
- nasogastric tube, chest tube, indwelling urinary catheter, and arterial line
- epicardial pacing wires
- pulmonary artery catheter.
■ Institute cardiac monitoring.
■ The evening before surgery, have the patient shower with antiseptic soap as ordered.
■ Restrict food and fluids after midnight as ordered.
■ Provide sedation as ordered.
■ Assist with pulmonary artery catheterization and insertion of arterial lines.

POSTTREATMENT CARE

■ Keep emergency resuscitative equipment immediately available.
■ Maintain arterial pressure within the limits set by the physician.
■ Adjust ordered I.V. medications according to facility protocol.
■ Maintain chest tube patency.
■ Administer medications as ordered.
■ Assist with weaning the patient from the ventilator as appropriate.
■ Promote chest physiotherapy.
■ Encourage coughing, deep breathing, and incentive spirometry use.
■ Assist the patient with range-of-motion (ROM) exercises.

Monitoring

■ Vital signs
■ Intake and output
■ Heart rate and rhythm
■ Heart sounds
■ Hemodynamic values
■ Complications
■ Nutritional status

■ Electrocardiogram
■ Arterial blood gas analysis
■ Breath sounds
■ Peripheral vascular status
■ Respiratory status
■ Cardiovascular status
■ Neurologic status
■ Renal function
■ Chest tube patency and drainage
■ Surgical wounds and dressings
■ Drainage
■ Electrolyte imbalances
■ Sternal stability

PATIENT TEACHING

Be sure to cover:
■ medications and possible adverse reactions
■ incentive spirometry
■ ROM exercises
■ incision care
■ signs and symptoms of infection, arterial reocclusion, and postpericardiotomy syndrome
■ how to identify and cope with postoperative depression
■ complications
■ when to notify the physician
■ dietary restrictions
■ activity restrictions
■ adequate rest periods
■ prescribed exercise program
■ smoking cessation
■ follow-up care
■ referral to the Mended Hearts Club and American Heart Association for information and support.

ENDARTERECTOMY, CAROTID

Overview

■ Surgical removal of atheromatous plaque from the inner lining of the carotid artery

■ Improves intracranial perfusion by increasing blood flow through the carotid artery

INDICATIONS
■ Reversible ischemic neurologic deficit
■ Completed stroke
■ Transient ischemic attack
■ High-grade asymptomatic or ulcerative lesions
■ Concurrent coronary artery disease

COMPLICATIONS
■ Blood pressure lability
■ Preoperative stroke
■ Temporary or permanent loss of carotid body function
■ Thrombosis
■ Respiratory distress
■ Wound infection
■ Ipsilateral vascular headache
■ Seizures
■ Intracerebral hemorrhage
■ Vocal cord paralysis
■ Transient or permanent neurologic deficit

Nursing interventions

PRETREATMENT CARE
■ Explain the treatment and preparation to the patient and his family.
■ Make sure the patient has signed an appropriate consent form.
■ Explain postoperative care and equipment.
■ Perform a complete neurologic assessment.
■ Assist with any invasive procedures as appropriate.
■ Obtain a baseline electroencephalogram before the patient is anesthetized as ordered.

POSTTREATMENT CARE
■ Perform a neurologic assessment every hour for the first 24 hours; check extremity strength, fine hand movements, speech, orientation, and level of consciousness.
■ Obtain an electrocardiogram if the patient experiences chest pain or arrhythmias.

Monitoring
■ Vital signs
■ Intake and output
■ Heart rate and rhythm
■ Neurologic status
■ Respiratory status
■ Surgical wound and dressings
■ Drainage
■ Cervical edema
■ Infection
■ Seizures

PATIENT TEACHING
Be sure to cover:
■ medications and possible adverse reactions
■ surgical wound care
■ signs and symptoms of infection
■ complications
■ when to notify the physician
■ risk factor modification, including:
– smoking cessation
– lipid lowering therapy
– weight reduction
– control of hypertension and diabetes mellitus
– regular exercise regimen
■ follow-up care
■ management of neurologic, sensory, or motor deficits
■ referral to a home health care agency as indicated.

HEART VALVE REPLACEMENT

Overview

■ Excision of a diseased heart valve and replacement with a mechanical or biological valve prosthesis

■ Usually involves a medial sternotomy approach

■ Alternatively, may involve a minimally invasive-port access approach, which eliminates the need for a large, invasive median sternotomy incision

INDICATIONS

■ Severe aortic valvular stenosis or insufficiency

■ Severe mitral valvular stenosis or insufficiency

COMPLICATIONS

■ Periprosthetic care
■ Cardiac arrhythmias
■ Hemorrhage
■ Coagulopathy
■ Stroke
■ Prosthetic valve endocarditis
■ Valve dysfunction or failure
■ Renal failure
■ Pulmonary embolism
■ Thromboembolism

Nursing interventions

PRETREATMENT CARE

■ Explain the treatment and preparation to the patient and his family.

■ Make sure the patient has signed an appropriate consent form.

■ Explain postoperative care and equipment.

■ Obtain results of laboratory studies, including blood typing and crossmatching.

POSTTREATMENT CARE

■ Administer medications as ordered.

■ Assist with temporary epicardial pacing as indicated.

■ Maintain mean arterial pressure within prescribed guidelines (usually between 70 and 100 mm Hg in an adult).

■ Maintain the chest tube system as ordered.

■ Administer I.V. fluids and blood products as ordered.

■ Perform chest physiotherapy.

■ Assist with weaning from the mechanical ventilator as indicated.

■ Encourage coughing, turning, and deep breathing.

■ Encourage the use of incentive spirometry.

■ Assist with early ambulation.

Monitoring

■ Vital signs
■ Intake and output
■ Daily weight
■ Complications
■ Cardiovascular status
■ Heart rate and rhythm
■ Heart sounds, including prosthetic valve sounds
■ Hemodynamic values
■ Respiratory status
■ Arterial blood gas analysis
■ Laboratory test results
■ Surgical wound and dressings
■ Abnormal bleeding
■ Drainage
■ Sternal stability

PATIENT TEACHING

Be sure to cover:

■ medications and possible adverse reactions
■ surgical wound care
■ signs and symptoms of infection
■ signs and symptoms of postpericardiotomy syndrome
■ complications
■ when to notify the physician
■ anticoagulant therapy
■ infective endocarditis prophylaxis
■ abnormal bleeding
■ balancing activity with rest
■ prescribed dietary restrictions
■ prescribed activity restrictions
■ prescribed exercise program
■ follow-up care

- importance of informing all health care providers of the prosthetic valve
- importance of wearing medical identification.

IMPLANTABLE CARDIOVERTER-DEFIBRILLATOR

Overview

- An implanted electronic device (also called an ICD) that monitors the heart for bradycardia, ventricular tachycardia, and fibrillation and delivers shocks or paced beats when indicated
- Stores information and electrocardiograms (ECGs) and tracks treatments and their outcome
- Allows information retrieval to evaluate the device's function and battery status and to adjust the settings
- Depending on the model, may deliver bradycardia pacing (both single- and dual-chamber), antitachycardia pacing, cardioversion, and defibrillation (see *Understanding the ICD*)

INDICATIONS

- Cardiac arrhythmias refractory to drug therapy, surgery, or catheter ablation
- Therapy for atrial arrhythmias such as atrial fibrillation

COMPLICATIONS

- Infection
- Venous thrombosis and embolism
- Pneumothorax
- Pectoral or diaphragmatic muscle stimulation
- Arrhythmias
- Cardiac tamponade
- Heart failure
- Lead dislodgment

UNDERSTANDING THE ICD

The implantable cardioverter-defibrillator (ICD) has a programmable pulse generator and lead system that monitors the heart's activity, detects ventricular arrhythmias and other tachyarrhythmias, and responds with appropriate therapies. The range of therapies includes antitachycardia and antibradycardia pacing, cardioversion, and defibrillation. Newer ICDs can also pace the atrium and ventricle.

Implantation of the ICD is similar to that of a permanent pacemaker. The cardiologist positions the lead (or leads) transvenously in the endocardium of the right ventricle (and the right atrium, if both chambers require pacing). The lead connects to a generator box implanted in the right or left upper chest near the clavicle.

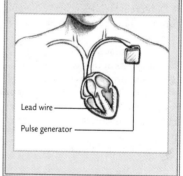

Lead wire

Pulse generator

- ICD malfunction, resulting in untreated ventricular fibrillation and cardiac arrest

Nursing interventions

PRETREATMENT CARE

- Explain the treatment and preparation to the patient and his family.

■ Make sure the patient has signed an appropriate consent form.
■ Obtain baseline vital signs and a 12-lead ECG.
■ Evaluate the patient's radial and pedal pulses.
■ Assess the patient's mental status.
■ Restrict food and fluids before the procedure as ordered.
■ Explain postoperative care.
■ If the patient is monitored, document and report any arrhythmias.
■ Administer medications as ordered, and prepare to assist with medical procedures (such as defibrillation) if indicated.

POSTTREATMENT CARE

■ Obtain a printed status report verifying the ICD type and model, status (on or off), detection rates, and therapies to be delivered (such as pacing, antitachycardia pacing, cardioversion, and defibrillation).
■ Don't remove the occlusive dressing for the first 24 hours without a physician's order.
■ After the first 24 hours, begin passive range-of-motion exercises if ordered, and progress as tolerated.
■ If the patient experiences cardiac arrest, initiate cardiopulmonary resuscitation and advanced cardiac life support.

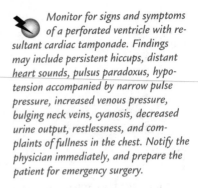 *For external defibrillation, use anteroposterior paddle placement; don't place paddles directly over the pulse generator.*

Monitoring

■ Vital signs
■ Intake and output
■ Heart rate and rhythm
■ Complications
■ Surgical incision and dressings
■ Drainage
■ Infection

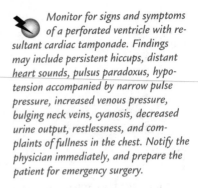 *Monitor for signs and symptoms of a perforated ventricle with resultant cardiac tamponade. Findings may include persistent hiccups, distant heart sounds, pulsus paradoxus, hypotension accompanied by narrow pulse pressure, increased venous pressure, bulging neck veins, cyanosis, decreased urine output, restlessness, and complaints of fullness in the chest. Notify the physician immediately, and prepare the patient for emergency surgery.*

PATIENT TEACHING

Be sure to cover:
■ medications and possible adverse reactions
■ signs and symptoms of infection
■ complications
■ when to notify the physician
■ importance of wearing medical alert identification that indicates ICD placement and of carrying ICD information at all times
■ what to do in an emergency, such as calling 911 and having a family member perform cardiopulmonary resuscitation if the ICD fails
■ avoidance of placing excessive pressure over the insertion site or moving or jerking the area, until the physician approves
■ prescribed activity restrictions
■ what to expect when the ICD discharges
■ notifying the physician when the ICD discharges
■ importance of informing airline personnel and health care workers who perform diagnostic tests (such as computed tomography scans and magnetic resonance imaging) of ICD presence
■ possible disruption of the ICD by electrical or electronic devices
■ follow-up care.

TYPES OF TEMPORARY PACEMAKERS

Temporary pacemakers come in three types: transcutaneous, transvenous, and epicardial. They're used to pace the heart after cardiac surgery, during cardiopulmonary resuscitation, and when sinus arrest, symptomatic sinus bradycardia, or complete heart block occurs.

Transcutaneous pacemaker
Completely noninvasive and easily applied, a transcutaneous pacemaker proves especially useful in an emergency. To perform pacing with the device, the physician places electrodes on the skin directly over the heart and connects them to a pulse generator.

Transvenous pacemaker
This balloon-tipped pacing catheter is inserted via the subclavian or jugular vein into the right ventricle. The procedure can be done at the bedside or in the cardiac catheterization laboratory. A transvenous pacemaker offers better control of the heartbeat than a transcutaneous pacemaker. However, electrode insertion takes longer, limiting its usefulness in emergencies.

Epicardial pacemaker
Implanted during open-heart surgery, an epicardial pacemaker permits rapid treatment of postoperative complications. During surgery, the physician attaches the leads to the heart and runs them out through the chest incision. Afterward, the leads are coiled on the patient's chest, insulated, and covered with a dressing. If pacing is needed, the leads are simply uncovered and attached to a pulse generator. When pacing is no longer needed, the leads can be removed under local anesthesia.

PACEMAKER INSERTION

Overview

- Pacemaker: battery-operated generator that controls heart rate by emitting timed electrical signals that trigger contraction of the heart muscle; may be temporary or permanent (see *Types of temporary pacemakers;* see also *Pacemaker coding systems,* page 230, *Pacemaker spikes,* page 231, and *When a temporary pacemaker malfunctions,* pages 232 and 233)
- In a new type of permanent pacemaker, the biventricular pacemaker, pacing leads are placed in the right and left ventricles, enabling both ventricles to be paced together. When used to treat patients with heart failure, these devices improve the activity tolerance of these patients.

INDICATIONS
Temporary pacemaker
- Emergency treatment of symptomatic bradycardia
- Bridge to permanent pacemaker implantation or to determine the effect of pacing on cardiac function
- Open-heart surgery

Permanent pacemaker
- Symptomatic bradycardia
- Advanced symptomatic atrioventricular block
- Sick sinus syndrome
- Sinus arrest

PACEMAKER CODING SYSTEMS

The capabilities of permanent pacemakers are described by a five-letter coding system, though typically only the first three letters are used.

First letter
The first letter identifies which heart chambers are paced. Here are the letters used to signify these options:
■ V = Ventricle
■ A = Atrium
■ D = Dual (ventricle and atrium)
■ 0 = None.

Second letter
The second letter signifies the heart chamber where the pacemaker senses the intrinsic activity:
■ V = Ventricle
■ A = Atrium
■ D = Dual
■ 0 = None.

Third letter
The third letter shows the pacemaker's response to the intrinsic electrical activity it senses in the atrium or ventricle:
■ T = Triggers pacing
■ I = Inhibits pacing
■ D = Dual; can be triggered or inhibited depending on the mode and where intrinsic activity occurs
■ 0 = None; doesn't change mode in response to sensed activity.

Fourth letter
The fourth letter denotes the pacemaker's programmability; it tells whether the pacemaker can be modified by an external programming device:
■ P = Basic functions programmable
■ M = Multiprogrammable parameters
■ C = Communicating functions such as telemetry
■ R = Rate responsiveness — rate adjusts to fit the patient's metabolic needs and achieve normal hemodynamic status
■ 0 = None.

Fifth letter
The fifth letter denotes the pacemaker's response to a tachyarrhythmia:
■ P = Pacing ability — the pacemaker's rapid burst paces the heart at a rate above its intrinsic rate to override the tachycardia source
■ S = Shock — an implantable cardioverter-defibrillator identifies ventricular tachycardia and delivers a shock to stop the arrhythmia
■ D = Dual ability to shock and pace
■ 0 = None.

■ Sinoatrial block
■ Stokes-Adams syndrome
■ Tachyarrhythmias
■ Arrhythmias caused by antiarrhythmic drugs

■ Arrhythmias
■ Cardiac tamponade
■ Heart failure
■ Pacemaker malfunction

COMPLICATIONS
■ Infection
■ Venous thrombosis, embolism
■ Pneumothorax
■ Pectoral or diaphragmatic muscle stimulation from the pacemaker

Nursing interventions

PRETREATMENT CARE
■ Explain the treatment and preparation to the patient and his family.
■ Make sure the patient has signed an appropriate consent form.

PACEMAKER SPIKES

Pacemaker impulses, the stimuli that travel from the pacemaker to the heart, are visible on the patient's electrocardiogram tracing as spikes. Whether large or small, the spikes appear above or below the isoelectric line. This example shows an atrial and a ventricular pacemaker spike.

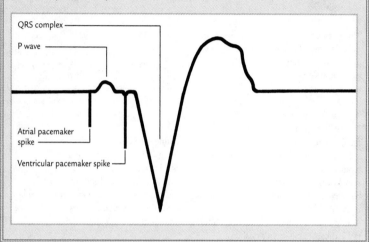

- Explain postoperative care.
- Obtain baseline vital signs and a 12-lead electrocardiogram.
- Restrict food and fluids as ordered.

POSTTREATMENT CARE
- Administer medications as ordered.
- Maintain continuous cardiac monitoring.
- Document the type of pacemaker inserted, lead system, pacemaker mode, and pacing guidelines.
- If the patient requires defibrillation, place paddles at least 4″ (10 cm) from the pulse generator; avoid anteroposterior paddle placement.
- After first 24 hours, begin passive range-of-motion exercises on the affected arm if ordered.

Monitoring
- Vital signs

- Intake and output
- Complications
- Surgical wound and dressing
- Drainage
- Abnormal bleeding
- Infection
- Cardiac arrhythmias
- Pacemaker function

PATIENT TEACHING
Be sure to cover:
- medications and adverse reactions
- complications and when to notify the physician
- incision care
- prescribed activity restrictions
- how to monitor the heart rate and rhythm
- avoidance of placing excessive pressure over the insertion site, making sudden moves, or extending arms over head for 8 weeks after discharge

WHEN A TEMPORARY PACEMAKER MALFUNCTIONS

Occasionally, a temporary pacemaker may fail to function appropriately. When this occurs, you'll need to take immediate action to correct the problem. Here you'll learn which steps to take when your patient's pacemaker fails to pace, capture, or sense intrinsic beats.

Failure to pace

This happens when the pacemaker either doesn't fire or fires too often. The pulse generator may not be working properly, or it may not be conducting the impulse to the patient.

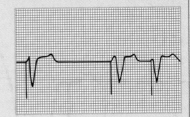

Nursing interventions

■ If the pacing or sensing indicator flashes, check the connections to the cable and the position of the pacing electrode in the patient (by X-ray). The cable may have come loose, or the electrode may have been dislodged, pulled out, or broken.
■ If the pulse generator is turned on but the indicators still aren't flashing, change the battery. If that doesn't help, use a different pulse generator.
■ Check the settings if the pacemaker is firing too rapidly. If they're correct or if altering them (according to facility policy or the physician's order) doesn't help, change the pulse generator.

Failure to capture

Here, you see pacemaker spikes but the heart isn't responding. This may be caused by changes in the pacing threshold from ischemia, an electrolyte imbalance (high or low potassium or magnesium levels), acidosis, an adverse reaction to a medication, a perforated ventricle, fibrosis, or the position of the electrode.

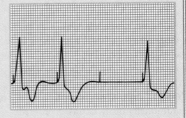

Nursing interventions

■ If the patient's condition has changed, notify the physician and ask him for new settings.
■ If pacemaker settings are altered by the patient or another, return them to their correct positions. Then make sure the face of the pacemaker is covered with a plastic shield. Tell the patient or others not to touch the dials.
■ If the heart isn't responding, try any or all of these suggestions: Carefully check all connections; increase the milliamperes slowly (according to facility policy or the physician's order); turn the patient on his left side, then on his right (if turning him to the left didn't help); schedule an anteroposterior or lateral chest X-ray to determine the position of the electrode.

WHEN A TEMPORARY PACEMAKER MALFUNCTIONS *(continued)*

Failure to sense intrinsic beats

This could cause ventricular tachycardia or ventricular fibrillation if the pacemaker fires on the vulnerable T wave. This could be caused by the pacemaker sensing an external stimulus as a QRS complex, which could lead to asystole, or by the pacemaker not being sensitive enough, which means it could fire anywhere within the cardiac cycle.

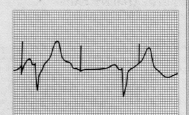

Nursing interventions

■ If the pacing is undersensing, turn the sensitivity control completely to the right. If it's oversensing, turn it slightly to the left.
■ If the pacemaker isn't functioning correctly, change the battery or the pulse generator.
■ Remove items in the room causing electromechanical interference (razors, radios, cautery devices, and so on).

Check the ground wires on the bed and other equipment for obvious damage. Unplug each piece and see if the interference stops. When you locate the cause, notify the staff engineer and ask him to check it.
■ If the pacemaker is still firing on the T wave and all else has failed, notify the physician and turn off the pacemaker. Make sure atropine is available in case the patient's heart rate drops. Be prepared to call a code and institute cardiopulmonary resuscitation if necessary.

■ prescribed diet and exercises
■ pacemaker identification
■ importance of informing medical personnel of the implanted pacemaker before certain diagnostic tests
■ how to test pacemaker function
■ follow-up care.

THROMBOLYTIC THERAPY

Overview

■ Administration of a thrombolytic drug (such as streptokinase, alteplase, anistreplase, or reteplase) to rapidly correct acute and extensive thrombotic disorders
■ Involves conversion of plasminogen to plasmin by thrombolytic drugs, which leads to lysis of thrombi, fibrinogen, and other plasma proteins

INDICATIONS

■ Thromboembolic disorders
■ Deep vein thrombosis
■ Peripheral arterial occlusion
■ Acute myocardial infarction
■ Acute pulmonary emboli
■ Failing or failed atrioventricular fistulas

COMPLICATIONS

■ Bleeding
■ Adverse reactions to the thrombolytic
■ Streptokinase resistance (with repeated use of this drug)
■ Arrhythmias

Nursing interventions

PRETREATMENT CARE
■ Explain the treatment and preparation to the patient and his family.
■ Make sure the patient has signed an appropriate consent form.
■ Explain postprocedure care.
■ Obtain samples for blood typing and crossmatching and for coagulation studies.
■ Obtain a baseline electrocardiogram and serum electrolyte, arterial blood gas, blood urea nitrogen, creatinine, and cardiac enzyme levels as ordered.

POSTTREATMENT CARE
■ Administer medications as ordered.
■ Minimize invasive procedures and venipunctures.
■ Administer anticoagulants as ordered.
■ Provide comfort measures.
■ Provide supplemental oxygen as ordered.
■ Restrict physical activity as ordered.

Monitoring
■ Vital signs
■ Intake and output
■ Hypersensitivity reactions
■ Abnormal bleeding
■ Heart rate and rhythm
■ Peripheral pulses
■ Motor and sensory function
■ Respiratory status
■ Coagulation studies

PATIENT TEACHING
Be sure to cover:
■ medications and possible adverse reactions
■ abnormal bleeding
■ signs and symptoms of thrombus formation and thromboembolic events
■ complications

■ when to notify the physician
■ prevention of thrombotic events
■ smoking cessation
■ follow-up care.

VALVULOPLASTY, BALLOON

Overview

■ Insertion of a balloon-tipped catheter through the femoral vein or artery and then into the heart, followed by repeated balloon inflation against the leaflets of a diseased heart valve
■ Enlarges the heart valve

INDICATIONS
■ Congenital valve defect
■ Valve calcification
■ Valvular stenosis secondary to rheumatic fever or aging
■ When the patient is a poor candidate for valve surgery

COMPLICATIONS
■ Valvular insufficiency
■ Embolism
■ Valve leaflet damage
■ Bleeding and hematoma at the arterial puncture site
■ Arrhythmias
■ Myocardial ischemia
■ Myocardial infarction
■ Circulatory insufficiency distal to the catheter entry site
■ Restenosis

Nursing interventions

PRETREATMENT CARE
■ Explain the treatment and preparation to the patient and his family.
■ Make sure the patient has signed an appropriate consent form.

- Restrict food and fluid intake as ordered.
- Explain postprocedure care.
- Obtain routine laboratory studies; report abnormal results.
- Make sure blood typing and cross-matching are completed.
- Palpate bilateral distal pulses (usually the dorsalis pedis or posterior tibial pulses) and mark them a skin marker.
- Obtain baseline vital signs.
- Assess baseline color, temperature, and sensation in the extremities.
- Administer a sedative as ordered.

If the patient is waiting for aortic aneurysm repair surgery, monitor for and immediately report signs and symptoms of acute dissection, such as sudden, excruciating chest or back pain, commonly described as tearing, ripping, or splitting. Other symptoms, resulting from involvement of major aortic branches, may include angina (coronary artery origin), neurologic deficits (carotid artery involvement), or limb ischemia (distal aorta compromise).

If the patient is waiting for aortic aneurysm repair surgery, be sure to watch for and immediately report the classic triad of shock, pulsatile mass, and abdominal or back pain, which highly suggests rupture.

POSTTREATMENT CARE

- Administer medications as ordered.
- Keep the affected leg straight as ordered.
- Elevate the head of the bed no more than 15 degrees as ordered.
- Immediately report diminished or absent peripheral pulses.
- If bleeding occurs, apply direct pressure and notify the physician.
- Provide I.V. fluids as ordered.
- After catheter removal, apply a pressure dressing as ordered.

Monitoring

- Vital signs
- Intake and output
- Heart rate and rhythm
- Heart sounds
- Puncture site and dressings
- Drainage
- Abnormal bleeding
- Vascular compromise
- Complications

PATIENT TEACHING

Be sure to cover:
- medications and possible adverse reactions
- prescribed activity restrictions
- abnormal bleeding
- signs and symptoms of valvular stenosis and insufficiency
- complications
- when to notify the physician
- follow-up care.

VASCULAR REPAIR

Overview

- May involve aneurysm resection, bypass grafting, embolectomy, or vein stripping
- Serves as the treatment of choice for damaged vessels

INDICATIONS

- Vessel damaged by an arteriosclerotic or thromboembolic disorder
- Aortic aneurysm
- Arterial occlusive disease
- Limb-threatening acute arterial occlusion
- Vessel trauma, infection, or congenital defect
- Vascular disease that doesn't respond to drug therapy or nonsurgical revascularization

COMPLICATIONS

- Vessel trauma
- Thrombus formation
- Embolism
- Hemorrhage
- Infection
- With bypass grafting: graft occlusion, narrowing, dilation, or rupture

Nursing interventions

PRETREATMENT CARE

- Explain the treatment and preparation to the patient and his family.
- Make sure the patient has signed an appropriate consent form.
- Explain postoperative care.
- Perform a complete vascular assessment.
- Obtain baseline vital signs.
- Evaluate pulses, noting any bruits.
- Restrict food and fluids as ordered.
- Administer sedation as ordered.

If the patient is awaiting surgery for aortic aneurysm repair, monitor for signs and symptom of acute dissection or rupture, and call the physician immediately if these appear. Emergency surgery may be necessary.

POSTTREATMENT CARE

- Administer medications as ordered.
- Position the patient as ordered.
- Explain recommended activity levels during the early recovery stage.
- Provide comfort measures.
- Use Doppler ultrasonography if peripheral pulses aren't palpable.
- As the patient's condition improves assist with weaning from the mechanical ventilator (if used).
- Encourage frequent coughing, turning, and deep breathing.
- Help with range-of-motion exercises.
- Provide incision care.
- Change dressings as ordered.

Monitoring

- Vital signs
- Intake and output
- Neurovascular status
- Heart rate and rhythm
- Hemodynamic values
- Complications
- Surgical wound and dressings
- Drainage
- Abnormal bleeding
- Infection

PATIENT TEACHING

Be sure to cover:

- medications and possible adverse reactions
- palpation and monitoring of peripheral pulses
- monitoring extremities for changes in temperature, sensation, and motor ability
- incision care
- signs and symptoms of infection
- complications
- when to notify the physician
- follow-up care
- smoking cessation
- risk factor modification.

PROCEDURES AND EQUIPMENT

ARTERIAL PRESSURE MONITORING: UNDERSTANDING THE ARTERIAL WAVEFORM

Normal arterial blood pressure produces a characteristic waveform, representing ventricular systole and diastole. The waveform has five distinct components: the anacrotic limb, systolic peak, dicrotic limb, dicrotic notch, and end diastole.

The *anacrotic limb* marks the waveform's initial upstroke, which results as blood is rapidly ejected from the ventricle through the open aortic valve into the aorta. The rapid ejection causes a sharp rise in arterial pressure, which appears as the waveform's highest point. This is called the *systolic peak*.

As blood continues into the peripheral vessels, arterial pressure falls, and the waveform begins a downward trend. This part is called *the dicrotic limb*. Arterial pressure usually will continue to fall until pressure in the ventricle is less than pressure in the aortic root. When this occurs, the aortic valve closes. This event appears as a small notch (the *dicrotic notch*) on the waveform's downside.

When the aortic valve closes, diastole begins, progressing until the aortic root pressure gradually descends to its lowest point. On the waveform, this is known as *end diastole*.

Normal arterial waveform

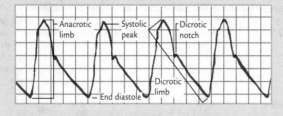

RECOGNIZING ABNORMAL ARTERIAL WAVEFORMS

Understanding a normal arterial waveform is relatively straightforward. However, an abnormal waveform is more difficult to decipher. Abnormal patterns and markings, however, may provide important diagnostic clues to the patient's cardiovascular status, or they may simply signal trouble in the monitor. Use this table to help you recognize and resolve waveform abnormalities.

Abnormality	Possible causes	Nursing interventions
Alternating high and low waves in a regular pattern		
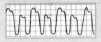	■ Ventricular bigeminy	■ Check the patient's electrocardiogram to confirm ventricular bigeminy. The tracing should reflect premature ventricular contractions every second beat.
Flattened waveform		
	■ Over-damped waveform or hypotensive patient	■ Check the patient's blood pressure with a sphygmomanometer. If you obtain a reading, suspect overdamping. Correct the problem by checking the pressure or the pressure bag and increasing, if necessary, or trying to aspirate the arterial line. If you succeed, flush the line. If the reading is very low or absent, suspect hypotension.
Slightly rounded waveform with consistent variations in systolic height		
	■ Patient on ventilator with positive end-expiratory pressure	■ Check the patient's systolic blood pressure regularly. The difference between the highest and lowest systolic pressure reading should be less than 10 mm Hg. If the difference exceeds that amount, suspect pulsus paradoxus, possibly from cardiac tamponade.
Slow upstroke		
	■ Aortic stenosis	■ Check the patient's heart sounds for signs of aortic stenosis and notify the physician.
Diminished amplitude on inspiration		
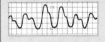	■ Pulsus paradoxus, possibly from cardiac tamponade, constrictive pericarditis, or lung disease	■ Note systolic pressure during inspiration and expiration. If inspiratory pressure is at least 10 mm Hg less than expiratory pressure, call the physician. ■ If you're also monitoring pulmonary artery pressure, observe for a diastolic plateau. This occurs when the mean central venous pressure (right atrial pressure), mean pulmonary artery pressure, and mean pulmonary artery wedge pressure are within 5 mm Hg of one another.

CARDIAC MONITORING:
POSITIONING MONITORING LEADS

This chart shows the correct electrode positions for some of the monitoring leads you'll commonly use. For each lead, you'll see electrode placement for a five-leadwire system, a three-leadwire system, and a telemetry system.

In the two-hardwire systems, the electrode positions for one lead may be identical to the electrode positions for another lead. In this case, you simply change the lead selector switch to the setting that corresponds to the lead you want. In some cases, you'll need to reposition the electrodes.

In the telemetry system, you can create the same lead with two electrodes that you do with three, simply by eliminating the ground electrode.

The illustrations below use these abbreviations: RA, right arm; LA, left arm; RL, right leg; LL, left leg; C, chest; and G, ground.

Five-leadwire system	Three-leadwire system	Telemetry system
Lead I		
Lead II		
Lead III		
Lead MCL$_1$		
Lead MCL$_6$		

THE LOOK OF MONITOR PROBLEMS

The following illustrations present the most commonly encountered monitor problems, including how to identify them, the possible causes, and possible interventions.

Waveform	Possible cause	Interventions
Artifact (waveform interference) 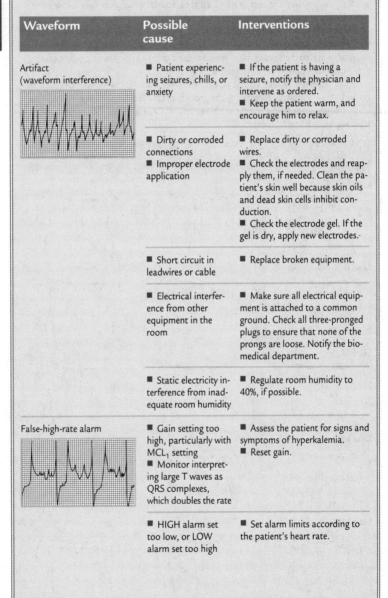	■ Patient experiencing seizures, chills, or anxiety	■ If the patient is having a seizure, notify the physician and intervene as ordered. ■ Keep the patient warm, and encourage him to relax.
	■ Dirty or corroded connections ■ Improper electrode application	■ Replace dirty or corroded wires. ■ Check the electrodes and reapply them, if needed. Clean the patient's skin well because skin oils and dead skin cells inhibit conduction. ■ Check the electrode gel. If the gel is dry, apply new electrodes.
	■ Short circuit in leadwires or cable	■ Replace broken equipment.
	■ Electrical interference from other equipment in the room	■ Make sure all electrical equipment is attached to a common ground. Check all three-pronged plugs to ensure that none of the prongs are loose. Notify the biomedical department.
	■ Static electricity interference from inadequate room humidity	■ Regulate room humidity to 40%, if possible.
False-high-rate alarm	■ Gain setting too high, particularly with MCL_1 setting ■ Monitor interpreting large T waves as QRS complexes, which doubles the rate	■ Assess the patient for signs and symptoms of hyperkalemia. ■ Reset gain.
	■ HIGH alarm set too low, or LOW alarm set too high	■ Set alarm limits according to the patient's heart rate.

THE LOOK OF MONITOR PROBLEMS (continued)

Waveform	Possible cause	Interventions
Weak signals 	■ Improper electrode application	■ Reapply the electrodes.
	■ QRS complex too small to register	■ Reset gain so that the height of the complex is greater than 1 mV. ■ Try monitoring the patient on another lead.
	■ Wire or cable failure	■ Replace any faulty wires or cables.
Wandering baseline 	■ Patient restless	■ Encourage the patient to relax.
	■ Chest wall movement during respiration	■ Make sure that tension on the cable isn't pulling the electrode away from the patient's body.
	■ Improper electrode application; electrode positioned over bone	■ Reposition improperly placed electrodes.
Fuzzy baseline (electrical interference) 	■ Electrical interference from other equipment in the room (60-cycle interference)	■ Ensure that all electrical equipment is attached to a common ground. ■ Check all three-pronged plugs to make sure none of the prongs are loose. Notify the biomedical department.
	■ Improper grounding of the patient's bed	■ Ensure that the bed ground is attached to the room's common ground.
	■ Electrode malfunction	■ Replace the electrodes.
Baseline (no waveform) 	■ Improper electrode placement (perpendicular to axis of heart)	■ Reposition improperly placed electrodes. ■ Assess the patient to be sure it's an equipment problem and not asystole.
	■ Electrode disconnected ■ Dry electrode gel	■ Check if electrodes are disconnected. ■ Check electrode gel. If the gel is dry, apply new electrodes.
	■ Wire or cable failure	■ Replace any faulty wires or cables.

Using an automated external defibrillator

It's estimated that 70% of sudden cardiac arrests are due to ventricular fibrillation (VF). An automated external defibrillator, or AED, is a defibrillator that can detect VF and rapid ventricular tachycardia (VT). After these rhythms are detected, the fully automated AED charges itself and delivers a shock. This reduces the time required for defibrillation.

Speedy defibrillation is the most important determinant of survival in a patient with VF. The longer it takes for defibrillation to occur, the less likely it becomes for defibrillation to be able to convert VF to a rhythm with a pulse. Defibrillation should occur before CPR is started in an unresponsive and pulseless patient unless a defibrillator isn't immediately available or if the AED indicates that the heart rhythm detected, such as asystole, shouldn't be shocked.

Types of AEDs

There are two basic types of AEDs: semiautomated (or shock-advisory) and fully automated. A semiautomated AED signals that the patient has a shockable arrhythmia (VF or pulseless VT with a rate greater than a preset rate set by the manufacturer), but the nurse must push the button for defibrillation to occur. The fully automated AED assesses the heart rhythm and automatically defibrillates if it detects VF or rapid VT — it requires only that the operator attach the defibrillatory pads and turn on the device.

Using a semiautomated AED

Until the Advanced Cardiac Life Support (ACLS) team arrives, follow this procedure if your patient is unresponsive.

■ First, assess the patient. If he's unresponsive, not breathing, and pulseless, call for help as you get an AED and attach it to the patient. Start CPR if there's a delay in obtaining or attaching the AED.

■ Turn on the power to the AED. Place one electrode pad on the chest, just below the right clavicle. Place the other pad at the cardiac apex to the left of the nipple line with the center of the electrode in the midaxillary line. The standard anterior-posterior positions may also be used as an acceptable alternative approach.

■ Press the button to analyze the patient's heart rhythm. If the AED indicates that the patient has a shockable rhythm, make sure everyone is clear of the bed, and push the shock button.

■ Defibrillate up to three times, if indicated. If the AED indicates that no further shocks are required, check for spontaneous pulse and respirations. Otherwise, check for pulse and breathing after the third defibrillation.

■ If there's no pulse, perform CPR for 1 minute, then check the pulse. If it's still absent, press the AED button to analyze the rhythm. If the AED indicates that the patient has a shockable rhythm, defibrillate up to three times, if indicated.

■ Continue this sequence until either shock is no longer advised (in which case, continue CPR), the pulse returns (in which case, assess vital signs, support airway and breathing, and provide appropriate medications for blood pressure and heart rate and rhythm), or until the ACLS team arrives.

BIPHASIC DEFIBRILLATORS

Most facility defibrillators are monophasic; they deliver a single current of electricity that travels in one direction between the two pads or paddles on the patient's chest. To be effective, they require a high amount of electric current.

Recently, new biphasic defibrillators have been introduced into facilities. Pad or paddle placement is the same as with the monophasic defibrillator. The difference is that the electric current discharged from the pads or paddles travels in a positive direction for a specified duration and then reverses and flows in a negative direction for the remaining time of the electrical discharge. It delivers two currents of electricity and lowers the defibrillation threshold of the heart muscle, making it possible to successfully defibrillate ventricular fibrillation (VF) with smaller amounts of energy. Instead of 200 joules, an initial shock of 150 joules is usually effective. The biphasic defibrillator is able to adjust for differences in impedance or the resistance of the current through the chest. This helps reduce the number of shocks needed to terminate VF. Biphasic technology utilizes lower energy levels and fewer shocks, and thus reduces the damage to the myocardial muscle. Biphasic defibrillators, when used at the clinically appropriate energy level, may be used for defibrillation and — when placed in the synchronized mode — for synchronized cardioversion.

HOW THE INTRA-AORTIC BALLOON PUMP WORKS

Made of polyurethane, the intra-aortic balloon is attached to an external pump console by means of a large-lumen catheter. The illustrations here show the direction of blood flow when the pump inflates and deflates the balloon.

Balloon inflation
The balloon inflates as the aortic valve closes and diastole begins. Diastole increases perfusion to the coronary arteries.

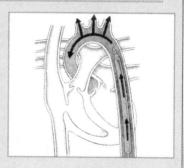

Balloon deflation
The balloon deflates before ventricular ejection, when the aortic valve opens. This permits ejection of blood from the left ventricle against a lowered resistance. As a result, aortic end-diastolic pressure and afterload decrease and cardiac output rises.

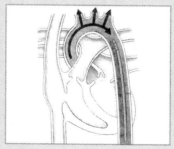

INTERPRETING INTRA-AORTIC BALLOON WAVEFORMS

During intra-aortic balloon counterpulsation, you can use electrocardiogram and arterial pressure waveforms to determine whether the balloon pump is functioning properly.

Normal inflation-deflation timing

Balloon inflation occurs after aortic valve closure; deflation, during isovolumetric contraction, just before the aortic valve opens. In a properly timed waveform, like the one shown at right, the inflation point lies at or slightly above the dicrotic notch. Both inflation and deflation cause a sharp V. Peak diastolic pressure exceeds peak systolic pressure; peak systolic pressure exceeds assisted peak systolic pressure.

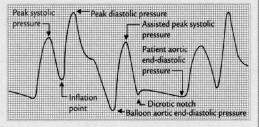

Early inflation

With *early inflation,* the inflation point lies before the dicrotic notch. Early inflation dangerously increases myocardial stress and decreases cardiac output.

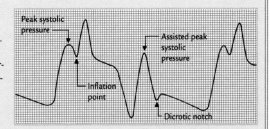

Early deflation

With *early deflation,* a U shape appears and peak systolic pressure is less than or equal to assisted peak systolic pressure. This won't decrease afterload or myocardial oxygen consumption.

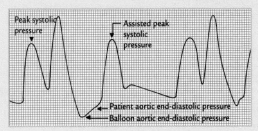

INTERPRETING INTRA-AORTIC BALLOON WAVEFORMS *(continued)*

Late inflation

With *late inflation*, the dicrotic notch precedes the inflation point, and the notch and the inflation point create a W shape. This can lead to a reduction in peak diastolic pressure, coronary and systemic perfusion augmentation time, and augmented coronary perfusion pressure.

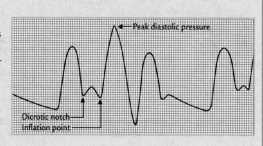

Late deflation

With *late deflation*, peak systolic pressure exceeds assisted peak systolic pressure. This increases afterload, myocardial oxygen consumption, cardiac workload, and preload. It occurs when the balloon has been inflated for too long.

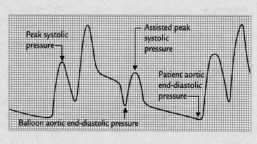

TROUBLESHOOTING INTRA-AORTIC BALLOON PUMPS

Problem	Possible causes	Interventions
High gas leak (automatic mode only)	■ Balloon leakage or abrasion	■ Check for blood in the tubing. ■ Stop pumping. ■ Notify the physician to remove the balloon.
	■ Condensation in extension tubing, volume limiter disk, or both	■ Remove condensate from tubing and volume limiter disk. ■ Refill, autopurge, and resume pumping.
	■ Kink in balloon catheter or tubing	■ Check catheter and tubing for kinks and loose connections; straighten and tighten any found. ■ Refill and resume pumping.

(continued)

TROUBLESHOOTING INTRA-AORTIC BALLOON PUMPS *(continued)*

Problem	Possible causes	Interventions
High gas leak (automatic mode only) *(continued)*	■ Tachycardia	■ Change wean control to 1:2 or operate on "manual" mode. ■ Keep in mind that alarms are off when pump is in manual mode. ■ Autopurge balloon every 1 to 2 hours, and monitor balloon pressure waveform closely.
	■ Malfunctioning or loose volume limiter disk	■ Replace or tighten disk. ■ Refill, autopurge, and resume pumping.
	■ System leak	■ Perform leak test.
Balloon line block (in automatic mode only)	■ Kink in balloon or catheter	■ Check catheter and tubing for kinks and loose connections; straighten and tighten any found. ■ Refill and resume pumping.
	■ Balloon catheter not unfurled; sheath or balloon positioned too high	■ Notify physician immediately to verify placement. ■ Anticipate need for repositioning or manual inflation of balloon.
	■ Condensation in tubing, volume limiter disk, or both	■ Remove condensate from tubing and volume limiter disk. ■ Refill, autopurge, and resume pumping.
	■ Balloon too large for aorta	■ Decrease volume control percentage by one notch.
	■ Malfunctioning volume limiter disk or incorrect volume limiter disk size	■ Replace volume limiter disk. ■ Refill, autopurge, and resume pumping.
No ECG trigger	■ Inadequate signal	■ Adjust ECG gain, and change lead or trigger mode.
	■ Lead disconnected	■ Replace lead.
	■ Improper ECG input mode (skin or monitor) selected	■ Adjust ECG input to appropriate mode (skin or monitor).
No atrial pressure trigger	■ Arterial line damped	■ Flush line.
	■ Arterial line open to atmosphere	■ Check connections on arterial pressure line.

TROUBLESHOOTING INTRA-AORTIC BALLOON PUMPS *(continued)*

Problem	Possible causes	Interventions
Trigger mode change	■ Trigger mode changed while pumping	■ Resume pumping.
Irregular heart rhythm	■ Patient experiencing arrhythmia, such as atrial fibrillation or ectopic beats	■ Change to R or QRS sense (if necessary to accommodate irregular rhythm). ■ Notify physician of arrhythmia.
Erratic atrio-ventricular (AV) pacing	■ Demand for paced rhythm occurring when in AV sequential trigger mode	■ Change to pacer reject trigger or QRS sense.
Noisy ECG signal	■ Malfunctioning leads	■ Replace leads. ■ Check ECG cable.
	■ Electrocautery in use	■ Switch to atrial pressure trigger.
Internal trigger	■ Trigger mode set on internal 80 beats/ minute	■ Select alternative trigger if patient has a heartbeat or rhythm. ■ Keep in mind that internal trigger is used only during cardiopulmonary bypass or cardiac arrest.
Purge incomplete	■ Off button pressed during autopurge, interrupted purge cycle	■ Initiate autopurging again, or initiate pumping.
High fill pressure	■ Malfunctioning volume limiter disk ■ Occluded vent line or valve	■ Replace volume limiter disk. ■ Refill, autopurge, and resume pumping. ■ Attempt to resume pumping. ■ If unsuccessful, notify physician and contact manufacturer.
No balloon drive	■ No volume limiter disk ■ Tubing disconnected	■ Insert volume limiter disk, and lock securely in place. ■ Reconnect tubing. ■ Refill, autopurge, and pump.
Low volume percentage	■ Volume control percentage not 100%	■ Assess cause of decreased volume, and reset, if necessary.
Incorrect timing	■ Inflate and deflate controls set incorrectly	■ Place inflate and deflate controls at set mid-point ■ Reassess timing and readjust

PA CATHETER: FROM BASIC TO COMPLEX

Depending on the intended uses, a pulmonary artery (PA) catheter may be simple or complex. The basic PA catheter has a distal and proximal lumen, a thermistor, and a balloon inflation gate valve. The *distal lumen,* which exists in the pulmonary artery, monitors PA pressure. Its hub is usually marked DISTAL or is color-coded yellow. The *proximal lumen* exists in the right atrium or vena cava, depending on the size of the patient's heart. It monitors right atrial pressure and can be used as the injected solution lumen for cardiac output determination and infusing solutions. The proximal lumen hub is usually marked PROXIMAL or is color-coded blue.

The *thermistor,* located about 1½" (4 cm) from the distal tip, measures temperature (aiding core temperature evaluation) and allows cardiac output measurement. The thermistor connector attaches to a cardiac output connector cable, then to a cardiac output monitor. Typically, it's color-coded red.

The *balloon inflation gate valve* is used for inflating the balloon tip with air. A stopcock connection, typically color-coded red, may be used.

Additional lumens

Some PA catheters have additional lumens used to obtain other hemodynamic data or permit certain interventions. For instance, a *proximal infusion port,* which exits in the right atrium or vena cava, allows additional fluid administration. A *right ventricular lumen,* exiting in the right ventricle, allows fluid administration, right ventricular pressure measurement, or use of a temporary ventricular pacing lead.

Some catheters have additional right atrial and right ventricular lumens for atrioventricular pacing. A *right ventricular ejection fraction test-response thermistor,* with PA and right ventricular sensing electrodes, allows volumetric and ejection fraction measurements. Fiber-optic filaments, such as those used in pulse oximetry, exit into the pulmonary artery and permit measurement of continuous mixed venous oxygen saturation.

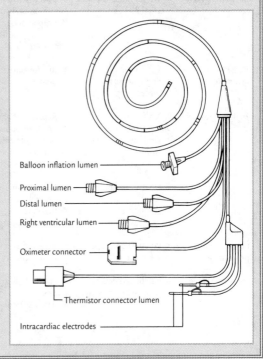

Balloon inflation lumen

Proximal lumen

Distal lumen

Right ventricular lumen

Oximeter connector

Thermistor connector lumen

Intracardiac electrodes

NORMAL PA WAVEFORMS

During pulmonary artery (PA) catheter insertion, the monitor shows various waveforms as the catheter advances through the heart chambers.

Right atrium

When the catheter tip enters the right atrium, the first heart chamber on its route, a waveform like the one shown at right appears on the monitor. Note the two small upright waves. The *a* waves represent right ventricular end-diastolic pressure, and the *v* waves, right atrial filling.

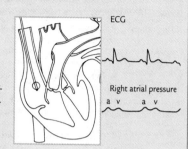

Right ventricle

As the catheter tip reaches the right ventricle, you'll see a waveform with sharp systolic upstrokes and lower diastolic dips.

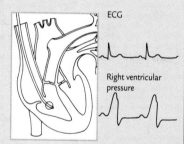

Pulmonary artery

The catheter then floats into the pulmonary artery, causing a waveform like the one shown at right. Note that the upstroke is smoother than on the right ventricular waveform. The dicrotic notch indicates pulmonic valve closure.

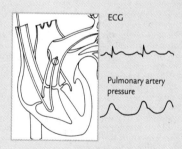

PAWP

Floating into a distal branch of the pulmonary artery, the balloon wedges where the vessel becomes too narrow for it to pass. The monitor now shows a pulmonary artery wedge pressure (PAWP) waveform, with two small upright waves. The *a* wave represents left ventricular end-diastolic pressure; the *v* wave represents left atrial filling. The balloon is then deflated and the catheter is left in the pulmonary artery.

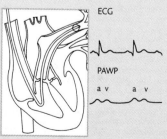

TROUBLESHOOTING
PULMONARY ARTERY CATHETERS

Problem	Possible causes	Interventions
No waveform	■ Transducer not open to the catheter	■ Check the stopcock, and make sure that it's open to the patient. ■ Reevaluate waveform.
	■ Transducer or monitor improperly set up	■ Recheck all connections and components of the system to ensure that they're set up properly. ■ Rebalance the transducer. ■ Replace the system, if necessary.
	■ Clotted catheter tip	■ Attempt to aspirate the clot with a syringe, if facility policy permits. ■ If successful, flush the line. ■ Don't attempt to flush if the clot can't be aspirated; notify the physician.
Overdamped waveform	■ Air in the line	■ Check the system for air. ■ Aspirate air, or force it through a stopcock port.
	■ Clotted catheter tip	■ Attempt to aspirate the clot with a syringe according to facility policy. ■ If successful, flush the line. ■ Don't attempt to flush if the clot can't be aspirated; notify the physician.
	■ Catheter tip lodged against vessel wall	■ Reposition the catheter by gently rotating it or pulling it back slightly according to facility policy. ■ Reposition the patient, if necessary. ■ Ask the patient to cough and breathe deeply to help move the catheter.
Noisy or erratic waveforms	■ Incorrectly positioned catheter	■ Anticipate need for a chest X-ray to verify catheter position. ■ Reposition catheter by gently rotating it or pulling it back slightly, according to facility policy. ■ Reposition the patient, if necessary. ■ Ask the patient to cough and breathe deeply to help move the catheter.
	■ Loose connections	■ Check all connections, and tighten as necessary.
	■ Faulty electrical circuit	■ Check to make sure that the power supply is turned on. ■ Reconnect the transducer to the monitor as necessary.

TROUBLESHOOTING
PULMONARY ARTERY CATHETERS *(continued)*

Problem	Possible causes	Interventions
Erratic waveform	■ Catheter fling	■ Reposition the patient according to facility policy. ■ Shorten tubing, if possible.
False pressure readings	■ Improper calibration or positioning of the transducer	■ Recalibrate the system. ■ Relevel the transducer.
Arrhythmia	■ Catheter irritation of ventricular endocardium or heart valves	■ Confirm arrhythmia via ECG. ■ Notify the physician. ■ Administer antiarrhythmics as ordered.
Ventricular waveform tracing	■ Catheter migration into the right ventricle	■ Inflate the balloon with 1.5 cc of air to move the catheter into the pulmonary artery. ■ If unsuccessful, notify the physician to reposition the catheter.
Continuous pulmonary artery wedge pressure (PAWP) waveform	■ Catheter migration or inflated balloon	■ Reposition the patient. ■ Ask the patient to cough and breathe deeply to help move the catheter. ■ If unsuccessful, notify the physician to reposition the catheter. Obtain portable chest X-ray as ordered. ■ Keep the balloon inflated for no longer than two respiratory cycles or 15 seconds in order to prevent.
Missing PAWP waveform	■ Catheter malposition	■ Reposition the patient. ■ Ask the patient to cough and breathe deeply to help move the catheter.
	■ Inadequate air in balloon tip	■ Reinflate the balloon, wait for balloon to deflate passively, and then instill the correct amount of air.
	■ Ruptured balloon	■ Note the balloon competence (resistance during inflation). ■ Keep in mind that the syringe's plunger should spring back after the balloon inflates. ■ Check for blood leaking from the balloon. ■ If ruptured, turn the patient to his left side, tape the balloon inflation port, and notify the physician.

HEMODYNAMIC VARIABLES

Parameter	Normal value	Formula
Mean arterial pressure (MAP)	70 to 105 mm Hg	$\dfrac{\text{Systolic blood pressure (BP)} + 2\,(\text{Diastolic BP})}{3}$
Central venous pressure (CVP; right atrial pressure [RAP])	2 to 6 cm H_2O; 2 to 8 mm Hg	N/A
Right ventricular pressure	20 to 30 mm Hg (systolic) 0 to 8 mm Hg (diastolic)	N/A
Pulmonary artery pressure (PAP)	20 to 30 mm Hg (systolic; PAS) 8 to 15 mm Hg (diastolic; PAD) 10 to 20 mm Hg (mean; PAM)	N/A
Pulmonary artery wedge pressure (PAWP)	4 to 12 mm Hg	N/A
Cardiac output (CO)	4 to 8 L/minute	Heart rate (HR) $\times$ stroke volume (SV)

Causes of high values	Potential causes of low values
■ Vasoconstriction ■ Use of inotropic agents ■ Polycythemia ■ Cardiogenic or hypovolemic shock ■ Atherosclerosis	■ Vasodilation ■ Moderate hypoxemia ■ Anemia ■ Nitrate drug therapy ■ Calcium channel blocker therapy ■ Septic shock ■ Neurogenic shock ■ Anaphylactic shock
■ Fluid overload ■ Pericardial tamponade ■ Pulmonary hypertension ■ Heart failure ■ Left ventricular myocardial infarction (MI) (could be high normal to elevated range) ■ Right ventricular MI ■ Pulmonary embolism ■ Cardiogenic shock	■ Dehydration ■ Hypovolemia ■ Diuretic therapy ■ Hemorrhage ■ Arrhythmias ■ Third-space fluid shifting
■ Fluid overload ■ Pulmonary hypertension	■ Dehydration ■ Diuretic therapy ■ Hemorrhage ■ Arrhythmias ■ Third-space fluid shifting
■ Hypertension ■ Vasoconstriction ■ Pulmonary edema ■ Pulmonary hypertension	■ Dehydration ■ Diuretic therapy ■ Calcium channel blocker therapy ■ Pulmonary embolism
■ Hypertension ■ Fluid overload ■ Pulmonary hypertension ■ Mitral valve regurgitation ■ Left-sided heart failure ■ MI ■ Cardiac tamponade	■ Dehydration ■ Hypovolemia ■ Pulmonary embolism ■ MI ■ Vasodilation ■ Diuretic therapy ■ Afterload reduction
■ Sepsis	■ Irregularities in heart rate ■ Hypovolemia ■ Pulmonary hypertension ■ Pericardial tamponade ■ MI ■ Pulmonary embolism ■ Decreased contractility ■ Decreased preload or increased afterload

(continued)

HEMODYNAMIC VARIABLES *(continued)*

Parameter	Normal value	Formula
Cardiac index (CI)	2.5 to 4 L/minute/m²	$\dfrac{CO}{\text{Body surface area}}$
Stroke volume (SV)	60 to 100 ml/beat	$\dfrac{CO}{HR}$
Stroke volume index	30 to 60 ml/beat/m²	$\dfrac{SV}{BSA}$
Systemic vascular resistance	900 to 1,200 dynes/sec/cm⁻⁵	$\dfrac{MAP - RAP \times 80}{CO}$
Systemic vascular resistance index	1,360 to 2,200 dynes/sec/cm⁻⁵/m²	$\dfrac{MAP - RAP \times 80}{CI}$

Causes of high values	Potential causes of low values
■ Sepsis	■ Irregularities in heart rate ■ Hypovolemia ■ Heart failure ■ Pulmonary embolism ■ Pulmonary hypertension ■ MI ■ Cardiac tamponade ■ Decreased contractility ■ Decreased preload or increased afterload
■ Positive inotropic drug therapy ■ Exercise ■ Bradycardia	■ Cardiac tamponade ■ Widespread vasodilation ■ Arrhythmias ■ Tachycardia
■ Bradyarrhythmias ■ Positive inotropic drug therapy	■ Hypovolemic shock ■ Vasodilation ■ Cardiogenic shock
■ Cardiogenic shock ■ Hypovolemic shock ■ Pericardial tamponade ■ Pulmonary embolism ■ Vasopressor therapy ■ Systemic hypertension ■ MI	■ Septic shock ■ Anaphylaxis ■ Vasodilator therapy ■ Cirrhosis ■ Arteriovenous fistulas ■ Thyrotoxicosis
■ Positive inotropic drug therapy ■ Polycythemia ■ Vasoconstriction ■ Cardiogenic shock ■ MI ■ Hypovolemic shock ■ Pericardial tamponade ■ Pulmonary embolism ■ Heart failure	■ Anemia ■ Nitrate therapy ■ Calcium channel blocker therapy ■ Septic shock ■ Neurogenic shock ■ Anaphylactic shock ■ Moderate hypoxemia

DRUGS

ANTIARRHYTHMICS

Drug	Indications	Adverse effects*
TYPE IA		
Disopyramide (Norpace, Norpace CR)	■ Premature ventricular contractions (PVCs) (unifocal, multifocal, or coupled); ventricular tachycardia; conversion of atrial fibrillation, atrial flutter, and paroxysmal atrial tachycardia to normal sinus rhythm	■ Hypotension, heart failure, heart block, arrhythmias ■ Blurred vision, dry eyes or nose ■ Cholestatic jaundice
Procainamide (Procanbid, Pronestyl, Pronestyl-SR)	■ Symptomatic PVCs; life-threatening ventricular tachycardia ■ Maintenance of normal sinus rhythm after conversion of atrial flutter ■ Prevention of atrial fibrillation or paroxysmal atrial tachycardia ■ Treatment of malignant hyperthermia	■ Seizures ■ Hypotension, ventricular asystole, bradycardia, AV block, ventricular fibrillation (after parenteral use) ■ Thrombocytopenia, neutropenia (especially with sustained-release forms), agranulocytosis ■ Maculopapular rash, urticaria, pruritus, flushing, angioneurotic edema ■ Lupuslike syndrome (especially after prolonged administration)
Quinidine gluconate (Quinaglute Dura-tabs, Quinalan); **quinidine sulfate** (Quinidex Extentabs, Quinora)	■ Atrial flutter or fibrillation conversion ■ Paroxysmal supraventricular tachycardia (PSVT) ■ Premature atrial contractions, PVCs, paroxysmal AV junctional rhythm or atrial or ventricular tachycardia, maintenance of cardioversion ■ Malaria (when quinine dihydrochloride is unavailable)	■ Vertigo, headache, ataxia ■ PVCs, ventricular tachycardia, atypical ventricular tachycardia (torsades de pointes), hypotension, complete AV block, tachycardia, electrocardiogram (ECG) changes (particularly widening of QRS complex and QT and PR intervals) ■ Tinnitus ■ Diarrhea, nausea, vomiting ■ Hemolytic anemia, thrombocytopenia, agranulocytosis ■ Hepatotoxicity ■ Acute asthmatic attack, respiratory arrest ■ Angioedema, cinchonism

* Common or life-threatening only

Special considerations

■ Contraindicated in patients with cardiogenic shock or second- or third-degree heart block in the absence of an artificial pacemaker, in congenital QT prolongation, and in sick sinus syndrome.
■ Monitor serum electrolyte and drug levels; may decrease serum potassium and glucose levels and increase cholesterol and triglyceride levels.
■ Patients with atrial flutter or fibrillation should be digitalized before disopyramide administration to ensure that enhanced atrioventricular (AV) conduction doesn't lead to ventricular tachycardia.
■ Monitor for signs of developing heart block, such as QRS-complex widening by more than 25% or QT-interval lengthening by more than 25% above baseline.

■ Contraindicated in patients with complete, second-, or third-degree heart block in the absence of an artificial pacemaker; and in patients with myasthenia gravis or systemic lupus erythematosus. Also contraindicated in patients with atypical ventricular tachycardia (torsades de pointes) because procainamide may aggravate this condition.
■ Administer cardiac glycoside before beginning procainamide therapy when treating atrial fibrillation and flutter because ventricular rate may accelerate because of vagolytic effects on the AV node.
■ Monitor blood pressure and ECG continuously during I.V. administration. Watch for prolonged QT interval and QRS complex (50% or greater widening), heart block, or increased arrhythmias. When these ECG signs appear, stop drug and monitor the patient closely.

■ Contraindicated in patients with intraventricular conduction defects, cardiac glycoside toxicity when AV conduction is grossly impaired, abnormal rhythms caused by escape mechanisms, and a history of drug-induced torsades de pointes or QT syndrome.
■ When drug is used to treat atrial tachyarrhythmias, ventricular rate may be accelerated from anticholinergic effects of drug on the AV node. Previous treatment with a cardiac glycoside will prevent this.
■ Monitor the ECG, especially when giving large doses. Quinidine-induced cardiotoxicity causes conduction defects (50% widening of the QRS complex), ventricular tachycardia or flutter, frequent PVCs, and complete AV block. When these signs appear, stop the drug and monitor the patient closely.

(continued)

ANTIARRHYTHMICS (continued)

Drug	Indications	Adverse effects*
TYPE IB		
Lidocaine hydrochloride (Xylocaine HCl)	■ Ventricular arrhythmias from myocardial infarction (MI), cardiac manipulation, or cardiac glycosides ■ Status epilepticus	■ Confusion, tremor, stupor, restlessness, light-headedness, hallucinations ■ Bradycardia, cardiac arrest, hypotension, new or worsened arrhythmias, asystole ■ Tinnitus, blurred or double vision ■ Respiratory arrest, status asthmaticus ■ Anaphylaxis
Mexiletine (Mexitil)	■ Treatment of documented life-threatening arrhythmias	■ New or worsened cardiac arrhythmias ■ Nausea, vomiting, diarrhea, heartburn ■ Rash ■ Tremors ■ Visual disturbances
Tocainide (Tonocard)	■ Treatment of life-threatening ventricular arrhythmias	■ Light-headedness, tremor, vertigo ■ Hypotension, new or worsened arrhythmias, heart failure, bradycardia ■ Nausea, vomiting ■ Blood dyscrasia ■ Hepatitis ■ Respiratory arrest, pulmonary fibrosis, pneumonitis
TYPE IC		
Flecainide (Tambocor)	■ Sustained ventricular tachycardia ■ PSVT, paroxysmal atrial fibrillation or flutter in patients without structural heart disease	■ Headache, light-headedness, syncope ■ New or worsened arrhythmias, heart failure, cardiac arrest, palpitations ■ Blurred vision and other visual disturbances ■ Dyspnea

* Common or life-threatening only

Special considerations

■ Contraindicated in patients hypersensitive to amide-type local anesthetics and in those with Stokes-Adams syndrome, Wolff-Parkinson-White syndrome, and severe degrees of sinoatrial (SA), AV, or intraventricular block in the absence of an artificial pacemaker. Also contraindicated in patients with inflammation or infection in puncture region, septicemia, severe hypertension, spinal deformities, and neurologic disorders.

■ In many severely ill patients, be alert for seizures, which may be the first sign of toxicity. However, severe reactions are usually preceded by somnolence, confusion, and paresthesia. Regard all signs and symptoms of toxicity as serious, and promptly reduce dosage or discontinue therapy. Continued infusion could lead to seizures and coma. Give oxygen through a nasal cannula, if not contraindicated. Keep oxygen and cardiopulmonary resuscitation equipment handy.

■ Monitor the patient for signs of excessive depression of cardiac conductivity (such as sinus node dysfunction, prolonged PR-interval, QRS complex widening, and appearance or exacerbation of arrhythmias). If they occur, reduce dosage or discontinue drug.

■ Contraindicated in patients with heart failure, cardiogenic shock, hypotension, or second- or third-degree heart block.

■ Be alert for fine tremor, usually in the hand. This is an early sign of toxicity that can progress to dizziness and later to ataxia and nystagmus as blood levels increase.

■ When changing from lidocaine to mexiletine, stop the infusion with the first dose of mexiletine. Keep the infusion line open until the arrhythmia appears to be satisfactorily controlled.

■ Monitor drug levels; therapeutic levels range from 0.75 to 2 µg/ml.

■ Contraindicated in patients hypersensitive to lidocaine or other amide-type local anesthetics and in those with second- or third-degree AV block in the absence of a pacemaker.

■ Drug is considered an oral lidocaine and may be used to ease transition from I.V. lidocaine to oral antiarrhythmic therapy.

■ Monitor blood levels; therapeutic levels range from 4 to 10 µg/ml.

■ Observe the patient for tremors, a possible sign that the maximum safe dose has been reached.

■ Contraindicated in patients with cardiogenic shock, second- or third-degree AV block, or right bundle-branch block with a left hemiblock (in the absence of an artificial pacemaker). Drug has proarrhythmic effects in patients with atrial fibrillation or flutter; therefore, it isn't recommended for these patients.

■ Drug has been linked to excessive mortality or nonfatal cardiac arrest rate in national multicenter trials. Restrict use to those patients in whom benefits outweigh risks.

■ Drug is a strong negative inotrope and may cause or worsen heart failure, especially in those with cardiomyopathy, heart failure, or low ejection fraction.

■ Before giving drug, correct any hypokalemia or hyperkalemia, which may alter drug effects.

■ Monitor serum levels; adverse effects increase when trough serum levels exceed 0.7 µg/ml.

■ Drug may increase acute and chronic endocardial pacing thresholds and may suppress ventricular escape rhythms.

(continued)

ANTIARRHYTHMICS *(continued)*

Drug	Indications	Adverse effects*

TYPE IC *(continued)*

Drug	Indications	Adverse effects*
Propafenone (Rythmol)	■ Suppression of documented life-threatening ventricular arrhythmias	■ Drowsiness ■ Bradycardia, heart failure, proarrhythmic events (ventricular tachycardia, PVCs, ventricular fibrillation) ■ Nausea, vomiting

TYPE II

Drug	Indications	Adverse effects*
Esmolol hydrochloride (Brevibloc)	■ Supraventricular tachycardia (SVT) ■ Intraoperative and postoperative tachycardia and hypertension ■ Acute myocardial ischemia	■ Dizziness ■ Hypotension ■ Nausea ■ Bronchospasm
Propranolol hydrochloride (Inderal)	■ Hypertension ■ Management of angina pectoris ■ Supraventricular, ventricular, and atrial arrhythmias; tachyarrhythmias due to excessive catecholamine action during anesthesia, hyperthyroidism, and pheochromocytoma ■ Reduction in post-MI mortality ■ Hypertrophic subaortic stenosis	■ Fatigue, lethargy ■ Bradycardia, hypotension, heart failure, worsening of AV block ■ Agranulocytosis ■ Bronchospasm

TYPE III

Drug	Indications	Adverse effects*
Amiodarone hydrochloride (Cordarone, Pacerone)	■ Recurrent ventricular fibrillation and unstable ventricular tachycardia; atrial fibrillation; angina; hypertrophic cardiomyopathy ■ Supraventricular arrhythmias	■ Malaise, fatigue ■ Bradycardia, hypotension, arrhythmias, heart failure, heart block, sinus arrest, asystole ■ Corneal microdeposits ■ Nausea, vomiting ■ Coagulation abnormalities, pancytopenia, neutropenia ■ Hepatic failure ■ Severe pulmonary toxicity (pneumonitis, alveolitis), organizing pneumonia, pleuritis ■ Photosensitivity

* Common or life-threatening only

Special considerations

■ Contraindicated in patients with severe or uncontrolled heart failure; cardiogenic shock; SA, AV, or intraventricular disorders of impulse conduction in the absence of a pacemaker; bradycardia; marked hypotension; bronchospastic disorders; or electrolyte imbalance.
■ Be prepared to individualize dosage because propafenone pharmacokinetics are complex.

■ Contraindicated in patients with sinus bradycardia, heart block greater than first-degree, cardiogenic shock, or overt heart failure.
■ Don't use the 2,500-mg ampule for direct I.V. injection.
■ Don't mix the drug with 5% sodium bicarbonate injection USP; they're incompatible.
■ Diluted solutions of esmolol are stable for at least 24 hours at room temperature.
■ To convert to other antiarrhythmic therapy after control has been achieved with esmolol, reduce infusion rate by half 30 minutes after giving first dose of other drug. If, after the second dose of the other drug, a satisfactory response is maintained for 1 hour, discontinue esmolol.

■ Contraindicated in patients with bronchial asthma, sinus bradycardia and heart block greater than first-degree, cardiogenic shock, and heart failure (unless failure is secondary to a tachyarrhythmia that can be treated with propranolol).
■ Monitor serum glucose level; drug may mask signs of hypoglycemia.

■ Contraindicated in patients with severe SA node disease resulting in bradycardia. Unless an artificial pacemaker is present, drug is contraindicated in patients with second- or third-degree AV block and in those in whom bradycardia has caused syncope.
■ Use with caution in patients already receiving antiarrhythmics, beta-adrenergic blockers, and calcium channel blockers. Use of amiodarone and ritonavir is contraindicated. Use cautiously with amprenavir.
■ Decrease digoxin, quinidine, phenytoin, and procainamide doses during amiodarone therapy to avoid toxicity.
■ When mixed in dextrose 5% in water (D_5W), be aware that amiodarone is incompatible with aminophylline, cefazolin, heparin, and sodium bicarbonate.
■ Administer solutions containing 2 mg/ml or more via a central venous catheter. Use an in-line filter and three-step process: rapid loading dose, slow loading dose, and maintenance infusion.

(continued)

ANTIARRHYTHMICS *(continued)*

Drug	Indications	Adverse effects*
TYPE III *(continued)*		
Dofetilide (Tikosyn)	■ Maintenance of normal sinus rhythm in patients with symptomatic atrial fibrillation or atrial flutter for more than 1 week; conversion of atrial fibrillation and atrial flutter to normal sinus rhythm	■ Headache, dizziness, syncope, stroke ■ Ventricular fibrillation, ventricular tachycardia, torsades de pointes, bradycardia, cardiac arrest, sudden death, MI ■ Angioedema
Ibutilide fumarate (Corvert)	■ Rapid conversion of atrial fibrillation or atrial flutter of recent onset to sinus rhythm	■ Sustained ventricular tachycardia, AV block, QT-interval prolongation, bradycardia
Sotalol (Betapace, Betapace AF)	■ Documented, life-threatening ventricular arrhythmias (Betapace) ■ Maintenance of normal sinus rhythm (delay in time to recurrence of atrial fibrillation/atrial flutter [AFIB/AFL]) in patients with symptomatic AFIB/AFL who are currently in sinus rhythm (Betapace AF)	■ Bradycardia, palpitations, chest pain, arrhythmias, heart failure, AV block, proarrhythmic events (ventricular tachycardia, PVCs, ventricular fibrillation) ■ Nausea, vomiting ■ Dyspnea, bronchospasm
TYPE IV		
Verapamil hydrochloride (Calan, Calan SR, Covera-HS, Verelan, Verelan PM)	■ Management of Prinzmetal's or variant angina or unstable or chronic stable angina pectoris ■ SVT ■ Control of ventricular rate in digitalized patients with chronic atrial flutter or fibrillation ■ Prophylaxis of repetitive paroxysmal supraventricular tachycardia ■ Hypertension	■ Dizziness ■ Transient hypotension, heart failure, pulmonary edema, bradycardia, AV block, ventricular asystole, ventricular fibrillation ■ Constipation

* Common or life-threatening only

Special considerations

■ Contraindicated in patients with creatinine clearance less than 20 ml/minute and in those with congenital or acquired long QT interval syndrome. Don't use in patients with baseline QT interval greater than 440 msec (500 msec in patients with ventricular conduction abnormalities).
■ The patient must be in a facility equipped with ECG monitoring and a staff trained in managing ventricular arrhythmias for at least 3 days; or, the patient must be monitored for a minimum of 12 hours after pharmacologic or electrical conversions to normal sinus rhythm, whichever is longer.
■ Withhold class I or III antiarrhythmics for at least three half-lives before starting drug.

■ Contraindicated in patients with a history of polymorphic ventricular tachycardia such as torsades de pointes.
■ Correct hypokalemia and hypomagnesemia before therapy begins to reduce the potential for proarrhythmia.
■ Admixtures of the product, with approved diluents, are chemically and physically stable for 24 hours at room temperature and for 48 hours at refrigerated temperatures.
■ Monitor the patient's ECG continuously throughout drug administration and for at least 4 hours afterward or until QT interval has returned to baseline because drug can induce or worsen ventricular arrhythmias in some patients. Longer monitoring is required if arrhythmic activity is noted.

■ Contraindicated in patients with severe sinus node dysfunction, sinus bradycardia, second- and third-degree AV block in the absence of an artificial pacemaker, congenital or acquired long-QT syndrome, cardiogenic shock, uncontrolled heart failure, and bronchial asthma.
■ Monitor serum electrolyte levels regularly, especially if the patient is receiving diuretics. Electrolyte imbalances, such as hypokalemia or hypomagnesemia, may enhance QT interval prolongation and increase risk of serious arrhythmias such as torsades de pointes.
■ Adjust dosage slowly, allowing 3 days (or five to six doses if the patient is receiving once-daily doses) between dose increments for adequate monitoring of QT intervals and for drug plasma levels to reach a steady state.

■ Contraindicated in patients with severe left ventricular dysfunction, cardiogenic shock, second- or third-degree AV block or sick sinus syndrome except in presence of functioning pacemaker, atrial flutter or fibrillation and accessory bypass tract syndrome, severe heart failure (unless secondary to verapamil therapy), and severe hypotension. In addition, I.V. verapamil is contraindicated in patients receiving I.V. beta-adrenergic blockers and in those with ventricular tachycardia.
■ If verapamil is added to therapy of the patient receiving digoxin, anticipate a reduction in digoxin dosage by half and monitor subsequent serum drug levels.
■ Stop disopyramide 48 hours before starting verapamil, and don't resume until 24 hours after verapamil has been stopped.

(continued)

ANTIARRHYTHMICS *(continued)*

Drug	Indications	Adverse effects*
MISCELLANEOUS		
Adenosine (Adenocard)	■ Conversion of PSVT to sinus rhythm	■ Facial flushing ■ Blurred vision, throat tightness ■ Groin pressure ■ Chest pressure, dyspnea, shortness of breath, hyperventilation
Digoxin (Lanoxin)	■ Heart failure, atrial fibrillation and flutter, paroxysmal atrial tachycardia	■ Fatigue, generalized muscle weakness, agitation, hallucinations, dizziness ■ Arrhythmias (most commonly, conduction disturbances with or without AV block, PVCs, and supraventricular arrhythmias) that may lead to increased severity of heart failure and hypotension ■ Yellow-green halos around visual images, blurred vision, light flashes, photophobia, diplopia ■ Anorexia, nausea

* Common or life-threatening only

DRUGS AND THE QT INTERVAL

Many drugs can prolong the QT interval, especially when combined with substances that affect the metabolism of the drug. This QT interval prolongation can lead to torsades de pointes, a lifethreatening polymorphic ventricular tachycardia. The list here shows some drugs that may affect the QT interval.

Anesthetic
■ Halothane

Antiarrhythmics
■ Disopyramide
■ Procainamide
■ Quinidine
■ Amiodarone
■ Sotalol

Antibiotics
■ Azithromycin
■ Clarithromycin
■ Erythromycin
■ Metronidazole
(with alcohol)
■ Moxifloxacin

Special considerations

■ Contraindicated in patients with second- or third-degree heart block or sick sinus syndrome, unless an artificial pacemaker is present, because adenosine decreases conduction through the AV node and may produce first-, second-, or third-degree heart block. These effects are usually transient; however, patients in whom significant heart block develops after a dose of adenosine shouldn't receive additional doses.
■ Don't use in atrial fibrillation or atrial flutter.
■ Don't use solutions that aren't clear.
■ Use Adenocard cautiously in patients with previous history of ventricular fibrillation or those taking digoxin and verapamil.
■ Monitor ECG rhythm during administration; drug may cause short-lasting first-, second-, or third-degree heart block or asystole.
■ Don't confuse adenosine phosphate with adenosine (Adenocard).

■ Contraindicated in patients with digoxin-induced toxicity, ventricular fibrillation, or ventricular tachycardia unless caused by heart failure.
■ Watch for ECG changes, including increased PR interval and depression of ST segment; drug may cause false-positive ST-T changes on an ECG during exercise testing.

Antidepressants
■ Amitriptyline
■ Clomipramine
■ Imipramine
■ Dothiepin
■ Doxepin

Antifungals
■ Fluconazole (in cirrhosis)
■ Ketoconazole

Antimalarials
■ Chloroquine
■ Mefloquine

Antipsychotics
■ Risperidone
■ Fluphenazine
■ Haloperidol
■ Clozapine
■ Thioridazine
■ Ziprasidone
■ Pimozide
■ Droperidol

Antivirals
■ Nelfinavir

Other drugs
■ Probucol

INFUSION FLOW RATES

Epinephrine infusion rates
Mix 1 mg in 250 ml (4 mcg/ml).

Dose (mcg/minute)	Infusion rate (ml/hour)
1	15
2	30
3	45
4	60
5	75
6	90
7	105
8	120
9	135
10	150
15	225
20	300
25	375
30	450
35	525
40	600

Isoproterenol infusion rates
Mix 1 mg in 250 ml (4 mcg/ml).

Dose (mcg/minute)	Infusion rate (ml/hour)
0.5	8
1	15
2	30
3	45
4	60
5	75
6	90
7	105
8	120
9	135
10	150
15	225
20	300
25	375
30	450

Dobutamine infusion rates
Mix 250 mg in 250 ml of dextrose 5% in water (D_5W) (1,000 mcg/ml). Determine infusion rate in ml/hour using ordered dose and patient's weight in pounds or kilograms.

Dose (mcg/ kg/minute)	lb	88	99	110	121	132	143
	kg	40	45	50	55	60	65
2.5		6	7	8	8	9	10
5		12	14	15	17	18	20
7.5		18	20	23	25	27	29
10		24	27	30	33	36	39
12.5		30	34	38	41	45	49
15		36	41	45	50	54	59
20		48	54	60	66	72	78
25		60	68	75	83	90	98
30		72	81	90	99	108	117
35		84	95	105	116	126	137
40		96	108	120	132	144	156

Nitroglycerin infusion rates

Determine the infusion rate in ml/hour using the ordered dose and the concentration of the drug solution.

Dose (mcg/minute)	25 mg/250 ml (100 mcg/ml)	50 mg/250 ml (200 mcg/ml)	100 mg/250 ml (400 mcg/ml)
5	3	2	1
10	6	3	2
20	12	6	3
30	18	9	5
40	24	12	6
50	30	15	8
60	36	18	9
70	42	21	10
80	48	24	12
90	54	27	14
100	60	30	15
150	90	45	23
200	120	60	30

154	165	176	187	198	209	220	231	242
70	75	80	85	90	95	100	105	110
11	11	12	13	14	14	15	16	17
21	23	24	26	27	29	30	32	33
32	34	36	38	41	43	45	47	50
42	45	48	51	54	57	60	63	66
53	56	60	64	68	71	75	79	83
63	68	72	77	81	86	90	95	99
84	90	96	102	108	114	120	126	132
105	113	120	128	135	143	150	158	165
126	135	144	153	162	171	180	189	198
147	158	168	179	189	200	210	221	231
168	180	192	204	216	228	240	252	264

(continued)

INFUSION FLOW RATES *(continued)*

Dopamine infusion rates

Mix 400 mg in 250 ml of D_5W (1,600 mcg/ml). Determine the infusion rate in ml/hour using the ordered dose and the patient's weight in pounds or kilograms.

Dose (mcg/ kg/minute)	lb	88	99	110	121	132	143
	kg	40	45	50	55	60	65
2.5		4	4	5	5	6	6
5		8	8	9	10	11	12
7.5		11	13	14	15	17	18
10		15	17	19	21	23	24
12.5		19	21	23	26	28	30
15		23	25	28	31	34	37
20		30	34	38	41	45	49
25		38	42	47	52	56	61
30		45	51	56	62	67	73
35		53	59	66	72	79	85
40		60	68	75	83	90	98
45		68	76	84	93	101	110
50		75	84	94	103	113	122

Nitroprusside infusion rates

Mix 50 mg in 250 ml of D_5W (200 mcg/ml). Determine the infusion rate in ml/hour using the ordered dose and the patient's weight in pounds or kilograms.

Dose (mcg/ kg/minute)	lb	88	99	110	121	132	143
	kg	40	45	50	55	60	65
0.3		4	4	5	5	5	6
0.5		6	7	8	8	9	10
1		12	14	15	17	18	20
1.5		18	20	23	25	27	29
2		24	27	30	33	36	39
3		36	41	45	50	54	59
4		48	54	60	66	72	78
5		60	68	75	83	90	98
6		72	81	90	99	108	117
7		84	95	105	116	126	137
8		96	108	120	132	144	156
9		108	122	135	149	162	176
10		120	135	150	165	180	195

154	165	176	187	198	209	220	231
70	75	80	85	90	95	100	105
7	7	8	8	8	9	9	10
13	14	15	16	17	18	19	20
20	21	23	24	25	27	28	30
26	28	30	32	34	36	38	39
33	35	38	40	42	45	47	49
39	42	45	48	51	53	56	59
53	56	60	64	68	71	75	79
66	70	75	80	84	89	94	98
79	84	90	96	101	107	113	118
92	98	105	112	118	125	131	138
105	113	120	128	135	143	150	158
118	127	135	143	152	160	169	177
131	141	150	159	169	178	188	197

154	165	176	187	198	209	220	231	242
70	75	80	85	90	95	100	105	110
6	7	7	8	8	9	9	9	10
11	11	12	13	14	14	15	16	17
21	23	24	26	27	29	30	32	33
32	34	36	38	41	43	45	47	50
42	45	48	51	54	57	60	63	66
63	68	72	77	81	86	90	95	99
84	90	96	102	108	114	120	126	132
105	113	120	128	135	143	150	158	165
126	135	144	153	162	171	180	189	198
147	158	168	179	189	200	210	221	231
168	180	192	204	216	228	240	252	264
189	203	216	230	243	257	270	284	297
210	225	240	255	270	285	300	315	330

INOTROPIC AND VASOPRESSOR AGENTS

Drug	Indications	Adverse effects*
Dobutamine hydrochloride (Dobutrex)	■ Increase in cardiac output in short-term treatment of cardiac decompensation caused by depressed contractility	■ Increased heart rate, hypertension, premature ventricular contractions (PVCs) ■ Asthmatic episodes ■ Anaphylaxis
Dopamine hydrochloride (Intropin)	■ Adjunct in shock to increase cardiac output, blood pressure, and urine flow ■ Short-term treatment of severe, refractory, chronic heart failure	■ Hypotension, bradycardia ■ Anaphylactic reactions
Epinephrine (Adrenalin Chloride)	■ Bronchospasm, hypersensitivity reactions, anaphylaxis ■ Restoration of cardiac rhythm in cardiac arrest	■ Nervousness, tremor, headache, drowsiness, cerebral hemorrhage, stroke ■ Palpitations, hypertension, ventricular fibrillation, shock, arrhythmias ■ Nausea, vomiting
Inamrinone lactate (Inocor)	■ Short-term management of heart failure ■ Cardiac life support in patients in whom other preferred drugs can't be used for pump failure and acute pulmonary edema	■ Arrhythmias ■ Thrombocytopenia ■ Hypersensitivity reactions (pericarditis, ascites, myositis vasculitis, pleuritis)

* Common or life-threatening only

Special considerations

- Contraindicated in patients with idiopathic hypertrophic subaortic stenosis.
- Dobutamine is incompatible with alkaline solution (sodium bicarbonate).
- Don't mix with or give through same I.V. line as heparin, hydrocortisone, cefazolin, or penicillin.
- The concentration of infusion solution shouldn't exceed 5,000 mcg/ml; use the solution within 24 hours. Rate and duration of infusion depend on patient response.
- Monitor serum electrolytes, especially potassium.
- Most patients experience an increase of 10 to 20 mm Hg in systolic blood pressure; some show an increase of 50 mm Hg or more. Most also experience an increase in heart rate of 5 to 15 beats/minute; some show increases of 30 or more beats/minute.

- Contraindicated in patients with uncorrected tachyarrhythmias, pheochromocytoma, or ventricular fibrillation.
- Use cautiously in patients with occlusive vascular disease, cold injuries, diabetic endarteritis, and arterial embolism; in those taking monoamine oxidase inhibitors; and in pregnant women.
- Reduce dosage gradually because severe hypotension may result in abrupt withdrawal of infusion. Administer I.V. fluids, as ordered, to expand blood volume.
- Don't mix other drugs in dopamine solutions. Discard solutions after 24 hours.
- Give drug in a large vein to prevent the possibility of extravasation.
- If extravasation occurs, stop the infusion and infiltrate the site promptly with 10 to 15 ml saline containing 5 to 10 mg phentolamine. Use syringe with a fine needle, and infiltrate area liberally with phentolamine solution.

- Contraindicated in patients with angle-closure glaucoma, shock (other than anaphylaxis), organic brain damage, cardiac dilation, arrhythmias, coronary insufficiency, or cerebral arteriosclerosis.
- Contraindicated in patients with sulfite allergies (some commercial products contain sulfites), except when epinephrine is being used for treatment of serious allergic reactions or other emergencies.
- Use with extreme caution in patients with long-standing bronchial asthma and emphysema in whom degenerative heart disease has developed. Also use cautiously in elderly patients and in those with hyperthyroidism, cardiovascular disease, hypertension, psychoneurosis, and diabetes.
- Administer breathing treatment with first symptoms of bronchospasm. Patient should use the fewest number of inhalations that provide relief. To prevent excessive dosage, at least 1 or 2 minutes should elapse before taking additional inhalations of epinephrine. Dosage requirements vary.

- Contraindicated in patients with severe aortic or pulmonic valvular disease (in place of surgical intervention) and patients in the acute phase of a myocardial infarction.
- Keep in mind that inamrinone is prescribed primarily for patients who haven't responded to therapy with cardiac glycosides, diuretics, and vasodilators.
- Administer drug as supplied, or dilute in normal or half-normal saline solution to concentration of 1 to 3 mg/ml. Don't dilute with solutions containing dextrose because a slow chemical reaction occurs over 24 hours. Inamrinone can be injected into running dextrose infusions through Y-connector or directly into tubing. Use diluted solution within 24 hours.
- Don't administer furosemide in I.V. lines containing inamrinone because a chemical reaction occurs immediately.
- Monitor platelet counts. A count below 150,000/µl necessitates dosage reduction.

(continued)

INOTROPIC AND VASOPRESSOR AGENTS *(continued)*

Drug	Indications	Adverse effects*
Milrinone lactate (Primacor)	■ Short-term I.V. therapy for heart failure	■ Nonsustained ventricular tachycardia, sustained ventricular tachycardia, ventricular fibrillation ■ Thrombocytopenia
Norepinephrine bitartrate* (Levophed) *formerly levarterenol bitartrate	■ Maintenance of blood pressure in acute hypotensive states ■ GI bleeding	■ Bradycardia, severe hypertension, arrhythmias ■ Asthmatic episodes ■ Anaphylaxis
Phenylephrine hydrochloride (Neo-Synephrine)	■ Hypotensive emergencies during spinal anesthesia ■ Mild to moderate hypotension ■ Paroxysmal supraventricular tachycardia ■ Adjunct in the treatment of severe hypotension or shock	■ Headache ■ Bradycardia, arrhythmias, PVCs, palpitations, tachycardia ■ Asthmatic episodes ■ Anaphylaxis, decreased organ perfusion (with prolonged use)

Special considerations

- Contraindicated in patients with severe aortic or pulmonic valvular disease (in place of surgical correction) and in patients in the acute phase of an MI.
- Use cautiously in patients with atrial fibrillation or flutter.
- Be sure to dilute milrinone further before I.V. administration. Acceptable diluents include half-normal saline solution, normal saline solution, and dextrose 5% in water.
- Don't administer furosemide in an I.V. line that contains milrinone.

- Contraindicated in patients with mesenteric or peripheral vascular thrombosis, profound hypoxia, hypercapnia, or hypotension resulting from blood volume deficit and during cyclopropane and halothane anesthesia.
- To treat extravasation, infiltrate site promptly with 10 to 15 ml saline solution containing 5 to 10 mg phentolamine, using a fine needle.
- Observe the patient constantly during norepinephrine administration. Obtain baseline blood pressure and pulse before therapy, and repeat every 2 minutes until stable. Repeat every 5 minutes during administration.

- Injectable form is contraindicated in those with severe hypertension or ventricular tachycardia.
- Use injectable form cautiously in patients with severe atherosclerosis, bradycardia, partial heart block, myocardial disease, or allergy to sulfites.
- Give I.V. through large veins, and monitor flow rate. To treat extravasation ischemia, infiltrate site promptly and liberally with 10 to 15 ml saline solution containing 5 to 10 mg phentolamine through fine needle. Topical nitroglycerin has also been used.
- During I.V. administration, monitor pulse, blood pressure, and central venous pressure every 2 to 5 minutes.

7

RESPIRATORY CARE

ASSESSMENT

RESPIRATORY SYSTEM: NORMAL FINDINGS

Inspection
- Chest configuration is symmetrical side-to-side.
- Anteroposterior diameter is less than the transverse diameter, with a 1:2 to 5:7 ratio in an adult.
- Chest shape is normal, with no deformities, such as barrel chest, kyphosis, retraction, sternal protrusion, or depressed sternum.
- Costal angle is less than 90 degrees, with the ribs joining the spine at a 45-degree angle.
- Respirations are quiet and unlabored, with no use of accessory neck, shoulder, or abdominal muscles. You should also see no intercostal, substernal, or supraclavicular retractions.
- Chest wall expands symmetrically during respirations.
- Adult respiratory rate is normal, at 16 to 20 breaths/minute. Expect some variation depending on your patient's age.
- Respiratory rhythm is regular, with expiration taking about twice as long as inspiration. Men and children breathe diaphragmatically, whereas women breathe thoracically.

- Skin color matches the rest of the body's complexion.

Palpation
- Skin is warm and dry.
- No tender spots or bulges in the chest are detectable.

Percussion
- Resonant percussion sounds can be heard over the lungs.

Auscultation
- Loud, high-pitched bronchial breath sounds can be heard over the trachea.
- Intense, medium-pitched bronchovesicular breath sounds can be heard over the mainstem bronchi, between the scapulae, and below the clavicles.
- Soft, breezy, low-pitched vesicular breath sounds can be heard over most of the peripheral lung fields.

RESPIRATORY ASSESSMENT LANDMARKS

These illustrations show common landmarks used in respiratory assessment.

Anterior view

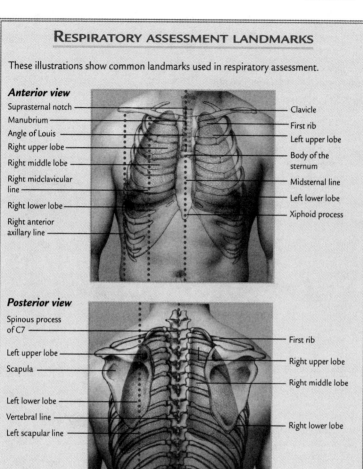

Suprasternal notch
Manubrium
Angle of Louis
Right upper lobe
Right middle lobe
Right midclavicular line
Right lower lobe
Right anterior axillary line

Clavicle
First rib
Left upper lobe
Body of the sternum
Midsternal line
Left lower lobe
Xiphoid process

Posterior view

Spinous process of C7
Left upper lobe
Scapula
Left lower lobe
Vertebral line
Left scapular line

First rib
Right upper lobe
Right middle lobe
Right lower lobe

RESPIRATORY CARE

PALPATING THE CHEST

To palpate the chest, place the palm of your hand (or hands) lightly over the thorax, as shown. Palpate for tenderness, alignment, bulging, and retractions of the chest and intercostal spaces. Assess the patient for crepitus, especially around drainage sites. Repeat this procedure on the patient's back.

Next, use the pads of your fingers, as shown, to palpate the front and back of the thorax. Pass your fingers over the ribs and any scars, lumps, lesions, or ulcerations. Note the skin temperature, turgor, and moisture. Also note tenderness and bony or subcutaneous crepitus. The muscles should feel firm and smooth.

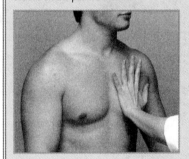 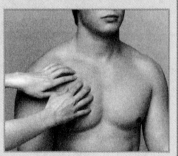

CHECKING FOR TACTILE FREMITUS

When you check the back of the thorax for tactile fremitus, ask the patient to fold his arms across his chest. This movement shifts the scapulae out of the way.

What to do
Check for tactile fremitus by lightly placing your open palms on both sides of the patient's back, as shown, without touching his back with your fingers. Ask the patient to repeat the phrase "ninety-nine" loud enough to produce palpable vibrations. Then palpate the front of the chest using the same hand positions.

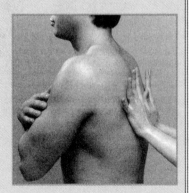

What the results mean
Vibrations that feel more intense on one side than the other indicate tissue consolidation on that side. Less intense vibrations may indicate emphysema, pneumothorax, or pleural effusion. Faint or no vibrations in the upper posterior thorax may indicate bronchial obstruction or a fluid-filled pleural space.

PERCUSSING THE CHEST

To percuss the chest, hyperextend the middle finger of your left hand if you're right-handed or the middle finger of your right hand if you're left-handed. Place your hand firmly on the patient's chest. Use the tip of the middle finger of your dominant hand — your right hand if you're right-handed, left hand if you're left-handed — to tap on the middle finger of your other hand just below the distal joint (as shown).

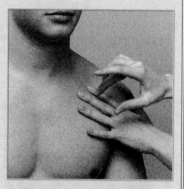

The movement should come from the wrist of your dominant hand, not your elbow or upper arm. Keep the fingernail you use for tapping short so you won't hurt yourself. Follow the standard per-cussion sequence over the front and back chest walls.

PERCUSSION SOUNDS

Use this chart to help you become more comfortable with percussion and to interpret percussion sounds quickly. Learn the different percussion sounds by practicing on yourself, your patients, and any other person willing to help.

Sound	Description	Clinical significance
Flat	Short, soft, high-pitched, extremely dull, found over the thigh	Consolidation, as in atelectasis and extensive pleural effusion
Dull	Medium in intensity and pitch, moderate length, thudlike, found over the liver	Solid area, as in pleural effusion
Resonant	Long, loud, low-pitched, hollow	Normal lung tissue
Hyperresonant	Very loud, lower-pitched, found over the stomach	Hyperinflated lung, as in emphysema or pneumothorax
Tympanic	Loud, high-pitched, moderate length, musical, drumlike, found over a puffed-out cheek	Air collection, as in a gastric air bubble or air in the intestines

PERCUSSION SEQUENCES

Follow these percussion sequences to distinguish between normal and abnormal sounds in the patient's lungs. Remember to compare sound variations from one side with the other as you proceed. Carefully describe abnormal sounds you hear and include their locations. You'll follow the same sequences for auscultation.

Anterior

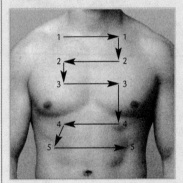

Posterior

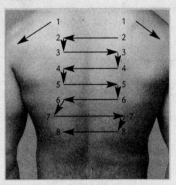

QUALITIES OF NORMAL BREATH SOUNDS

Use this chart to help you become more comfortable with percussion and to interpret percussion sounds quickly. Learn the different percussion sounds by practicing on yourself, your patients, and any other person willing to help.

Breath sound	Quality	Inspiration-expiration ratio	Location
Tracheal	Harsh, high-pitched	I < E	Over trachea
Bronchial	Loud, high-pitched	I > E	Next to trachea
Bronchovesicular	Medium in loudness and pitch	I = E	Next to sternum, between scapula
Vesicular	Soft, low-pitched	I > E	Remainder of lungs

COMPARING ABNORMAL BREATH SOUNDS

Sound	Description	Cause
Crackles	Light crackling, popping, intermittent, nonmusical sounds, like hairs being rubbed together, heard on inspiration or expiration, may further be classified as fine (high-pitched) or coarse (low-pitched)	Air moving through fluid-filled airways, especially in smaller airways and alveoli, such as with heart failure, pulmonary edema, pneumonia, pulmonary fibrosis, also alveoli popping open in atelectasis, in elderly patients
Pleural friction rub	Low-pitched, continual, superficial, squeaking or grating sound, like pieces of sandpaper being rubbed together, heard on inspiration and expiration	Inflamed parietal and visceral pleural linings rubbing together such as with pleuritis
Rhonchi	Low-pitched, snoring, monophonic, sounds, also called *sonorous wheeze*, heard primarily on expiration, but may be heard throughout the respiratory cycle	Air moving through secretions in larger airways, usually clear with coughing such as with chronic bronchitis
Stridor	High-pitched, monophonic crowing sound heard on inspiration, commonly louder in the neck than over the chest wall	Air moving through partial upper airway obstruction from swollen, inflamed tissue or foreign body, such as with laryngospasm, laryngeal edema from irritated airway, smoke inhalation, allergic reaction, foreign body; it's a medical emergency and requires immediate treatment
Wheezes	High-pitched, continual, musical or whistling sound, commonly called *sibilant wheeze*, heard predominately on expiration, but may be heard on inspiration and expiration	Air moving through a narrowed or partially obstructed airway caused by swelling, secretions or tumor, such as with asthma, chronic bronchitis, emphysema

RESPIRATORY CARE

RESPIRATORY SYSTEM:
INTERPRETING YOUR FINDINGS

Your assessment will reveal a group of findings that may lead you to suspect a particular disorder. This chart shows some common groups of findings for signs and symptoms of the respiratory system, along with their probable causes.

Sign or symptom and findings	Probable cause
COUGH	
■ Nonproductive cough ■ Pleuritic chest pain ■ Dyspnea ■ Tachypnea ■ Anxiety ■ Decreased vocal fremitus ■ Tracheal deviation toward the affected side	Atelectasis
■ Productive cough with small amounts of purulent (or mucopurulent), blood-streaked sputum or large amounts of frothy sputum ■ Dyspnea ■ Anorexia ■ Fatigue ■ Weight loss ■ Wheezing ■ Clubbing	Lung cancer
■ Nonproductive cough ■ Dyspnea ■ Pleuritic chest pain ■ Decreased chest motion ■ Pleural friction rub ■ Tachypnea ■ Tachycardia ■ Flatness on percussion ■ Egophony	Pleural effusion
DYSPNEA	
■ Acute dyspnea ■ Tachypnea ■ Crackles and rhonchi in both lung fields ■ Intercostal and suprasternal retractions ■ Restlessness ■ Anxiety ■ Tachycardia	Acute respiratory distress syndrome

RESPIRATORY SYSTEM:
INTERPRETING YOUR FINDINGS *(continued)*

Sign or symptom and findings	Probable cause

DYSPNEA *(continued)*

■ Progressive exertional dyspnea ■ A history of smoking ■ Barrel chest ■ Accessory muscle hypertrophy ■ Diminished breath sounds ■ Pursed-lip breathing ■ Prolonged expiration ■ Anorexia ■ Weight loss	Emphysema
■ Acute dyspnea ■ Pleuritic chest pain ■ Tachycardia ■ Decreased breath sounds ■ Low-grade fever ■ Dullness on percussion ■ Cool, clammy skin	Pulmonary embolism

HEMOPTYSIS

■ Sputum ranging in color from pink to dark brown ■ Productive cough ■ Dyspnea ■ Chest pain ■ Crackles on auscultation ■ Chills ■ Fever	Pneumonia
■ Frothy, blood-tinged pink sputum ■ Severe dyspnea ■ Orthopnea ■ Gasping ■ Diffuse crackles ■ Cold, clammy skin ■ Anxiety	Pulmonary edema
■ Blood-streaked or blood-tinged sputum ■ Chronic productive cough ■ Fine crackles after coughing ■ Dyspnea ■ Dullness to percussion ■ Increased tactile fremitus	Pulmonary tuberculosis

(continued)

RESPIRATORY SYSTEM: INTERPRETING YOUR FINDINGS (continued)

Sign or symptom and findings	Probable cause
HEMOPTYSIS (continued)	
■ Sudden onset of wheezing ■ Stridor ■ Dry, paroxysmal cough ■ Gagging ■ Hoarseness ■ Decreased breath sounds ■ Dyspnea ■ Cyanosis	Aspiration of a foreign body
■ Audible wheezing on expiration ■ Prolonged expiration ■ Apprehension ■ Intercostal and supraclavicular retractions ■ Rhonchi ■ Nasal flaring ■ Tachypnea	Asthma
■ Wheezing ■ Coarse crackles ■ Hacking cough that later becomes productive ■ Dyspnea ■ Barrel chest ■ Clubbing ■ Edema ■ Weight gain	Chronic bronchitis

DIAGNOSTIC TESTS

ARTERIAL BLOOD GAS ANALYSIS

Overview

■ Used to evaluate gas exchange in the lungs

■ Partial pressure of arterial oxygen (PaO_2): the amount of oxygen crossing the alveolar capillary membrane and the concentration of arterial oxygen in the blood

■ Partial pressure of arterial carbon dioxide ($PaCO_2$): the concentration of arterial carbon dioxide in the blood; reflects the adequacy of alveolar ventilation and respiratory response to acid-base balance

■ pH: the hydrogen ion (H^+) concentration, indicating acidity or alkalinity of the blood

■ Bicarbonate (HCO_3^-): a measure of the metabolic component of acid-base balance

■ Arterial oxygen saturation (SaO_2): the ratio of the amount of oxygen in the blood combined with hemoglobin to the total amount of oxygen that the hemoglobin can carry

PURPOSE

■ To evaluate efficiency of pulmonary gas exchange

■ To assess integrity of the ventilatory control system

■ To determine acid-base balance (see *Understanding acid-base disorders,* page 284)

■ To monitor response to respiratory therapy

■ To monitor pathophysiologic changes influencing ventilatory effort or gas exchange

PATIENT PREPARATION

■ Make sure the patient has signed an appropriate consent form.

■ Restriction of food or fluids isn't necessary before the test.

■ Explain that the study requires an arterial blood sample and that brief cramping or throbbing pain may be felt at the puncture site.

■ Before the puncture, evaluate the arterial blood supply to the hand by performing the Allen test. (See *Performing Allen's test,* page 285.)

■ Note and report all allergies.

Teaching points

Be sure to cover:

■ the purpose of the study and how it's done

■ who will perform the arterial puncture, where, and when

■ that the procedure takes less than 10 minutes.

POSTPROCEDURE CARE

■ Apply direct manual pressure to the puncture site for 3 to 5 minutes or until hemostasis is obtained.

■ Apply a sterile dressing.

Monitoring

■ Vital signs

■ Peripheral vascular status

■ Bleeding or hematoma formation at the puncture site

Observe for signs of circulatory impairment, such as swelling, discoloration, pain, numbness, or tingling in the extremity used for the puncture.

PRECAUTIONS

■ Exposing the sample to air affects PaO_2 and $PaCO_2$, interfering with accurate results.

■ Failure to comply with correct sample handling procedures will adversely affect the test results.

■ Venous blood in the sample will render lower PaO_2 and elevate $PaCO_2$.

■ Drugs including bicarbonates, ethacrynic acid, hydrocortisone, metolazone, prednisone, and thiazides may elevate $PaCO_2$.

■ Drugs including acetazolamide, methicillin, nitrofurantoin, and tetracycline may decrease $PaCO_2$.

■ Wait at least 20 minutes before drawing arterial blood gas in the following situations:

– after initiating, changing, or discontinuing oxygen therapy

– after initiating or changing settings of mechanical ventilation

– after extubation.

COMPLICATIONS

■ Hematoma

■ Bleeding

■ Infection

■ Thrombosis

■ Nerve damage

UNDERSTANDING ACID-BASE DISORDERS

Disorder and ABG findings	Possible causes	Signs and symptoms
Respiratory acidosis (excess carbon dioxide retention) pH < 7.35 HCO_3^- > 26 mEq/L (if compensating) $PaCO_2$ > 45 mm Hg	■ Central nervous system depression from drugs, injury, or disease ■ Asphyxia ■ Hypoventilation from pulmonary, cardiac, musculoskeletal, or neuromuscular disease	■ Diaphoresis, headache, tachycardia, confusion, restlessness, apprehension, flushed face
Respiratory alkalosis (excess carbon dioxide excretion) pH > 7.45 HCO_3^- < 22 mEq/L (if compensating) $PaCO_2$ < 35 mm Hg	■ Hyperventilation from anxiety, pain, or improper ventilator settings ■ Respiratory stimulation from drugs, disease, hypoxia, fever, or high room temperature ■ Gram-negative bacteremia	■ Rapid, deep respirations; paresthesia; light-headedness; twitching; anxiety; fear
Metabolic acidosis (bicarbonate loss, acid retention) pH < 7.35 HCO_3^- < 22 mEq/L $PaCO_2$ < 35 mm Hg (if compensating)	■ Bicarbonate depletion from diarrhea ■ Excessive production of organic acids from hepatic disease, endocrine disorders, shock, or drug intoxication ■ Inadequate excretion of acids from renal disease	■ Rapid, deep breathing; fruity breath; fatigue; headache; lethargy; drowsiness; nausea; vomiting; coma (if severe); abdominal pain
Metabolic alkalosis (bicarbonate retention, acid loss) pH > 7.45 HCO_3^- > 26 mEq/L $PaCO_2$ > 45 mm Hg (if compensating)	■ Loss of hydrochloric acid from prolonged vomiting or gastric suctioning ■ Loss of potassium from increased renal excretion (as in diuretic therapy) or steroids ■ Excessive alkali ingestion	■ Slow, shallow breathing; hypertonic muscles; restlessness; twitching; confusion; irritability; apathy; tetany; seizures; coma (if severe)

Interpretation

NORMAL FINDINGS

■ PaO_2: 80 to 100 mm Hg
■ $PaCO_2$: 35 to 45 mm Hg
■ pH: 7.35 to 7.45
■ SaO_2: 95% to 100%
■ HCO_3^-: 22 to 26 mEq/L

ABNORMAL RESULTS

■ Low PaO_2 and SaO_2 levels in combination with a high $PaCO_2$ suggest conditions that impair respiratory function or obstruct the bronchioles such as mucous plugging.
■ Low PaO_2 and SaO_2, with a normal $PaCO_2$ suggest impaired diffusion between alveoli and blood, or an arteri-

PERFORMING ALLEN'S TEST

Don't obtain an arterial blood gas specimen from the radial artery until you assess collateral arterial blood supply using Allen's test.

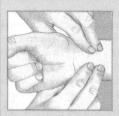 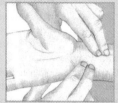 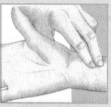

Direct the patient to close his hand while you occlude his radial and ulnar arteries for 10 to 30 seconds, watching for the hand to blanch.

Tell the patient to open his hand.

Release pressure on the ulnar artery. Color should return to the patient's hand in 15 seconds. If the color doesn't return, select another site for an arterial puncture.

ovenous shunt that permits blood to bypass the lungs.

BRONCHOSCOPY

Overview

■ Direct visualization of the larynx, trachea, and bronchi using a rigid or fiber-optic bronchoscope
■ Flexible fiber-optic bronchoscope: allows a better view of the segmental and subsegmental bronchi with less risk of trauma
■ Large, rigid bronchoscope: used to remove foreign objects, excise endobronchial lesions, and control massive hemoptysis; requires general anesthesia
■ A brush, biopsy forceps, or a catheter may be passed through bronchoscope for obtaining specimens for cytologic or microbiologic examination

PURPOSE

■ To allow visual examination of tumors, obstructions, secretions, or foreign bodies in the tracheobronchial tree
■ To diagnose bronchogenic carcinoma, tuberculosis, interstitial pulmonary disease, and fungal or parasitic pulmonary infections
■ To obtain specimens for microbiological and cytologic examination
■ To locate bleeding sites in the tracheobronchial tree
■ To remove foreign bodies, malignant or benign tumors, mucous plugs, and excessive secretions from the tracheobronchial tree

PATIENT PREPARATION

■ Make sure the patient has signed an appropriate consent form.
■ Note all allergies.
■ Instruct the patient to fast for 6 to 12 hours before the test.

- Obtain results of preprocedure studies; report any abnormal results.
- Obtain baseline vital signs.
- An I.V. sedative may be given.
- Remove the patient's dentures.

Teaching points

Be sure to cover:
- the test's purpose and how it's done
- who will perform the test and where
- that the test takes 45 to 60 minutes
- that the airway isn't blocked
- that hoarseness, loss of voice, hemoptysis, and sore throat may occur.

POSTPROCEDURE CARE

- Position a conscious patient in semi-Fowler's position.
- Position an unconscious patient on one side, with the head of the bed slightly elevated to prevent aspiration.
- Instruct the patient to spit out saliva rather than swallow it.
- Observe for bleeding.
- Resume the patient's usual diet, beginning with sips of clear liquid or ice chips, when the gag reflex returns.
- Provide lozenges or a soothing liquid gargle to ease discomfort when the gag reflex returns.
- Check follow-up chest X-ray to ensure no pneumothorax.

Monitoring

- Vital signs
- Characteristics of sputum
- Respiratory status

    Immediately report subcutaneous crepitus around the patient's face, neck, or chest because these may indicate tracheal or bronchial perforation or pneumothorax.

    Watch for and immediately report symptoms of respiratory difficulty associated with laryngeal edema or laryngospasm, such as laryngeal stridor and dyspnea.

PRECAUTIONS

- Check the patient's history for hypersensitivity to the anesthetic.
- Failure to observe pretest dietary restrictions may result in aspiration.
- Failure to place the specimens in the appropriate containers or to send them to the laboratory immediately may interfere with accurate test results.
- Bronchoscopy findings must be correlated with clinical signs and symptoms and radiographic and cytologic findings.

COMPLICATIONS

- Tracheal or bronchial perforation
- Hypoxemia
- Cardiac arrhythmias
- Bleeding
- Infection
- Bronchospasm
- Laryngeal edema

Interpretation

NORMAL FINDINGS

- The bronchi appear structurally similar to the trachea.
- The right bronchus is slightly larger and more vertical than the left.
- Smaller segmental bronchi branch off from the main bronchi.

ABNORMAL RESULTS

- Structural abnormalities of the bronchial wall suggest inflammation, ulceration, tumors, and enlargement of submucosal lymph nodes.
- Structural abnormalities of endotracheal origin suggest stenosis, compression, ectasia, and diverticulum.
- Structural abnormalities of the trachea or bronchi suggest calculi, foreign bodies, masses, and paralyzed vocal cords.
- Abnormal results of tissue and cell studies suggest interstitial pulmonary

disease, infection, carcinoma, and tuberculosis.

CHEST RADIOGRAPHY

Overview

- A noninvasive and relatively inexpensive study
- X-ray beams penetrate the chest and react on specially sensitized film; air is radiolucent, so thoracic structures appear as different densities on the film
- Commonly known as chest X-ray

PURPOSE

- To establish a baseline for future comparison
- To detect pulmonary disorders such as pneumonia
- To detect mediastinal abnormalities such as tumors
- To verify correct placement of pulmonary artery catheters, endotracheal (ET) tubes, and chest tubes
- To determine location of swallowed or aspirated radiopague foreign bodies
- To determine location and size of lesions
- To evaluate response to interventions such as diuretic therapy

PATIENT PREPARATION

- Make sure the patient has signed an appropriate consent form.
- Restriction of food and fluids isn't necessary before the test.
- Move cardiac monitoring cables, oxygen tubing, I.V. tubing, pulmonary artery catheter lines, and other equipment out of the radiographic field.
- Explain that the patient will be asked to take a deep breath and hold it momentarily while the film is being exposed.

Teaching points

Be sure to cover:
- the purpose of the study
- who will perform the test
- that the test takes less than 5 minutes.

POSTPROCEDURE CARE

- Check that no tubes have been dislodged during positioning.

PRECAUTIONS

- Chest radiography is usually contraindicated during the first trimester of pregnancy.
- Whenever possible, place a lead apron over the patient's abdomen to protect the gonads.
- To avoid radiation exposure, leave the area or wear lead shielding while the films are being exposed.
- Portable films may be less reliable than stationary radiographs.
- Inability to take a full inspiration will decrease the quality of radiographs.

COMPLICATIONS

- Potential for dislodging tubes or wires, such as the ET tube or pacemaker wires during positioning

Interpretation

NORMAL FINDINGS
Trachea

- There's a visible midline in the anterior mediastinal cavity.
- It has a translucent, tubelike appearance.

Heart

- It's visible in the anterior left mediastinal cavity.
- It appears solid because of its blood content.

Aortic knob
- It's visible as water density.
- It's formed by the aortic arch.

Mediastinum (mediastinal shadow)
- It's visible as the space between the lungs.
- It has a shadowy appearance, widening at the hilum.

Ribs
- They're visible as thoracic cavity encasement.

Spine
- It has a visible midline in the posterior chest that's best seen on a lateral view.

Clavicles
- They're visible in the upper thorax.
- They're intact and equidistant in properly centered films.

Hila (lung roots)
- They're visible above the heart.
- They're found where pulmonary vessels, bronchi, and lymph nodes join the lungs.
- They appear as small, white, bilateral branching densities.

Mainstem bronchus
- It's visible as part of the hila.
- It has a translucent, tubelike appearance.

Bronchi
- They aren't usually visible.

Lung fields
- They aren't usually visible, except for blood vessels.

Hemidiaphragm
- It's rounded and visible.

- The right side is 1 to 2 cm higher than the left side.

ABNORMAL RESULTS
Deviations from normal findings should be correlated with additional tests and physical findings.
- Deviation of trachea from midline suggests possible tension pneumothorax or pleural effusion.
- Right heart hypertrophy suggests possible cor pulmonale or heart failure.
- A tortuous aortic knob suggests atherosclerosis.
- Gross widening of the mediastinum suggests neoplasm or aortic aneurysm.
- A break or misalignment of bones suggests fracture.
- Visible bronchi suggest bronchial pneumonia.
- Flattening of the diaphragm suggests emphysema or asthma.
- Irregular, patchy infiltrates in the lung fields suggest pneumonia.

COMPUTED TOMOGRAPHY OF THE THORAX

Overview

- Provides cross-sectional views of the chest and three-dimensional information as opposed to two-dimensional information provided by chest X-ray
- I.V. contrast agent used if differentiating vessels from adjacent structures is necessary
- Used to detect small differences in tissue density
- Also known as CT of the thorax or chest

PURPOSE
- To locate suspected neoplasms

■ To differentiate coin-sized calcified lesions (indicating tuberculosis) from tumors
■ To revaluate mediastinal lymph nodes (with contrast)
■ To evaluate aortic aneurysms (with contrast)
■ To evaluate the severity of lung disease such as emphysema
■ To aid in planning radiation treatment

PATIENT PREPARATION
■ Make sure the patient has signed an appropriate consent form.
■ Note and report all allergies.
■ Ensure adequate hydration, especially in case of decreased renal function.
■ Restriction of food and fluids before the test is necessary with the use of contrast enhancement as ordered.
■ Stress the need to remain still during the test because movement can limit test accuracy. The patient may experience minimal discomfort because of lying still.
■ Explain the importance of following breathing instructions.
■ Warn about transient discomfort from the needle puncture and a warm or flushed feeling if an I.V. contrast medium is used.
■ Explain that the equipment may be noisy.

Teaching points
Be sure to cover:
■ the purpose of the study and how it's done
■ who will perform the test and where
■ that the test takes 1 hour
■ that radiation exposure is minimal.

POSTPROCEDURE CARE
■ Watch for signs of delayed hypersensitivity to the contrast agent, including pruritus, urticaria, and respiratory distress.
■ Encourage fluid intake if a contrast agent was used.
■ Resume normal diet and activity unless otherwise ordered.

PRECAUTIONS
■ CT of the thorax is contraindicated during pregnancy.
■ I.V. contrast agent is contraindicated in people with a history of hypersensitivity reactions to iodine, shellfish, or radiographic contrast agents or a history of renal insufficiency.
■ Inability to lie still during scanning may interfere with accurate diagnosis and require repetition of the test, which increases radiation exposure.
■ An obese patient may exceed the weight limit of the scanning table.

COMPLICATIONS
■ Adverse reaction to the iodinated contrast media
■ Extravasation of I.V. contrast media

Interpretation

NORMAL FINDINGS
■ Black areas on a thoracic CT scan indicate air; white areas indicate bone.
■ Shades of gray correspond to fluid, fat, and soft-tissue densities.

ABNORMAL RESULTS
■ Well-circumscribed or poorly defined areas of slightly lower density than normal parenchyma suggest possible primary and metastatic neoplasms.
■ Relatively low-density, homogeneous areas, usually with well-defined borders, suggest possible abscesses.
■ Sharply defined round or oval structures, with densities lower than abscesses and neoplasms, suggest cysts.

RESPIRATORY CARE

■ Structural abnormalities suggest possible disorders including:
- aortic aneurysm
- enlarged lymph nodes
- pleural effusion
- bronchiectasis
- emphysema.

LUNG PERFUSION SCAN

Overview

■ Produces a visual image of pulmonary blood flow after I.V. injection of a radiopharmaceutical
■ Human serum albumin microspheres (particles) or macroaggregated albumin, bonded to technetium, possibly used

PURPOSE

■ To assess arterial perfusion of the lungs
■ To detect pulmonary emboli
■ To evaluate pulmonary function

PATIENT PREPARATION

■ Make sure the patient has signed an appropriate consent form.
■ Note and report all allergies.
■ Restriction of food and fluids isn't necessary before the test.
■ Stress the importance of lying still during imaging.

Teaching points

Be sure to cover:
■ the purpose of the study and how it's performed
■ who will perform the test and where
■ that the test takes about 30 minutes
■ that the amount of radioactivity is minimal.

POSTPROCEDURE CARE

■ Apply warm soaks if a hematoma develops at the injection site.

PRECAUTIONS

■ Lung perfusion scan is contraindicated in hypersensitivity to the radiopharmaceutical.

COMPLICATIONS

■ Sensitivity to the radiopharmaceutical

Interpretation

NORMAL FINDINGS

■ Hot spots (areas of high uptake) indicate normal blood perfusion.
■ The uptake pattern is uniform.

ABNORMAL RESULTS

■ Cold spots (areas of low uptake) indicate poor perfusion, suggesting an embolism.
■ Decreased regional blood flow, without vessel obstruction, suggests possible pneumonitis.

LUNG VENTILATION SCAN

Overview

■ A nuclear scan performed after inhalation of air mixed with radioactive gas
■ Differentiates areas of ventilated lung from areas of underventilated lungs

PURPOSE

■ To diagnose pulmonary emboli when used in combination with lung perfusion scan
■ To identify areas of the lung that are capable of ventilation

- To evaluate regional respiratory function
- To locate regional hypoventilation

PATIENT PREPARATION

- Make sure the patient has signed an appropriate consent form.
- Note and report all allergies.
- Restriction of food or fluids isn't necessary before the test.
- Stress the importance of lying still during imaging.
- Explain that the patient wears a tight-fitting mask during the study.

Teaching points

Be sure to cover:
- the purpose of the study and how it's done
- who will perform the test and where
- that the test takes 15 to 30 minutes.

POSTPROCEDURE CARE

- Reinstate any oxygen therapy previously ordered.

Monitoring

- Vital signs
- Respiratory status

PRECAUTIONS

- Leaks in the closed system of radioactive gas can contaminate the surrounding atmosphere.

COMPLICATIONS

- Panic attacks from wearing the tight-fitting mask

Interpretation

NORMAL FINDINGS

- Gas should be equally distributed in both lungs.

ABNORMAL RESULTS

- Unequal gas distribution in both lungs suggests poor ventilation or air-

way obstruction in areas with low radioactivity.
- When performed with a lung perfusion scan, vascular obstruction with normal ventilation suggests decreased perfusion such as in pulmonary embolism.
- Both ventilation and perfusion abnormalities suggests possible parenchymal disease.

PULMONARY ANGIOGRAPHY

Overview

- Radiographic examination of the pulmonary circulation after injection of a radiopaque contrast agent into the pulmonary artery or one of its branches
- May be used to diagnose pulmonary embolism when lung ventilation perfusion scans are indeterminate
- May be performed to administer local thrombolytic therapy in patients with pulmonary embolism (PE)
- Also known as *pulmonary arteriography*

PURPOSE

- To detect pulmonary embolism in a symptomatic patient with an equivocal lung scan
- To evaluate pulmonary circulation abnormalities
- To provide accurate preoperative evaluation of patients with shunt physiology caused by congenital heart disease
- To treat identified PE with thrombolysis

PATIENT PREPARATION

- Make sure the patient has signed an appropriate consent form.
- Note and report all allergies.

- Check the patient's history for hypersensitivity to iodine, seafood, or iodinated contrast agents.
- Check for and report history of anticoagulation.
- Check for and report history of renal insufficiency.
- Note and inform the physician of abnormal laboratory results.
- Discontinue heparin infusion 3 to 4 hours before the test as ordered.
- Fasting is required for 8 hours before the test or as ordered.
- Explain the need to use a local anesthetic.
- Warn about a possible urge to cough, flushed feeling, or salty taste for 3 to 5 minutes after the injection.

Teaching points
Be sure to cover:
- the purpose of the study and how it's done
- who will perform the test and where
- that the test takes about 1½ to 2 hours
- that the patient will be monitored during the study.

POSTPROCEDURE CARE
- Maintain bed rest as ordered.
- Resume usual diet as ordered.
- Restart anticoagulation as ordered.
- Encourage oral fluid intake, or administer I.V. fluids as ordered to help eliminate the contrast agent.

Monitoring
- Vital signs
- Intake and output
- Catheter insertion site
- Bleeding
- Infection
- Hematoma formation
- Renal function studies
- Adverse reaction to contrast agent

Observe the site for bleeding and swelling. If these occur, maintain pressure at the insertion site for at least 10 minutes and notify the radiologist.

PRECAUTIONS
- Pulmonary angiography is contraindicated during pregnancy.
- Ventricular arrhythmias may be caused by passage of the catheter through the heart chambers.

Complications

- Myocardial perforation or rupture
- Ventricular arrhythmias and conduction defects
- Acute renal failure
- Bleeding and hematoma formation
- Infection
- Adverse reaction to contrast agent
- Cardiac valve damage
- Right-sided heart failure

Interpretation

NORMAL FINDINGS
- The contrast agent should flow symmetrically and without interruption through the pulmonary circulation.

ABNORMAL RESULTS
- Interruption of blood flow and filling defects suggests possible acute pulmonary embolism.
- Arterial webs, stenoses, irregular occlusions, wall-scalloping, and "pouching" defects (a concave edge of thrombus facing the opacified lumen) suggest chronic pulmonary embolism.

PULMONARY FUNCTION TESTS

Overview

■ Evaluation of pulmonary function through a series of spirometric measurements
■ Also known as *PFTs*

PURPOSE

■ To assess effectiveness of a specific therapeutic regimen
■ To differentiate between obstructive and restrictive pulmonary disease
■ To evaluate pulmonary status before surgery
■ To stage a disease process
■ To determine disability
■ To assess diffusion capacity

PATIENT PREPARATION

■ Make sure the patient has signed an appropriate consent form.
■ Note and report all allergies.
■ Withhold bronchodilators for 8 hours as ordered.
■ Stress the need to avoid a heavy meal before the tests.
■ Stress the need to avoid smoking for 12 hours before the tests.
■ Provide reassurance that the procedure is painless and the patient can rest between tests.

Teaching points

Be sure to cover:
■ the purpose of the study and how it's done
■ who will perform the test and where
■ that the study takes 1 to 2 hours.
■ Accuracy of the study may be diminished with chest pain, abdominal pain, or cough.

Pulmonary function tests may be contraindicated in patients with acute coronary insufficiency, angina, or recent myocardial infarction. Watch for respiratory distress, changes in pulse rate and blood pressure, coughing, and bronchospasm in these patients.

COMPLICATIONS

■ Respiratory distress
■ Bronchospasm
■ Physical exhaustion

Interpretation

NORMAL FINDINGS

■ Normal values are predicted for each patient based on age, height, weight, and gender and are expressed as a percentage:
  – Tidal volume (V_T) is 5 to 7 mg/kg of body weight.
  – Expiratory reserve volume (ERV) is 25% of vital capacity (VC).
  – Inspiratory capacity (IC) is 75% of VC.
  – Forced expiratory volume $(FEV)_1$ is 83% of VC after 1 second.
  – FEV_2 is 94% of VC after 2 seconds.
  – FEV_3 is 97% of VC after 3 seconds.

ABNORMAL RESULTS

■ FEV_1 less than 80% suggests obstructed pulmonary disease.
■ FEV_1/forced vital capacity (FVC) ratio greater than 80% suggests restrictive pulmonary disease.
■ Decreased V_T suggests possible restrictive disease.
■ Decreased minute volume (MV) suggests possible disorders such as pulmonary edema.
■ Increased MV suggests possible acidosis, exercise, or low compliance states.
■ Reduced carbon dioxide response suggests possible emphysema, myxedema, obesity, hypoventilation syndrome, or sleep apnea.
■ Residual volume greater than 35% of total lung capacity (TLC) after

maximal expiratory effort suggests obstructive disease.
- Decreased IC suggests restrictive disease.
- Increased functional residual suggests possible obstructive pulmonary disease.
- Low TLC suggests restrictive disease.
- High TLC suggests obstructive disease.
- Decreased FVC suggests flow resistance from obstructive disease or from restrictive disease.
- Low forced expiratory flow suggests obstructive disease of the small and medium-sized airways.
- Decreased peak expiratory flow rate suggests upper airway obstruction.
- Decreased diffusing capacity for carbon monoxide suggests possible interstitial pulmonary disease.

THORACENTESIS

Overview

- Performed diagnostically to obtain samples of pleural fluid for analysis, or therapeutically to relieve respiratory symptoms caused by the accumulation of excess pleural fluid
- Samples are examined for color, consistency, pH, glucose and protein content, cellular composition, and the enzymes lactate dehydrogenase (LD) and amylase; also examined cytologically for malignant cells and cultured for pathogens
- Risk of puncturing the lung, liver, or spleen: reduced by locating the fluid before thoracentesis, by physical examination and chest X-ray or ultrasonography
- Also known as *pleural fluid aspiration*

PURPOSE

- To provide pleural fluid samples to determine the cause and nature of pleural effusion
- To provide symptomatic relief with large pleural effusion

PATIENT PREPARATION

- Make sure the patient has signed an appropriate consent form.
- Note and report all allergies.
- Record baseline vital signs.
- Food and fluids may be restricted if sedation will be used.
- Explain to the patient that pleural fluid may be located by chest X-ray or ultrasound study.
- Explain that a local anesthetic will be used. Warn about a stinging sensation felt on injection of the anesthetic and some pressure during withdrawal of the fluid.
- Instruct the patient to avoid coughing, deep breathing, or moving during the test to minimize the risk of injury to the lung.

Teaching points

Be sure to cover:
- the purpose of the study and how it's done
- who will perform the test and where
- that the study takes about 1 hour.

POSTPROCEDURE CARE

- Elevate the head of the bed to facilitate breathing.
- Obtain a chest X-ray as ordered.

Tell the patient to immediately report difficulty breathing. Immediately report signs and symptoms of pneumothorax, tension pneumothorax, and pleural fluid reaccumulation.

Monitor the patient for reexpansion pulmonary edema, a rare but serious complication of thoracentesis. Thoracentesis should be halted if the pa-

tient has sudden chest tightness or coughing.

Monitoring
- Vital signs
- Pulse oximetry
- Breath sounds
- Puncture site and dressings
- Subcutaneous emphysema
- Pleural pressure

PRECAUTIONS
■ Supplemental oxygen is administered and close pulse oximetry is monitored during thoracentesis.

Thoracentesis is contraindicated in patients with uncorrected bleeding disorders or anticoagulant therapy. The benefits of the procedure should outweigh the risks for a patient taking an anticoagulant with an International Normalized Ratio of 1.5 to 2.5.

■ Note the patient's temperature and use of antimicrobial therapy.

Pleural fluid for pH determination must be collected anaerobically, heparinized, kept on ice, and analyzed promptly.

COMPLICATIONS
- Laceration of intercostal vessels
- Pneumothorax
- Mediastinal shift
- Reexpansion pulmonary edema
- Bleeding and infection

Interpretation

NORMAL FINDINGS
■ The pleural cavity should maintain negative pressure and contain less than 50 ml of serous fluid.

ABNORMAL RESULTS
■ Bloody fluid suggests possible hemothorax, malignancy, or traumatic tap.
■ Milky fluid suggests chylothorax.
■ Fluid with pus suggests empyema.
■ Transudative effusion suggests heart failure, hepatic cirrhosis, or renal disease.
■ Exudative effusion suggests lymphatic drainage abstraction, infections, pulmonary infarctions, and neoplasms.
■ Positive cultures suggest infection.
■ Predominating lymphocytes suggest tuberculosis or fungal or viral effusions.
■ Elevated LD levels in a nonpurulent, nonhemolyzed, nonbloody effusion suggest possible malignant tumor.
■ Pleural fluid glucose levels that are 30 to 40 mg/dl lower than blood glucose levels may indicate cancer, bacterial infection, or metastasis.
■ Increased amylase suggests pleural effusions associated with pancreatitis.

RESPIRATORY CARE

DISEASES

ACUTE RESPIRATORY DISTRESS SYNDROME

Overview

DESCRIPTION
■ A form of pulmonary edema; may be difficult to recognize

■ Hallmark sign includes hypoxemia despite increased supplemental oxygen
■ A four-stage syndrome; can rapidly progress to intractable and fatal hypoxemia
■ Little or no permanent lung damage occurring in patients who recover

■ May coexist with disseminated intravascular coagulation (DIC)
■ Also known as *shock, stiff, white, wet,* or *Da Nang lung* and *ARDS*

PATHOPHYSIOLOGY
■ Increased permeability of the alveolocapillary membranes that allows fluid to accumulate in the lung interstitium, alveolar spaces, and small airways, causing the lung to stiffen
■ Ventilation that's impaired, reducing oxygenation of pulmonary capillary blood
■ Elevated capillary pressure that increases interstitial and alveolar edema
■ Alveolar closing pressure that then exceeds pulmonary pressures
■ Closure and collapse of the alveoli

CAUSES
■ Indirect or direct lung trauma (most common)
■ Anaphylaxis
■ Aspiration of gastric contents
■ Diffuse pneumonia (especially viral)
■ Drug overdose
■ Idiosyncratic drug reaction
■ Inhalation of noxious gases
■ Near-drowning
■ Oxygen toxicity
■ Coronary artery bypass grafting
■ Hemodialysis
■ Leukemia
■ Acute miliary tuberculosis
■ Pancreatitis
■ Thrombotic thrombocytopenic purpura
■ Uremia
■ Venous air embolism

COMPLICATIONS
■ Metabolic acidosis
■ Respiratory acidosis
■ Cardiac arrest

Assessment

HISTORY
■ Dyspnea, especially on exertion

PHYSICAL FINDINGS
Stage I
■ Shortness of breath, especially on exertion
■ Normal to increased respiratory and pulse rates
■ Diminished breath sounds

Stage II
■ Respiratory distress
■ Use of accessory muscles
■ Pallor, anxiety, and restlessness
■ Dry cough with thick, frothy sputum
■ Bloody, sticky secretions
■ Cool, clammy skin
■ Tachycardia and tachypnea
■ Elevated blood pressure
■ Basilar crackles

Stage III
■ Breathing rate more than 30 breaths/minute
■ Tachycardia with arrhythmias
■ Labile blood pressure
■ Productive cough
■ Pale, cyanotic skin
■ Crackles and rhonchi possible

Stage IV
■ Acute respiratory failure with severe hypoxia
■ Deteriorating mental status
■ May become comatose
■ Pale, cyanotic skin
■ Lack of spontaneous respirations
■ Bradycardia with arrhythmias
■ Hypotension
■ Metabolic and respiratory acidosis

TEST RESULTS
Laboratory
- Arterial blood gas (ABG) analysis initially showing a reduced partial pressure of arterial oxygen (Pao_2) (less than 60 mm Hg) and a decreased partial pressure of arterial carbon dioxide ($Paco_2$) (less than 35 mm Hg)
- ABG analysis later showing increased $Paco_2$ (more than 45 mm Hg) and decreased bicarbonate levels (less than 22 mEq/L) and decreased Pao_2 despite oxygen therapy
- Gram stain and sputum culture and sensitivity showing infectious organism
- Blood cultures revealing infectious organisms
- Toxicology tests showing drug ingestion
- Increased serum amylase in pancreatitis

Imaging
- Chest X-rays may show early bilateral infiltrates; in later stages, a ground-glass appearance and, eventually, "whiteouts" of both lung fields.

Diagnostic procedures
- Pulmonary artery catheterization may show a pulmonary artery wedge pressure of 12 to 18 mm Hg.

Treatment

GENERAL
- Treatment of the underlying cause
- Correction of electrolyte and acid-base imbalances

For mechanical ventilation
- Target low tidal volumes; use of increased respiratory rates
- Target plateau pressures less than or equal to 40 cm H_2O

DIET
- Fluid restriction
- Tube feedings
- Parenteral nutrition

ACTIVITY
- Bed rest
- Prone positioning

MEDICATION
- Humidified oxygen
- Bronchodilators
- Diuretics

For mechanical ventilation
- Sedatives
- Narcotics
- Neuromuscular blocking agents
- Short course of high-dose corticosteroids if fatty emboli or chemical injury
- Sodium bicarbonate if severe metabolic acidosis
- Fluids and vasopressors if hypotensive
- Antimicrobials if nonviral infection

SURGERY
- Possible tracheostomy

MONITORING
- Vital signs
- Hemodynamics
- Intake and output
- Respiratory status
- Mechanical ventilator settings
- Sputum characteristics
- Level of consciousness
- Breath sounds
- Daily weight
- ABG results
- Pulse oximetry
- Cardiac rate and rhythm
- Serum electrolyte results
- Response to treatment
- Complications, such as cardiac arrhythmias, DIC, GI bleeding, infec-

tion, malnutrition, and pneumothorax
- Nutritional status

Because positive end-expiratory pressure (PEEP) may lower cardiac output, check for hypotension, tachycardia, and decreased urine output. To maintain PEEP, suction only as needed.

ASTHMA

Overview

DESCRIPTION
- Involves episodic, reversible airway obstruction resulting from bronchospasms, increased mucus secretions, and mucosal edema
- Signs and symptoms that range from mild wheezing and dyspnea to life-threatening respiratory failure
- Signs and symptoms of bronchial airway obstruction that may or may not persist between acute episodes
- A chronic reactive airway disorder

PATHOPHYSIOLOGY
- Tracheal and bronchial linings overreact to various stimuli, causing episodic smooth-muscle spasms that severely constrict the airways.
- Mucosal edema and thickened secretions further block the airways.
- Immunoglobulin (Ig) E antibodies, attached to histamine-containing mast cells and receptors on cell membranes, initiate intrinsic asthma attacks.
- When exposed to an antigen such as pollen, the IgE antibody combines with the antigen. On subsequent exposure to the antigen, mast cells degranulate and release mediators.
- The mediators cause the bronchoconstriction and edema of an asthma attack.

- During an asthma attack, expiratory airflow decreases, trapping gas in the airways and causing alveolar hyperinflation.
- Atelectasis may develop in some lung regions.
- The increased airway resistance initiates labored breathing.

CAUSES
- Sensitivity to specific external allergens or from internal, nonallergenic factors

In extrinsic asthma (atopic asthma)
- Pollen
- Animal dander
- House dust or mold
- Kapok or feather pillows
- Food additives containing sulfites and any other sensitizing substance

In intrinsic asthma (nonatopic asthma)
- Emotional stress
- Genetic factors

In bronchoconstriction
- Hereditary predisposition
- Sensitivity to allergens or irritants such as pollutants
- Viral infections
- Drugs, such as aspirin, beta-adrenergic blockers, and nonsteroidal anti-inflammatory drugs
- Psychological stress
- Cold air
- Exercise

COMPLICATIONS
- Status asthmaticus
- Respiratory failure
- Death

Assessment

HISTORY
- Intrinsic asthma is often preceded by severe respiratory tract infections, especially in adults.
- Irritants, emotional stress, fatigue, endocrine changes, temperature and humidity variations, and exposure to noxious fumes may aggravate intrinsic asthma attacks.
- An asthma attack may begin dramatically, with simultaneous onset of severe, multiple symptoms, or insidiously, with gradually increasing respiratory distress.
- Exposure to a particular allergen is followed by a sudden onset of dyspnea and wheezing and by tightness in the chest accompanied by a cough that produces thick, clear, or yellow sputum.

PHYSICAL FINDINGS
- Visibly dyspneic
- Ability to speak only a few words before pausing for breath
- Use of accessory respiratory muscles
- Diaphoresis
- Increased anteroposterior thoracic diameter
- Hyperresonance
- Tachycardia; tachypnea; mild systolic hypertension
- Inspiratory and expiratory wheezes
- Prolonged expiratory phase of respiration
- Diminished breath sounds
- Cyanosis, confusion, and lethargy indicate the onset of life-threatening status asthmaticus and respiratory failure

TEST RESULTS
Laboratory
- Arterial blood gas (ABG) analysis revealing hypoxemia
- Increased serum IgE levels from an allergic reaction
- Complete blood count with differential showing increased eosinophil count

Imaging
- Chest X-rays may show hyperinflation with areas of focal atelectasis.

Diagnostic procedures
- Pulmonary function tests (PFTs) may show decreased peak flows and forced expiratory volume in 1 second, low-normal or decreased vital capacity, and increased total lung and residual capacities.
- Skin testing may identify specific allergens.
- Bronchial challenge testing shows the clinical significance of allergens identified by skin testing.

Other
- Pulse oximetry measurements may show decreased oxygen saturation.

Treatment

GENERAL
- Prevention by avoiding precipitating factors (see *Averting an asthma attack,* page 300)
- Desensitization to specific antigens
- Prompt treatment for status asthmaticus to prevent progression to fatal respiratory failure

DIET
- Fluid replacement

ACTIVITY
- As tolerated

MEDICATION
- Bronchodilators (see *Using a metered-dose inhaler,* page 301)
- Corticosteroids

AVERTING AN ASTHMA ATTACK

This flowchart shows pathophysiologic changes that occur with asthma. Treatments and interventions show where the physiologic cascade would be altered to stop an asthma attack.

Exposure to allergens and causative factors

Avoidance of allergens
Allergy injections
Reduction of causative factors
(stress-reduction classes)
Corticosteroids

Immunoglobulin E stimulation

Mast cell degranulation

Mast cell stabilizers

Histamine
Leukotrienes
Prostaglandins
Bradykinins

Antihistamines

Mucus secretion
Inflammation
Bronchospasm

Bronchodilators

Wheezing and narrowing of airways

Airway obstruction

Key: ✳ = treatment

- Histamine antagonists
- Leukotriene antagonists
- Anticholinergic bronchodilators
- Low-flow oxygen
- Antibiotics
- Heliox trial (before intubation)
- I.V. magnesium sulfate (controversial)

The patient with increasingly severe asthma that doesn't respond to drug therapy is usually admitted for treatment with corticosteroids, epinephrine, and sympathomimetic aerosol sprays. He may require endotracheal intubation and mechanical ventilation.

MONITORING

- Vital signs
- Intake and output
- Severity of asthma
- Signs and symptoms of theophylline toxicity
- Breath sounds
- ABG results
- PFT results
- Pulse oximetry
- Complications of corticosteroids
- Level of anxiety

BRONCHITIS, CHRONIC

Overview

DESCRIPTION

- Form of chronic obstructive pulmonary disease
- Characterized by excessive production of tracheobronchial mucus with a cough for at least 3 months each year for 2 consecutive years
- Severity that's linked to the amount of cigarette smoke or other pollutants inhaled and inhalation duration
- Respiratory tract infections that typically exacerbate the cough and related symptoms
- Few patients with chronic bronchitis develop significant airway obstruction

PATHOPHYSIOLOGY

- Results in hypertrophy and hyperplasia of the bronchial mucous glands, increased goblet cells, ciliary damage, squamous metaplasia of the columnar epithelium, and chronic leukocytic and lymphocytic infiltration of bronchial walls.
- Additional effects include widespread inflammation, airway narrowing, and mucus within the airways—all producing resistance in the small airways and, in turn, a severe ventilation-perfusion imbalance.

USING A METERED-DOSE INHALER

When instructing your patient about proper metered-dose inhaler (MDI) use, include these points:

- Shake the MDI well before use.
- Exhale normally. Then place the mouthpiece in your mouth and close your lips around it.
- Begin slow, steady inspirations through your mouth until your lungs feel full.
- While inhaling slowly, squeeze firmly on the MDI to deliver the dose while continuing to breathe in one deep steady breath, not several shallow ones.
- Hold your breath for several seconds before exhaling.
- Exhale slowly through pursed lips.
- Gargle with normal saline solution, if desired.

Note: When using an extender or a spacer device, follow the same routine as described above, with the MDI mouthpiece inserted in one end of the spacer and the other end placed in the mouth. Many spacers are equipped with a small whistle that sounds if the dose is being inhaled too fast.

CAUSES

- Cigarette smoking
- Possible genetic predisposition
- Environmental pollution
- Organic or inorganic dusts and noxious gas exposure

COMPLICATIONS

- Cor pulmonale
- Pulmonary hypertension
- Right ventricular hypertrophy
- Acute respiratory failure

Assessment

HISTORY
- Long-time smoker
- Frequent upper respiratory tract infections
- Productive cough
- Exertional dyspnea
- Cough, initially prevalent in winter, but gradually becoming year-round
- Increasingly severe coughing episodes
- Worsening dyspnea

PHYSICAL FINDINGS
- Cough producing copious gray, white, or yellow sputum
- Cyanosis, also called a *blue bloater*
- Accessory respiratory muscle use
- Tachypnea
- Substantial weight gain
- Pedal edema
- Jugular vein distention
- Wheezing
- Prolonged expiratory time
- Rhonchi

TEST RESULTS
Laboratory
- Arterial blood gas analysis showing decreased partial pressure of oxygen and normal or increased partial pressure of carbon dioxide
- Sputum culture revealing how many microorganisms and neutrophils

Imaging
- Chest X-ray may show hyperinflation and increased bronchovascular markings.

Diagnostic procedures
- Pulmonary function tests show increased residual volume, decreased vital capacity and forced expiratory flow, and normal static compliance and diffusing capacity.

Other
- Electrocardiography may show atrial arrhythmias; peaked P waves in leads II, III, and aV_F; and right ventricular hypertrophy.

Treatment

GENERAL
- Smoking cessation
- Avoidance of air pollutants
- Chest physiotherapy
- Ultrasonic or mechanical nebulizer treatments

DIET
- Adequate fluid intake
- High-calorie, protein-rich

ACTIVITY
- As tolerated with frequent rest periods

MEDICATION
- Oxygen
- Antibiotics
- Bronchodilators
- Corticosteroids
- Diuretics

SURGERY
- Tracheostomy in advanced disease

MONITORING
- Vital signs
- Intake and output
- Sputum production
- Respiratory status
- Breath sounds
- Daily weight
- Edema
- Response to treatment

EMPHYSEMA

Overview

DESCRIPTION
■ Characterized by exertional dyspnea
■ One of several diseases usually labeled collectively as chronic obstructive pulmonary disease or chronic obstructive lung disease

PATHOPHYSIOLOGY
■ Recurrent inflammation associated with the release of proteolytic enzymes from lung cells causes abnormal, irreversible enlargement of the air spaces distal to the terminal bronchioles.
■ This enlargement leads to the destruction of alveolar walls, which results in a breakdown of elasticity.

CAUSES
■ Genetic deficiency of alpha$_1$-antitrypsin
■ Cigarette smoking

COMPLICATIONS
■ Recurrent respiratory tract infections
■ Cor pulmonale
■ Respiratory failure
■ Peptic ulcer disease
■ Spontaneous pneumothorax
■ Pneumomediastinum

Assessment

HISTORY
■ Long-time smoker
■ Shortness of breath
■ Chronic cough
■ Anorexia and weight loss
■ Malaise

PHYSICAL FINDINGS
■ Barrel chest
■ Pursed-lip breathing
■ Use of accessory muscles
■ Cyanosis
■ Clubbed fingers and toes
■ Tachypnea
■ Decreased tactile fremitus
■ Decreased chest expansion
■ Hyperresonance
■ Decreased breath sounds
■ Crackles
■ Inspiratory wheeze
■ Prolonged expiratory phase with grunting respirations
■ Distant heart sounds

TEST RESULTS
Laboratory
■ Arterial blood gas analysis showing decreased partial pressure of oxygen; partial pressure of carbon dioxide normal until late in the disease
■ Red blood cell count showing an increased hemoglobin level late in the disease

Imaging
■ Chest X-ray may show:
– a flattened diaphragm
– reduced vascular markings at the lung periphery
– overaeration of the lungs
– a vertical heart
– enlarged anteroposterior chest diameter
– large retrosternal air space.

Diagnostic procedures
■ Pulmonary function tests typically show:
– increased residual volume and total lung capacity
– reduced diffusing capacity
– increased inspiratory flow.
■ Electrocardiography may show tall, symmetrical P waves in leads II, III, and aV_F; a vertical QRS axis; and signs of right ventricular hypertrophy late in the disease.

Treatment

GENERAL
- Chest physiotherapy
- Possible transtracheal catheterization and home oxygen therapy

DIET
- Adequate hydration
- High-protein, high-calorie

ACTIVITY
- As tolerated

MEDICATION
- Bronchodilators
- Anticholinergics
- Mucolytics
- Corticosteroids
- Antibiotics
- Oxygen

SURGERY
- Chest tube insertion for pneumothorax

MONITORING
- Vital signs
- Intake and output
- Daily weight
- Complications
- Respiratory status
- Activity tolerance

LUNG CANCER

Overview

DESCRIPTION
- Tumors arising from the respiratory epithelium
- Most common types are epidermoid (squamous cell), adenocarcinoma, small-cell (oat cell), and large-cell (anaplastic)

- Most common site is wall or epithelium of bronchial tree
- For most patients, prognosis is poor, depending on extent of cancer when diagnosed and cells' growth rate (only about 13% of patients with lung cancer survive 5 years after diagnosis)

PATHOPHYSIOLOGY
- Individuals with lung cancer demonstrate bronchial epithelial changes progressing from squamous cell alteration or metaplasia to carcinoma in situ.
- Tumors originating in the bronchi are thought to be more mucus producing.
- Partial or complete obstruction of the airway occurs with tumor growth, resulting in lobar collapse distal to the tumor.
- Early metastasis occurs to other thoracic structures, such as hilar lymph nodes or the mediastinum.
- Distant metastasis occurs to the brain, liver, bone, and adrenal glands.

CAUSES
- Exact cause unclear

RISK FACTORS
- Tobacco smoking
- Exposure to carcinogenic and industrial air pollutants (asbestos, arsenic, chromium, coal dust, iron oxides, nickel, radioactive dust, and uranium)
- Genetic predisposition

COMPLICATIONS
- Spread of primary tumor to intrathoracic structures
- Tracheal obstruction
- Esophageal compression with dysphagia
- Phrenic nerve paralysis with hemidiaphragm elevation and dyspnea

- Sympathetic nerve paralysis with Horner's syndrome
- Spinal cord compression
- Lymphatic obstruction with pleural effusion
- Hypoxemia
- Anorexia and weight loss, sometimes leading to cachexia, digital clubbing, and hypertrophic osteoarthropathy
- Neoplastic and paraneoplastic syndromes, including Pancoast's syndrome and syndrome of inappropriate secretion of antidiuretic hormone

Assessment

HISTORY
- Possibly no symptoms
- Exposure to carcinogens
- Coughing
- Hemoptysis
- Shortness of breath
- Hoarseness
- Fatigue

PHYSICAL FINDINGS
- Dyspnea on exertion
- Finger clubbing
- Edema of the face, neck, and upper torso
- Dilated chest and abdominal veins (superior vena cava syndrome)
- Weight loss
- Enlarged lymph nodes
- Enlarged liver
- Decreased breath sounds
- Wheezing
- Pleural friction rub

TEST RESULTS
Laboratory
- Cytologic sputum analysis showing diagnostic evidence of pulmonary malignancy
- Abnormal liver function tests, especially with metastasis

Imaging
- Chest X-rays show advanced lesions and can show a lesion up to 2 years before signs and symptoms appear; findings may indicate tumor size and location.
- Contrast studies of the bronchial tree (chest tomography, bronchography) demonstrate size and location as well as spread of lesion.
- Bone scan is used to detect metastasis.
- Computed tomography of the brain is used to detect metastasis.

Diagnostic procedures
- Bronchoscopy can be used to identify the tumor site. Bronchoscopic washings provide material for cytologic and histologic study.
- Needle biopsy of the lungs (relies on biplanar fluoroscopic visual control to locate peripheral tumors before withdrawing a tissue specimen for analysis) allows firm diagnosis in 80% of patients.
- Tissue biopsy of metastatic sites (including supraclavicular and mediastinal nodes and pleura) is used to assess disease extent. Based on histologic findings, staging describes the disease's extent and prognosis and is used to direct treatment.
- Thoracentesis allows chemical and cytologic examination of pleural fluid.
- Gallium scans of the liver and spleen help to detect metastasis.

Treatment

GENERAL
- Various combinations of surgery, radiation therapy, and chemotherapy to improve prognosis
- Palliative (most treatments)
- Preoperative and postoperative radiation therapy
- Laser therapy (investigational)

DIET
- Well-balanced

ACTIVITY
- As tolerated per breathing capacity

MEDICATION
- Chemotherapy drug combinations
- Immunotherapy (investigational)

SURGERY
- Partial removal of lung (wedge resection, segmental resection, lobectomy, radical lobectomy)
- Total removal of lung (pneumonectomy, radical pneumonectomy)

MONITORING
- Chest tube function and drainage
- Postoperative complications
- Wound site
- Vital signs
- Sputum production
- Hydration and nutrition
- Oxygenation
- Pain control

PNEUMONIA

Overview

DESCRIPTION
- Acute infection of the lung parenchyma that impairs gas exchange
- May be classified by etiology, location, or type

PATHOPHYSIOLOGY
- A gel-like substance forms as microorganisms and phagocytic cells break down.
- This substance consolidates within the lower airway structure.
- Inflammation involves the alveoli, alveolar ducts, and interstitial spaces surrounding the alveolar walls.
- In lobar pneumonia, inflammation starts in one area and may extend to the entire lobe. In bronchopneumonia, it starts simultaneously in several areas, producing patchy, diffuse consolidation. In atypical pneumonia, inflammation is confined to the alveolar ducts and interstitial spaces.

CAUSES
Bacterial and viral pneumonia
- Chronic illness and debilitation
- Cancer
- Abdominal and thoracic surgery
- Atelectasis
- Bacterial or viral respiratory infections
- Chronic respiratory disease
- Influenza
- Smoking
- Malnutrition
- Alcoholism
- Sickle cell disease
- Tracheostomy
- Exposure to noxious gases
- Aspiration
- Immunosuppressive therapy

Aspiration pneumonia
- Advanced age
- Debilitation
- Nasogastric tube feedings
- Impaired gag reflex
- Poor oral hygiene
- Decreased level of consciousness

COMPLICATIONS
- Septic shock
- Hypoxemia
- Respiratory failure
- Empyema
- Bacteremia
- Endocarditis
- Pericarditis
- Meningitis
- Lung abscess
- Death

Assessment

HISTORY
Bacterial pneumonia
■ Sudden onset of:
- Pleuritic chest pain
- Cough
- Purulent sputum production
- Chills

Viral pneumonia
■ Nonproductive cough
■ Constitutional symptoms
■ Fever

Aspiration pneumonia
■ Fever
■ Weight loss
■ Malaise

PHYSICAL FINDINGS
■ Fever
■ Sputum production
■ Dullness over the affected area
■ Crackles, wheezing, or rhonchi
■ Decreased breath sounds
■ Decreased fremitus

TEST RESULTS
Laboratory
■ Complete blood count showing leukocytosis
■ Positive blood cultures for causative organism
■ Arterial blood gas (ABG) values showing hypoxemia
■ Fungal or acid-fast bacilli cultures identifying the etiologic agent
■ Assay for legionella-soluble antigen in urine detecting presence of antigen
■ Sputum culture, Gram stain, and smear revealing the infecting organism

Imaging
■ Chest X-rays generally show patchy or lobar infiltrates.

Diagnostic procedures
■ Bronchoscopy or transtracheal aspiration specimens identify the etiologic agent.

Other
■ Pulse oximetry may reveal decreased oxygen saturation.

Treatment

GENERAL
■ Mechanical ventilation (positive end-expiratory pressure) for respiratory failure

DIET
■ High-calorie
■ Adequate fluids

ACTIVITY
■ Bed rest

MEDICATION
■ Antibiotics
■ Humidified oxygen
■ Antitussives
■ Analgesics
■ Bronchodilators

SURGERY
■ Drainage of parapneumonic pleural effusion or lung abscess

MONITORING
■ Vital signs
■ Intake and output
■ Daily weight
■ Sputum production
■ Respiratory status
■ Breath sounds
■ Pulse oximetry
■ ABG values

RESPIRATORY CARE

Pneumothorax

Overview

Description
- Accumulation of air or gas between the parietal and visceral pleurae, leading to lung collapse
- Amount of trapped air or gas determines the degree of lung collapse
- Most common pneumothorax types: open, closed, and tension

Pathophysiology
- Air accumulates and separates the visceral and parietal pleurae.
- Negative pressure is eliminated, affecting elastic recoil forces.
- The lung recoils and collapses toward the hilus.
- In open pneumothorax, atmospheric air flows directly into the pleural cavity, collapsing the lung on the affected side.
- In closed pneumothorax, air enters the pleural space from within the lung, increasing pleural pressure and preventing lung expansion.
- In tension pneumothorax, air in the pleural space is under higher pressure than air in the adjacent lung. Air enters the pleural space from a pleural rupture only on inspiration. This air pressure exceeds barometric pressure, causing compression atelectasis. Increased pressure may displace the heart and great vessels and cause mediastinal shift.

Causes
Open pneumothorax
- Penetrating chest injury
- Central venous catheter insertion
- Chest surgery
- Transbronchial biopsy
- Thoracentesis
- Percutaneous lung biopsy

Closed pneumothorax
- Blunt chest trauma
- Rib fracture
- Clavicle fracture
- Congenital bleb rupture
- Emphysematous bullae rupture
- Barotrauma
- Erosive tubercular or cancerous lesions
- Interstitial lung disease

Tension pneumothorax
- Penetrating chest wound
- Lung or airway puncture from positive-pressure ventilation
- Mechanical ventilation after chest injury
- High positive end-expiratory pressures, causing rupture of alveolar blebs
- Chest tube occlusion or malfunction

Complications
- Fatal pulmonary and circulatory impairment

Assessment

History
- Possibly asymptomatic (with small pneumothorax)
- Sudden, sharp, pleuritic pain
- Pain that worsens with chest movement, breathing, and coughing
- Shortness of breath

Physical findings
- Asymmetrical chest wall movement
- Overexpansion and rigidity on the affected side
- Possible cyanosis
- Subcutaneous emphysema
- Hyperresonance on the affected side
- Decreased or absent breath sounds on the affected side
- Decreased tactile fremitus over the affected side

Tension pneumothorax
- Distended jugular veins
- Pallor
- Anxiety
- Tracheal deviation away from the affected side
- Weak, rapid pulse
- Hypotension
- Tachypnea
- Cyanosis

(See *Understanding tension pneumothorax.*)

TEST RESULTS
Laboratory
- Arterial blood gas analysis possibly showing hypoxemia

Imaging
- Chest X-rays may show air in the pleural space and, possibly, a mediastinal shift.

Other
- Pulse oximetry may show decreased oxygen saturation.

Treatment

GENERAL
- Conservative treatment of spontaneous pneumothorax with no signs of increased pleural pressure, less than 30% lung collapse, and no obvious physiologic compromise

DIET
- As tolerated

ACTIVITY
- Bed rest

MEDICATION
- Oxygen
- Analgesics

UNDERSTANDING TENSION PNEUMOTHORAX

In tension pneumothorax, air accumulates intrapleurally and can't escape. As intrapleural pressure increases, the ipsilateral lung is affected and also collapses.

On inspiration, the mediastinum shifts toward the unaffected lung, impairing ventilation.

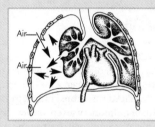

On expiration, the mediastinal shift distorts the vena cava and reduces venous return.

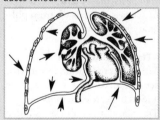

SURGERY
- Thoracotomy, pleurectomy for recurring spontaneous pneumothorax
- Repair of traumatic pneumothorax

OTHER
- Chest tube insertion

MONITORING
- Vital signs
- Intake and output
- Respiratory status

- Breath sounds
- Chest tube system
- Complications
- Pneumothorax recurrence

Watch for signs and symptoms of tension pneumothorax, which can be fatal. These include anxiety, hypotension, tachycardia, tachypnea, and cyanosis.

PULMONARY EMBOLISM

Overview

DESCRIPTION
- Obstruction of the pulmonary arterial bed occurring when a mass (such as a dislodged thrombus) lodges in the main pulmonary artery or branch, partially or completely obstructing it
- Most thrombi originate in deep veins of the leg
- Can be asymptomatic, but sometimes causes rapid death from pulmonary infarction

PATHOPHYSIOLOGY
- Thrombus formation results from vascular wall damage, venous stasis, or blood hypercoagulability.
- Trauma, clot dissolution, sudden muscle spasm, intravascular pressure changes, or peripheral blood flow changes can cause the thrombus to loosen or fragmentize.
- The thrombus (now an embolus) floats to the heart's right side and enters the lung through the pulmonary artery. There, the embolus may dissolve, continue to fragmentize, or grow.
- By occluding the pulmonary artery, the embolus prevents alveoli from producing enough surfactant to maintain alveolar integrity. Alveoli collapse and atelectasis develops.

- If the embolus enlarges, it may occlude most or all of the pulmonary vessels and cause death.

CAUSES
- Deep vein thrombosis
- Pelvic, renal, and hepatic vein thrombosis
- Right heart thrombus
- Upper extremity thrombosis
- Atrial fibrillation
- Valvular heart disease
- Rarely, other types of emboli, such as bone, air, fat, amniotic fluid, tumor cells, or a foreign body

RISK FACTORS
Various disorders and treatments (see *Who's at risk for pulmonary embolism*)

COMPLICATIONS
- Pulmonary infarction
- Pulmonary hypertension
- Embolic extension
- Hepatic congestion and necrosis
- Pulmonary abscess
- Shock
- Acute respiratory distress syndrome
- Massive atelectasis
- Right-sided heart failure
- Ventilation-perfusion mismatch
- Death

Assessment

HISTORY
- Predisposing factors
- Shortness of breath for no apparent reason
- Pleuritic pain or angina

PHYSICAL FINDINGS
- Tachycardia
- Low-grade fever
- Weak, rapid pulse
- Hypotension
- Productive cough, possibly with blood-tinged sputum

WHO'S AT RISK FOR PULMONARY EMBOLISM?

Many disorders and treatments heighten the risk for pulmonary embolism. At particular risk are surgical patients. The anesthetic used during surgery can injure lung vessels, and surgery or prolonged bed rest can promote venous stasis, which compounds the risk.

Predisposing disorders

- Lung disorders, especially chronic types
- Cardiac disorders
- Infection
- Diabetes mellitus
- History of thromboembolism, thrombophlebitis, or vascular insufficiency
- Sickle cell disease
- Autoimmune hemolytic anemia
- Polycythemia
- Osteomyelitis
- Long-bone fracture
- Manipulation or disconnection of central lines

Venous stasis

- Prolonged bed rest or immobilization
- Obesity
- Over age 40
- Burns
- Recent childbirth
- Orthopedic casts

Venous injury

- Surgery, particularly of the legs, pelvis, abdomen, or thorax
- Leg or pelvic fractures or injuries
- I.V. drug abuse
- I.V. therapy

Increased blood coagulability

- Cancer
- Use of high-estrogen hormonal contraceptives

- Warmth, tenderness, and edema of the lower leg
- Restlessness
- Transient pleural friction rub
- Crackles
- S_3 and S_4 gallop with increased intensity of the pulmonic component of S_2
- With a large embolus: cyanosis, syncope, distended jugular veins

TEST RESULTS
Laboratory
- Arterial blood gas (ABG) values showing hypoxemia
- Elevated D-dimer level

Imaging
- Lung ventilation perfusion scan shows a ventilation-perfusion mismatch.
- Pulmonary angiography shows a pulmonary vessel filling defect or an abrupt vessel ending and reveals the location and extent of pulmonary embolism.
- Chest X-rays may show a small infiltrate or effusion.
- Spiral chest computed tomography scan may show central pulmonary emboli.

Diagnostic procedures
- Electrocardiography may reveal right axis deviation and right bundle-branch block; it may also show atrial fibrillation.

Treatment

GENERAL
- Maintenance of adequate cardiovascular and pulmonary function
- Mechanical ventilation

DIET
- Possible fluid restriction

ACTIVITY
- Bed rest during the acute phase

MEDICATION
- Oxygen therapy
- Thrombolytics
- Anticoagulation
- Corticosteroids (controversial)
- Diuretics
- Antiarrhythmics
- Vasopressors (for hypotension)
- Antibiotics (for septic embolus)

SURGERY
- Vena caval interruption
- Vena caval filter placement
- Pulmonary embolectomy

MONITORING
- Vital signs
- Intake and output
- Respiratory status
- Pulse oximetry
- ABG values
- Deep vein thrombosis
- Complications
- Coagulation study results
- Abnormal bleeding
- Stools for occult blood

PULMONARY HYPERTENSION

Overview

DESCRIPTION
- Occurs in a primary form (rare) and a secondary form
- In both forms, resting systolic pulmonary artery pressure (PAP) above 30 mm Hg and mean PAP above 18 mm Hg
- In primary or idiopathic form, increased PAP and pulmonary vascular resistance for no obvious cause
- Primary form also known as *PPH*

PATHOPHYSIOLOGY
- In PPH, the intimal lining of the pulmonary arteries thickens for no apparent reason. This narrows the artery and impairs distensibility, increasing vascular resistance.
- Secondary pulmonary hypertension occurs from hypoxemia caused by conditions involving alveolar hypoventilation, vascular obstruction, or left-to-right shunting.

CAUSES
Primary pulmonary hypertension
- Unknown
- Possible hereditary factors
- Possible altered autoimmune mechanisms

Secondary pulmonary hypertension
- Chronic obstructive pulmonary disease
- Sarcoidosis
- Diffuse interstitial pneumonia
- Malignant metastases
- Scleroderma
- Use of some diet drugs
- Obesity
- Sleep apnea
- Hypoventilation syndromes
- Kyphoscoliosis
- Pulmonary embolism
- Vasculitis
- Left atrial myxoma
- Congenital cardiac defects
- Mitral stenosis

COMPLICATIONS
- Cor pulmonale
- Heart failure

- Cardiac arrest
- Death

Assessment

HISTORY
- Shortness of breath with exertion
- Weakness, fatigue
- Pain during breathing
- Near-syncope

PHYSICAL FINDINGS
- Ascites
- Jugular vein distention
- Peripheral edema
- Restlessness and agitation
- Mental status changes
- Decreased diaphragmatic excursion
- Apical impulse displaced beyond midclavicular line
- Right ventricular lift
- Reduced carotid pulse
- Hepatomegaly
- Tachycardia
- Systolic ejection murmur
- Widely split S_2
- S_3 and S_4
- Hypotension
- Decreased breath sounds
- Tubular breath sounds

TEST RESULTS
Laboratory
- Arterial blood gas (ABG) values showing hypoxemia

Imaging
- Ventilation-perfusion lung scan may show a ventilation-perfusion mismatch.
- Pulmonary angiography may reveal filling defects in the pulmonary vasculature.

Diagnostic procedures
- Electrocardiography may reveal right axis deviation.

- Pulmonary artery catheterization shows increased PAP, with systolic pressure above 30 mm Hg; increased pulmonary artery wedge pressure; decreased cardiac output; and decreased cardiac index.
- Pulmonary function tests may show decreased flow rates and increased residual volume or reduced total lung capacity.
- Echocardiography may show valvular heart disease or atrial myxoma.

Other
- Lung biopsy may show tumor cells.

Treatment

DIET
- Low-sodium
- Fluid restriction (in right-sided heart failure)

ACTIVITY
- Bed rest during acute phase

MEDICATION
- Oxygen therapy
- Cardiac glycosides
- Diuretics
- Vasodilators
- Calcium channel blockers
- Bronchodilators
- Beta-adrenergic blockers
- Epoprostenol

SURGERY
- Heart-lung transplantation if indicated

MONITORING
- Vital signs
- Intake and output
- Daily weight
- Respiratory status
- Signs and symptoms of right-sided heart failure
- Heart rhythm

- ABG values
- Hemodynamic values

TUBERCULOSIS

Overview

DESCRIPTION
- An acute or chronic infection characterized by pulmonary infiltrates and the formation of granulomas with caseation, fibrosis, and cavitation
- Prognosis excellent with proper treatment
- Also known as *TB*

PATHOPHYSIOLOGY
- Multiplication of the bacillus *Mycobacterium tuberculosis* causes an inflammatory process where deposited.
- A cell-mediated immune response follows, usually containing the infection within 4 to 6 weeks.
- The T-cell response results in the formation of granulomas around the bacilli, making them dormant. This confers immunity to subsequent infection.
- Bacilli within granulomas may remain viable for many years, resulting in a positive purified protein derivative or other skin test for TB.
- Active disease develops in 5% to 15% of those infected.
- Transmission occurs when an infected person coughs or sneezes, spreading infected droplets.

CAUSES
- Exposure to *M. tuberculosis*
- Sometimes, exposure to other strains of mycobacteria

RISK FACTORS
- Close contact with newly diagnosed TB patient
- History of prior TB
- Multiple sexual partners
- Recent immigration from Africa, Asia, Mexico, or South America
- Gastrectomy
- History of silicosis, diabetes, malnutrition, cancer, Hodgkin's disease, or leukemia
- Drug and alcohol abuse
- Residence in mental health facility
- Nursing home residence
- Immunosuppression and use of corticosteroids
- Prison residence
- Homelessness

COMPLICATIONS
- Massive pulmonary tissue damage
- Respiratory failure
- Bronchopleural fistulas
- Pneumothorax
- Pleural effusion
- Pneumonia
- Infection of other body organs by small mycobacterial foci
- Liver involvement disease secondary to drug therapy

Assessment

HISTORY
In primary infection
- May be asymptomatic after a 4- to 8-week incubation period
- Weakness and fatigue
- Anorexia
- Weight loss
- Low-grade fever
- Night sweats

In reactivated infection
- Chest pain
- Productive cough for blood, or mucopurulent or blood-tinged sputum
- Low-grade fever

PHYSICAL FINDINGS
- Dullness over the affected area
- Crepitant crackles

- Bronchial breath sounds
- Wheezes
- Whispered pectoriloquy

TEST RESULTS
Laboratory
- Positive tuberculin skin test reaction in both active and inactive TB
- Stains and cultures of sputum, cerebrospinal fluid, urine, drainage from abscess, or pleural fluid showing heat-sensitive, nonmotile, aerobic, and acid-fast bacilli

Imaging
- Chest X-rays show nodular lesions, patchy infiltrates, cavity formation, scar tissue, and calcium deposits.
- Computed tomography or magnetic resonance imaging scans show presence and extent of lung damage or support the diagnosis.

Diagnostic procedures
- Bronchoscopy specimens show heat-sensitive, nonmotile, aerobic, acid-fast bacilli in specimens.

Treatment

GENERAL
- After 2 to 4 weeks, disease is no longer infectious; patient can resume normal activities while continuing to take medication.

DIET
- Well-balanced, high-calorie

ACTIVITY
- Rest, initially

MEDICATION
- Antitubercular therapy for at least 6 months with daily oral doses of:
  - isoniazid
  - rifampin
  - pyrazinamide
  - ethambutol, added in some cases.
- Second-line drugs include:
  - capreomycin
  - streptomycin
  - aminosalicylic acid (para-aminosalicylic acid)
  - pyrazinamide
  - cycloserine.

SURGERY
- For some complications

MONITORING
- Vital signs
- Intake and output
- Daily weight
- Complications
- Adverse reactions
- Visual acuity if taking ethambutol
- Liver and kidney function tests

TREATMENTS

THORACOTOMY

Overview

- Surgical incision into the thoracic cavity, most commonly performed to remove part or all of a lung and thus spare healthy lung tissue from disease
- May involve pneumonectomy, lobectomy, segmental resection, or wedge resection
- Exploratory thoracotomy: done to evaluate the chest and pleural space for chest trauma and tumors

■ Decortication: removal or stripping of the fibrous membrane covering the visceral pleura; helps reexpand the lung in empyema

■ Thoracoplasty: removes part or all of one rib to reduce chest cavity size, decreasing the risk of mediastinal shift; may be done when tuberculosis has reduced lung volume

INDICATIONS

■ To locate and examine thoracic abnormalities

■ To perform a biopsy

■ To remove diseased lung tissue

COMPLICATIONS

■ Hemorrhage

■ Infection

■ Tension pneumothorax

■ Bronchopleural fistula

■ Empyema

■ Persistent air space that the remaining lung tissue doesn't expand to fill

Nursing interventions

PRETREATMENT CARE

■ Explain the treatment and preparation to the patient and his family.

■ Make sure the patient has signed an appropriate consent form.

■ Explain postoperative care.

■ Arrange for laboratory studies and tests; report abnormal results.

■ Withhold food and fluids as ordered.

POSTTREATMENT CARE

■ Administer medications as ordered.

■ After pneumonectomy, make sure the patient lies only on the operative side or his back until stabilized.

■ Make sure chest tubes are patent and functioning.

■ Provide comfort measures.

■ Encourage coughing, deep breathing, and incentive spirometry use.

■ Have the patient splint the incision as needed.

■ Perform passive range-of-motion (ROM) exercises, progressing to active ROM exercises.

■ Perform incision care and dressing changes as ordered.

Monitoring

■ Vital signs

■ Intake and output

■ Complications

■ Respiratory status

■ Breath sounds

■ Surgical wound and dressings

■ Drainage

■ Abnormal bleeding

Monitor for and immediately report dyspnea, chest pain, hypotension, irritating cough, vertigo, syncope, anxiety, subcutaneous emphysema, or tracheal deviation from the midline. These findings indicate tension pneumothorax.

PATIENT TEACHING

Be sure to cover:

■ medications and possible adverse reactions

■ coughing and deep-breathing techniques

■ incentive spirometry

■ incision care and dressing changes

■ signs and symptoms of infection

■ complications

■ when to notify the physician

■ monitoring of sputum characteristics

■ ROM exercises

■ prescribed physical activity restrictions

■ ways to prevent infection

■ smoking cessation

■ wound care and dressing change care

■ home health care as needed

■ follow-up care.

TRACHEOTOMY

Overview

- Surgical creation of an opening into the trachea through the neck
- May be permanent or temporary

INDICATIONS

- Prolonged mechanical ventilation
- To prevent aspiration in an unconscious or paralyzed patient
- Upper airway obstruction caused by trauma, burns, epiglottitis, or a tumor
- To remove lower tracheobronchial secretions in a patient who can't clear them

COMPLICATIONS

- Hemorrhage
- Edema
- Aspiration of secretions
- Pneumothorax
- Subcutaneous emphysema
- Infection
- Airway obstruction
- Hypoxia
- Arrhythmias

Nursing interventions

PRETREATMENT CARE

- Explain the treatment and preparation to the patient and his family.
- Make sure the patient has signed an appropriate consent form.
- Obtain appropriate supplies or a tracheotomy tray.
- Devise an appropriate communication system.
- Obtain samples for arterial blood gas (ABG) analysis and other required diagnostic tests; report abnormal results.

POSTTREATMENT CARE

- Administer medications as ordered.

EMERGENCY TRACHEOSTOMY EQUIPMENT

In the event that the patient coughs or pulls out his tracheostomy tube, emergency equipment needs to be readily available. A sterile tracheal dilator can be used to keep the stoma open and the airway patent until a new tube can be inserted. The following equipment should be at the patient's bedside:

Sterile tracheal dilator or sterile hemostat # sterile obturator that fits the tracheostomy tube in use # extra sterile tracheostomy tube and obturator in appropriate size # suction equipment and supplies (Keep these supplies in full view in the patient's room at all times for easy access in case of emergency. Consider taping an emergency sterile tracheostomy tube in a sterile wrapper to the head of the bed for easy access in an emergency.)

- Keep a sterile tracheostomy tube with obturator (including a tube one size smaller) at the bedside. (See *Emergency tracheostomy equipment.*)
- Turn the patient every 2 hours and provide chest physiotherapy.
- Provide oxygen and humidification as ordered.
- Suction the airway as indicated.
- Monitor cuff pressures as ordered (usually should measure less than 25 cm H_2O [18 mm Hg]). (See *Deflating and inflating a tracheostomy cuff,* page 318.)
- Provide comfort measures.
- Perform incision care and dressing changes as ordered.

Monitoring

- Vital signs

RESPIRATORY CARE

DEFLATING AND INFLATING A TRACHEOSTOMY CUFF

As part of tracheostomy care, you may be required to deflate and inflate a tracheostomy cuff. If so, gather a 5-ml or 10-ml syringe, padded hemostat, and stethoscope and follow these steps:

1. Read the cuff manufacturer's instruction because cuff types and procedures vary.

2. Assess the patient's condition, explain the procedure to him, and reassure him. Wash your hands thoroughly.

3. Help the patient into semi-Fowler's position, if possible, or place him in a supine position so secretions above the cuff site will be pushed up into his mouth if he's receiving positive-pressure ventilation.

4. Suction the oropharyngeal cavity to prevent pooled secretions from descending into the trachea after cuff deflation.

5. Release the padded hemostat clamping the cuff inflation tubing, if a hemostat is present.

6. Insert a 5-ml or 10-ml syringe into the cuff pilot balloon and very slowly withdraw all air from the cuff. Leave the syringe attached to the tubing for later reinflation of the cuff.

7. Remove ventilation device. Suction the lower airway through existing tube to remove all secretions, and then reconnect the patient to the ventilation device.

8. Maintain cuff deflation for the prescribed time. Observe the patient for adequate ventilation, and suction as necessary. If the patient has difficulty breathing, reinflate the cuff immediately by depressing the syringe plunger very slowly. Use a stethoscope to listen over the trachea for the air leak, and then inject the least amount of air needed to achieve an adequate tracheal seal.

9. When inflating the cuff, you may use the minimal-leak technique or the minimal occlusive-volume technique to help gauge the proper inflation point.

10. If you're inflating the cuff using cuff pressure measurement, be careful not to exceed 25 mm Hg.

11. After you've inflated the cuff, if the tubing doesn't have a one-way valve at the end, clamp the inflation line with a padded hemostat (to protect the tubing) and remove the syringe.

12. Check for a minimal-leak cuff seal. You shouldn't feel air coming from the patient's mouth, nose, or tracheostomy site, and a conscious patient shouldn't be able to speak. Be alert for air leaks from the cuff itself.

13. Note the exact amount of air used to inflate the cuff to detect tracheal malacia if more air is consistently needed.

14. Make sure the patient is comfortable and can easily reach the call button and communication aids.

15. Properly clean or dispose of all equipment, supplies, and trash according to your facility's policy. Replenish used supplies and make sure all necessary emergency supplies are at the bedside.

- Intake and output
- Respiratory status
- Breath sounds
- Pulmonary secretions
- Surgical wound and dressings
- Drainage
- Abnormal bleeding
- Complications
- ABG values
- Pulse oximetry values
- Tracheostomy tube cuff pressures
- Edema

PATIENT TEACHING

Be sure to cover:
- medications and possible adverse reactions
- tracheostomy and tube care
- protection of the stoma from water
- use of a foam filter over the stoma in winter
- signs and symptoms of infection
- complications
- when to notify the physician
- proper disposal of expelled secretions
- follow-up care.

COMMERCIAL CHEST DRAINAGE SYSTEM

This illustration depicts a commercial, disposable chest drainage system that combines drainage collection, water seal, and suction control in one unit.

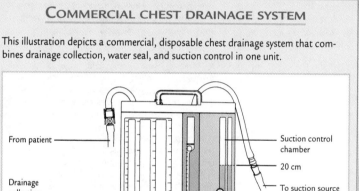

From patient

Drainage collection chambers

Suction control chamber

20 cm

To suction source or air

Water seal chamber

CHEST DRAINAGE: CHECKING FOR LEAKS

When attempting to locate a leak, try:
- clamping the chest tube momentarily at various points along its length, beginning at the tube's proximal end and working down toward the drainage system
- paying special attention to the seal around the connections
- pushing any loose connections back together and taping them securely.

The bubbling will stop when a clamp is placed between the air leak and the water seal. If you clamp along the tube's entire length and the bubbling doesn't stop, you'll probably need to replace the drainage unit because it may be cracked.

CHEST DRAINS

Problem	Interventions
Patient rolling over on drainage tubing, causing obstruction	■ Reposition the patient, and remove kinks in the tubing. ■ Auscultate for decreased breath sounds, and percuss for dullness, which indicates a fluid accumulation, or for hyperresonance, which indicates an air accumulation.
Dependent loops in tubing trapping fluids and preventing effective drainage	■ Make sure the chest drainage unit sits below the patient's chest level. If necessary, raise the bed slightly to increase the gravity flow. Remove kinks in the tubing. ■ Monitor the patient for decreased breath sounds, and percuss for dullness.
No drainage appearing in collection chamber	■ If draining blood or other fluid, suspect a clot or obstruction in the tubing. Gently milk the tubing to expel the obstruction, if your facility's policy permits. ■ Monitor the patient for lung-tissue compression caused by accumulated pleural fluid.
Substantial increase in bloody drainage, indicating possible active bleeding or drainage of old blood	■ Monitor the patient's vital signs. Look for an increased pulse rate, decreased blood pressure, and orthostatic changes that may indicate acute blood loss. ■ Measure drainage every 15 to 30 minutes to determine if it's occurring continuously or in one gush as a result of position changes. Report drainage greater than 200 ml in 1 hour.
No bubbling in suction-control chamber	■ Check for obstructions in the tubing. Make sure all connections are tight. ■ Check that the suction apparatus is turned on. Increase the suction slowly until you see gentle bubbling.
Loud, vigorous bubbling in suction-control chamber	■ Turn down the suction source until bubbling is just visible.
Constant bubbling in water-seal chamber	■ Assess the chest drainage unit and tubing for an air leak. ■ If an air leak isn't noted in the external system, notify the physician immediately. Leaking and trapping of air in the pleural space can result in a tension pneumothorax.
Evaporation causing water level in suction-control chamber to drop below desired –20 cm H_2O	■ Using a syringe and needle, add water or normal saline solution through a resealable diaphragm on the back of the suction-control chamber.

CHEST DRAINS (continued)

Problem	Interventions
Trouble breathing immediately after special procedure; chest drainage unit improperly placed on the patient's bed, interfering with drainage.	■ Raise the head of the bed and reposition the unit so that gravity promotes drainage. ■ Perform a quick respiratory assessment, and take the patient's vital signs. Make sure enough water is in the water-seal and suction-control chambers.
As bed lowers, chest drainage unit caught under bed; tubing comes apart and becomes contaminated	■ Clamp the chest tube proximal to the latex connecting tubing. ■ Insert the distal end of the chest tube into a jar of sterile water or saline until the end is 2 to 4 cm below the top of the water. Unclamp the chest tube. ■ Have another nurse obtain a new closed chest drainage system, and set it up. ■ Attach the chest tube to the new unit. ■ To prevent a tension pneumothorax (which may occur when clamping stops air and fluid from escaping), never leave the chest tube clamped for more than 1 minute.

REMOVING A CHEST TUBE

After the patient's lung has reexpanded, you may assist the physician in removing the chest tube. First, obtain the patient's vital signs and perform a respiratory assessment. After explaining the procedure to the patient, administer an analgesic, as ordered, 30 minutes before tube removal. Then follow the steps listed here:

■ Place the patient in semi-Fowler's position or on his unaffected side.

■ Place a linen-saver pad under the affected side to protect the bed linen from drainage and to provide a place to put the chest tube after removal.

■ Put on clean gloves and remove the chest tube dressings, being careful not to dislodge the chest tube. Discard soiled dressings.

■ The physician puts on sterile gloves, holds the chest tube in place with sterile forceps, and cuts the suture anchoring the tube.

■ Make sure the chest tube is securely clamped, and then instruct the patient to perform Valsalva's maneuver by exhaling fully and bearing down. Valsalva's maneuver effectively increases intrathoracic pressure.

■ The physician holds an airtight dressing, usually petroleum gauze, so that he can cover the insertion site with it immediately after removing the tube. After he removes the tube and covers the insertion site, secure the dressing with tape. Be sure to cover the dressing completely with tape to make it as airtight as possible.

■ Dispose of the chest tube, soiled gloves, and equipment according to your facility's policy.

■ Take the patient's vital signs as ordered, and assess the depth and quality of his respirations. Assess him carefully for signs and symptoms of pneumothorax, subcutaneous emphysema, or infection.

HOW ETco$_2$ MONITORING WORKS

The optical portion of an end-tidal carbon dioxide (ETco$_2$) monitor contains an infrared light source, a sample chamber, a special carbon dioxide (CO$_2$) filter, and a photodetector. The infrared light passes through the sample chamber and is absorbed in varying amounts, depending on the amount of CO$_2$ the patient has just exhaled. The photodetector measures CO$_2$ content and relays this information to the microprocessor in the monitor, which displays the CO$_2$ value and waveform.

The CO$_2$ waveform, or capnogram, produced in ETco$_2$ monitoring reflects the course of CO$_2$ elimination during exhalation. A normal capnogram (as show below) consists of several segments, which reflect the various stages of exhalation and inhalation.

Normally, any gas eliminated from the airway during early exhalation is dead-space gas that hasn't undergone exchange at the alveolocapillary membrane. Measurements taken during this period contain no CO$_2$. As exhalation continues, CO$_2$ concentration rises sharply and rapidly. The sensor now detects gas that has undergone exchange producing measurable quantities of CO$_2$.

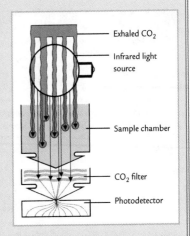

Exhaled CO$_2$

Infrared light source

Sample chamber

CO$_2$ filter

Photodetector

The final stages of alveolar emptying occur during late exhalation. During the alveolar plateau phase, CO$_2$ concentration rises more gradually because alveolar emptying is more constant.

The point at which ETco$_2$ value is derived is the end of exhalation, when CO$_2$ concentration peaks. Unless an alveolar plateau is present, this value doesn't accurately estimate alveolar CO$_2$. During inhalation, the CO$_2$ concentration declines sharply to zero.

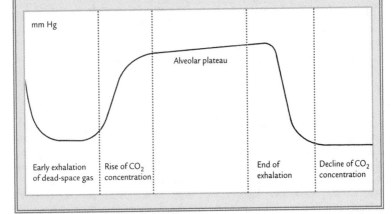

mm Hg

Alveolar plateau

Early exhalation of dead-space gas | Rise of CO$_2$ concentration | End of exhalation | Decline of CO$_2$ concentration

DISPOSABLE ETco₂ DETECTOR: ANALYZING CO₂ LEVELS

Depending on which end-tidal carbon dioxide (ETCO₂) detector you use, the meaning of color changes within the detector dome may differ from the analysis for the Easy Cap detector described here.

■ The rim of the Easy Cap is divided into four segments (clockwise from the top): CHECK, A, B, and C. The CHECK segment is solid purple, signifying the absence of CO₂.

■ The numbers in the other sections range from 0.03 to 5, indicating the percentage of exhaled CO₂. The color should fluctuate during ventilation from purple (section A) during inspiration to yellow (section C) at the end of expiration. This indicates that the ETCO₂ levels are adequate (above 2%).

■ An end-expiratory color change from the C range to the B range may be the first sign of hemodynamic instability.

■ During cardiopulmonary resuscitation (CPR), an end-expiratory color change from the A or B range to the C range may mean the return of spontaneous ventilation.

■ During prolonged cardiac arrest, inadequate pulmonary perfusion leads to

Color indications on detector dome

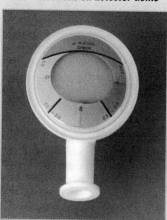

inadequate gas exchange. The patient exhales little or no CO₂, so the color stays in the purple range even with proper intubation. Ineffective CPR also leads to inadequate pulmonary perfusion.

RESPIRATORY CARE

DISPOSABLE ETco₂ DETECTOR GUIDELINES

When using a disposable end-tidal carbon dioxide ($ETco_2$) detector, check the instructions and ensure ideal working conditions for the device. In addition, follow the guidelines detailed here.

Humidity, moisture, and heat

■ Watch for changes indicating that the $ETco_2$ detector's precision is decreasing—for example, sluggish color changes from breath. A detector normally may be used for approximately 2 hours. However, using it with a ventilator that delivers high-humidity ventilation may shorten its life span to no more than 15 minutes.

■ Don't use the detector with a heated humidifier or nebulizer.

■ Keep the detector protected from secretions, which would render the device useless. If secretions enter the dome, remove and discard the detector.

■ Use a heat and moisture exchanger to protect the detector. In some detectors, this filter fits between the endotracheal (ET) tube and the detector.

■ If using a heat and moisture exchanger, remember that it will increase your patient's breathing effort. Be alert for increased resistance and breathing difficulties and remove the exchanger, if necessary.

Additional precautions

■ Instilling epinephrine through the ET tub can damage the detector's indictor (color may stay yellow). If this happens, discard the device.

■ Never reuse a disposable $ETco_2$ detector; it's intended for one-time, one-patient use only.

LARYNGOSCOPE TECHNIQUES

You may need to vary your laryngoscope technique during intubation depending on the type of blade used.

Curved blade

If you use a curved blade, apply upward traction with the tip of the blade in the vallecula. This displaces the epiglottis anteriorly.

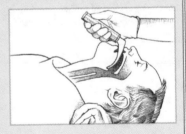

Straight blade

If you use a straight blade, elevate the epiglottis anteriorly, exposing the opening of the glottis.

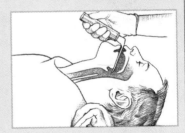

THREE METHODS TO SECURE AN ET TUBE

Before taping an endotracheal (ET) tube in place, make sure the patient's face is clean, dry, and free from beard stubble. If possible, suction his mouth and dry the tube just before taping. Also, check the reference mark on the tube to ensure correct placement. After taping, always check for bilateral breath sounds to ensure that the tube hasn't been displaced by manipulation.

To tape the tube securely, use one of these three methods.

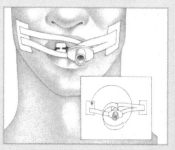

Method 1

Cut two 2″ (5.1-cm) strips and two 15″ (38.1-cm) strips of 1″ cloth adhesive tape. Then cut a 13″ (33-cm) slit in one end of each 15″ strip (as shown below).

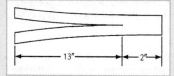

Apply compound benzoin tincture to the patient's cheeks. Place the 2″ strips on his cheeks, creating a new surface on which to anchor the tape securing the tube. When frequent retaping is necessary, this helps preserve the patient's skin integrity. If the patient's skin is excoriated or at risk, you can use a transparent semipermeable dressing to protect the skin.

Apply the benzoin tincture to the tape on the patient's face and to the part of the tube where you'll be applying the tape. On the side of the mouth where the tube will be anchored, place the unslit end of the long tape on top of the tape on the patient's cheek.

Wrap the top half of the tape around the tube twice, pulling the tape tightly around the tube. Then, directing the tape over the patient's upper lip, place the end of the tape on his other cheek. Cut off excess tape. Use the lower half of the tape to secure an oral airway, if necessary (as shown above).

Or twist the lower half of the tape around the tube twice and attach it to the original cheek (as shown below). Taping in opposite directions places equal traction on the tube.

If you've taped in an oral airway or are concerned about the tube's stability, apply the other 15″ strip of tape in the same manner, starting on the other side of the patient's face. If the tape around the tube is too bulky, use only the upper part of the tape and cut off the lower part. If the patient has copious oral secretions, seal the tape by cutting a 1″ piece of paper tape, coating it with benzoin tincture, and placing the paper tape over the adhesive tape.

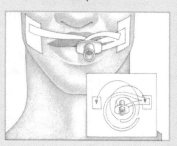

(continued)

RESPIRATORY CARE

RESPIRATORY CARE

THREE METHODS TO SECURE AN **ET** TUBE *(continued)*

Method 2

Cut one piece of 1″ cloth adhesive tape long enough to wrap around the patient's head and overlap in front. Then cut an 8″ (20.3-cm) piece of tape and center it on the longer piece, sticky sides together. Next, cut a 5″ (12.7-cm) slit in each end of the longer tape (as shown below).

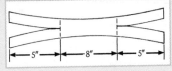

Apply benzoin tincture to the patient's cheeks, under his nose, and under his lower lip. (Don't spray benzoin directly on his face because the vapors can be irritating if inhaled and can also harm his eyes.)

Place the top half of one end of the tape under the patient's nose and wrap the lower half around the ET tube. Place the lower half of the other end of the tape along his lower lip and wrap the top half around the tube (as shown below).

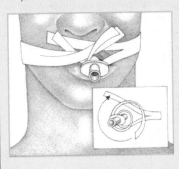

Method 3

Cut a tracheostomy tie in two pieces, one a few inches longer than the other, and cut two 6″ (15.2-cm) pieces of 1″ cloth adhesive tape. Then cut a 2″ slit in one end of both pieces of tape. Fold back the other end of the tape ½″ (1.3 cm) so that the sticky sides are together, and cut a small hole in it (as shown below).

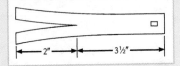

Apply benzoin tincture to the part of the ET tube that will be taped. Wrap the split ends of each piece of tape around the tube, one piece on each side. Overlap the tape to secure it.

Apply the free ends of the tape to both sides of the patient's face. Then insert tracheostomy ties through the holes in the tape and knot the ties (as shown below).

Bring the longer tie behind the patient's neck. Knotting the ties on the side prevents him from lying on the knot and developing a pressure ulcer.

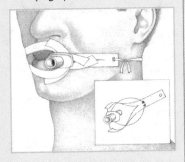

MECHANICAL VENTILATION GLOSSARY

Assist-control mode: The assist-control mode allows the ventilator to deliver a preset rate; however, the patient can initiate additional breaths, which trigger the ventilator to deliver the preset tidal volume at positive pressure.

Continuous positive airway pressure (CPAP): The CPAP setting prompts the ventilator to deliver positive pressure to the airway throughout the respiratory cycle. It works only on patients who can breathe spontaneously.

Control mode: The control mode allows the ventilator to deliver a preset tidal volume at a fixed rate regardless of whether or not the patient is breathing spontaneously.

Fraction of inspired oxygen (FIO_2): The FIO_2 is the amount of oxygen delivered to the patient by the ventilator. The dial or digital display on the ventilator that sets this percentage is labeled by the term oxygen concentration or oxygen percentage.

I:E ratio: The I:E ratio compares the duration of inspiration with the duration of expiration. The I:E ratio of normal, spontaneous breathing is 1:2, meaning that expiration is twice as long as inspiration.

Inspiratory flow rate (IFR): The IFR denotes the tidal volume delivered within a certain time. Its value can range from 20 to 120 L/minute.

Minute ventilation or minute volume (V_E): The V_E measurement results from the multiplication of respiratory rate and tidal volume.

Peak inspiratory pressure (PIP): Measured by the pressure manometer on the ventilator, the PIP reflects the amount of pressure required to deliver a preset tidal volume.

Positive end-expiratory pressure (PEEP): In the PEEP mode, the ventilator is triggered to apply positive pressure at the end of each expiration to increase the area for oxygen exchange by helping to inflate and keep open collapsed alveoli.

Pressure support ventilation (PSV): The PSV mode allows the ventilator to apply a preset amount of positive pressure when the patient inspires spontaneously. PSV increases tidal volume while decreasing the patient's breathing workload. This may be used during weaning trials.

Respiratory rate: The respiratory rate is the number of breaths per minute delivered by the ventilator; also called frequency.

Sensitivity setting: The sensitivity setting determines the amount of effort the patient must exert to trigger the inspiratory cycle.

Sigh volume: The sigh volume is a ventilator-delivered breath that's 1½ times as large as the patient's tidal volume.

Synchronized intermittent mandatory ventilation (SIMV): The SIMV allows the ventilator to deliver a preset number of breaths at a specific tidal volume. The patient may supplement these mechanical ventilations with his own breaths, in which case the tidal volume and rate are determined by his own inspiratory ability.

Tidal volume (V_T): V_T refers to the volume of air delivered to the patient with each cycle, usually 12 to 15 cc/kg.

VENTILATOR MODES

Positive pressure ventilators are categorized as volume or pressure ventilators and have a variety of modes and options. Volume modes include controlled ventilation (CV) or controlled mandatory ventilation (CMV), assist-control (A/C) or assisted mandatory ventilation (AMV), and intermittent mandatory ventilation (IMV) and synchronized intermittent mandatory ventilation (SIMV). Pressure modes include pressure support ventilation (PSV), pressure controlled ventilation (PCV), and pressure-controlled/inverse ratio ventilation (PC/IRV).

Volume modes
CV or CMV

In this mode, the ventilator supplies all of the patient's ventilation. The respiratory rate, tidal volume (V_T), inspiratory time, and any positive end-expiratory pressure (PEEP) are preset. This mode is usually used when the patient is unable to initiate spontaneous breaths, such as when he's paralyzed from a spinal cord injury or neuromuscular disease, or chemically paralyzed with neuromuscular blocking agents.

A/C or AMV

In the A/C or AMV mode, the basic respiratory rate is set along with the V_T, inspiratory time, and PEEP but the patient is allowed to breathe faster than the preset rate. The sensitivity is set so that when the patient initiates a spontaneous breath, a full V_T is delivered, so that all breaths whether triggered by the patient or delivered at the set rate are the same V_T. If the patient tires and his drive to breathe is negated, the ventilator continues to deliver breaths at the preset rate.

IMV or SIMV

IMV and SIMV modes require that the respiratory rate, V_T, inspiratory time, sensitivity, and PEEP are preset. Mandatory breaths are delivered at a set rate and V_T. In between the mandatory breaths, the patient can breathe spontaneously at his own rate and V_T. The V_T of these spontaneous breaths can vary because they're determined by the patient's ability to generate negative pressure in his chest. With SIMV, the ventilator synchronizes the mandatory breaths with the patient's own inspirations.

Pressure modes
PSV

The PSV mode augments the inspiration of the spontaneous breathing patient. The inspiratory pressure level, PEEP, and sensitivity are preset. When the patient initiates a breath, the breath is delivered at the preset pressure level and is maintained throughout inspiration. The V_T, respiratory rate, and inspiratory time are determined by the patient.

PCV or PC/IRV

In PCV mode inspiratory pressure, inspiratory time, respiratory rate, and PEEP are preset. V_T will vary with the patient's airway pressure and compliance. PC/IVR combines pressure-limited ventilation with an inverse ratio of inspiration to expiration. In this mode, the inspiratory pressure, respiratory rate, inspiratory time (1:1, 2:1, 3:1, or 4:1), and PEEP are preset. Both of these modes may be used in patients with acute respiratory distress syndrome.

RESPONDING TO VENTILATOR ALARMS

Signal	Possible cause	Interventions
Low-pressure alarm	■ Tube disconnected from ventilator ■ Endotracheal (ET) tube displaced above vocal cords or tracheostomy tube extubated ■ Leaking tidal volume from low cuff pressure (from an underinflated or ruptured cuff or a leak in the cuff or one-way valve) ■ Ventilator malfunction ■ Leak in ventilator circuitry (from loose connection or hole in tubing, loss of temperature-sensitive device, or cracked humidification jar)	■ Reconnect the tube to the ventilator. ■ Check the tube placement and reposition, if needed. If extubation or displacement has occurred, ventilate the patient manually and call the physician immediately. ■ Listen for a whooshing sound around the tube, indicating an air leak. If you hear one, check the cuff pressure. If you can't maintain pressure, call the physician; he may need to insert a new tube. ■ Disconnect the patient from the ventilator and ventilate him manually, if necessary. Obtain another ventilator. ■ Make sure all connections are intact. Check for holes or leaks in the tubing and replace, if necessary. Check the humidification jar and replace, if cracked.
High-pressure alarm	■ Increased airway pressure or decreased lung compliance caused by worsening disease ■ Patient biting on oral ET tube ■ Secretions in airway ■ Condensate in large-bore tubing ■ Intubation of right mainstem bronchus ■ Patient coughing, gagging, or attempting to talk ■ Chest wall resistance ■ Failure of high-pressure relief valve ■ Bronchospasm	■ Auscultate the lungs for evidence of increasing lung consolidation, barotrauma, or wheezing. Call the physician, if indicated. ■ Insert a bite block if needed. ■ Look for secretions in the airway. To remove them, suction the patient or have him cough. ■ Check tubing for condensate and remove any fluid. ■ Check tube position. If it has slipped, call the physician; he may need to reposition it. ■ If the patient fights the ventilator, the physician may order a sedative or neuromuscular blocking agent. ■ Reposition the patient to see if doing so improves chest expansion. If repositioning doesn't help, administer the prescribed analgesic. ■ Have the faulty equipment replaced. ■ Assess the patient for the cause. Report to the physician and treat the patient, as ordered.

RESPIRATORY CARE

CRITERIA FOR WEANING

Successful weaning depends on the patient's ability to breathe on his own.

This means that the patient must have a spontaneous respiratory effort that can maintain ventilation, a stable cardiovascular system, and sufficient respiratory muscle strength and level of consciousness to sustain spontaneous breathing.

Pulmonary function criteria include:
■ minute ventilation less than or equal to 10 L/minute, indicating that the patient is breathing at a stable rate with adequate tidal volume
■ negative inspiratory force greater than or equal to –20 cm H_2O, indicating the patient's ability to initiate respirations independently
■ maximum voluntary ventilation greater than or equal to twice the resting minute volume, indicating the patient's ability to sustain maximal respiratory effort
■ tidal volume of 5 to 10 ml/kg, indicating the patient's ability to ventilate lungs adequately
■ partial pressure of arterial oxygen (Pao_2) less than or equal to 60 mm Hg (50 mm Hg or the ability to maintain baseline levels if the patient has chronic lung disease)
■ arterial pH ranging from 7.35 to 7.45 (or normal for the patient)
■ partial pressure of arterial carbon dioxide less than or equal to 45 mm Hg (or normal for the patient)

■ arterial pH ranging from 7.35 to 7.45 (or normal for the patient)
■ fractional concentration of inspired oxygen less than or equal to 0.4.
  Other criteria include:
■ adequate natural airway or functioning tracheostomy
■ ability to cough and mobilize secretions
■ successful withdrawal of any neuromuscular blocker such as pancuronium bromide
■ clear or clearing chest X-ray
■ absence of infection, acid-base or electrolyte imbalance, hyperglycemia, arrhythmia, renal failure, anemia, fever, or excessive fatigue.

Ultimately, after being weaned, the patient should demonstrate:
■ respiratory rate less than 24 breaths/minute
■ heart rate and blood pressure within 15% of his baseline
■ tidal volume of at least 3 to 5 ml/kg
■ arterial pH greater than 7.35
■ Pao_2 maintained at greater than 60 mm Hg
■ Pao_2 maintained at less than 45 mm Hg
■ oxygen saturation maintained at greater than 90%
■ absence of cardiac arrhythmias
■ absence of accessory muscle use.

METHODS OF WEANING

The three most commonly used methods of weaning are described here. In patients receiving long-term mechanical, intermittent mandatory ventilation with or without pressure support, ventilation is used.

Intermittent mandatory ventilation

With intermittent mandatory ventilation (IMV), breaths produced by the ventilator are gradually decreased, allowing the patient to breath independently. Decreasing ventilator-produced breaths allows the patient to increase his respiratory muscle strength and endurance. As the number of ventilator breaths decrease, the patient increase the number of spontaneous breaths until he's breathing independently.

Pressure support ventilation

Pressure support ventilation (PSV) is often used as an adjunct to IMV in the weaning process. In this method, a set burst of pressure is applied during inspiration with the patient's normal breathing pattern. PSV helps to decrease the patient's work of breathing, thereby allowing him to build up respiratory muscle strength. As the patient's strength improves, PSV is gradually decreased.

T-piece

Weaning via a T-piece is commonly used for patients requiring short-term mechanical ventilation. A T-piece is attached to the end of the endotracheal tube. The patient is then disconnected from the ventilator and allowed to initiate spontaneous breaths. In the beginning, the amount of time the patient is off the ventilator is short, possibly 1 to 12 minutes. The time off the ventilator is gradually increased until the patient is breathing independently. During the weaning process, the patient receives supplemental oxygen therapy at or above the concentration that he was receiving while on the ventilator.

This method is sometimes used for patients receiving long-term mechanical ventilation. In these situations, the patient is weaned during the day and placed back on the ventilator when fatigue occurs, and during the night for rest.

RESPIRATORY CARE

RESPIRATORY CARE

USING A BAG-MASK DEVICE

Place the mask over the patient's face so that the apex of the triangle covers the bridge of the nose and the base lies between the lower lip and chin.

Make sure that the patient's mouth remains open underneath the mask. Attach the bag to the mask and to the tubing leading to the oxygen source.

Or, if the patient has a tracheostomy or endotracheal tube in place, remove the mask from the bag and attach the device directly to the tube.

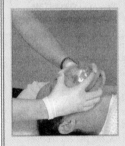
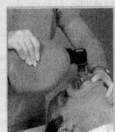
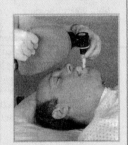

INSERTING A NASOPHARYNGEAL AIRWAY

First, hold the airway beside the patient's face to make sure it's the proper size (as shown top right). It should be slightly smaller than the patient's nostril diameter and slightly longer than the distance from the tip of his nose to his earlobe.

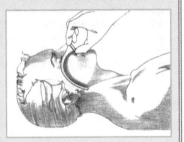

To insert the airway, hyperextend the patient's neck (unless contraindicated). Then push up the tip of his nose and pass the airway into his nostril (as shown bottom right). Avoid pushing against any resistance to prevent tissue trauma and airway kinking.

To check for correct airway placement, first close the patient's mouth. Then place your finger over the tube's opening to detect air exchange. Also, depress the patient's tongue with a tongue blade and look for the airway tip behind the uvula.

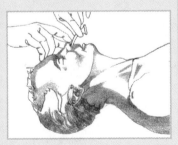

INSERTING AN ORAL AIRWAY

Unless this position is contraindicated, hyperextend the patient's head (as shown below) before using either the cross-finger or tongue blade insertion method.

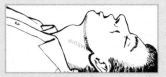

To insert an oral airway using the cross-finger method, place your thumb on the patient's lower teeth and your index finger on his upper teeth. Gently open his mouth by pushing his teeth apart (as shown below).

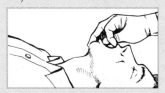

Insert the airway upside down to avoid pushing the tongue toward the pharynx, and slide it over the tongue toward the back of the mouth. Rotate the airway as it approaches the posterior wall of the pharynx so that it points downward (as shown below).

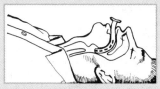

To use the tongue blade technique, open the patient's mouth and depress his tongue with the blade. Guide the airway over the back of the tongue as you did for the cross-finger technique.

HOW OXIMETRY WORKS

The pulse oximeter allows noninvasive monitoring of the percentage of arterial saturated by oxygen, or arterial oxygen saturation (SpO_2) levels, by measuring the absorption (amplitude) of light waves as they pass through areas of the body that are highly perfused by arterial blood. Oximetry is also used to monitor pulse rate and amplitude.

Light-emitting diodes in a transducer (photodetector) attached to the patient's body (shown below on the index finger) send red and infrared light beams through tissue. The photodetector records the relative amount of each color absorbed by arterial blood and transmits the data to a monitor, which displays the information with each heartbeat. If the SpO_2 level or pulse rate varies from preset limits, the monitor triggers visual and audible alarms.

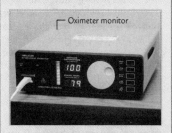
Oximeter monitor

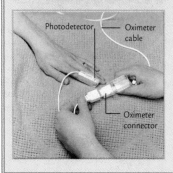
Photodetector — Oximeter cable
Oximeter connector

Factors affecting pulse oximetry readings

Oximetry may be intermittent or continuous and is used to monitor arterial oxygen saturation. Normal oxygen saturation levels are 95% to 100% for adults. Lower levels may indicate hypoxemia and warrant intervention.

Certain factors can interfere with accuracy. For example, an elevated bilirubin level may falsely lower oxygen saturation readings, whereas elevated carboxyhemoglobin or methemoglobin levels can falsely elevate oxygen saturation readings.

Certain intravascular substances, such as lipid emulsions and dyes, can also prevent accurate readings. Other interfering factors include excessive light (such as from phototherapy or direct sunlight), excessive patient movement, excessive ear pigment, hypothermia, hypotension, and vasoconstriction.

Some acrylic nails and certain colors of nail polish may interfere with readings (blue, green, black, and brown-red may interfere).

Troubleshooting pulse oximeter problems

To maintain a continuous display of arterial oxygen saturation (SpO_2) levels, you need to keep the monitoring site clean and dry. Make sure the skin doesn't become irritated from adhesives used to keep disposable probes in place. You may need to change the site if this happens. Disposable probes that irritate the skin can be replaced by nondisposable models that don't need tape.

A common problem with pulse oximeters is failure of the device to obtain a signal. If this happens, *first check the patient's vital signs*. If they're sufficient to produce a signal, check for the following problems.

Poor connection
Check that the sensors are properly aligned. Make sure that wires are intact and securely fastened and that the pulse oximeter is plugged into a power source.

Inadequate or intermittent blood flow to the site
Check the patient's pulse rate and capillary refill time and take corrective action if blood flow to the site is decreased. This may require you to loosen restraints, remove tight-fitting clothes, take off a blood pressure cuff, or check arterial and I.V. lines. If none of these interventions works, you may need to find an alternate site. Finding a site with proper circulation may be a challenge when the patient is receiving vasoconstrictive drugs.

Equipment malfunction
Remove the pulse oximeter from the patient and attempt to obtain an SpO_2 level on yourself or another healthy person. If you're able to obtain a normal value, the equipment is functioning properly.

SPUTUM COLLECTION:
ATTACHING SPECIMEN TRAP TO SUCTION CATHETER

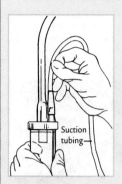

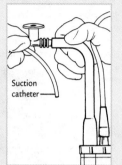

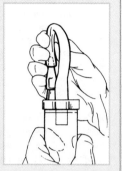

Wearing gloves, push the suction tubing onto the male adapter of the in-line trap.

Insert the suction catheter into the rubber tubing of the trap, as shown.

After suctioning, disconnect the in-line trap from the suction tubing and catheter. To seal the container, connect the rubber tubing to the male adapter of the trap.

CLOSED TRACHEAL SUCTIONING

The closed tracheal suction system can ease removal of secretions and reduce patient complications. Consisting of a sterile suction catheter in a clear plastic sleeve, the system permits the patient to remain connected to the ventilator during suctioning.

As a result, the patient can maintain the tidal volume, oxygen concentration, and positive end-expiratory pressure

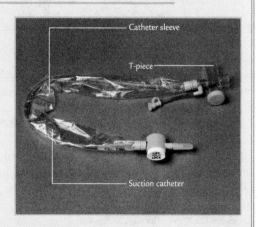

(continued)

CLOSED TRACHEAL SUCTIONING *(continued)*

delivered by the ventilator while being suctioned. In turn, this reduces the occurrence of suction-induced hypoxemia.

Another advantage of this system is a reduced risk of infection, even when the same catheter is used many times. The caregiver doesn't need to touch the catheter, and the ventilator circuit remains closed.

Implementation

To perform the procedure, gather a closed suction control valve, a T-piece to connect the artificial airway to the ventilator breathing circuit, and a catheter sleeve that encloses the catheter and has connections at each end for the control valve and the T-piece. Then follow these steps:

■ Remove the closed suction system from its wrapping. Attach the control valve to the connecting tubing.
■ Depress the thumb suction control valve, and keep it depressed while setting the suction pressure to the desired level.
■ Connect the T-piece to the ventilator breathing circuit, making sure that the irrigation port is closed; then connect the T-piece to the patient's endotracheal or tracheostomy tube (as shown below).

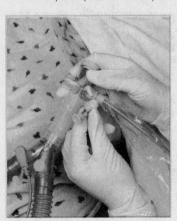

■ With one hand keeping the T-piece parallel the patient's chin, use the thumb and index finger of the other hand to advance the catheter through the tube and into the patient's tracheobronchial tree (as shown below).

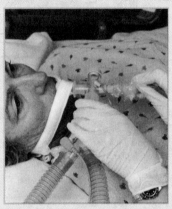

■ It may be necessary to gently retract the catheter sleeve as you advance the catheter.
■ While continuing to hold the T-piece and control valve, apply intermittent suction and withdraw the catheter until it reaches its fully extended length in the sleeve. Repeat the procedure as necessary.
■ After you've finished suctioning, flush the catheter by maintaining suction while slowly introducing normal saline solution or sterile water into the irrigation port.
■ Place the thumb control valve in the off position.
■ Dispose of and replace the suction equipment and supplies according to your facility's policy.
■ Change the closed suction system every 24 hours to minimize the risk of infection.

S̄vo₂ MONITORING EQUIPMENT

The mixed venous oxygen saturation (S̄vo₂) monitoring system consists of a flow-directed pulmonary artery (PA) catheter with fiber-optic filaments, an optical module, and a co-oximeter. The co-oximeter displays a continuous digital S̄vo₂ value; the strip recorder prints a permanent record.

Catheter insertion follows the same technique as with any thermodilution flow-directed PA catheter. The distal lumen connects to an external PA pressure monitoring system; the proximal or central venous pressure lumen connects to another monitoring system or to a continuous-flow administration unit; and the optical module connects to the co-oximeter unit.

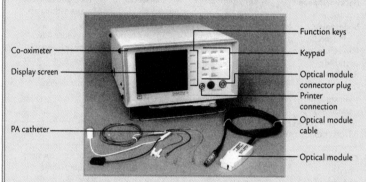

Co-oximeter

Display screen

PA catheter

Function keys

Keypad

Optical module connector plug

Printer connection

Optical module cable

Optical module

Normal S̄vo₂ waveform

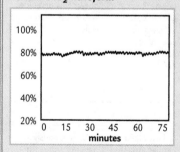

S̄vo₂ with patient activities

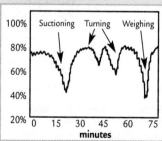

Suctioning   Turning   Weighing

S̄vo₂ with PEEP and Fio₂ changes

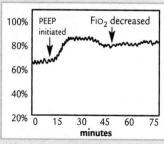

PEEP initiated

Fio₂ decreased

DRUGS

ANTI-INFLAMMATORY AGENTS

Drug	Indication	Adverse reactions	Special considerations
INHALED CORTICOSTEROIDS			
Beclomethasone (Qvar); **budesonide** (Pulmicort); **flunisolide** (Aerobid); **fluticasone** (Flovent); **triamcinolone** (Azmacort)	■ Long-term asthma control	■ Hoarseness, dry mouth, wheezing, bronchospasm, oral candidiasis	■ Not for treatment of acute asthma attacks. ■ To reduce adverse effects, use a spacer. ■ Rinse mouth after use to prevent oral fungal infection.
MAST CELL STABILIZERS			
Cromolyn (Intal); **nedocromil** (Tilade)	■ Adjunct treatment for asthma prophylaxis and prevention of bronchoconstriction with exposure to known allergens, such as exercise and cold air; prevents the release of type 1 allergic reaction mediators	■ Wheezing, cough, bronchospasm (after inhalation of dry powder), irritated throat, rash, urticaria, angioedema, eosinophilic pneumonia	■ Not for treatment of acute asthma attacks. ■ Stop if eosinophilic pneumonia develops. ■ Use with caution in children.
SYSTEMIC CORTICOSTEROIDS			
Dexamethasone (Decadron); **methylprednisolone** (Medrol); **prednisone** (Deltasone)	■ Used for anti-inflammatory effects in acute respiratory failure, acute respiratory distress syndrome, and chronic obstructive pulmonary disease (COPD) ■ Used for anti-inflammatory and immunosuppressive effects in asthma	■ Heart failure, cardiac arrhythmias, edema, circulatory collapse, thromboembolism, pancreatitis, peptic ulcer	■ Use cautiously in patients with recent myocardial infarction, hypertension, renal disease, and GI ulcer. Monitor blood pressure and blood glucose levels.

BRONCHODILATORS

Drug	Indication	Adverse reactions	Special considerations
SHORT-ACTING INHALED BETA$_2$-ADRENERGIC AGONISTS			
Albuterol (Proventil); **pirbuterol** (Maxair)	■ Short-acting beta$_2$-adrenergic agonists for relief of acute symptoms with asthma and bronchospasm	■ Paradoxical bronchospasm, tachycardia, palpitations, tremor, hyperactivity	■ Warn the patient about the possibility of paradoxical bronchospasm and, if it occurs, to stop taking the drug and seek medical treatment. ■ Elderly patients may require a lower dose. ■ Monitor respiratory status, vital signs, and cardiac rhythm.
Terbutaline (Brethine)	■ Bronchospasm	■ Cardiac arrhythmias, palpitations, tremor, paradoxical bronchospasm	■ Use cautiously in patients with cardiovascular disorders, diabetes, seizures, and hyperthyroidism.
ALPHA- AND BETA-ADRENERGIC AGONIST			
Epinephrine (Adrenalin)	■ Relaxes bronchial smooth muscle by stimulating beta$_2$ receptors, used for bronchospasm, hypersensitivity reaction, anaphylaxis, asthma	■ Ventricular fibrillation, palpitations, tachycardia, cerebral hemorrhage	■ Use cautiously in elderly patients and patients with long-standing asthma and emphysema with degenerative heart disease. ■ Monitor respiratory status, vital signs, and cardiac rhythm. ■ Contraindicated in patients with angle-closure glaucoma, coronary insufficiency, and cerebral arteriosclerosis.

(continued)

BRONCHODILATORS *(continued)*

Drug	Indication	Adverse reactions	Special considerations

LONG-ACTING BETA$_2$-ADRENERGIC AGONIST

Drug	Indication	Adverse reactions	Special considerations
Salmeterol (Serevent)	■ Maintenance treatment of asthma and COPD	■ Ventricular arrhythmias, palpitations, tachycardia, bronchospasm	■ Not for treatment of acute asthma attacks. ■ Tell the patient that acute symptoms must be treated with a short-acting beta$_2$-adrenergic agent. ■ Warn the patient about the possibility of paradoxical bronchospasm and, if it occurs, to stop taking the drug and seek medical treatment. ■ Use with caution in elderly patients with cardiovascular disease.

ANTICHOLINERGIC AGENTS

Drug	Indication	Adverse reactions	Special considerations
Ipratropium (Atrovent)	■ Bronchospasm associated with chronic bronchitis and emphysema	■ Bronchospasm, chest pain, palpitations, and nervousness	■ Because of delayed onset of bronchodilation, not recommended for acute respiratory distress. ■ Use cautiously in patients with angle-closure glaucoma, bladder neck obstruction, and prostatic hypertrophy. ■ Monitor respiratory status, vital signs, and cardiac rhythm.

NEUROMUSCULAR BLOCKING AGENTS

Drug and indications	Adverse effects*	Special considerations
DEPOLARIZING		
Succinylcholine (Anectine) ■ Adjunct to general anesthesia to aid endotracheal (ET) intubation ■ Induction of skeletal muscle paralysis during surgery or mechanical ventilation	■ Bradycardia, arrhythmias, cardiac arrest ■ Postoperative muscle pain ■ Respiratory depression, apnea, bronchoconstriction ■ Malignant hyperthermia, increased intraocular pressure, flushing	■ Contraindicated in patients with history of malignant hyperthermia, myopathies associated with creatinine phosphokinase, acute angle-closure glaucoma, and penetrating eye injuries. ■ Monitor the patient for histamine release and resulting hypotension and flushing.
NONDEPOLARIZING		
Atracurium besylate (Tracrium) ■ Adjunct to general anesthesia, to facilitate ET intubation, and to provide skeletal muscle relaxation during surgery or mechanical ventilation	■ Flushing, bradycardia ■ Prolonged dose-related apnea, bronchospasm, laryngospasm ■ Anaphylaxis	■ Drug doesn't affect consciousness or relieve pain. Be sure to keep the patient sedated. Have emergency respiratory support readily available. ■ Drug has little or no effect on heart rate and doesn't counteract or reverse the bradycardia caused by anesthetics or vagal stimulation. Thus, bradycardia is seen more frequently with atracurium than with other neuromuscular blocking agents. Pretreatment with anticholinergics (atropine or glycopyrrolate) is advised. ■ Use drug only if ET intubation, administration of oxygen under positive pressure, artificial respiration, and assisted or controlled ventilation are immediately available. ■ Use a peripheral nerve stimulator to monitor responses during intensive care unit administration; it may be used to detect residual paralysis during recovery and to avoid atracurium overdose.

*Common or life-threatening only

(continued)

RESPIRATORY CARE

NEUROMUSCULAR BLOCKING AGENTS *(continued)*

Drug and indications	Adverse effects*	Special considerations

NONDEPOLARIZING *(continued)*

Cisatracurium besylate
(Nimbex)
■ Adjunct to general anesthesia, to facilitate ET intubation, and to provide skeletal muscle relaxation during surgery or mechanical ventilation in the coronary care unit (CCU)
■ Maintenance of neuromuscular blockade in the CCU

■ Drug isn't compatible with propofol injection or ketorolac injection for Y-site administration. Drug is acidic and also may not be compatible with an alkaline solution having a pH greater than 8.5, such as barbiturate solutions for Y-site administration. Don't dilute in lactated Ringer's injection because of chemical instability.
■ Drug isn't recommended for rapid sequence ET intubation because of its intermediate onset of action.
■ In patients with neuromuscular disease (myasthenia gravis and myasthenic syndrome), watch for possible prolonged neuromuscular block. The use of a peripheral nerve stimulator and a dose not exceeding 0.02 mg/kg is recommended to assess the level of neuromuscular block and to monitor dosage requirements.
■ Burn patients may develop resistance to nondepolarizing neuromuscular blockers; they may need dosage increases and may exhibit shortened duration of action.
■ Monitor the patient's acid-base balance and electrolyte levels. Acid-base or serum electrolyte abnormalities may potentiate or antagonize the action of cisatracurium.

Vecuronium bromide
(Norcuron)
■ Adjunct to anesthesia, to facilitate intubation, and to provide skeletal muscle relaxation during surgery or mechanical ventilation

■ Prolonged, dose-related respiratory insufficiency or apnea

■ Administer by rapid I.V. injection or I.V. infusion. Don't give I.M.
■ Diluent supplied by manufacturer contains benzyl alcohol, which isn't intended for use in neonates.
■ Recovery time may double in patients with cirrhosis or cholestasis.
■ Assess baseline serum electrolyte levels, acid-base balance, and renal and hepatic function before administration.

*Common or life-threatening only

SEDATIVES

Drug and indications	Adverse effects*	Special considerations
Midazolam (Versed) ■ Preoperative sedation (to induce sleepiness or drowsiness and relieve apprehension) ■ Conscious sedation ■ Continuous infusion for sedation of intubated and mechanically ventilated patients as a component of anesthesia or during treatment in a critical care setting ■ Sedation, anxiolysis, and amnesia before diagnostic, therapeutic, or endoscopic procedures or before induction of anesthesia	■ Pain ■ Cardiac arrest ■ Nausea ■ Hiccups, decreased respiratory rate, apnea, respiratory arrest	■ Contraindicated in patients with acute angle-closure glaucoma and in those experiencing shock, coma, or acute alcohol intoxication. ■ Use cautiously in patients with uncompensated acute illnesses, in elderly or debilitated patients, and in patients with myasthenia gravis or neuromuscular disorders and pulmonary disease. ■ Closely monitor cardiopulmonary function; continuously monitor patients who have received midazolam to detect potentially life-threatening respiratory depression. ■ Have emergency respiratory equipment readily available. Laryngospasm and bronchospasm, although rare, may occur. ■ Midazolam can be mixed in the same syringe with morphine, meperidine, atropine, and scopolamine. Solution is stable for 30 minutes. Solutions compatible with midazolam include dextrose 5% in water (D_5W), normal saline solution, and lactated Ringer's solution
Propofol (Diprivan) ■ Induction and maintenance of sedation in mechanically ventilated patients	■ Hypotension, bradycardia ■ Hyperlipidemia ■ Apnea	■ Contraindicated in patients hypersensitive to propofol or components of the emulsion, including soybean oil, egg lecithin, and glycerol. Because drug is administered as an emulsion, administer cautiously to patients with a disorder of lipid metabolism (such as pancreatitis, primary hyperlipoproteinemia, and diabetic hyperlipidemia). Use cautiously if the patient is receiving lipids as part of a total parenteral nutrition infusion; I.V. lipid dose may need to be reduced. Use cautiously in elderly or debilitated patients and in those with circulatory disorders. ■ Although the hemodynamic effects of drug can vary, its major effect in patients maintaining spontaneous ventilation is arterial hypotension (arterial pressure can decrease as much as 30%) with little or no change in heart rate and cardiac output. However, significant depression of cardiac output may occur in patients undergoing assisted or controlled positive pressure ventilation. ■ Don't mix propofol with other drugs or blood products. If it's to be diluted before infusion, use only D_5W and don't dilute to a concentration of less than 2 mg/ml. After dilution, drug appears to be more stable in glass containers than in plastic. ■ If used for sedation of a mechanically ventilated patient, wake him every 24 hours.

*Common or life-threatening only

RESPIRATORY CARE

8

GASTROINTESTINAL CARE

ASSESSMENT

GI SYSTEM: NORMAL FINDINGS

- Skin is free from vascular lesions, jaundice, surgical scars, and rashes.
- Faint venous patterns (except in thin patients) are apparent.
- Abdomen is symmetrical, with a flat, round, or scaphoid contour.
- Umbilicus is positioned midway between the xiphoid process and the symphysis pubis, with a flat or concave hemisphere.
- No variations in the color of the patient's skin are detectable.
- No bulges are apparent.
- The abdomen moves with respiration.
- Pink or silver-white striae from pregnancy or weight loss may be apparent.

Auscultation
- High-pitched, gurgling bowel sounds are heard every 5 to 15 seconds through the diaphragm of the stethoscope in all four quadrants of the abdomen.
- Vascular sounds are heard through the bell of the stethoscope.
- A venous hum is heard over the inferior vena cava.
- No bruits, murmurs, friction rubs, or other venous hums are apparent.

Percussion
- Tympany is the predominant sound over hollow organs including the stomach, intestines, bladder, abdominal aorta, and gallbladder.
- Dullness can be heard over solid masses including the liver, spleen, pancreas, kidneys, uterus, and a full bladder.

Palpation
- No tenderness or masses are detectable.
- Abdominal musculature is free from tenderness and rigidity.
- No guarding, rebound tenderness, distention, or ascites are detectable.
- The liver is unpalpable, except in children. (If palpable, liver edge is regular, sharp, and nontender and felt no more than ¾″ [1.9 cm] below the right costal margin.)
- The spleen is unpalpable.
- The kidneys are unpalpable, except in thin patients or those with a flaccid abdominal wall. (You'll typically feel the right kidney before you feel the left one. When palpable, the kidney is solid and firm.)

ABDOMINAL QUADRANTS

To perform a systematic GI assessment, visualize the abdominal structures by mentally dividing the abdomen into four quadrants, as shown below.

Right upper quadrant
- Right lobe of liver
- Gallbladder
- Pylorus
- Duodenum
- Head of the pancreas
- Hepatic flexure of the colon
- Portions of the ascending and transverse colon

Left upper quadrant
- Left lobe of the liver
- Stomach
- Body of the pancreas
- Splenic flexure of the colon
- Portions of the transverse and descending colon

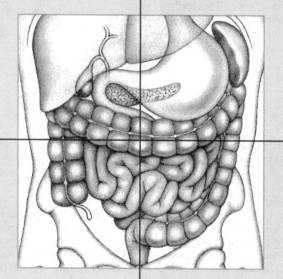

Right lower quadrant
- Cecum and appendix
- Portion of the ascending colon

Left lower quadrant
- Sigmoid colon
- Portion of the descending colon

PALPATING AND HOOKING THE LIVER

These illustrations show the correct hand positions for palpating and hooking the liver.

Palpating the liver
■ Place the patient in the supine position. Standing at his right side, place your left hand under his back at the approximate location of the liver.
■ Place your right hand slightly below the mark you made earlier at the liver's upper border. Point the fingers of your right hand toward the patient's head just under the right costal margin.
■ As the patient inhales deeply, gently press in and up on the abdomen until the liver brushes under your right hand. The edge should be smooth, firm, and somewhat round. Note any tenderness.

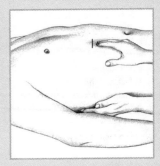

ELICITING ABDOMINAL PAIN

Rebound tenderness and the iliopsoas and obturator signs can indicate conditions, such as appendicitis and peritonitis. You can elicit these signs of abdominal pain, as illustrated here.

Rebound tenderness
Help the patient into a supine position with his knees flexed to relax the abdominal muscles. Place your hands gently on the right lower quadrant at McBurney's point—located about midway between the umbilicus and the anterior superior iliac spine.

Slowly and deeply dip your fingers into the area; then release the pressure in a quick, smooth motion. Pain on release—rebound tenderness—is a positive sign. The pain may radiate to the umbilicus. *Caution:* Don't repeat this maneuver to minimize the risk of rupturing an inflamed appendix.

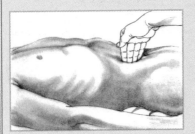

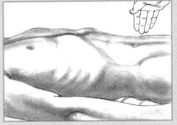

Hooking the liver

■ Hooking is an alternate way of palpating the liver. To hook the liver, stand next to the patient's right shoulder, facing his feet. Place your hands side by side, and hook your fingertips over the right costal margin, below the lower mark of dullness.

■ Ask the patient to take a deep breath as you push your fingertips in and up. If the liver is palpable, you may feel its edge as it slides down in the abdomen as he breathes in.

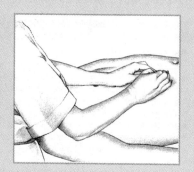

Iliopsoas sign

Help the patient into a supine position with his legs straight. Instruct him to raise his right leg upward as you exert slight pressure with your hand.

Repeat the maneuver with the left leg. When testing either leg, increased abdominal pain is a positive result, indicating irritation of the psoas muscle.

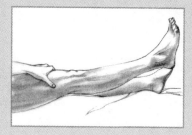

Obturator sign

Help the patient into a supine position with his right leg flexed 90 degrees at the hip and knee. Hold the leg just above the knee and at the ankle; then rotate the leg laterally and medially. Pain in the hypogastric region is a positive sign, indicating irritation of the obturator muscle.

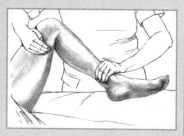

GI SYSTEM: INTERPRETING YOUR FINDINGS

Your assessment will reveal a group of findings that may lead you to suspect a particular disorder. The chart below shows some common groups of findings for signs and symptoms of the GI system, along with their probable causes.

Sign or symptom and findings	Probable cause
ABDOMINAL PAIN	
■ Localized abdominal pain, described as steady, gnawing, burning, aching, or hungerlike, high in the midepigastrium, slightly off center, usually on the right ■ Pain begins 2 to 4 hours after a meal ■ Ingestion of food or antacids brings relief ■ Changes in bowel habits ■ Heartburn or retrosternal burning	Duodenal ulcer
■ Pain and tenderness in the right or left lower abdominal quadrant, may become sharp and severe on standing or stooping ■ Abdominal distention ■ Mild nausea and vomiting ■ Occasional menstrual irregularities ■ Slight fever	Ovarian cyst
■ Referred, severe upper abdominal pain, tenderness, and rigidity that diminish with inspiration ■ Fever, shaking chills, achiness ■ Blood-tinged or rusty sputum ■ Dry, hacking cough ■ Dyspnea	Pneumonia
DIARRHEA	
■ Soft, unformed stools or watery diarrhea that may be foul-smelling or grossly bloody ■ Abdominal pain, cramping, and tenderness ■ Fever	*Clostridium difficile* infection
■ Diarrhea occurs within several hours of ingesting milk or milk products ■ Abdominal pain, cramping, and bloating ■ Borborygmi ■ Flatus	Lactose intolerance
■ Recurrent bloody diarrhea with pus or mucus ■ Hyperactive bowel sounds ■ Cramping lower abdominal pain ■ Occasional nausea and vomiting	Ulcerative colitis

GI SYSTEM: INTERPRETING YOUR FINDINGS *(continued)*

Sign or symptom and findings	Probable cause
HEMATOCHEZIA	
■ Moderate to severe rectal bleeding ■ Epistaxis ■ Purpura	Coagulation disorders
■ Bright-red rectal bleeding with or without pain ■ Diarrhea or ribbon-shaped stools ■ Stools may be grossly bloody ■ Weakness and fatigue ■ Abdominal aching and dull cramps	Colon cancer
■ Chronic bleeding with defecation ■ Painful defecation	Hemorrhoids
NAUSEA AND VOMITING	
■ Nausea and vomiting follow or accompany abdominal pain ■ Pain progresses rapidly to severe, stabbing pain in the right lower quadrant (McBurney's sign) ■ Abdominal rigidity and tenderness ■ Constipation or diarrhea ■ Tachycardia	Appendicitis
■ Nausea and vomiting of undigested food ■ Diarrhea ■ Abdominal cramping ■ Hyperactive bowel sounds ■ Fever	Gastroenteritis
■ Nausea and vomiting ■ Headache with severe, constant, throbbing pain ■ Fatigue ■ Photophobia ■ Light flashes ■ Increased noise sensitivity	Migraine headache

DIAGNOSTIC TESTS

BARIUM ENEMA

Overview

- Radiographic examination of the large intestine after rectal instillation of barium sulfate (single-contrast technique), or barium sulfate and air (double-contrast technique)
- History of altered bowel habits; lower abdominal pain; or passage of blood, mucus, or pus in stools

PURPOSE

- Aids in diagnosing colorectal cancer and inflammatory bowel disease
- To detect polyps, diverticula, and changes in the large intestine
- To define the extent of inflammatory diseases

PATIENT PREPARATION

- Make sure the patient has signed an appropriate consent form.
- Note all allergies.
- Administer a bowel preparation as ordered.
- Dairy products are restricted (liquid diet 24 hours before the test).
- Instruct the patient to drink five 8-oz (240-ml) glasses of clear liquids in the 12 to 24 hours before the test to ensure adequate hydration.
- Withhold breakfast before the procedure; clear liquids allowed if the test is scheduled for late afternoon.
- Warn the patient that cramps or the urge to defecate may be experienced as the barium or air is introduced into the intestine.
- Explain that the anal sphincter should be tightly contracted against the rectal tube to hold the tube in position and prevent the barium from leaking.

Various diets, laxatives, and cleansing enemas may be used, but some conditions, such as ulcerative colitis and active GI bleeding, may preclude the use of laxatives and enemas.

POSTPROCEDURE CARE

- Encourage extra oral fluid intake to prevent dehydration and help eliminate the barium.
- Administer a mild cathartic or an enema because barium retention can cause intestinal obstruction or fecal impaction.

Monitoring

- Vital signs
- Intake and output
- Stools
- Abdominal distension
- Bowel sounds

PRECAUTIONS

- Flexible sigmoidoscopy provides the best view of the rectosigmoid region, where most colon cancers occur.
- Barium enema should precede barium swallow and the upper GI and small-bowel series because retained barium in the GI tract may interfere with subsequent radiographic studies.
- Contraindications include fulminant ulcerative colitis associated with systemic toxicity and megacolon, suspected bowel perforation, and pregnancy.
- Barium enema is performed cautiously with bowel obstruction, acute inflammatory conditions, acute vascular insufficiency of the bowel, acute fulminant bloody diarrhea, and suspected pneumatosis cystoides intestinalis.

COMPLICATIONS
- Perforation of the colon
- Water intoxication
- Barium granulomas
- Intraperitoneal and extraperitoneal extravasation of barium

Interpretation

NORMAL FINDINGS
Single-contrast test
- Intestine is uniformly filled with barium and colonic haustral markings are clearly apparent.
- Intestinal walls collapse as the barium is expelled.
- Mucosa has a regular, feathery appearance on the postevacuation film.

Double-contrast test
- Intestine is uniformly distended with air, with a thin layer of barium providing detail of the mucosal pattern.

ABNORMAL RESULTS
- Localized filling defects, with transition between normal and necrotic mucosa, suggest carcinoma.
- Diffuse inflammatory lesions originating in the anal region and ascending through the intestine suggest ulcerative colitis.
- Diffuse inflammatory lesions originating in the cecum and terminal ileum and then descending through the intestine suggest granulomatous colitis.
- Structural abnormalities suggest many possible disorders, such as saccular adenomatous polyps, broad-based villous polyps, intussusception, sigmoid volvulus, and sigmoid torsion.

CHOLECYSTOGRAPHY, ORAL

Overview

- Radiographic examination of the gallbladder after administration of contrast medium
- Indicated for patients with symptoms of biliary tract disease
- Commonly performed to confirm gallbladder disease

PURPOSE
- To detect gallstones
- To aid diagnosis of inflammatory disease and tumors of gallbladder

PATIENT PREPARATION
- Make sure the patient has signed an appropriate consent form.
- Note and report all allergies.
- Instruct the patient to eat a meal containing fat at noon the day before the test as ordered to stimulate release of bile from the gallbladder.
- Instruct the patient to eat a fat-free meal in the evening as ordered to inhibit gallbladder contraction and to promote bile accumulation.
- The patient may have nothing to eat or drink, except water, after the evening meal.
- Give the patient an oral contrast agent (usually tablets) as ordered 2 to 3 hours after the evening meal.

Examine any vomitus or diarrhea for undigested tablets. If noted, notify the physician and the radiography department.

- Administer an enema the morning of the test if ordered.

Teaching points
Be sure to cover:
- the purpose of the study and how it's done

POSTPROCEDURE CARE

■ If the test results are normal, the patient may resume his usual diet as ordered.

■ If gallstones are discovered, the physician orders an appropriate diet, usually fat-restricted, to help prevent acute attacks.

■ If oral cholecystography must be repeated, the low-fat diet must be continued until a definitive diagnosis can be made.

PRECAUTIONS

■ Oral cholecystography should precede barium studies to prevent retained barium from interfering with subsequent radiograph films.

■ Oral cholecystography is contraindicated in patients with severe renal or hepatic damage, and in those with a hypersensitivity to iodine, seafood, or other contrast media.

■ Oral cholecystography is contraindicated in pregnant patients because of possible teratogenic effects of radiation.

COMPLICATIONS

■ Adverse reaction to contrast medium

Interpretation

NORMAL FINDINGS

■ Opacification of the gallbladder is normal.

■ The gallbladder appears pear-shaped with smooth, thin walls.

ABNORMAL RESULTS

■ Filling defects may indicate gallstones.

■ Fixed defects may indicate polyps or a benign tumor.

■ Failed or faint opacification may indicate inflammatory disease, such as cholecystitis, with or without gallstones.

■ Failure of the gallbladder to contract following stimulation by a fatty meal may indicate cholecystitis or common bile duct obstruction.

COLONOSCOPY

Overview

■ Visual examination of the lining of the large intestine with a flexible fiber-optic endoscope

■ Indicated for patients with a history of constipation or diarrhea, persistent rectal bleeding, or lower abdominal pain, and for colorectal cancer screening

■ Performed as either an inpatient or outpatient procedure

PURPOSE

■ To detect and evaluate inflammatory and ulcerative bowel disease

■ To locate the origin of lower GI bleeding

■ To aid diagnosis of colonic strictures and benign or malignant lesions

■ To evaluate the colon for postoperative recurrence of polyps or malignant lesions

PATIENT PREPARATION

■ Make sure the patient has signed an appropriate consent form.

■ Note and report all allergies.

■ A clear liquid diet is required for 24 to 48 hours before the test.

■ Be sure the patient has nothing by mouth after midnight.

■ Administer bowel preparation as ordered the day before the test.

■ The large intestine must be thoroughly cleaned to be clearly visible.

■ Warn the patient that an urge to defecate may be experienced when the scope is inserted and advanced.
■ Explain that air is introduced through the colonoscope to distend the intestinal wall and facilitate the test.
■ Explain that I.V. sedation will be administered.

Teaching points
Be sure to cover:
■ the test's purpose and how it's done.

POSTPROCEDURE CARE
■ Provide a safe environment until the patient has recovered from sedation.
■ Resume a usual diet as ordered.

If a polyp has been removed, inform the patient that there may be some blood in his stool and that he should report excessive bleeding immediately.

Monitoring
■ Vital sign
■ Respiratory status
■ Level of consciousness
■ Abdominal distension
■ Bowel sounds
■ Bleeding
■ Stools

Observe the patient closely for signs of bowel perforation: malaise, rectal bleeding, abdominal pain and distention, fever, and mucopurulent drainage. Notify the physician immediately if such signs develop.

Watch closely for adverse effects of the sedative, such as respiratory depression, hypotension, bradycardia, and confusion. Have emergency resuscitation equipment immediately available as well as a narcotic antagonist such as naloxone.

PRECAUTIONS
■ Colonoscopy is contraindicated in pregnancy and in patients who have recently had an acute myocardial infarction or abdominal surgery.
■ Colonoscopy is contraindicated in patients who have ischemic bowel disease, acute diverticulitis, peritonitis, fulminant granulomatous colitis, fulminant ulcerative colitis, or a perforated viscus.
■ Patients shouldn't drive, operate any machinery, or ingest alcohol for 24 hours after sedation.
■ Poor bowel preparation greatly impairs visual examination
■ Retained barium from previous diagnostic studies impairs accurate visual examination.
■ Acute colonic hemorrhage interferes with the examination.
■ Fixation of the sigmoid colon from inflammatory bowel disease, surgery, or radiation therapy may inhibit passage of the colonoscope.

COMPLICATIONS
■ Perforation of the large intestine
■ Excessive bleeding from a biopsy or polypectomy site
■ Retroperitoneal emphysema

Interpretation

NORMAL FINDINGS
■ The large intestine mucosa beyond the sigmoid colon appears light pink and is marked by semilunar folds and deep tubular pits.
■ Blood vessels are visible beneath the intestinal mucosa, which glistens from mucus secretion.

ABNORMAL RESULTS
■ Structural abnormalities detected by colonoscopy alone suggest diverticular disease or lower GI bleeding.

GASTROINTESTINAL CARE

SPIRAL CT

Noncontrast spiral, or helical, computed tomography (CT) has many advantages. It has replaced excretory pyelography as first-line imaging for suspected acute renal colic. It enables accurate diagnosis of flank pain in less than 1 minute and efficient calculation of stone size. Contrast agents are avoided, so this eliminates any complications caused by the agents. Imaging results aren't affected by operator experience, which is another advantage over excretory pyelography. Preliminary studies show a 94% to 100% overall diagnostic accuracy rate.

Spiral CT aids in the differential diagnosis of abdominal aortic aneurysms, masses in the adnexal uteri, appendicitis, diverticulitis, gallstones, and hernias.

■ Structural abnormalities detected by colonoscopy, in conjunction with histologic and cytologic test results, may indicate: proctitis, granulomatous and ulcerative colitis, Crohn's disease, or malignant and benign lesions.

COMPUTED TOMOGRAPHY OF THE ABDOMEN AND PELVIS

Overview

■ Form of X-ray that creates cross-sectional images in various body planes
■ Computed tomography (CT) of abdomen: includes the area between the dome of the diaphragm and iliac crests

■ Pelvic CT: includes the area between the iliac crests and the perineum
■ In males, pelvic viscera include the bladder and prostate
■ In females, pelvic viscera include the bladder and adnexa
■ CT of abdomen performed with or without CT of pelvis
■ Spiral CT scans of the abdomen and pelvis also possible (see *Spiral CT*)

PURPOSE
■ To evaluate soft tissue and organs of the abdomen, pelvis, and retroperitoneal space
■ To evaluate inflammatory disease
■ To aid staging of neoplasms
■ To evaluate trauma
■ To detect tumors, cysts, hemorrhage, or edema
■ To evaluate response to chemotherapy

PATIENT PREPARATION
■ Make sure the patient has signed an appropriate consent form.
■ Note and report all allergies.
■ Restriction of food and fluids before the test is usually required.
■ Stress the need to remain still during testing because movement can limit the test's accuracy. The patient may experience minimal discomfort because of lying still.
■ Warn about transient discomfort from the needle puncture and a warm or flushed feeling or metallic taste if an I.V. contrast medium is used.
■ Inform the patient that clacking sounds are heard as the table is moved into the scanner.

Teaching points
Be sure to cover:
■ the purpose of the study and how it's done

POSTPROCEDURE CARE
■ Normal diet and activities may be resumed unless otherwise ordered.

PRECAUTIONS
■ CT of the abdomen and pelvis isn't usually recommended during pregnancy because of potential risk to the fetus.
■ Check the patient's history for hypersensitivity to shellfish, iodine, or iodinated contrast media, and document such reactions on the patient's chart.
■ Inform the physician of any sensitivity so that prophylactic medications may be ordered; the physician may choose not to use contrast enhancement.

COMPLICATIONS
■ Adverse reaction to iodinated contrast medium

Interpretation

NORMAL FINDINGS
■ Organs are normal in size and position.
■ There are no masses or other abnormalities.

ABNORMAL RESULTS
■ Well-circumscribed or poorly-defined areas of slightly lower density than normal parenchyma suggest possible primary and metastatic neoplasms.
■ Relatively low-density, homogeneous areas, usually with well-defined borders, suggest possible abscesses.
■ Sharply defined round or oval structures, with densities less than that of abscesses and neoplasms, suggest cysts.
■ Dilatation of the biliary ducts suggests obstructive disease from tumor or calculi.

ENDOSCOPIC RETROGRADE CHOLANGIO-PANCREATOGRAPHY

Overview

■ Radiographic examination of the pancreatic ducts and hepatobiliary tree after injection of contrast medium into the duodenal papilla
■ Also known as ERCP

PURPOSE
■ To evaluate obstructive jaundice
■ To diagnose cancer of the duodenal papilla, pancreas, and biliary ducts
■ To locate calculi and stenosis in pancreatic ducts and hepatobiliary tree

PATIENT PREPARATION
■ Make sure the patient has signed an appropriate consent form.
■ Note and report all allergies.
■ Administer a sedative as ordered.
■ Instruct the patient to fast before the study as ordered.
■ Explain the use of a local anesthetic spray to suppress the gag reflex and the use of a mouth guard to protect the teeth.
■ Provide reassurance that oral insertion of the endoscope doesn't obstruct breathing and that the patient remains conscious during the procedure.

Teaching points
Be sure to cover:
■ the purpose of the study and how it's done.

GASTROINTESTINAL CARE

POSTPROCEDURE CARE
■ Withhold food and fluids until the gag reflex returns; resume diet as ordered.
■ Provide soothing lozenges and warm saline gargles for sore throat.

Monitoring
■ Vital signs
■ Cardiac rhythm
■ Pulse oximetry
■ Level of consciousness
■ Abdominal distention and bowel sounds
■ Adverse drug reactions
■ Signs and symptoms of:
– Perforation
– Respiratory depression
– Urinary retention
– Ascending cholangitis
– Pancreatitis

PRECAUTIONS
■ Inform the physician about hypersensitivity to iodine, seafood, or iodinated contrast media.
■ The procedure is contraindicated in:
– pregnancy
– stricture or obstruction of the esophagus or duodenum
– acute pancreatitis or cholangitis
– severe cardiorespiratory disease.

Emergency resuscitation equipment and a benzodiazepine and narcotic antagonist should be immediately available during the test.

COMPLICATIONS
■ Ascending cholangitis
■ Pancreatitis
■ Adverse drug reactions
■ Cardiac arrhythmias
■ Perforation of the bowel
■ Respiratory depression

Interpretation

NORMAL FINDINGS
■ Duodenal papilla appears as a small red or pale erosion protruding into the lumen.
■ Pancreatic and hepatobiliary ducts usually join and empty through the duodenal papilla; separate orifices are sometimes present.
■ Contrast agent uniformly fills the pancreatic duct, hepatobiliary tree, and gallbladder.

ABNORMAL RESULTS
■ Hepatobiliary tree tilling defects, strictures, or irregular deviations suggest possible biliary cirrhosis, primary sclerosing cholangitis, calculi, or cancer of the bile ducts.
■ Filling defects, strictures, and irregular deviations of pancreatic duct suggest possible pancreatic cysts and pseudocysts, pancreatic tumors, chronic pancreatitis, pancreatic fibrosis, calculi, or papillary stenosis.

PARACENTESIS

Overview

■ A method of obtaining samples of ascitic fluid for diagnostic and therapeutic purposes by insertion of a trocar and cannula through the abdominal wall
■ May be performed using image-guidance
■ Four-quadrant tap: aspiration of fluid from each quadrant of the abdomen to verify abdominal trauma and need for surgery
■ Peritoneal fluid analysis: examination of gross appearance, red blood cell and white blood cell counts, cytologic studies, microbiological studies for bacteria and fungi, and determina-

tions of protein, glucose, amylase, ammonia, and alkaline phosphatase levels

PURPOSE
- To determine cause of ascites
- To detect abdominal trauma
- To remove accumulated ascitic fluid

PATIENT PREPARATION
- Make sure the patient has signed an appropriate consent form.
- Note and report all allergies.
- Restriction of food and fluids before the test isn't necessary.
- Inform the patient that a local anesthetic will be used.

Teaching points
Be sure to cover:
- the purpose of the study and how it's done.

POSTPROCEDURE CARE
- Resume previous activity as ordered.
- Administer I.V. infusions and albumin as ordered.

Monitoring
- Vital signs
- Intake and output
- Puncture site and drainage
- Daily weight
- Daily abdominal girth measurement
- Bleeding
- Infection
- Hematuria, which may indicate bladder trauma.
- Serum electrolyte (especially sodium) and protein levels

If a large amount of fluid was removed, watch for signs of vascular collapse (tachycardia, tachypnea, hypotension, dizziness, and mental status changes).

Watch for signs and symptoms of hemorrhage and shock and for increasing pain and abdominal tenderness. These may indicate a perforated intestine or, depending on the site of the tap, puncture of the inferior epigastric artery, hematoma of the anterior cecal wall, or rupture of the iliac vein or bladder.

Observe the patient with severe hepatic disease for signs of hepatic coma, which may result from loss of sodium and potassium accompanying hypovolemia. Watch for mental status changes, drowsiness, and stupor. Such a patient is also prone to uremia, infection, hemorrhage, and protein depletion.

PRECAUTIONS
- Paracentesis is contraindicated in pregnancy and in bleeding tendencies.

COMPLICATIONS
- Bleeding, hemorrhage
- Infection
- Bladder trauma
- Shock
- Perforated intestine
- Inferior epigastric artery puncture
- Anterior cecal wall hematoma
- Iliac vein rupture

Interpretation

NORMAL FINDINGS
- Peritoneal fluid is odorless and clear to pale yellow.

ABNORMAL RESULTS
- Milk-colored fluid may indicate chylous ascites.
- Bloody fluid may indicate:
  – benign or malignant tumor
  – hemorrhagic pancreatitis
  – perforated intestine or duodenal ulcer.
- Cloudy or turbid fluid may indicate peritonitis or an infectious process.

■ Gram-positive cocci commonly indicate primary peritonitis; gram-negative organisms indicate secondary peritonitis.

■ Fungi may indicate histoplasmosis, candidiasis, or coccidioidomycosis.

ULTRASONOGRAPHY OF THE GALLBLADDER AND BILIARY SYSTEM

Overview

■ Focused beam of high-frequency sound waves passes into the right upper quadrant of the abdomen, creating echoes that vary with changes in tissue density

■ Images reveal the size, shape, structure, and position of gallbladder and biliary system

■ Has largely replaced oral cholecystography because it doesn't expose the patient to radiation and doesn't require contrast enhancement; oral cholecystography is performed when ultrasonography is inconclusive

■ Ultrasound of gallbladder is procedure of choice for evaluating jaundice and for emergency diagnosis of patients with signs of acute cholecystitis such as right upper quadrant pain with or without local tenderness

■ When ultrasonography fails to clearly define the site of biliary obstruction: necessitates percutaneous transhepatic cholangiography or endoscopic retrograde cholangiopancreatography

PURPOSE

■ To confirm diagnosis of cholelithiasis

■ To diagnose acute cholecystitis

■ To distinguish between obstructive and nonobstructive jaundice

PATIENT PREPARATION

■ Make sure the patient has signed an appropriate consent form.

■ Note and report all allergies.

■ Provide a fat-free meal in the evening before the study.

■ Fasting is required for 8 to 12 hours before the procedure, if possible; this promotes accumulation of bile in the gallbladder and enhances ultrasonic visualization.

Teaching points

Be sure to cover:
■ the purpose of the test.

POSTPROCEDURE CARE

■ Resume the patient's normal diet.

■ Remove the lubricating jelly from the patient's skin.

PRECAUTIONS

■ Fasting before the study prevents the excretion of bile in the gallbladder.

COMPLICATIONS

■ None known

Interpretation

NORMAL FINDINGS

■ The normal gallbladder is sonolucent; it appears circular on transverse scans and pear-shaped on longitudinal scans.

■ Although the gallbladder's size varies, its outer walls normally appear sharp and smooth.

ABNORMAL RESULTS

■ Mobile, echogenic areas, usually associated with an acoustic shadow, suggests gallstones within the gallbladder lumen or the biliary system.

■ When the gallbladder is shrunken or fully impacted with gallstones, inadequate bile may make gallstone detection difficult and the gallbladder itself may fail to be visualized. In this case, the presence of an acoustic shadow in the gallbladder fossa suggests cholelithiasis.

■ An acoustic shadow in the cystic and common bile ducts suggests possible choledocholithiasis.

■ Fixed echogenic areas within the gallbladder lumen suggests possible polyps or tumors; polyps usually appear as sharply defined, echogenic areas; carcinoma appears as a poorly defined mass commonly associated with a thickened gallbladder wall.

■ A fine layer of echoes that slowly gravitates to the dependent portion of the gallbladder as the patient changes position, suggests biliary sludge within the gallbladder lumen.

■ An enlarged gallbladder with thickened, double-rimmed walls, usually accompanied by gallstones within the lumen, suggests acute cholecystitis.

■ A contracted gallbladder with thickened walls suggests chronic cholecystitis.

■ A dilated biliary system and, usually, a dilated gallbladder suggests obstructive jaundice.

UPPER GI AND SMALL-BOWEL SERIES

Overview

■ Involves fluoroscopic examination of esophagus, stomach, and small intestine after ingestion of barium sulfate, a contrast agent

■ As barium passes through digestive tract, fluoroscopy shows peristalsis and the mucosal contours of organs; spot films record significant findings

■ Indicated for patients who have upper GI symptoms (difficulty swallowing, regurgitation, burning or gnawing epigastric pain), signs of small-bowel disease (diarrhea, weight loss), and signs of GI bleeding (hematemesis, melena)

■ Can be used to detect various mucosal abnormalities; many patients need biopsy afterward to rule out cancer or distinguish specific inflammatory diseases

■ Oral cholecystography, barium enema, and routine X-rays: should always precede this test because retained barium clouds anatomic detail on X-ray films

PURPOSE

■ To detect hiatal hernia, diverticula, and varices

■ To aid diagnosis of strictures, ulcers, tumors, regional enteritis, and malabsorption syndrome

■ To detect motility disorders

PATIENT PREPARATION

■ Make sure the patient has signed an appropriate consent form.

■ Note and report all allergies.

■ Withhold oral medications after midnight and anticholinergics and narcotics for 24 hours as ordered because these drugs affect small intestine motility.

■ Withhold antacids, histamine-2–receptor antagonists, and proton pump inhibitors as ordered if gastric reflux is suspected.

■ Instruct the patient to maintain a low-residue diet for 2 or 3 days before the test and to fast and avoid smoking after midnight before the test.

■ Inform the patient that the barium mixture has a milkshake consistency and chalky taste; although flavored, the patient may find the taste unpleasant; 16 to 20 oz (480 to 600 ml) are needed for a complete examination.

■ Warn the patient that the abdomen may be compressed to ensure proper coating of the stomach or intestinal walls with barium or to separate overlapping bowel loops.

Teaching points

Be sure to cover:
- the purpose of the study and how it's done.

POSTPROCEDURE CARE

- Make sure additional X-rays haven't been ordered before allowing the patient food, fluids, and oral medications.
- Instruct the patient to drink plenty of fluid (unless contraindicated) to help eliminate the barium.
- Administer a cathartic or enema as ordered.
- Inform him that his stool will be light-colored for 24 to 72 hours.
- Because barium retention in the intestine may cause obstruction or fecal impaction, notify the physician if the patient doesn't pass barium within 2 to 3 days.
- Tell the patient to advise the physician of abdominal fullness or pain or a delay in return to brown stools.

Monitoring

- Vital signs
- Intake and output
- Bowel movements
- Abdominal distention
- Bowel sounds

PRECAUTIONS

- Upper GI and small-bowel series is contraindicated in patients with obstruction or perforation of the GI tract because barium may intensify the obstruction or seep into the abdominal cavity.
- If a perforation is suspected, Gastrografin (a water-soluble contrast medium) may be used instead of barium.

- Upper GI and small-bowel series is contraindicated in pregnant patients because of the possible teratogenic effects of radiation.

COMPLICATIONS

- Bowel obstruction
- Fecal impaction

Interpretation

NORMAL FINDINGS

- After the barium suspension is swallowed, it pours over the base of the tongue into the pharynx, and is propelled by a peristaltic wave through the entire length of the esophagus in about 2 seconds.
- The bolus evenly fills and distends the lumen of the pharynx and esophagus, and the mucosa appears smooth and regular.
- When the peristaltic wave reaches the base of the esophagus, the cardiac sphincter opens, allowing the bolus to enter the stomach; this is followed by closing of the cardiac sphincter.
- As barium enters the stomach, it outlines the characteristic longitudinal folds called rugae, which are best observed using the double-contrast technique.
- When the stomach is completely filled with barium its outer contour appears smooth and regular without evidence of flattened, rigid areas suggesting intrinsic or extrinsic lesions.
- After barium enters the stomach it quickly empties into the duodenal bulb through relaxation of the pyloric sphincter.
- Although the mucosa of the duodenal bulb is relatively smooth, circular folds become apparent as barium enters the duodenal loop; these folds deepen and become more numerous in the jejunum. Barium temporarily

lodges between these folds, producing a speckled pattern on the X-ray film.
- As barium enters the ileum, the circular folds become less prominent and, except for their broadness, resemble those in the duodenum.
- The diameter of the small intestine tapers gradually from the duodenum to the ileum.

ABNORMAL RESULTS
- Structural abnormalities of the esophagus suggest possible strictures, tumors, hiatal hernia, diverticula, varices, and ulcers.
- Dilatation of the esophagus suggests possible benign strictures.
- Erosive changes in the esophageal mucosa suggest possible malignant strictures.
- Filling defects in the column of barium suggest possible esophageal tumors; malignant esophageal tumors change the mucosal contour.
- Narrowing of the distal esophagus strongly suggests achalasia (cardiospasm).
- Backflow of barium from the stomach into the esophagus suggests gastric reflux.

- Filling defects in the stomach, which usually disrupt peristalsis, suggest malignant tumors, usually adenocarcinomas.
- Outpouchings of the gastric mucosa that generally don't affect peristalsis suggest benign tumors, such as adenomatous polyps and leiomyomas.
- Evidence of partial or complete healing, characterized by radiating folds extending to the edge of the ulcer crater, suggests benign ulcers.
- Radiating folds that extend beyond the ulcer crater to the edge of the mass suggest malignant ulcers.
- Edematous changes in the mucosa of the antrum or duodenal loop, or dilation of the duodenal loop suggest possible pancreatitis or pancreatic carcinoma.
- Edematous changes, segmentation of the barium column, and flocculation in the small intestine suggest possible malabsorption syndrome.
- Filling defects of the small intestine suggest possible Hodgkin's disease and lymphosarcoma.

DISEASES

APPENDICITIS

Overview

DESCRIPTION
- Most common major abdominal surgical disease
- Inflammation of the vermiform appendix
- Fatal if left untreated; gangrene and perforation develop within 36 hours

PATHOPHYSIOLOGY
- Mucosal ulceration triggers inflammation, which temporarily obstructs the appendix.
- Obstruction causes mucus outflow, increasing pressure in the distended appendix; the appendix then contracts.
- Bacteria multiply and inflammation and pressure increase, restricting blood flow and causing thrombus and abdominal pain.

CAUSES
- Foreign body
- Neoplasm
- Mucosal ulceration
- Fecal mass
- Stricture
- Barium ingestion
- Viral infection

RISK FACTORS
- Adolescent male

COMPLICATIONS
- Wound infection
- Intra-abdominal infection
- Fecal fistula
- Intestinal obstruction
- Incisional hernia
- Peritonitis (most common)
- Death

Assessment

HISTORY
- Abdominal pain that's initially generalized, then localizes in the right lower abdomen (McBurney's point)
- Anorexia
- Nausea, vomiting

PHYSICAL FINDINGS
- Low-grade fever, tachycardia
- Adjusts posture to decrease pain
- Guarding
- Normoactive bowel sounds, with possible constipation or diarrhea
- Rebound tenderness and spasm of the abdominal muscles
- Rovsing's sign
- Psoas sign
- Obturator sign
- Absent abdominal tenderness or flank tenderness with retrocecal or pelvic appendix

TEST RESULTS
Laboratory
- White blood cell count moderately elevated, with increased numbers of immature cells

Imaging
- Abdominal or transvaginal ultrasound showing appendiceal inflammation
- Barium enema revealing nonfilling appendix
- Abdominal computed tomography scan demonstrating suspected perforation or abscess

Treatment

GENERAL
- Delaying surgery until antibiotic therapy has been initiated, if an abscess is suspected

DIET
- Nothing by mouth until after surgery, then gradual return to regular diet

ACTIVITY
- Early postoperative ambulation

MEDICATION
- I.V. fluids
- Analgesics
- Antibiotics preoperatively and if peritonitis develops

SURGERY
- Appendectomy

MONITORING
After surgery
- Vital signs
- Intake and output
- Pain relief
- Bowel sounds, passing of flatus, or bowel movements
- Wound healing

CHOLELITHIASIS, CHOLECYSTITIS, AND RELATED DISORDERS

Overview

DESCRIPTION
Cholelithiasis
- Leading biliary tract disease
- Formation of calculi (gallstones) in the gallbladder
- Prognosis usually good with treatment, unless infection occurs

Cholecystitis
- Related disorder that arises from formation of gallstones
- Gallbladder becomes acutely or chronically inflamed
- Usually caused by a gallstone lodged in the cystic duct
- Acute form most common during middle age
- Chronic form most common among elderly persons
- Prognosis good with treatment

Choledocholithiasis
- Related disorder that arises from formation of gallstones
- Partial or complete biliary obstruction due to gallstones lodged in the common bile duct
- Prognosis good unless infection occurs

Cholangitis
- Related disorder that arises from formation of gallstones
- Infected bile duct
- Commonly associated with choledocholithiasis
- Nonsuppurative cholangitis usually responds rapidly to antibiotic treatment
- Suppurative cholangitis has a poor prognosis unless surgery to correct obstruction and drain infected bile is performed promptly

Gallstone ileus
- Related disorder that arises from formation of gallstones
- Obstruction of the small bowel by a gallstone
- Most common in elderly persons
- Prognosis good with surgery

PATHOPHYSIOLOGY
- Calculi formation in the biliary system causes obstruction.
- Obstruction of hepatic duct leads to intrahepatic retention of bile; increased release of bilirubin into the bloodstream occurs.
- Obstruction of cystic duct leads to inflammation of the gallbladder; increased gallbladder contraction and peristalsis occurs.
- Obstruction of bile causes impairment of digestion and absorption of lipids.

CAUSES
- Calculi formation; type of disorder that develops depends on where in the gallbladder or biliary tract the calculi collect
- Acute cholecystitis also a result of conditions that alter gallbladder's ability to fill or empty (trauma, reduced blood supply to the gallbladder, prolonged immobility, chronic dieting, adhesions, prolonged anesthesia, and opioid abuse)

RISK FACTORS
- High-calorie, high-cholesterol diet
- Associated with obesity
- Elevated estrogen levels from hormonal contraceptive use, postmenopausal hormone-replacement therapy, or pregnancy

■ Diabetes mellitus, ileal disease, hemolytic disorders, hepatic disease (cirrhosis), or pancreatitis
■ Rapid weight loss

COMPLICATIONS
Cholelithiasis
■ Cholangitis
■ Cholecystitis
■ Choledocholithiasis
■ Gallstone ileus

Cholecystitis
■ Gallbladder complications, such as empyema, hydrops or mucocele, and gangrene
■ Chronic cholecystitis and cholangitis

Choledocholithiasis
■ Cholangitis
■ Obstructive jaundice
■ Pancreatitis
■ Secondary biliary cirrhosis

Cholangitis
■ Septic shock
■ Death

Gallstone ileus
■ Bowel obstruction

Assessment

HISTORY
■ Gallbladder disease may produce no symptoms (even when X-rays reveal gallstones)
■ Acute cholelithiasis, acute cholecystitis, and choledocholithiasis produce symptoms of classic gallbladder attack

Gallbladder attack
■ Sudden onset of severe steady or aching pain in the midepigastric region or the right upper abdominal quadrant

■ Pain radiating to the back, between the shoulder blades or over the right shoulder blade, or just to the shoulder area
■ Attack occurring after eating a fatty meal or a large meal after fasting for an extended time
■ Attack occurring in the middle of the night
■ Nausea, vomiting, and chills
■ Low-grade fever
■ History of milder GI symptoms that preceded the acute attack; indigestion, vague abdominal discomfort, belching, and flatulence after eating meals or snacks rich in fats

PHYSICAL FINDINGS
Gallbladder attack
■ Severe pain
■ Pallor
■ Diaphoresis
■ Low-grade fever (high in cholangitis)
■ Exhaustion
■ Jaundice (chronic)
■ Dark-colored urine and clay-colored stools
■ Tachycardia
■ Tenderness over the gallbladder, which increases on inspiration (Murphy's sign)
■ Palpable, painless, sausagelike mass (calculus-filled gallbladder without ductal obstruction)
■ Hypoactive bowel sounds

TEST RESULTS
Laboratory
■ Blood studies possibly revealing elevated levels of serum alkaline phosphatase, lactate dehydrogenase, aspartate aminotransferase, icteric index, and total bilirubin; white blood cell count slightly elevated during cholecystitis attack

Imaging

■ Plain abdominal X-rays show gallstones if they contain enough calcium to be radiopaque.

■ Ultrasonography of the gallbladder confirms cholelithiasis in most patients and distinguishes between obstructive and nonobstructive jaundice; calculi as small as 2 mm can be detected.

■ Oral cholecystography confirms the presence of gallstones, although this test is gradually being replaced by ultrasonography.

■ Technetium-labeled iminodiacetic acid scan of the gallbladder indicates cystic duct obstruction and acute or chronic cholecystitis if the gallbladder can't be seen.

Diagnostic procedures

■ Percutaneous transhepatic cholangiography, imaging performed under fluoroscopic guidance supports the diagnosis of obstructive jaundice and is used to visualize calculi in the ducts.

Treatment

GENERAL

■ Endoscopic retrograde cholangiopancreatography to visualize and remove calculi

■ Lithotripsy

DIET

■ Low-fat

■ Nothing by mouth if surgery required

ACTIVITY

■ As tolerated

■ Avoid heavy lifting or contact sports for 6 weeks after surgery

MEDICATION

■ Gallstone dissolution therapy

■ Vitamin supplements

■ Bile salts

■ Analgesics

■ Antispasmodics

■ Anticholinergics

■ Antiemetics

■ Antibiotics

SURGERY

■ Most common treatment for gallbladder and duct disease

■ May include cholecystectomy (laparoscopic or abdominal), cholecystectomy with operative cholangiography, choledochostomy, or exploration of the common bile duct

MONITORING

■ Vital signs

■ Intake and output

■ Pain control

After surgery

■ Signs and symptoms of bleeding, infection, or atelectasis

■ Wound site

■ Drain function and drainage

■ Bowel function

■ T-tube patency and drainage

CIRRHOSIS

Overview

DESCRIPTION

■ Chronic hepatic disease

■ Several types exist

PATHOPHYSIOLOGY

■ Diffuse destruction and fibrotic regeneration of hepatic cells occurs.

■ Necrotic tissue yields to fibrosis.

■ Liver structure and normal vasculature are altered.

■ Blood and lymph flow are impaired.

■ Hepatic insufficiency occurs.

GASTROINTESTINAL CARE

CAUSES

Laënnec's or micronodular cirrhosis (alcoholic or portal cirrhosis)

- Chronic alcoholism
- Malnutrition

Postnecrotic or macronodular cirrhosis

- Complication of viral hepatitis
- Possible after exposure to such liver toxins as arsenic, carbon tetrachloride, and phosphorus

Biliary cirrhosis

- Prolonged biliary tract obstruction or inflammation

Idiopathic cirrhosis (cryptogenic)

- No known cause
- Sarcoidosis
- Chronic inflammatory bowel disease

RISK FACTORS

- Alcoholism
- Toxins
- Biliary obstruction
- Hepatitis
- Metabolic disorders

COMPLICATIONS

- Portal hypertension
- Bleeding esophageal varices
- Hepatic encephalopathy
- Hepatorenal syndrome
- Death

Assessment

HISTORY

- Chronic alcoholism
- Malnutrition
- Viral hepatitis
- Exposure to liver toxins such as arsenic

- Prolonged biliary tract obstruction or inflammation

In early stage

- Vague signs and symptoms
- Abdominal pain
- Diarrhea, constipation
- Fatigue
- Nausea, vomiting
- Muscle cramps

With disease progression

- Chronic dyspepsia
- Constipation
- Pruritus
- Weight loss
- Bleeding tendency, such as frequent nosebleeds, easy bruising, and bleeding gums

PHYSICAL FINDINGS

- Telangiectasis on the cheeks
- Spider angiomas on the face, neck, arms, and trunk
- Gynecomastia
- Umbilical hernia
- Distended abdominal blood vessels
- Ascites
- Testicular atrophy
- Menstrual irregularities
- Palmar erythema
- Clubbed fingers
- Thigh and leg edema
- Ecchymosis
- Anemia
- Jaundice
- Palpable, large, firm liver with a sharp edge (early finding)
- Enlarged spleen
- Asterixis
- Slurred speech, paranoia, hallucinations

TEST RESULTS
Laboratory

- Elevated levels of liver enzymes, such as alanine aminotransferase, aspartate aminotransferase, total serum

bilirubin, and indirect bilirubin; decreased total serum albumin and protein levels; prolonged prothrombin time; decreased hemoglobin, hematocrit, and serum electrolyte levels; deficient vitamins A, C, and K
■ Increased urine levels of bilirubin and urobilinogen; decreased fecal urobilinogen levels

Imaging
■ Abdominal X-rays show liver and spleen size and cysts or gas in the biliary tract or liver; liver calcification; and massive ascites.
■ Computed tomography and liver scans are used to determine liver size, identify liver masses, and visualize hepatic blood flow and obstruction.

Diagnostic procedures
■ Liver biopsy is the definitive test for cirrhosis, revealing hepatic tissue destruction and fibrosis.
■ Esophagogastroduodenoscopy reveals bleeding esophageal varices, stomach irritation or ulceration, and duodenal bleeding and irritation.

Treatment

GENERAL
■ Removal or alleviation of underlying cause
■ Paracentesis
■ Esophageal balloon tamponade
■ Sclerotherapy
■ I.V. fluids
■ Blood transfusion

DIET
■ Restricted sodium consumption
■ Restricted fluid intake
■ No alcohol

ACTIVITY
■ Frequent rest periods as needed

HOW THE LEVEEN SHUNT WORKS

Intractable ascites resulting from chronic liver disease can be controlled by draining ascitic fluid from the abdominal cavity into the superior vena cava, using the LeVeen peritoneovenous shunt. The shunt consists of a peritoneal tube, a venous tube, and a one-way pressure-sensitive valve that controls fluid flow.

Operation is simple. As the patient inhales, pressure within his abdomen increases while pressure in his superior vena cava decreases. This pressure differential causes the shunt's valve to open, allowing ascitic fluid to drain from the abdominal cavity into the superior vena cava. When the patient exhales, superior vena cava pressure rises and intra-abdominal pressure falls; this pressure differential forces the valve shut, stopping fluid flow.

The valve's one-way design prevents blood from backing into the tubing, reducing the risk of clotting and shunt occlusion. It also prevents the valve from opening if superior vena cava pressure remains higher than intra-abdominal pressure, as commonly occurs in patients with heart failure. This reduces the risk of fluid overload in the vascular system.

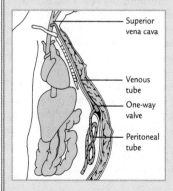

Superior vena cava

Venous tube

One-way valve

Peritoneal tube

MEDICATION
- Vitamin and nutritional supplements
- Antacids
- Potassium-sparing diuretics
- Beta-adrenergic blockers and vasopressin
- Ammonia detoxicant
- Antiemetics

SURGERY
- May be required to divert ascites into venous circulation; if so, a peritoneovenous shunt is used (see *How the LeVeen shunt works,* page 367)
- Portal-systemic shunts

MONITORING
- Vital signs
- Complete blood count, electrolytes
- Hydration and nutritional status
- Abdominal girth
- Weight
- Bleeding tendencies
- Skin integrity
- Changes in mentation, behavior

CROHN'S DISEASE

Overview

DESCRIPTION
- Inflammatory bowel disease that may affect any part of the GI tract
- Extends through all layers of the intestinal wall; may involve regional lymph nodes and mesentery

PATHOPHYSIOLOGY
- Crohn's disease involves slow, progressive inflammation of the bowel.
- Lymphatic obstruction is caused by enlarged lymph nodes.
- Edema, mucosal ulceration, fissures, and abscesses occur.

- Elevated patches of closely packed lymph follicles (Peyer's patches) develop in the small intestinal lining.
- Fibrosis occurs, thickening the bowel wall and causing stenosis.
- Inflamed bowel loops adhere to other diseased or normal loops.
- The diseased bowel becomes thicker, shorter, and narrower.

CAUSES
- Exact cause unknown
- Contributing factors include lymphatic obstruction and infection

RISK FACTORS
- History of allergies
- Immune disorders
- Genetic predisposition

COMPLICATIONS
- Anal fistula
- Perineal abscess
- Fistulas of the bladder or vagina or to the skin in an old scar area
- Intestinal obstruction
- Perforation
- Nutritional deficiencies caused by malabsorption and maldigestion

Assessment

HISTORY
- Gradual onset of signs and symptoms, marked by periods of remission and exacerbation
- Fatigue and weakness
- Fever, flatulence, nausea
- Steady, colicky, or cramping abdominal pain that usually occurs in the right lower abdominal quadrant
- Diarrhea that may worsen after emotional upset or ingestion of poorly tolerated foods, such as milk, fatty foods, and spices
- Weight loss

Physical findings
■ Possible soft or semiliquid stool, usually without gross blood
■ Right lower abdominal quadrant tenderness
■ Possible abdominal mass, indicating adherent loops of bowel

Test results
Laboratory
■ Occult blood in stools
■ Increased white blood cell count and erythrocyte sedimentation rate
■ Decreased serum potassium, calcium, magnesium, and hemoglobin
■ Hypoglobulinemia from intestinal protein loss

Imaging
■ X-rays of the small bowel may show irregular mucosa, ulceration, and stiffening.
■ Barium enema reveals the string sign (segments of stricture separated by normal bowel) and may also show fissures and narrowing of the lumen.

Diagnostic procedures
■ Sigmoidoscopy and colonoscopy show patchy areas of inflammation and may also reveal the characteristic coarse irregularity (cobblestone appearance) of the mucosal surface.
■ Biopsy reveals granulomas in up to one-half of all specimens.

Treatment

General
■ Stress reduction

Diet
■ Avoidance of foods that worsen diarrhea
■ Avoidance of raw fruits and vegetables if blockage occurs

■ Adequate caloric, protein, and vitamin intake
■ Parenteral nutrition if necessary

Activity
■ Reduced physical activity

Medication
■ Corticosteroids
■ Immunosuppressant agents
■ Sulfonamides
■ Anti-inflammatory agents
■ Antibacterial and antiprotozoal agents
■ Antidiarrheals
■ Opioid analgesics
■ Vitamin supplements
■ Antispasmodics

Surgery
■ Indicated for acute intestinal obstruction
■ Colectomy with ileostomy

Monitoring
■ Abdominal pain and distention
■ Vital signs, daily weight
■ Intake and output, including amount of stool
■ Pneumaturia
■ Serum electrolytes and glucose, hemoglobin, and stools for occult blood
■ Catheter insertion site, especially with total parenteral nutrition
■ Signs of infection or obstruction
■ Bleeding, especially with steroid use

GASTROINTESTINAL CARE

ESOPHAGEAL CANCER

Overview

Description
■ Esophageal tumors usually fungating and infiltrating and nearly always fatal

- Common sites of metastasis are liver and lungs
- Includes two types of malignant tumors: squamous cell carcinoma and adenocarcinoma

Pathophysiology
- Most esophageal cancers are poorly differentiated squamous cell carcinomas (50% occur in the lower portion of the esophagus; 40% in the middle portion; 10% in the upper or cervical esophagus).
- Adenocarcinomas occur less frequently and are contained to the lower third of the esophagus.
- The tumor partially constricts the lumen of the esophagus.
- Regional metastasis occurs early by way of submucosal lymphatics, often fatally invading adjacent vital intrathoracic organs. (If the patient survives primary extension, the liver and lungs are the usual sites of distant metastases; unusual metastasis sites include the bone, kidneys, and adrenal glands.)
- The prognosis for esophageal cancer is grim: 5-year survival rates occur in fewer than 5% of cases and most patients die within 6 months of diagnosis.

Causes
- Unknown

Risk factors
- Chronic irritation from heavy smoking
- Excessive use of alcohol
- Stasis-induced inflammation, as in achalasia or stricture
- Previous head and neck tumors
- Nutritional deficiency, such as in untreated sprue and Plummer-Vinson syndrome

Complications
- Direct invasion of adjoining structures
- Inability to control secretions
- Obstruction of the esophagus
- Loss of lower esophageal sphincter control (may result in aspiration pneumonia)

Assessment

History
- Feeling of fullness, pressure, indigestion, or substernal burning
- Dysphagia and weight loss; the degree of dysphagia varies, depending on the extent of disease
- Hoarseness
- Pain on swallowing or pain that radiates to the back
- Anorexia, vomiting, and regurgitation of food

Physical findings
- Chronic cough (possibly from aspiration)
- Cachexia and dehydration

Test results
Imaging
- X-rays of the esophagus, with barium swallow and motility studies, are used to delineate structural and filling defects and reduced peristalsis.
- Computed tomography scan may help to diagnose and monitor esophageal lesions.
- Magnetic resonance imaging permits evaluation of the esophagus and adjacent structures.

Diagnostic procedures
- Esophagoscopy, punch and brush biopsies, and exfoliative cytologic tests confirm esophageal tumors.
- Bronchoscopy (usually performed after an esophagoscopy) may reveal

tumor growth in the tracheobronchial tree.

■ Endoscopic ultrasonography of the esophagus combines endoscopy and ultrasound technology to measure the depth of penetration of the tumor.

Treatment

GENERAL
■ Surgery and other treatments to relieve disease effects because esophageal cancer usually advanced when diagnosed
■ Palliative therapy used to keep esophagus open:
– Dilatation of the esophagus
– Laser therapy
– Radiation therapy
– Placement of metal stent to bypass the tumor

DIET
■ Liquid to soft, as tolerated
■ High-calorie supplements

ACTIVITY
■ No restrictions

MEDICATION
■ Chemotherapy and radiation therapy
■ Analgesics

SURGERY
■ Radical surgery to excise tumor and resect esophagus or stomach and esophagus
■ Gastrostomy or jejunostomy

OTHER
■ Endoscopic laser treatment and bipolar electrocoagulation
■ Monitoring

Postoperatively
■ Vital signs
■ Hydration and nutritional status

■ Electrolyte levels
■ Intake and output
■ Postoperative complications
■ Swallowing ability
■ Pain control

GASTRIC CANCER

Overview

DESCRIPTION
■ Classified according to gross appearance (polypoid, ulcerating, ulcerating and infiltrating, or diffuse)
■ Prognosis depends on stage of disease at time of diagnosis (5-year survival rate about 15%)

PATHOPHYSIOLOGY
■ The most commonly affected areas of the stomach are the pylorus and antrum.
■ The remaining areas affected in order of descending frequency are the lesser curvature of the stomach, the cardia, the body of the stomach, and the greater curvature of the stomach.
■ Rapid metastasis occurs to the regional lymph nodes, omentum, liver, and lungs.

CAUSES
■ Unknown

RISK FACTORS
■ Gastritis with gastric atrophy
■ People with type A blood (10% increased risk)
■ Family history of gastric cancer
■ Smoked foods, pickled vegetables, and salted fish and meat
■ High alcohol consumption
■ Smoking

COMPLICATIONS
■ Malnutrition
■ GI obstruction

- Iron deficiency anemia
- Metastasis

Assessment

HISTORY
- Back, epigastric, or retrosternal pain not relieved with nonprescription medications
- Vague feeling of fullness, heaviness, and moderate abdominal distention after meals
- Weight loss, nausea, vomiting
- Weakness and fatigue
- Dysphagia

PHYSICAL FINDINGS
- Palpable mass
- Palpable lymph nodes, especially the supraclavicular and axillary nodes
- Other assessment findings that depend on extent of disease and location of metastasis

TEST RESULTS
Laboratory
- Complete blood count possibly showing iron deficiency anemia
- Liver function studies possibly elevated with metastatic spread of tumor to liver
- Carcinoembryonic antigen radioimmunoassay possibly elevated

Imaging
- Barium X-rays of the GI tract with fluoroscopy shows changes that suggest gastric cancer.

Diagnostic procedures
- Gastroscopy with fiber-optic endoscope is used to help to rule out other diffuse gastric mucosal abnormalities by allowing direct visualization.
- Gastroscopic biopsy permits evaluation of gastric mucosal lesions.

Other
- Gastric acid stimulation test discloses whether the stomach secretes acid properly.

Treatment

GENERAL
- Radiation therapy combined with chemotherapy (not indicated preoperatively because it may damage viscera and impede healing)

DIET
- Based on extent of disorder
- Parenteral feeding with inability to consume adequate calories

ACTIVITY
- No restrictions

MEDICATION
- Chemotherapy
- Antiemetics
- Sedatives and tranquilizers
- Opioid analgesics

SURGERY
- Excision of lesion with appropriate margins (in more than one-third of patients)
- Gastroduodenostomy
- Gastrojejunostomy
- Partial gastric resection
- Total gastrectomy (If metastasis has occurred, the omentum and spleen may have to be removed.)

MONITORING
- Pain control
- Vital signs
- Hydration and nutritional status
- Nasogastric tube function and drainage
- Wound site
- Postoperative complications
- Effects of medications

GASTROESOPHAGEAL REFLUX DISEASE

Overview

DESCRIPTION
- Backflow of gastric or duodenal contents, or both, into the esophagus and past the lower esophageal sphincter (LES), without associated belching or vomiting
- Reflux of gastric acid, causing acute epigastric pain, usually after a meal
- Popularly called heartburn
- Also called GERD

PATHOPHYSIOLOGY
- Reflux occurs when LES pressure is deficient or pressure in the stomach exceeds LES pressure. The LES relaxes and gastric contents regurgitate into the esophagus.
- The degree of mucosal injury is based on the amount and concentration of refluxed gastric acid, proteolytic enzymes, and bile acids.

CAUSES
- Pyloric surgery (alteration or removal of the pylorus), which allows reflux of bile or pancreatic juice
- Hiatal hernia with incompetent sphincter
- Any condition or position that increases intra-abdominal pressure

RISK FACTORS
- Any agent that lowers LES pressure: acidic and fatty food, alcohol, cigarettes, anticholinergics (atropine, belladonna)
- Nasogastric intubation for more than 4 days

COMPLICATIONS
- Reflux esophagitis
- Esophageal stricture
- Esophageal ulcer
- Barrett's esophagus (metaplasia and possible increased risk of neoplasm)
- Anemia from esophageal bleeding
- Reflux aspiration leading to chronic pulmonary disease

Assessment

HISTORY
- Minimal or no symptoms in one-third of patients
- Heartburn that typically occurs 1½ to 2 hours after eating
- Heartburn that worsens with vigorous exercise, bending, lying down, wearing tight clothing, coughing, constipation, and obesity
- Reported relief by using antacids or sitting upright
- Regurgitation without associated nausea or belching
- Feeling of fluid accumulation in the throat without a sour or bitter taste
- Chronic pain radiating to the neck, jaws, and arms that may mimic angina pectoris
- Nocturnal hypersalivation and wheezing

PHYSICAL FINDINGS
- Odynophagia (sharp substernal pain on swallowing), possibly followed by a dull substernal ache
- Bright red or dark brown blood in vomitus
- Laryngitis and morning hoarseness
- Chronic cough

TEST RESULTS
Imaging
- Barium swallow with fluoroscopy shows evidence of recurrent reflux.

Diagnostic procedures
- Esophageal acidity test shows degree of gastroesophageal reflux.

■ Gastroesophageal scintillation testing shows reflux.

■ Esophageal manometry reveals abnormal LES pressure and sphincter incompetence.

■ Acid perfusion (Bernstein) test result confirms esophagitis.

■ Esophagoscopy and biopsy results confirm pathologic changes in the mucosa.

Treatment

GENERAL
■ Modification of lifestyle
■ Positional therapy
■ Removal of cause

DIET
■ Weight reduction
■ Avoidance of dietary causes
■ Avoidance of eating 2 hours before sleep

ACTIVITY
■ No restrictions

MEDICATION
■ Antacids
■ Cholinergics
■ Histamine-2–receptor antagonists
■ Proton pump inhibitors

SURGERY
■ Hiatal hernia repair
■ Vagotomy or pyloroplasty

MONITORING
After surgery
■ Respiratory status
■ Pain
■ Intake and output
■ Vital signs
■ Chest tube drainage

HEPATITIS, VIRAL

Overview

DESCRIPTION
■ Fairly common systemic disease
■ Marked by hepatic cell destruction, necrosis, and autolysis, leading to anorexia, jaundice, and hepatomegaly
■ In most patients, hepatic cells eventually regenerate with little or no residual damage, allowing recovery
■ Complications more likely with old age and serious underlying disorders
■ Prognosis poor if edema and hepatic encephalopathy develop
■ Six types recognized (A, B, C, D, E, and G), and a seventh suspected

PATHOPHYSIOLOGY
■ Hepatic inflammation caused by virus leads to diffuse injury and necrosis of hepatocytes.
■ Hypertrophy and hyperplasia of Kupffer cells and sinusoidal lining cells occurs.
■ Bile obstruction may occur.

CAUSES
■ Infection with the causative viruses for each of six major forms of viral hepatitis

Type A
■ Transmittal by the fecal-oral or parenteral route
■ Ingestion of contaminated food, milk, or water

Type B
■ Transmittal by contact with contaminated human blood, secretions, and stool

Type C
■ Transmittal primarily by sharing of needles by I.V. drug users, through blood transfusions, or tattoo needles

Type D
■ Found only in patients with an acute or a chronic episode of hepatitis B

Type E
■ Transmittal by parenteral route and often water-borne

Type G
■ Thought to be blood-borne, with transmission similar to that of hepatitis B and C

COMPLICATIONS
■ Life-threatening fulminant hepatitis
■ Death
■ Chronic active hepatitis (in hepatitis B)
■ Syndrome resembling serum sickness, characterized by arthralgia or arthritis, rash, and angioedema; can lead to misdiagnosis of hepatitis B as rheumatoid arthritis or lupus erythematosus (in hepatitis B)
■ Primary liver cancer (in hepatitis B or C)
■ In hepatitis D, mild or asymptomatic form of hepatitis B that flares into severe, progressive chronic active hepatitis and cirrhosis

Assessment

HISTORY
■ Revelation of a source of transmission

Prodromal stage
■ Patient easily fatigued, with generalized malaise
■ Anorexia, mild weight loss
■ Depression
■ Headache, photophobia

■ Weakness
■ Arthralgia, myalgia
■ Nausea or vomiting
■ Changes in the senses of taste and smell

Clinical jaundice stage
■ Pruritus
■ Abdominal pain or tenderness
■ Indigestion
■ Anorexia
■ Possible jaundice of sclerae, mucous membranes, and skin

Posticteric stage
■ Most symptoms decreasing or subsided

PHYSICAL FINDINGS
Prodromal stage
■ Fever (100° to 102° F [37.8° to 38.9° C])
■ Dark-colored urine
■ Clay-colored stools

Clinical jaundice stage
■ Rashes, erythematous patches, or hives
■ Abdominal tenderness in the right upper quadrant
■ Enlarged and tender liver
■ Splenomegaly
■ Cervical adenopathy

Posticteric stage
■ Decrease in liver enlargement

TEST RESULTS
Laboratory
■ In suspected viral hepatitis, hepatitis profile routinely performed; result identifying antibodies specific to the causative virus and establishing the type of hepatitis:
– Type A — Detection of an antibody to hepatitis A (anti-HAV) confirming the diagnosis

– Type B – The presence of hepatitis B surface antigens (HBsAg) and hepatitis B antibodies (anti-HBs) confirming the diagnosis

– Type C – Diagnosis depends on serologic testing for the specific antibody one or more months after the onset of acute illness; until then, diagnosis principally established by obtaining negative test results for hepatitis A, B, and D

– Type D – Detection of intrahepatic delta antigens or immunoglobulin (Ig) M antidelta antigens in acute disease (or IgM and IgG in chronic disease) establishing the diagnosis

– Type E – Detection of hepatitis E antigens supporting the diagnosis; however, diagnosis possibly also ruling out hepatitis C

– Type G – Detection of hepatitis G ribonucleic acid supporting the diagnosis; (serologic assays are being developed)

■ Additional findings from liver function studies supporting the diagnosis:

– Serum aspartate aminotransferase and serum alanine aminotransferase levels increased in the prodromal stage of acute viral hepatitis

– Serum alkaline phosphatase levels slightly increased

– Serum bilirubin levels elevated; levels possibly remaining elevated late in the disease, especially with severe disease

– Prothrombin time (PT) prolonged; (PT more than 3 seconds longer than normal indicating severe liver damage)

– White blood cell counts commonly revealing transient neutropenia and lymphopenia followed by lymphocytosis

Diagnostic procedures
■ Liver biopsy shows chronic hepatitis.

Treatment

GENERAL
For HCV
■ Aimed at clearing hepatitis C virus (HCV) from the body, stopping or slowing of hepatic damage, and symptom relief

DIET
■ Largest meal in morning because nausea intensifies as day progresses
■ Small, high-calorie, high-protein meals (reduced protein intake if signs of precoma – lethargy, confusion, mental changes – develop)
■ Parenteral feeding (if appropriate)

ACTIVITY
■ Frequent rest periods as needed
■ Avoidance of contact sports and strenuous activity

MEDICATION
■ Standard immunoglobulin
■ Vaccine
■ Interferon alfa-2b
■ Antiemetics
■ Cholestyramine

SURGERY
■ Possible liver transplant

MONITORING
■ Hydration and nutritional status
■ Daily weight
■ Intake and output
■ Stool for color, consistency, amount, and frequency
■ Signs of complications

IRRITABLE BOWEL SYNDROME

Overview

DESCRIPTION
- Common condition marked by chronic or periodic diarrhea alternating with constipation
- Accompanied by straining and abdominal cramps
- Initial episodes early in life and late teens to twenties
- Prognosis is good
- Also known as spastic colon, spastic colitis, mucous colitis

PATHOPHYSIOLOGY
- The precise etiology is unclear.
- It involves a change in bowel motility, reflecting an abnormality in the neuromuscular control of intestinal smooth muscle.

CAUSES
- Anxiety and stress
- Dietary factors, such as fiber, raw fruits, coffee, alcohol, and foods that are cold, highly seasoned, or laxative in nature

Other possible triggers
- Hormones
- Laxative abuse
- Allergy to certain foods or drugs
- Lactose intolerance

COMPLICATIONS
- Diverticulitis and colon cancer
- Chronic inflammatory bowel disease

Assessment

HISTORY
- Chronic constipation, diarrhea, or both

- Lower abdominal pain (typically in the left lower quadrant) usually relieved by defecation or passage of gas
- Stools are small with visible mucus or small, pasty, and pencil-like stools instead of diarrhea
- Dyspepsia
- Abdominal bloating
- Heartburn
- Faintness and weakness
- Contributing psychological factors, such as a recent stressful life change, that may have triggered or aggravated symptoms
- Anxiety and fatigue

PHYSICAL FINDINGS
- Normal bowel sounds
- Tympany over a gas-filled bowel

TEST RESULTS
- Assessment involves studies to rule out other, more serious disorders.

Laboratory
- Negative stool examination for occult blood, parasites, and pathogenic bacteria
- Normal complete blood count, serologic tests, serum albumin, and erythrocyte sedimentation rate

Imaging
- Barium enema may reveal colonic spasm and a tubular appearance of the descending colon. It's also used to rule out certain other disorders, such as diverticula, tumors, and polyps.

Diagnostic procedures
- Sigmoidoscopy may disclose spastic contractions.

Treatment

GENERAL
- Stress management
- Lifestyle modifications

DIET
■ Based on the patient's symptoms
■ Initially, an elimination diet
■ Avoidance of sorbitol, nonabsorbable carbohydrates, and lactose-containing foods
■ Increased dietary bulk
■ Increased fluid intake

ACTIVITY
■ Regular exercise

MEDICATION
■ Anticholinergic, antispasmodic drugs
■ Antidiarrheals
■ Laxatives
■ Antiemetics
■ Simethicone
■ Mild tranquilizers
■ Tricyclic antidepressants

MONITORING
■ Weight
■ Diet
■ Bowel movements

LIVER CANCER

Overview

DESCRIPTION
■ Malignant cells growing in the tissues of the liver
■ Rapidly fatal, usually within 6 months
■ After cirrhosis, the leading cause of fatal hepatic disease
■ Liver metastasis occurring as solitary lesion (the first sign of recurrence after a remission)

PATHOPHYSIOLOGY
■ Most (90%) of primary liver tumors originate in the parenchymal cells and are hepatomas. Others originate in the intrahepatic bile ducts (cholangiomas).
■ Approximately 30% to 70% of patients with hepatomas also have cirrhosis.
■ Rare tumors include a mixed-cell type, Kupffer cell sarcoma, and hepatoblastoma
■ The liver is one of the most common sites of metastasis from other primary cancers.

CAUSES
■ Immediate cause unknown
■ Environmental exposure to carcinogens
■ Possibly androgens and oral estrogens
■ Hepatitis B and C viruses

RISK FACTORS
■ Cirrhosis
■ Excessive alcohol intake
■ Malnutrition

COMPLICATIONS
■ GI hemorrhage
■ Progressive cachexia
■ Liver failure

Assessment

HISTORY
■ Weight loss
■ Weakness, fatigue, and fever
■ Severe pain in the epigastrium or right upper quadrant

PHYSICAL FINDINGS
■ Jaundice
■ Dependent edema
■ Abdominal bruit, hum, or rubbing sound
■ Tender, nodular, enlarged liver
■ Ascites
■ Palpable mass in the right upper quadrant

TEST RESULTS
Laboratory
- Abnormal liver function studies
- Alpha-fetoprotein levels greater than 500 mcg/ml
- Abnormal electrolyte study results

Imaging
- Liver scan may show filling defects.
- Arteriography may define large tumors.

Diagnostic procedures
- Liver biopsy by needle or open biopsy reveals cancerous cells.

Treatment

GENERAL
- Radiation therapy (alone or with chemotherapy)

DIET
- High-calorie, low-protein

ACTIVITY
- Frequent rest periods
- Postoperative avoidance of heavy lifting and contact sports

MEDICATION
- Chemotherapeutic drugs

SURGERY
- Resection (lobectomy or partial hepatectomy)
- Liver transplantation

MONITORING
- Vital signs
- Hydration and nutritional status
- Weight
- Pain control
- Neurologic status
- Complete blood count; liver function tests
- Postoperative complications
- Wound site

PANCREATIC CANCER

Overview

DESCRIPTION
- Fourth most lethal type of carcinoma
- Carries a poor prognosis (most patients die within 1 year of diagnosis)

PATHOPHYSIOLOGY
- Pancreatic cancer is almost always adenocarcinoma.
- Nearly two-thirds of tumors appear in the head of the pancreas; islet cell tumors are rare.
- Two main tissue types form fibrotic nodes. Cylinder cells arise in ducts and degenerate into cysts; large, fatty, granular cells arise in parenchyma.

CAUSES
- Possible link to inhalation or absorption of carcinogens, which the pancreas then excretes (such as cigarette smoke, excessive fat and protein, food additives, and industrial chemicals)

RISK FACTORS
- Chronic pancreatitis
- Diabetes
- Chronic alcohol abuse
- Smoking
- Occupational exposure to chemicals

COMPLICATIONS
- Nutrient malabsorption
- Type 1 diabetes
- Liver and GI problems
- Mental status changes

Assessment

HISTORY
■ Colicky, dull, or vague intermittent epigastric pain, which may radiate to the right upper quadrant or dorso-lumbar area; unrelated to posture or activity and aggravated by meals
■ Anorexia, nausea, and vomiting
■ Rapid, profound weight loss

PHYSICAL FINDINGS
■ Jaundice
■ Large, palpable, well-defined mass in the subumbilical or left hypochondrial region
■ Abdominal bruit or pulsation

TEST RESULTS
Laboratory
■ Absence of pancreatic enzymes
■ Increased serum bilirubin
■ Possible increase in serum lipase and amylase levels
■ Prolonged thrombin time
■ Elevated levels of aspartate aminotransferase and alanine aminotransferase (if liver cell necrosis present)
■ Markedly elevated alkaline phosphatase level (in biliary obstruction)
■ Measurable serum insulin (if islet cell tumor present)
■ Hypoglycemia or hyperglycemia
■ Elevation in specific tumor markers for pancreatic cancer, including carcinoembryonic antigen, pancreatic oncofetal antigen, alpha-fetoprotein, and serum immunoreactive elastase I

Imaging
■ Barium swallow, retroperitoneal insufflation, cholangiography, and scintigraphy can locate the neoplasm and detect changes in the duodenum or stomach.
■ Ultrasonography and computed tomography scans can identify a mass.
■ Magnetic resonance imaging scan discloses tumor location and size.
■ Angiography reveals tumor vascularity.
■ Endoscopic retrograde cholangiopancreatography allows tumor visualization and specimen biopsy.

Diagnostic procedures
■ Percutaneous fine-needle aspiration biopsy may detect tumor cells.
■ Laparotomy with biopsy allows definitive diagnosis.

Treatment

GENERAL
■ Mainly palliative
■ May involve radiation therapy as adjunct to fluorouracil chemotherapy

DIET
■ Well-balanced, as tolerated
■ Small, frequent meals

ACTIVITY
■ Postoperative avoidance of lifting and contact sports
■ After recovery, no restriction

MEDICATION
■ Chemotherapy
■ Antibiotics
■ Anticholinergics
■ Antacids
■ Diuretics
■ Insulin
■ Analgesics
■ Pancreatic enzymes

SURGERY
■ Total pancreatectomy
■ Cholecystojejunostomy, choledochoduodenostomy, and choledochojejunostomy
■ Gastrojejunostomy
■ Whipple's operation or radical pancreatoduodenectomy

MONITORING
- Fluid balance and nutrition
- Abdominal girth, metabolic state, and daily weight
- Blood glucose levels
- Complete blood count
- Pain control

PERITONITIS

Overview

DESCRIPTION
- Inflammation of the peritoneum; may extend throughout the peritoneum or localize as an abscess
- Commonly decreases intestinal motility and causes intestinal distention with gas
- Lethal in 10% of cases, with bowel obstruction the usual cause of death
- Can be acute or chronic

PATHOPHYSIOLOGY
- Bacteria invade the peritoneum after inflammation and perforation of the GI tract.
- Fluid containing protein and electrolytes accumulates in the peritoneal cavity; normally transparent, the peritoneum becomes opaque, red, inflamed, and edematous.
- Infection may localize as an abscess rather than disseminate as a generalized infection.

CAUSES
- GI tract perforation (from appendicitis, diverticulitis, peptic ulcer, or ulcerative colitis)
- Bacterial or chemical inflammation

COMPLICATIONS
- Abscess
- Septicemia
- Respiratory compromise
- Bowel obstruction
- Shock

Assessment

HISTORY
Early phase
- Vague, generalized abdominal pain
- If localized: pain over a specific area (usually the inflammation site)
- If generalized: diffuse pain over the abdomen

With progression
- Increasingly severe and constant abdominal pain that increases with movement and respirations
- Possible referral of pain to shoulder or thoracic area
- Anorexia, nausea, and vomiting
- Inability to pass stools and flatus
- Hiccups

PHYSICAL FINDINGS
- Fever
- Tachycardia
- Hypotension
- Shallow breathing
- Signs of dehydration
- Positive bowel sounds (early); absent bowel sounds (later)
- Abdominal rigidity
- General abdominal tenderness
- Rebound tenderness
- Typical patient positioning: lying very still with knees flexed

TEST RESULTS
Laboratory
- Complete blood count showing leukocytosis

Imaging
- Abdominal X-rays show edematous and gaseous distention of the small and large bowel. With perforation of a visceral organ, X-rays show air in the abdominal cavity.
- Chest X-rays may reveal elevation of the diaphragm.

Diagnostic procedures
■ Paracentesis shows the nature of the exudate and permits bacterial culture testing.

Treatment

GENERAL
■ I.V. fluids
■ Nasogastric (NG) intubation

DIET
■ Nothing by mouth until bowel function returns
■ Gradual increase in diet
■ Parenteral nutrition if necessary

ACTIVITY
■ Bed rest until condition improves
■ Avoidance of lifting for at least 6 weeks postoperatively

MEDICATION
■ Antibiotics, based on infecting organism
■ Electrolyte replacement
■ Analgesics

SURGERY
■ Treatment of choice; procedure varies with the cause of peritonitis

MONITORING
■ Fluid and nutritional status
■ Pain control
■ Vital signs
■ NG tube function and drainage
■ Bowel function
■ Wound site
■ Signs and symptoms of dehiscence

Watch for signs and symptoms of abscess formation, including persistent abdominal tenderness and fever.

ULCERATIVE COLITIS

Overview

DESCRIPTION
■ Inflammatory, commonly chronic disease that causes ulcerations of the mucosa in the colon
■ Usually begins in the rectum and sigmoid colon and may extend upward into the entire colon
■ Rarely affects the small intestine, except for the terminal ileum
■ Produces congestion, edema (leading to mucosal friability), and ulcerations
■ Range of severity from mild, localized disorder to fulminant disease that causes many complications

PATHOPHYSIOLOGY
■ The disorder primarily involves the mucosa and the submucosa of the bowel.
■ Crypt abscesses and mucosal ulceration may occur.
■ The mucosa typically appears granular and friable.
■ The colon becomes a rigid, foreshortened tube.
■ In severe ulcerative colitis, areas of hyperplastic growth occur, with swollen mucosa surrounded by inflamed mucosa with shallow ulcers.
■ Submucosa and the circular and longitudinal muscles may be involved.

CAUSES
■ Etiology unknown
■ May be related to an abnormal immune response in the GI tract, possibly associated with genetic factors.

RISK FACTORS
■ Stress (may increase severity of an attack)

COMPLICATIONS

- Nutritional deficiencies
- Perineal sepsis
- Anal fissure, anal fistula
- Perirectal abscess
- Hemorrhage, anemia
- Toxic megacolon
- Cancer
- Coagulation defects
- Erythema nodosum on the face and arms
- Pyoderma gangrenosum on the legs and ankles
- Uveitis
- Pericholangitis, sclerosing cholangitis
- Cirrhosis
- Cholangiocarcinoma
- Ankylosing spondylitis
- Strictures
- Pseudopolyps, stenosis, and perforated colon leading to peritonitis and toxemia
- Arthritis

Assessment

HISTORY

- Remission and exacerbation of symptoms
- Mild cramping and lower abdominal pain
- Recurrent bloody diarrhea as often as 10 to 25 times daily
- Nocturnal diarrhea
- Fatigue and weakness
- Anorexia and weight loss
- Nausea and vomiting

PHYSICAL FINDINGS

- Liquid stools with visible pus, mucus, and blood
- Possible abdominal distention
- Abdominal tenderness
- Perianal irritation, hemorrhoids, and fissures

TEST RESULTS
Laboratory

- Stool specimen analysis revealing blood, pus, and mucus, but no pathogenic organisms
- Other supportive laboratory tests showing decreased serum levels of potassium, magnesium, hemoglobin, and albumin as well as leukocytosis and increased prothrombin time; elevated erythrocyte sedimentation rate correlating with the severity of the attack

Imaging

- Barium enema discloses the extent of disease and complications, such as strictures and carcinoma. This study isn't performed in a patient with active signs and symptoms.

Diagnostic procedures

- Sigmoidoscopy confirms rectal involvement in most cases by showing increased mucosal friability, decreased mucosal detail, and thick inflammatory exudates, edema, and erosions.
- Colonoscopy may be used to determine the extent of the disease and to evaluate the areas of stricture and pseudopolyps. This test isn't performed when the patient has active signs and symptoms.
- Biopsy, performed during colonoscopy, helps to confirm the diagnosis.

Treatment

GENERAL

- I.V. fluid replacement
- Blood transfusions (if needed)

DIET

- Nothing by mouth (if severe)
- Parenteral nutrition (with severe disease)
- Supplemental feedings

ACTIVITY
- Rest periods during exacerbations

MEDICATION
- Corticotropin and adrenal cortico-steroids
- Sulfasalazine
- Mesalamine
- Antispasmodics and antidiarrheals
- Fiber supplements

SURGERY
- Treatment of last resort
- Proctocolectomy with ileostomy
- Pouch ileostomy
- Ileoanal reservoir with loop ileostomy
- Colectomy (after 10 years of active disease)

MONITORING
- Response to treatment
- Fluid and electrolyte status
- Hemoglobin and hematocrit levels
- Complications

After surgery
- Vital signs
- Wound site
- Pain level
- Bowel function
- Nasogastric tube function and drainage
- Skin integrity

TREATMENTS

APPENDECTOMY

Overview

- Surgical removal of an inflamed vermiform appendix
- Prevents imminent rupture or perforation of the appendix
- May involve laparoscopy for diagnosis and appendix removal

INDICATIONS
- Acute appendicitis

COMPLICATIONS
- Infection
- Paralytic ileus

With perforation
- Local or general peritonitis
- Paralytic ileus
- Intestinal obstruction
- Abscess

Nursing interventions

PRETREATMENT CARE
- Explain the treatment and preparation to the patient and his family.
- Make sure the patient has signed an appropriate consent form.
- Administer prophylactic antibiotics as ordered.
- Administer I.V. fluids as ordered.
- Insert a nasogastric (NG) tube as ordered.
- Place the patient in Fowler's position.
- Avoid giving analgesics, cathartics, or enemas or applying heat to the abdomen.
- Provide reassurance.

POSTTREATMENT CARE
- Place the patient in Fowler's position after anesthesia wears off.
- Ensure the patency of drainage catheters and tubes.
- Encourage the patient to ambulate as soon as possible.

■ Encourage coughing, deep breathing, and frequent position changes.

■ Gradually resume oral intake after NG tube removal.

■ Assist with emergency treatment of peritonitis if needed.

Monitoring
■ Vital signs
■ Intake and output
■ Bowel sounds
■ Surgical wounds and dressings
■ Signs and symptoms of peritonitis
■ Drainage
■ Complications

PATIENT TEACHING
Be sure to cover:
■ medications and possible adverse reactions
■ signs and symptoms of infection
■ signs and symptoms of intestinal obstruction
■ complications
■ when to notify the physician
■ wound care
■ activity restrictions
■ follow-up care.

BOWEL RESECTION WITH OSTOMY

Overview

■ Excision of diseased bowel and creation of a stoma on the outer abdominal wall to allow feces elimination

■ Laparoscopic approach possible for both standard colostomy and end-ileostomy

INDICATIONS
■ Inflammatory bowel disease
■ Familial adenomatous polyposis
■ Diverticulitis
■ Advanced colorectal cancer

COMPLICATIONS
■ Hemorrhage
■ Sepsis
■ Ileus
■ Fluid and electrolyte imbalance
■ Skin excoriation
■ Pelvic abscess
■ With a Kock ileostomy: incompetent nipple valve
■ Psychological problems

Nursing interventions

PRETREATMENT CARE
■ Explain preoperative and postoperative procedures and equipment to the patient and his family.
■ Discuss postoperative analgesia.
■ Make sure the patient has signed an appropriate consent form.
■ Tell the patient what to expect for fecal drainage and bowel movement control.
■ Provide total parenteral nutrition as ordered.
■ Administer antibiotics and other medications as ordered.

Monitoring
■ Vital signs
■ Nutritional status
■ Fluid and electrolyte status
■ Intake and output
■ Daily weight

POSTTREATMENT CARE
■ Provide meticulous wound care.
■ Administer analgesics as ordered.
■ After an abdominoperineal resection, irrigate the perineal area as ordered.
■ If the patient has a Kock pouch with a catheter inserted in the stoma:
– connect the catheter to low intermittent suction or to straight drainage as ordered

– check catheter patency regularly, and irrigate with 20 to 30 ml of normal saline solution as ordered
– assess pouch drainage, and advance the patient's diet as ordered
– clamp and unclamp the pouch catheter to increase its capacity as ordered.
■ Encourage the patient to express feelings and concerns.
■ Arrange for a consultation with an enterostomal therapist if possible.
■ Arrange for the patient to meet with a well-adjusted ostomy patient if possible.

Monitoring
■ Vital signs
■ Intake and output
■ Dehydration
■ Electrolyte imbalance
■ Stoma drainage
■ Infection
■ Peritonitis or sepsis
■ Skin irritation and excoriation
■ Stoma appearance

Immediately report excessive blood or mucus draining from the stoma, which could indicate hemorrhage or infection.

PATIENT TEACHING
Be sure to cover:
■ medications and possible adverse reactions
■ ostomy type and function
■ ostomy appliances
■ resumption of sexual intercourse
■ stoma and skin care
■ dietary restrictions
■ importance of a high fluid intake
■ avoidance of alcohol, laxatives, and diuretics (unless approved by the physician)
■ bowel retraining
■ sitz baths (after abdominoperineal resection)

■ signs and symptoms of inflammation and infection
■ complications
■ when to notify the physician
■ follow-up care.

CHOLECYSTECTOMY

Overview

■ Surgical removal of the gallbladder
■ May be performed as an open abdominal surgical procedure or as a laparoscopic procedure

INDICATIONS
■ Gallbladder or biliary duct disease refractory to drug therapy, dietary changes, and other supportive treatments

COMPLICATIONS
■ Peritonitis
■ Postcholecystectomy syndrome
■ Atelectasis
■ Bile duct injury
■ Small bowel injury
■ Wound infection
■ Ileus
■ Urinary retention
■ Retained gallstones

Nursing interventions

PRETREATMENT CARE
■ Explain the treatment and preparation to the patient and his family.
■ Make sure the patient has signed an appropriate consent form.
■ Withhold oral intake as ordered.
■ Administer preoperative medications as ordered.

Abdominal approach
■ Tell the patient that:
– a nasogastric (NG) tube will be in place for 1 to 2 days and an abdominal

drain will be in place for 3 to 5 days after surgery

– a T tube may remain in place for up to 2 weeks

– the patient may be discharged with the T tube in place.

Laparoscopic approach
■ Tell the patient that:

– an indwelling urinary catheter will be inserted into the bladder

– an NG tube will be placed in the stomach

– tubes are usually removed in the postanesthesia room

– three small incisions will be covered with a small sterile dressing

– discharge may occur on the day of surgery or 1 day after.

POSTTREATMENT CARE
■ Administer medications as ordered.
■ Place the patient in low Fowler's position.
■ Attach the NG tube to low intermittent suction as ordered.
■ Report drainage greater than 500 ml after 48 hours.
■ Provide meticulous skin care, especially around drainage tube insertion sites.
■ After NG tube removal, introduce foods as ordered.
■ Clamp the T tube before and after each meal as ordered.
■ After laparoscopic cholecystectomy, start clear liquids as ordered when the patient has fully recovered from anesthesia.
■ Assist with early ambulation.
■ Encourage coughing and deep-breathing exercises.
■ Encourage incentive spirometry use.
■ Provide analgesics as ordered.

Monitoring
■ Vital signs
■ Intake and output

■ Complications
■ Postcholecystectomy syndrome
■ Respiratory status
■ Amount and characteristics of drainage
■ Surgical dressings
■ Position and patency of drainage tubes

PATIENT TEACHING
Be sure to cover:
■ medications and possible adverse reactions
■ coughing and deep-breathing exercises
■ T tube home care if applicable
■ signs and symptoms of biliary obstruction
■ signs and symptoms of infection
■ complications
■ when to notify the physician
■ follow-up care.

GASTRIC SURGERY

Overview

■ Surgery involving the stomach; the specific procedure depends on the location and extent of the disorder
■ Partial gastrectomy: excision of part of the stomach
■ Bilateral vagotomy: transection of the right and left vagus nerves, typically done to relieve ulcer symptoms and eliminate vagal nerve stimulation of gastric secretions
■ Pyloroplasty: incision of the pylorus and reconstruction of the pyloric channel, typically done to relieve pyloric obstruction or speed gastric emptying after vagotomy

INDICATIONS
■ Chronic ulcer disease
■ Cancer
■ Obstruction

- GI hemorrhage
- Perforated ulcer

COMPLICATIONS

- Hemorrhage
- Obstruction
- Dumping syndrome
- Paralytic ileus
- Perforation
- Vitamin B_{12} deficiency, anemia
- Atelectasis

Nursing interventions

PRETREATMENT CARE

- Preoperative preparation depends on the type of surgery. With emergency surgery, preparation may be limited.
- Explain the treatment and preparation to the patient and his family.
- Make sure the patient has signed an appropriate consent form.
- Stabilize the patient's fluid and electrolyte status as ordered.
- Obtain serum samples for hematologic studies.
- Begin I.V. fluid replacement and total parenteral nutrition (TPN) as ordered.
- Prepare the patient for abdominal X-rays as ordered.
- Explain postoperative care and equipment.

Monitoring

- Vital signs
- Intake and output
- Nutritional status
- Laboratory test results

POSTTREATMENT CARE

- Administer medications as ordered.
- Place the patient in low or semi-Fowler's position.

⚡ *Watch for hypotension, brady-cardia, and respiratory changes. These findings may signal hemorrhage and shock.*

- Administer tube feedings or TPN as ordered.
- Administer I.V. fluid and electrolyte replacement therapy as ordered.
- Encourage coughing, deep breathing, use of incentive spirometry, and position changes.

Monitoring

- Vital signs
- Intake and output
- Complications
- Nutritional status
- Laboratory test results
- Surgical wound site and dressings
- Abnormal bleeding
- Drainage
- Dehydration
- Bowel sounds
- Respiratory status

⚡ *Monitor for and report weak-ness, nausea, flatulence, and palpitations occurring within 30 minutes after a meal. These findings suggest that the patient has dumping syndrome.*

PATIENT TEACHING

Be sure to cover:
- medications and possible adverse reactions
- abnormal bleeding
- signs and symptoms of infection
- signs and symptoms of obstruction or perforation
- complications
- when to notify the physician
- coughing and deep-breathing exercises
- splinting of the incision
- surgical wound care
- dumping syndrome and its prevention
- dietary restrictions
- tube feedings if appropriate

- follow-up care
- stress-management techniques
- smoking cessation.

LAPAROSCOPY AND LAPAROTOMY

Overview

- Allow examination of the pelvic cavity and repair or removal of diseased or injured structures
- Laparoscopy (also called pelvic peritoneoscopy): insertion of a laparoscope (endoscope) through the abdominal wall near the umbilicus
- Laparotomy: a general term for any surgical incision made into the abdominal wall; called an exploratory laparotomy when the extent of abdominal injury or disease is unknown

INDICATIONS
Laparoscopy

- Certain abdominal surgical procedures such as cholecystectomy
- Tubal ligation
- Ovarian cyst aspiration
- Ovarian biopsy
- Graafian follicle aspiration
- Cauterization of endometrial implants
- Lysis of adhesions
- Oophorectomy
- Salpingectomy
- Detection of abnormalities, such as cysts, adhesions, fibroids, and infection
- Identification of the cause of pelvic pain
- Diagnosis of endometriosis, ectopic pregnancy, or pelvic inflammatory disease
- Evaluation of pelvic masses
- Examination of the fallopian tubes in an infertile patient

Laparotomy

- Extensive surgical repair
- Pelvic conditions untreatable by laparoscopy
- Resection of ovarian cysts containing endometrial tissue

COMPLICATIONS

- Infection
- Hemorrhage
- Other complications associated with the specific procedure performed

Nursing interventions

PRETREATMENT CARE

- Explain the treatment and preparation to the patient and her family.
- Make sure the patient has signed an appropriate consent form.
- Explain postoperative care.
- Restrict food and fluids as ordered.
- Obtain laboratory results and report abnormal findings to the physician.

POSTTREATMENT CARE

- Administer medications as ordered.
- Assess for abdominal pain and, if the patient had a laparoscopy, for abdominal cramps or shoulder pain.
- Provide comfort measures.
- Explain that bloating or abdominal fullness from laparoscopy will subside as gas is absorbed.

Monitoring

- Vital signs
- Intake and output
- Complications
- Abnormal bleeding
- Surgical wound and dressings
- Drainage
- Infection

PATIENT TEACHING

Be sure to cover:

GASTROINTESTINAL CARE

- medications and possible adverse reactions
- coughing and deep-breathing exercises
- use of incentive spirometry
- incision care
- signs and symptoms of infection
- complications
- when to notify the physician
- prescribed activity restrictions
- follow-up care.

PANCREATECTOMY

Overview

- Surgical removal of part or all of the pancreas
- May involve various types of resections, drainage procedures, and anastomoses to treat pancreatic diseases when more conservative techniques have failed
- Common resections include pancreatoduodenectomy or Whipple procedure that involve the removal of the head of the pancreas, the entire duodenum, a portion of the jejunum, the distal third of the stomach, and the lower half of the common bile duct, with the reestablishment of continuity of the biliary, pancreatic, and GI tract systems

INDICATIONS
- Pancreatic cancer
- Chronic pancreatitis
- Islet cell tumor or insulinoma

COMPLICATIONS
- Hemorrhage
- Fistula formation
- Abscess
- Common bile duct obstruction
- Pseudocyst
- Insulin dependence
- Paralytic ileus

Nursing interventions

PRETREATMENT CARE
- Explain the treatment and preparation to the patient and his family.
- Make sure the patient has signed an appropriate consent form.
- Explain postoperative care.
- Provide emotional support.
- Administer analgesics as ordered.
- Arrange for required diagnostic studies as ordered.
- Provide enteral or parenteral nutrition before surgery if ordered.
- Provide low-fat, high-calorie feedings as ordered.
- Administer oral hypoglycemic agents or insulin as ordered.
- Administer mechanical and antibiotic bowel preparation as well as prophylactic systemic antibiotics as ordered.
- Assist with nasogastric tube and indwelling urinary catheter insertion.

Monitoring
- Vital signs
- Intake and output
- Blood and urine glucose levels
- Withdrawal symptoms in patients with recent history of alcohol abuse
- Pulmonary status
- Liver dysfunction
- Liver function test results
- Coagulation study results

POSTTREATMENT CARE
- Administer medications as ordered.
- Administer plasma expanders and I.V. fluids as ordered.
- Administer oxygen as ordered.
- Encourage deep breathing, coughing, and incentive spirometry use.
- Maintain the patency of drainage tubes.
- Change dressings, and provide incision care as ordered.

■ Use a wound pouching system to contain drainage as needed.

 Monitor for and report absent bowel sounds, severe abdominal pain, vomiting, or fever. These findings may indicate a fistula or paralytic ileus.

Monitoring
■ Vital signs
■ Hemodynamic values
■ Intake and output
■ Nutritional status
■ Pulmonary status
■ Complications
■ Infection
■ Surgical wound and dressing
■ Abnormal bleeding
■ Drainage
■ Metabolic alkalosis or acidosis
■ Serum glucose and calcium levels
■ Bowel sounds

PATIENT TEACHING
Be sure to cover:
■ medications and possible adverse reactions
■ incision care
■ signs and symptoms of infection
■ complications
■ when to notify the physician
■ home blood glucose monitoring
■ how to recognize and manage hypoglycemia and hyperglycemia
■ prescribed dietary and activity restrictions
■ pancreatic enzyme replacement if necessary
■ follow-up care.

SPLENECTOMY

Overview
■ Surgical removal of the spleen

INDICATIONS
■ Hematologic disorders

■ Traumatic splenic rupture
■ Hypersplenism
■ Hereditary spherocytosis
■ Chronic idiopathic thrombocytopenic purpura
■ Hodgkin's disease

COMPLICATIONS
■ Bleeding
■ Infection
■ Pneumonia
■ Atelectasis

Nursing interventions

PRETREATMENT CARE
■ Explain the treatment and preparation to the patient and his family.
■ Make sure the patient has signed an appropriate consent form.
■ Report abnormal results of blood studies.
■ Administer blood products, vitamin K, or fresh frozen plasma as ordered.
■ Obtain vital signs, and perform a baseline respiratory assessment.
■ Notify the physician if you suspect respiratory infection; surgery may be delayed.
■ Explain postoperative care.

POSTTREATMENT CARE
■ Administer medications and I.V. fluids as ordered.
■ Assist with early ambulation.
■ Encourage coughing, deep breathing, and incentive spirometry use.
■ Administer analgesics as needed and ordered.
■ Provide comfort measures.
■ Provide incision care as ordered.
■ Change dressings as ordered.
■ Maintain patency of drains.

Monitoring
■ Vital signs
■ Intake and output
■ Complications

■ Surgical wound and dressings
■ Drainage
■ Abnormal bleeding
■ Hematologic studies
■ Infection

PATIENT TEACHING

Be sure to cover:
■ medications and potential adverse reactions

■ coughing and deep-breathing techniques
■ signs and symptoms of infection
■ complications
■ when to notify the physician
■ ways to prevent infection
■ incision care
■ follow-up care.

PROCEDURES AND EQUIPMENT

MEASURING NG TUBE LENGTH

To determine how long the nasogastric (NG) tube must be to reach the stomach, hold the end of the tube at the tip of the patient's nose. Extend the tube to the patient's earlobe and then down to the xiphoid process.

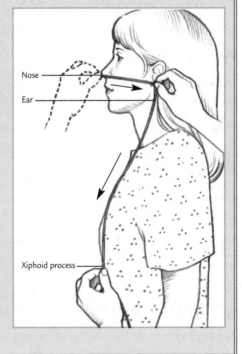

Nose

Ear

Xiphoid process

COMMON TYPES OF
NASOENTERIC-DECOMPRESSION TUBES

The type of nasoenteric-decompression tube chosen depends on the size of the patient and his nostrils, the estimated duration of intubation, and the reason for the procedure. Whichever tube is used, provide good mouth care, and check the patient's nares frequently for signs of irritation. If any are noted, retape the tube so that it doesn't cause tension and then lubricate the nostril. Alternatively, the tube may be inserted through the other nostril.

Most tubes are impregnated with a radiopaque mark so that placement can easily be confirmed by X-ray or other imaging technique. The most commonly used nasoenteric tubes are described here.

Cantor tube

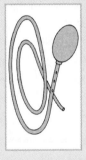

The Cantor tube is a 10′ (3 m)-long single-lumen tube with a balloon that can hold mercury at its distal tip. The tube may be used to relieve bowel obstructions and to aspirate intestinal contents.

Miller-Abbott tube

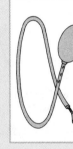

The Miller-Abbott tube is a 10′-long tube with two lumens: one for inflating the distal balloon with air and one for instilling mercury or water. Also used for bowel obstruction, the tube allows aspiration of intestinal contents.

Harris tube

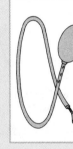

Measuring only 6′ (1.8 m) long, the Harris tube is a single-lumen tube that also ends with a balloon that holds mercury. Used primarily for treating a bowel obstruction, the tube allows lavage of the intestinal tract, usually with a Y-tube attached.

Dennis tube

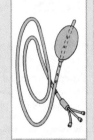

The Dennis tube is a 10′-long, three-lumen sump tube used to decompress the intestinal tract before or after GI surgery. Each lumen is marked to denote its use: irrigation, drainage, or balloon inflation.

TYPES OF NG TUBES

The physician will choose the type and diameter of nasogastric (NG) tube that best suits the patient's needs, including lavage, aspiration, enteral therapy, or stomach decompression. Choices may include the Levin and Salem sump tubes.

Levin tube

The Levin tube is a rubber or plastic tube with a single lumen, a length of 42″ to 50″ (106.5 to 127 cm), and holes at the tip and along the side.

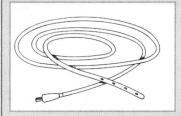

Salem sump tube

The Salem sump tube is a double-lumen tube made of clear plastic and has a blue sump port (pigtail) that allows atmospheric air to enter the patient's stomach. Thus, the tube floats freely and doesn't adhere to or damage gastric mucosa. The larger port of this 48″ (121.9-cm) tube serves as the main suction conduit. The tube has openings at 45, 55, 65, and 75 cm as well as a radiopaque line to verify placement.

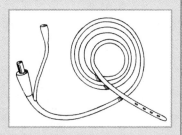

CLEARING A NASOENTERIC-DECOMPRESSION TUBE OBSTRUCTION

If your patient's nasoenteric-decompression tube appears to be obstructed, notify the physician right away. He may order measures such as those below to restore patency.

■ First, disconnect the tube from suction and irrigate with normal saline solution. Use gravity flow to help clear the obstruction unless ordered otherwise.
■ If irrigation doesn't reestablish patency, tug slightly on the tube to free it from the gastric mucosa because it may be against the intestinal wall.
■ If gentle tugging doesn't restore patency, the tube may be kinked. Before manipulating the tube to try to clear the obstruction, take the following precautions:

– Never reposition or irrigate a nasoenteric-decompression tube (without a physician's order) in a patient who has had GI surgery.
– Avoid manipulating a tube in a patient who had the tube inserted during surgery as this may disturb new sutures.
– Don't try to reposition a tube in a patient who was difficult to intubate (because of an esophageal stricture, for example).

TYPES OF ESOPHAGEAL TUBES

When working with patients who have an esophageal tube, remember the advantages of each type.

Sengstaken-Blakemore tube

This triple-lumen, double-balloon tube has a gastric aspiration port, which allows you to obtain drainage from below the gastric balloon and to instill medication.

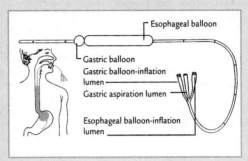

- Esophageal balloon
- Gastric balloon
- Gastric balloon-inflation lumen
- Gastric aspiration lumen
- Esophageal balloon-inflation lumen

Linton tube

This triple-lumen, single-balloon tube has a port for gastric aspiration and one for esophageal aspiration as well. Additionally, the Linton tube reduces the risk of esophageal necrosis because it doesn't have an esophageal balloon.

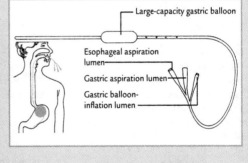

- Large-capacity gastric balloon
- Esophageal aspiration lumen
- Gastric aspiration lumen
- Gastric balloon-inflation lumen

Minnesota esophagogastric tamponade tube

This esophageal tube has four lumens and two balloons. The device provides pressure-monitoring ports for both balloons without the need for Y-connectors. One port is used for gastric suction and the other for esophageal suction.

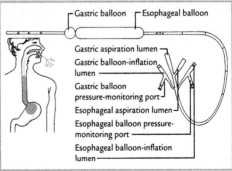

- Gastric balloon
- Esophageal balloon
- Gastric aspiration lumen
- Gastric balloon-inflation lumen
- Gastric balloon pressure-monitoring port
- Esophageal aspiration lumen
- Esophageal balloon pressure-monitoring port
- Esophageal balloon-inflation lumen

GASTROINTESTINAL CARE

HOW TO REINSERT A GASTROSTOMY FEEDING BUTTON

If your patient's gastrostomy feeding button pops out (with coughing, for example), it needs to be reinserted. Here are some steps to follow.

Prepare the equipment

Collect the feeding button, an obturator, and water-soluble lubricant. If the button is to be reinserted, wash it with soap and water and rinse it thoroughly.

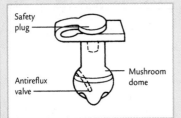

Safety plug

Antireflux valve

Mushroom dome

Insert the button

■ Check the depth of the patient's stoma to make sure you have a feeding button of the correct size.
■ Clean around the stoma.
■ Lubricate the obturator with a water-soluble lubricant, and distend the button several times to ensure patency of the antireflux valve within the button.
■ Lubricate the mushroom dome and the stoma.
■ Gently push the button through the stoma into the stomach.

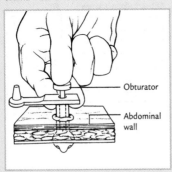

Obturator

Abdominal wall

■ Remove the obturator by gently rotating it as you withdraw it, to keep the antireflux valve from adhering to it.
■ If the valve sticks nonetheless, gently push the obturator back into the button until the valve closes.
■ After removing the obturator, make sure the valve is closed.
■ Next, close the flexible safety plug, which should be relatively flush with the skin surface.

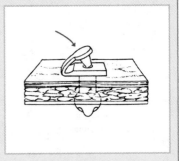

■ If you need to administer a feeding right away, open the safety plug and attach the feeding adapter and feeding tube.
■ Deliver the feeding as ordered.

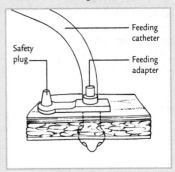

Safety plug

Feeding catheter

Feeding adapter

CARING FOR A PEG OR PEJ SITE

The exit site of a percutaneous endoscopic gastrostomy (PEG) or percutaneous endoscopic jejunostomy (PEJ) tube requires routine observation and care. Follow these care guidelines:

■ Change the dressing daily while the tube is in place
■ After removing the dressing, carefully slide the tube's outer bumper away from the skin (as shown at right, top) about ½″ (1.5 cm).
■ Examine the skin around the tube. Look for redness and other signs of infection or erosion.
■ Gently depress the skin surrounding the tube and inspect for drainage (as shown at right, bottom). Expect minimal wound drainage initially after implantation. This should subside in about 1 week.
■ Inspect the tube for wear and tear. (A tube that wears out will need replacement.)
■ Clean the site with the prescribed cleaning solution.
■ Apply povidone-iodine ointment over the exit site, according to your facility's guidelines.
■ Rotate the outer bumper 90 degrees (to avoid repeating the same tension on the same skin area), and slide the outer bumper back over the exit site.
■ If leakage appears at the PEG site, or if the patient risks dislodging the tube, apply a sterile gauze dressing over the site. Don't put sterile gauze underneath the outer bumper. Loosening the anchor this way allows the feeding tube free play, which could lead to wound abscess.
■ Write the date and time of the dressing change on the tape.

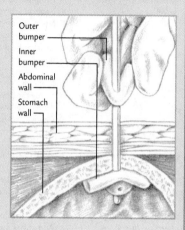

Outer bumper
Inner bumper
Abdominal wall
Stomach wall

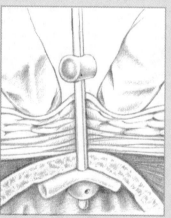

MANAGING TUBE FEEDING PROBLEMS

Complication	Intervention
Aspiration of gastric secretions	■ Discontinue feeding immediately. ■ Perform tracheal suction of aspirated contents, if possible. ■ Notify the physician. Prophylactic antibiotics and chest physiotherapy may be ordered. ■ Check tube placement before feeding to prevent complication.
Hyperglycemia	■ Monitor blood glucose levels. ■ Notify the physician of elevated levels. ■ Administer insulin, if ordered. ■ Change the formula to one with a lower sugar content, as ordered.
Tube obstruction	■ Flush the tube with warm water. If necessary, replace the tube. ■ Flush the tube with 50 ml of water after each feeding to remove excess sticky formula, which could occlude the tube.
Vomiting, bloating, diarrhea, or cramps	■ Reduce the flow rate. ■ Administer metoclopramide to increase GI motility. ■ Warm the formula to prevent GI distress. ■ For 30 minutes after feeding, position the patient on his right side with his head elevated to facilitate gastric emptying. ■ Notify the physician. He may want to reduce the amount of formula being given during each feeding.

APPLYING A SKIN BARRIER AND POUCH

Fitting a skin barrier and ostomy pouch properly can be done in a few steps. A commonly used, two-piece pouching system with flanges is depicted below.

Measure the stoma using a measuring guide.

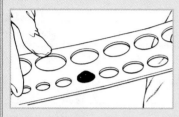

Trace the appropriate circle carefully on the back of the skin barrier.

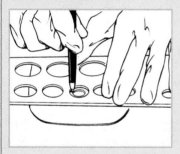

Cut the circular opening in the skin barrier. Bevel the edges to keep them from irritating the patient.

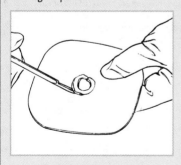

Remove the backing from the skin barrier and moisten it or apply barrier paste, as needed, along the edge of the circular opening.

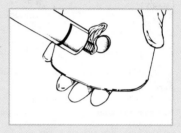

Center the skin barrier over the stoma, adhesive side down, and gently press it to the skin.

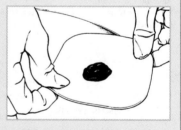

Gently press the pouch opening onto the ring until it snaps into place.

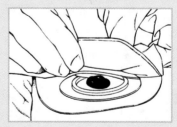

DRUGS

COMMONLY USED DRUGS FOR GI DISORDERS

Drugs	Indication
AMMONIA DETOXICANT	
Lactulose (Chronulac)	■ To prevent and treat portal-systemic encephalopathy in patients with severe hepatic disease (laxative effects increase clearance of nitrogenous products and decrease serum ammonia levels) ■ Also used as laxative to treat constipation
ANTACIDS	
Aluminum hydroxide (Alternagel)	■ To prevent and treat heartburn and acid indigestion; also, adjunct therapy for peptic ulcer disease
Aluminum hydroxide and magnesium hydroxide (Maalox)	■ To prevent and treat heartburn and acid indigestion; also, adjunct therapy for peptic ulcer disease
Calcium carbonate (Tums)	■ To prevent and treat heartburn and acid indigestion; also, adjunct therapy for peptic ulcer disease ■ Calcium supplement
ANTIDIURETIC HORMONE	
Vasopressin (Pitressin)	■ Vasopressin injection administered I.V. or intra-arterially into the superior mesenteric artery to treat acute, massive, GI hemorrhage (such as in peptic ulcer disease, ruptured esophageal varices, Mallory-Weiss Syndrome)

Adverse reactions	Special considerations
■ Abdominal cramps, diarrhea, flatulence	■ After giving through nasogastric (NG) tube, flush tube with water. ■ For administration by retention enema, patient should retain drug for 30 to 60 minutes. ■ Neomycin and other antibiotics may decrease effectiveness.
■ Constipation, intestinal obstruction, encephalopathy	■ Use cautiously in patients with renal disease. ■ May interfere with imaging techniques using technitium-99m (99m-TC) sodium pertechnetate ■ When giving through NG tube, flush with water after instilling.
■ Diarrhea, hypermagnesemia in patients with severe renal impairment	■ Not recommended for patients with renal disease ■ May interfere with imaging testing with 99m-TC sodium pertechnetate ■ Flush NG tube after instilling.
■ Nausea, vomiting, may cause hypercalcemia with excessive use	■ Use cautiously in patients with renal disease, cardiac disease, or sarcoidosis. ■ Monitor for hypercalcemia.
■ Angina, cardiac arrhythmias (bradycardia, heart block), cardiac arrest, water intoxication, seizures, bronchospasms, coronary thrombosis, mesenteric and small bowel infarction may occur with mesenteric artery intra-arterial infusion	■ Intra-arterial infusion requires angiographic catheter placement. ■ Monitor intake and output closely. ■ Watch for water intoxication (drowsiness, headache, confusion, anuria). ■ Monitor heart rhythm. ■ Use with caution in patients with coronary artery disease, heart failure, renal disease, asthma, and seizure disorders. ■ Use is contraindicated in patients with chronic nephritis. ■ Use with caution in elderly, preoperative, and postoperative patients.

GASTROINTESTINAL CARE

(continued)

COMMONLY USED DRUGS FOR GI DISORDERS *(continued)*

Drugs	Indication
ANTIEMETICS	
Dolasetron mesylate (Anzemet); **ondansetron hydrochloride** (Zofran)	■ To prevent and treat postoperative and cancer chemotherapy nausea and vomiting
Metoclopramide hydrochloride (Reglan)	■ To prevent and treat postoperative and cancer chemotherapy nausea and vomiting ■ To treat delayed gastric emptying secondary to diabetic gastroparesis
HISTAMINE-2 RECEPTOR ANTAGONISTS	
Famotidine (Pepcid)	■ To treat duodenal and gastric ulcers, gastroesophageal reflux disease (GERD), Zollinger-Ellison Syndrome
Ranitidine (Zantac)	■ To treat duodenal and gastric ulcers, GERD, Zollinger-Ellison Syndrome
PROTON PUMP INHIBITORSS	
Lansoprazole (Prevacid); **omeprazole** (Prilosec); **pantoprazole** (Protonix)	■ To treat duodenal and gastric ulcers, erosive esophagitis, GERD, Zollinger-Ellison Syndrome; to eradicate *Helicobacter pylori*

Adverse reactions	Special considerations
■ Diarrhea, arrhythmias, electrocardiogram changes (prolong PR, QT and widen QRS), liver test abnormalities, pruritus	■ Monitor heart rhythm. ■ Use with caution in patients with prolonged QT interval or with congenital QT syndrome. ■ Interaction with cytochrome P-450 drugs. ■ Monitor liver function.
■ Restlessness, anxiety, depression, suicidal ideation, seizures, bradycardia, bronchospasm, transient hypertension	■ Use with caution in patients with GI hemorrhage, mechanical obstruction and patients with pheochromocytoma seizures, depression, or hypertension.
■ Headache, palpitations, diarrhea, constipation	■ May cause irritation at I.V. site. ■ When giving through NG tube, flush tube after instilling. ■ Antacids may be administered concurrently.
■ Malaise, reversible confusion, depression or hallucinations, blurred vision, jaundice, leukopenia, angioedema	■ Antacids decrease ranitidine absorption; give 1 hour apart. ■ Use with caution in patients with renal or hepatic disease. ■ Monitor renal and liver function studies.
■ Diarrhea, abdominal pain, nausea, constipation, chest pain, dizziness, hyperglycemia	■ Use with caution in patients with severe liver disease. ■ Monitor liver function studies and blood glucose.

GASTROINTESTINAL CARE

9

GENITOURINARY CARE

ASSESSMENT

GENITOURINARY SYSTEM: NORMAL FINDINGS

Inspection
- No lesions, discoloration, or swelling is apparent on the skin over the kidney and bladder areas.
- No urethral discharge or ulcerations are apparent.
- Pubic area is free from lesions and parasites.

  Female:
- Labia majora are moist and free from lesions.
- Vaginal discharge is normal. (Discharge varies from clear and stretchy to white and opaque, depending on the menstrual cycle; odorless; and nonirritating to the mucosa).
- Cervix looks smooth and round.

  Male:
- Penis appears slightly wrinkled, with the color ranging from pink to dark brown, depending on the patient's skin color.
- Smegma is present.
- Urethral meatus is pink and smooth and located in the center of the glans.
- Scrotum is free from swelling and edema but has some sebaceous cysts.

Percussion
- No costovertebral angle tenderness is apparent.
- Tympany is heard over the empty bladder.

Palpation
- Kidneys are unpalpable, except in very thin and elderly patients.
- Bladder is unpalpable.

  Female:
- Labia feel soft, without swelling, hardness, or tenderness.
- Bartholin's glands are unpalpable.
- Vaginal wall has no nodularity, tenderness, or bulging.
- Cervix is smooth and firm, protrudes ¼" to 1¼" (0.5 to 3 cm) into the vagina, and is freely moveable in all directions.

  Male:
- Penis feels somewhat firm, with the skin smooth and movable.
- Testicles are equally sized, move freely in the scrotal sac, and feel firm, smooth, and rubbery.
- Epididymis is smooth, discrete, nontender, and free from swelling and induration.
- No inguinal or femoral hernias are apparent.
- Prostate gland is smooth and rubbery, is about the size of a walnut, and doesn't protrude into the rectal lumen.

Auscultation
- No bruits can be heard over the renal arteries.

PERCUSSING THE URINARY ORGANS

Percuss the kidneys and bladder using these techniques.

Kidney percussion

With the patient sitting upright, percuss each costovertebral angle (the angle over each kidney whose borders are formed by the lateral and downward curve of the lowest rib and the vertebral column). To perform indirect fist percussion, place your left palm over the costovertebral angle and gently strike it with your right fist. Normally, the patient will feel a thudding sensation or pressure during percussion.

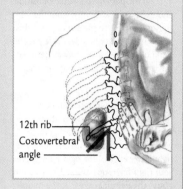

12th rib

Costovertebral angle

Bladder percussion

Using mediate percussion, percuss the area over the bladder, beginning 2″ (5 cm) above the symphysis pubis. To detect differences in sound, percuss toward the bladder's base. Percussion normally produces a tympanic sound. (Over a urine-filled bladder, it produces a dull sound.)

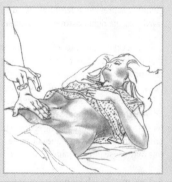

PALPATING THE URINARY ORGANS

In a normal adult, the kidneys usually aren't palpable because they're located deep within the abdomen. However, they may be palpable in a thin patient or in one with reduced abdominal muscle mass, and the right kidney, slightly lower than the left, may be easier to palpate altogether. Keep in mind that both kidneys descend with deep inhalation.

An adult's bladder may not be palpable either. However, if it's palpable, it normally feels firm and relatively smooth.

When palpating urinary organs, use bimanual palpation, beginning on the patient's right side and proceeding as follows.

(continued)

GENITOURINARY CARE

PALPATING THE URINARY ORGANS *(continued)*

Kidney palpation

1. Help the patient to a supine position, and expose the abdomen from the xiphoid process to the symphysis pubis. Standing at the right side, place your left hand under the back, midway between the lower costal margin and the iliac crest.

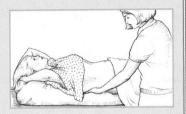

2. Next, place your right hand on the patient's abdomen, directly above your left hand. Angle this hand slightly toward the costal margin. To palpate the right lower edge of the right kidney, press your right fingertips about 1½″ (3.5 cm) above the right iliac crest at the midinguinal line; press your left fingertips upward into the right costovertebral angle.

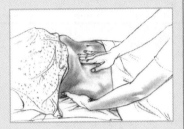

3. Instruct the patient to inhale deeply so that the lower portion of the right kidney can move down between your hands. If it does, note its shape and size. Normally, it feels smooth, solid, and firm, yet elastic. Ask the patient if palpation causes tenderness. (*Note:* Avoid using excessive pressure to palpate the kidney because this may cause intense pain.)

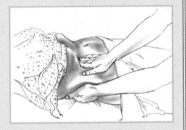

4. To assess the left kidney, move to the patient's left side, and position your hands as described above, but with this change: Place your right hand 2″ (5 cm) above the left iliac crest. Then apply pressure with both hands as the patient inhales. If the left kidney can be palpated, compare it with the right kidney; it should be the same size.

Bladder palpation

Before palpating the bladder, make sure the patient has voided. Then locate the edge of the bladder by pressing deeply in the midline 1″ to 2″ (2.5 to 5 cm) above the symphysis pubis. As the bladder is palpated, note its size and location, and check for lumps, masses, and tenderness. The bladder normally feels firm and relatively smooth. During deep palpation, the patient may report the urge to urinate—a normal response.

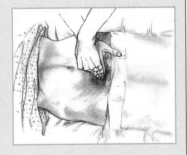

FEMALE GU SYSTEM: INTERPRETING YOUR FINDINGS

After you assess the patient, a group of findings may lead you to suspect a particular disorder. The chart below shows common groups of findings for the signs and symptoms of the female genitourinary (GU) system, along with their probable causes.

Sign or symptom and findings	Probable cause
DYSMENORRHEA	
■ Steady, aching pain that begins before menses and peaks at the height of menstrual flow; may occur between menstrual periods ■ Pain may radiate to the perineum or rectum ■ Premenstrual spotting ■ Dyspareunia ■ Infertility ■ Nausea and vomiting ■ Tender, fixed adnexal mass palpable on bimanual examination	Endometriosis
■ Severe abdominal pain ■ Fever ■ Malaise ■ Foul-smelling, purulent vaginal discharge ■ Menorrhagia ■ Cervical motion tenderness and bilateral adnexal tenderness on pelvic examination	Pelvic inflammatory disease
■ Cramping pain that begins with menstrual flow and diminishes with decreasing flow ■ Abdominal bloating ■ Breast tenderness ■ Depression ■ Irritability ■ Headache ■ Diarrhea	Premenstrual syndrome
DYSURIA	
■ Urinary frequency ■ Nocturia ■ Straining to void ■ Hematuria ■ Perineal or low-back pain ■ Fatigue ■ Low-grade fever	Cystitis
■ Dysuria throughout voiding ■ Bladder distention ■ Diminished urinary stream ■ Urinary frequency and urgency ■ Sensation of bloating or fullness in the lower abdomen or groin	Urinary system obstruction

(continued)

FEMALE GU SYSTEM: INTERPRETING YOUR FINDINGS *(continued)*

Sign or symptom and findings	Probable cause
DYSURIA *(continued)*	
■ Urinary urgency ■ Hematuria ■ Cloudy urine ■ Bladder spasms ■ Feeling of warmth or burning during urination	Urinary tract infection
URINARY INCONTINENCE	
■ Urge or overflow incontinence ■ Hematuria ■ Dysuria ■ Nocturia ■ Urinary frequency ■ Suprapubic pain from bladder spasms ■ Palpable mass on bimanual examination	Bladder cancer
■ Overflow incontinence ■ Painless bladder distention ■ Episodic diarrhea or constipation ■ Orthostatic hypotension ■ Syncope ■ Dysphagia	Diabetic neuropathy
■ Urinary urgency and frequency ■ Visual problems ■ Sensory impairment ■ Constipation ■ Muscle weakness ■ Emotional lability	Multiple sclerosis
VAGINAL DISCHARGE	
■ Profuse, white, curdlike discharge with a yeasty, sweet odor ■ Exudate may be lightly attached to the labia and vaginal walls ■ Vulvar redness and edema ■ Intense labial itching and burning ■ External dysuria	Candidiasis
■ Yellow, mucopurulent, odorless, or acrid discharge ■ Dysuria ■ Dyspareunia ■ Vaginal bleeding after douching or coitus	*Chlamydia* infection
■ Yellow or green, foul-smelling discharge that can be expressed from the Bartholin's or Skene's ducts ■ Dysuria ■ Urinary frequency and incontinence ■ Vaginal redness and swelling	Gonorrhea

MALE GU SYSTEM: INTERPRETING YOUR FINDINGS

After you assess the patient, a group of findings may lead you to suspect a particular disorder. The chart below shows common groups of findings for the signs and symptoms of the male genitourinary (GU) system, along with their probable causes.

Sign or symptom and findings	Probable cause
MALE GENITAL LESIONS	
■ Fluid-filled vesicles on the glans penis, foreskin, or penile shaft ■ Painful ulcers ■ Tender inguinal lymph nodes ■ Fever ■ Malaise ■ Dysuria	Genital herpes
■ Painless warts (tiny pink swellings that grow and become pedunculated) near the urethral meatus ■ Lesions spread to the perineum and the perianal area ■ Cauliflower appearance of multiple swellings	Genital warts
■ Sharply defined, slightly raised, scaling patches on the inner thigh or groin (bilaterally), or on the scrotum or penis ■ Severe pruritus	Tinea cruris (jock itch)
SCROTAL SWELLING	
■ Swollen scrotum that's soft or unusually firm ■ Bowel sounds may be auscultated in the scrotum	Hernia
■ Gradual scrotal swelling ■ Scrotum may be soft and cystic or firm and tense ■ Painless ■ Round, nontender scrotal mass on palpation ■ Glowing when transilluminated	Hydrocele
■ Scrotal swelling with sudden and severe pain ■ Unilateral elevation of the affected testicle ■ Nausea and vomiting	Testicular torsion
URETHRAL DISCHARGE	
■ Purulent or milky urethral discharge ■ Sudden fever and chills ■ Lower back pain ■ Myalgia ■ Perineal fullness ■ Arthralgia ■ Urinary frequency and urgency ■ Cloudy urine ■ Dysuria ■ Tense, boggy, very tender, and warm prostate palpated on digital rectal examination	Prostatitis

(continued)

MALE GU SYSTEM: INTERPRETING YOUR FINDINGS *(continued)*

Sign or symptom and findings	Probable cause

URETHRAL DISCHARGE *(continued)*

■ Opaque, gray, yellowish, or blood-tinged discharge that's painless ■ Dysuria ■ Eventual anuria	Urethral neoplasm
■ Scant or profuse urethral discharge that's either thin and clear, mucoid, or thick and purulent ■ Urinary hesitancy, frequency, and urgency ■ Dysuria ■ Itching and burning around the meatus	Urethritis

URINARY HESITANCY

■ Reduced caliber and force of urinary stream ■ Perineal pain ■ A feeling of incomplete voiding ■ Inability to stop the urine stream ■ Urinary frequency ■ Urinary incontinence ■ Bladder distention	Benign prostatic hyperplasia
■ Urinary frequency and dribbling ■ Nocturia ■ Dysuria ■ Bladder distention ■ Perineal pain ■ Constipation ■ Hard, nodular prostate palpated on digital rectal examination	Prostatic cancer
■ Dysuria ■ Urinary frequency and urgency ■ Hematuria ■ Cloudy urine ■ Bladder spasms ■ Costovertebral angle tenderness ■ Suprapubic, low back, pelvic, or flank pain ■ Urethral discharge	Urinary tract infection

DIAGNOSTIC TESTS

CYSTOMETRY

Overview

- Measures pressure and volume of fluid in the bladder during filling, storing, and voiding
- Used to assess neuromuscular function of bladder
- Results supported by results of other urologic tests, such as cystourethrography and excretory urography
- Also called CMG

PURPOSE

- To evaluate detrusor muscle function and tonicity
- To determine cause of bladder dysfunction
- To measure bladder reaction to thermal stimulation
- To detect the cause of involuntary bladder contractions and incontinence

PATIENT PREPARATION

- Make sure the patient has signed an appropriate consent form.
- Note and report all allergies.
- Check the medication history for drugs that may affect test results such as antihistamines.
- Restriction of food and fluids isn't necessary.
- Ask the patient to urinate before the test.
- Assess for signs and symptoms of urinary tract infection.

Teaching points

Be sure to cover:
- the test's purpose and how it's done.

POSTPROCEDURE CARE

- Administer a sitz bath or warm tub bath for discomfort.
- Encourage oral fluid intake (unless contraindicated) to relieve dysuria.
- Notify the physician if hematuria persists after the third voiding.
- Administer antibiotics as ordered.

Monitoring

- Vital signs
- Intake and output
- Hematuria
- Signs and symptoms of infection

PRECAUTIONS

- CMG is contraindicated in acute urinary tract infections.
- Straining with urination could cause ambiguous cystometric readings.
- Drugs, such as antihistamines, may interfere with bladder function and alter test results.
- Inability to urinate in a supine position will interfere with test results.

COMPLICATIONS

- Infection
- Bleeding

Interpretation

NORMAL FINDINGS

- Ability to start and stop micturition
- No residual urine
- Positive vesical sensation
- First urge to void at 150 to 200 ml
- Bladder capacity: 400 to 500 ml
- No bladder contractions
- Low intravesical pressure
- Positive bulbocavernosus reflex
- Positive saddle sensation test
- Positive ice water test

- Positive anal reflex
- Positive heat sensation and pain

Abnormal results

- Inability to stop micturition, early first urge to void, decreased bladder capacity, bladder contractions, increased intravesical pressure, and positive bethanechol sensitivity test suggest inhibited neurogenic bladder.
- Inability to start and stop micturition, residual urine, absent vesical sensation, absent first urge to void, decreased bladder capacity, bladder contractions, increased intravesical pressure, increased bulbocavernosus reflex, negative saddle sensation test, and absent heat sensation and pain suggest reflex neurogenic bladder.

Cystourethroscopy

Overview

- Allows visual examination of the bladder, urethra, ureter orifice, ureters, and prostate in males
- Combines two endoscopic techniques, cystoscopy and urethroscopy
- Uses a cystoscope to examine the bladder
- Uses a urethroscope, or panendoscope, to examine bladder neck and urethra
- The cystoscope and urethroscope pass through a common sheath inserted into the urethra to obtain the desired view
- Usually preceded by kidney-ureter-bladder radiography, excretory urography, and the bladder tumor antigen (BTA) urine test

Purpose

- To diagnose and evaluate urinary tract disorders by direct visualization of urinary structures

- To facilitate biopsy, lesion resection, removal of calculi, dilatation of a constricted urethra, and catheterization of the renal pelvis for pyelography

Patient preparation

- Make sure the patient has signed an appropriate consent form.
- Note and report all allergies.
- Administer a sedative if ordered.
- Instruct the patient to urinate.
- Food/fluid restriction is unnecessary unless general anesthesia ordered.

Teaching points

Be sure to cover:
- the test's purpose and how it's done
- who will perform the test and where
- that the test takes 20 to 30 minutes.

Postprocedure care

- Provide postoperative general anesthesia care as indicated.
- Encourage oral fluid intake and administer I.V. fluids as ordered.
- Administer analgesia as ordered.
- Administer antibiotics as ordered.

   Report flank or abdominal pain, chills, fever, an elevated white blood cell count, or low urine output to the physician immediately.
- Notify the physician if the patient doesn't void within 8 hours after the test or if bright red blood persists after three voidings.
- Instruct the patient to abstain from alcohol for 48 hours.
- As ordered, apply heat to the lower abdomen to relieve pain and muscle spasm and administer a warm sitz bath.

Monitoring

- Vital signs
- Intake and output
- Bleeding; hematuria
- Signs and symptoms of infection
- Bladder distention

PRECAUTIONS
- Cystourethroscopy is contraindicated in acute forms of urethritis, prostatitis, or cystitis and in bleeding disorders.

COMPLICATIONS
- Sepsis
- Infection
- Bleeding

Interpretation

NORMAL FINDINGS
- Urethra, bladder, and ureteral orifices appear normal in size, shape, and position.
- Mucosal lining of the lower urinary tract appears smooth and shiny.
- There's no evidence of erythema, cysts, or other abnormalities.
- There are no obstructions, tumors, or calculi in the bladder.

ABNORMAL RESULTS
- Structural abnormalities suggest various disorders, including enlarged prostate gland in older men, urethral strictures, calculi, tumors, diverticula, ulcers and polyps.

EXCRETORY UROGRAPHY

Overview

- Allows visualization of the renal parenchyma, calyces, and pelvis as well as the ureters, bladder and, in some cases, the urethra after I.V. administration of a contrast medium
- Also known as intravenous pyelography or IVP

PURPOSE
- To evaluate the structure and function of kidneys, ureters, and bladder
- To support a differential diagnosis of renovascular hypertension

PATIENT PREPARATION
- Make sure the patient has signed an appropriate consent form.
- Note and report all allergies, especially hypersensitivity to iodine, iodine-containing foods, or iodinated contrast media.
- Instruct the patient to fast for 8 hours before the test.
- Administer a laxative, if ordered, the night before the test.
- Obtain and report any abnormal results of renal function test, such as blood urea nitrogen and creatinine.
- Warn the patient that he might experience a transient burning sensation and metallic taste when the contrast agent is injected.

Teaching points
Be sure to cover:
- the test's purpose and how it's done
- who will perform the test and where
- that the test takes about 30 to 45 minutes.

POSTPROCEDURE CARE
- Observe for delayed reactions to the contrast medium.
- Continue I.V. fluids or provide oral fluids to promote hydration.

PRECAUTIONS
- Excretory urography is contraindicated in a patient with abnormal renal function.
- Antibiotics may be ordered if pyelonephritis is identified.
- Fecal matter, gas, or retained barium in the colon from a previous diagnostic study may interfere with results.

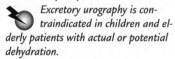 *Excretory urography is contraindicated in children and elderly patients with actual or potential dehydration.*

COMPLICATIONS

- Adverse reaction to contrast media
- Dehydration
- Impaired renal function

Interpretation

NORMAL FINDINGS

- Kidneys, ureters, and bladder show no gross evidence of soft- or hard-tissue lesions.
- Visualization of the contrast medium in the kidneys occurs promptly.
- Bilateral renal parenchyma and pelvicaliceal systems have normal conformity.
- There's no postvoiding mucosal abnormality and little residual urine.

ABNORMAL RESULTS

- Anatomic abnormalities may suggest:
  - renal and ureteral calculi
  - supernumerary or absent kidney
  - polycystic kidney disease
  - redundant pelvis or ureter
  - space-occupying lesions or tumors
  - renal, bladder, or ureteral hematoma, laceration, or trauma
  - hydronephrosis.

KIDNEY-URETER-BLADDER RADIOGRAPHY

Overview

- Used to survey the abdomen without requiring intact renal function
- Also known as a flat plate of the abdomen or KUB radiography

PURPOSE

- To evaluate the size, structure, and position of the kidneys and bladder
- To screen for abnormalities, such as calcifications, in the region of the kidneys, ureters, and bladder

PATIENT PREPARATION

- Make sure the patient has signed an appropriate consent form.
- Note and report all allergies.
- Restriction of food or fluids isn't necessary.

Teaching points

Be sure to cover:
- the test's purpose and how it's done
- who will perform the test and where
- that the test only takes a few minutes.

POSTPROCEDURE CARE

- No specific posttest care is necessary.

PRECAUTIONS

- The procedure shouldn't follow recent instillation of barium, which obscures the urinary system.
- A male patient should have gonadal shielding.
- A female patient's ovaries can't be shielded because they're too close to the kidneys, ureters, and bladder.

COMPLICATIONS

- None known

Interpretation

NORMAL FINDINGS

- Kidney shadows appear bilaterally, the right slightly lower than the left.
- Both kidneys should be approximately the same size, with the superior poles tilted slightly toward the vertebral column, paralleling the shadows of the psoas muscles.
- The bladder's shadow isn't as clearly visible as the kidneys' shadows.

ABNORMAL RESULTS

- Bilateral renal enlargement suggests possible polycystic kidney disease, multiple myeloma, lymphoma, amyloidosis, hydronephrosis, or compensatory renal hypertrophy.

■ Unilateral renal enlargement suggests possible tumor, cyst, or hydronephrosis.

PAPANICOLAOU TEST

Overview

■ Widely used for early detection of cervical cancer
■ Permits cytologic evaluation of the vaginal pool, prostatic secretions, urine, gastric secretions, cavity fluids, bronchial aspirates, sputum, and solid tumor cells obtained by fine-needle aspiration
■ Also known as a Pap test
■ ThinPrep Pap test: a relatively new tool for early detection of cervical cancer (see *ThinPrep Pap test*)

PURPOSE
■ To detect malignant cells
■ To detect inflammatory changes in tissue
■ To assess response to chemotherapy and radiation therapy
■ To detect viral, fungal and, occasionally, parasitic invasion

PATIENT PREPARATION
■ Make sure the patient has signed an appropriate consent form.
■ Note and report all allergies.
■ Schedule the study for midcycle of the menstrual cycle.
■ Advise the patient that she might experience slight discomfort from the speculum.
■ Explain the need to avoid activities that can wash away cellular deposits and change vaginal pH, including:
- sexual intercourse for 24 hours
- douching for 48 hours
- using vaginal creams or medications for 1 week.

THINPREP PAP TEST

In 1996, the United States Food and Drug Administration approved the ThinPrep Papanicolaou (Pap) test as a replacement for the conventional Pap test for cervical cancer screening.

Today, most laboratories in the United States can process the test, which is significantly more effective than the traditional test for detecting cervical abnormalities for many patient populations, and most insurance companies reimburse for it.

The ThinPrep Pap test has also been approved for testing for human papillomavirus, a sexually transmitted disease causally linked to cervical cancer, and can be used to diagnose *Chlamydia trachomatis* and *Neisseria gonorrhoeae*.

Teaching points
Be sure to cover:
■ the test's purpose and how it's done
■ who will perform the test and when
■ that the test takes 5 to 10 minutes.

POSTPROCEDURE CARE
■ If bleeding occurs, supply the patient with a sanitary napkin.
■ Schedule a return appointment for her next Pap test.

PRECAUTIONS
■ If vaginal or vulval lesions are present, scrapings taken directly from the lesion are preferred.
■ Preserve the slides immediately.

COMPLICATIONS
■ Bleeding

Interpretation

NORMAL FINDINGS
■ No malignant cells or abnormalities are present.

GENITOURINARY CARE

ABNORMAL RESULTS

■ Cells with relatively large nuclei, only small amounts of cytoplasm, abnormal nuclear chromatin patterns, and marked variation in size, shape, and staining properties, with prominent nucleoli suggests malignancy.
■ Atypical but nonmalignant cells suggest a benign abnormality.
■ Atypical cells may suggest dysplasia.

PROSTATE GLAND BIOPSY

Overview

■ Needle excision of a prostate tissue specimen for histologic examination
■ Three possible approaches: perineal, transrectal (usually for high prostatic lesions), or transurethral

PURPOSE

■ To confirm prostate cancer
■ To determine cause of prostatic hypertrophy

PATIENT PREPARATION

■ Make sure the patient has signed an appropriate consent form.
■ Note and report all allergies.
■ For a transrectal approach, administer enemas until the return is clear as ordered.
■ Administer antibiotics as ordered.
■ Administer a sedative before study as ordered.
■ Explain need for a local anesthetic.
■ Depending on the approach used, the patient may need to fast for 6 to 8 hours before the test.

Teaching points

Be sure to cover:
■ the test's purpose and how it's done
■ who will perform it and where
■ that it takes less than 30 minutes.

POSTPROCEDURE CARE

■ Administer analgesics as ordered.
■ Gradually resume normal diet and activity as tolerated.

Monitoring

■ Vital signs
■ Intake and output
■ Urinary retention
■ Bleeding
■ Infection
■ Biopsy site
■ Hematuria

Observe the biopsy site for and immediately report hematoma and signs of infection, such as redness, swelling, and pain.

PRECAUTIONS

■ Failure to obtain an adequate tissue specimen may affect accuracy of results.
■ Check the patient's history for reaction to anesthetics.

Watch for and immediately report urinary retention, frequency, or hematuria.

COMPLICATIONS

■ Bleeding into the prostatic urethra and bladder
■ Infection
■ Urinary retention

Interpretation

NORMAL FINDINGS

■ The prostate gland normally consists of a thin, fibrous capsule surrounding the stroma, which is made up of elastic and connective tissues and smooth-muscle fibers.
■ The epithelial glands, found in these tissues and muscle fibers, drain into the chief excreting ducts.
■ No cancer cells are present.

Abnormal results

■ Increased acid phosphatase levels suggest possible metastatic prostate cancer.

■ Low acid phosphatase levels suggest possible cancer that is confined to the prostatic capsule.

■ Histologic examination of the tissue reveals various possible disorders, including:

- prostate, rectal, and bladder cancer
- benign prostatic hyperplasia
- prostatitis
- tuberculosis
- lymphomas.

Renal angiography

Overview

■ Radiographic examination of renal vasculature and parenchyma after arterial injection of contrast medium

■ Follows standard aortography, showing variations in number, size, and condition of the main renal arteries and their relationship to the aorta

Purpose

■ To demonstrate renal vasculature configuration before surgery

■ To determine cause of renovascular hypertension

■ To evaluate chronic renal disease or renal failure

■ To investigate renal masses and renal trauma

■ To identify complications after a kidney transplant

■ To differentiate highly vascular tumors from avascular cysts

■ To define arterial supply in prospective renal donors

Patient preparation

■ Make sure the patient has signed an appropriate consent form.

■ Note and report all allergies, including hypersensitivity to iodine, seafood, or contrast media.

■ Evaluate peripheral pulse sites and mark them for postprocedure assessment.

■ Instruct the patient to fast for 8 hours before the test.

■ Tell the patient to drink extra fluids the day before the test and after the test to maintain adequate hydration.

■ Instruct the patient to use a laxative or enema the evening before the test.

■ Warn the patient that transient flushing, burning, and nausea may be experienced during injection of the contrast medium.

Teaching points

Be sure to cover:

■ the test's purpose and how it's done

■ who will perform the test and where

■ that the test takes about 1 hour.

Postprocedure care

■ Maintain bed rest with the affected leg straight at the hip as ordered.

■ If active bleeding or expanding hematoma occurs, apply direct manual pressure and notify the physician promptly.

■ Apply cold compresses to the puncture site to lessen edema and pain as ordered.

■ Encourage oral fluid intake to prevent nephrotoxicity from the contrast medium.

Monitoring

■ Vital signs

■ Intake and output

■ Puncture site

■ Bleeding; hematoma formation

■ Infection

■ Peripheral pulses

■ Neurovascular status of extremities

■ Renal function

■ Adverse reaction to contrast media

PRECAUTIONS
■ Renal angiography is contraindicated in:
- pregnancy
- hypersensitivity to contrast media
- uncorrected dehydration
- uncorrected coagulopathies.

COMPLICATIONS
■ Adverse reaction to contrast media
■ Bleeding
■ Hematoma formation
■ Infection
■ Arterial dissection
■ Vasovagal reactions
■ Nephrotoxicity
■ Thrombosis
■ Embolism
■ Vasospasm

Interpretation

NORMAL FINDINGS
■ Normal renal vascular tree and normal architecture of renal parenchyma are found.

ABNORMAL RESULTS
■ Hypervascular areas suggest possible renal tumors.
■ Clearly delineated, radiolucent masses suggest possible renal cysts.
■ Constriction in the blood vessel suggests possible vasospasm or renal artery stenosis.
■ Characteristic "beads-on-a-string appearance" suggests possible presence of alternating aneurysms and stenotic regions in renal artery dysplasia.
■ The appearance of absent or cut off blood vessels suggests possible renal infarction.
■ Abnormal widening of the artery suggests possible renal artery aneurysm.
■ Direct connection between the renal artery and renal vein suggests a renal arteriovenous fistula.

■ An increase in capsular vessels with abnormal intrarenal circulation suggests possible renal abscesses or inflammatory masses.
■ Intrarenal hematoma, parenchymal laceration, shattered kidney, and areas of infarction suggests possible renal trauma.

RENAL BIOPSY, PERCUTANEOUS

Overview

■ Needle aspiration of a core kidney tissue specimen for histologic examination
■ Provides valuable information about glomerular and tubular function
■ Ultrasound commonly used to direct biopsy toward the lower pole of the kidney, avoiding major vessels

PURPOSE
■ To aid diagnosis of diffuse renal parenchymal disease
■ To monitor progression of renal disease and assess effectiveness of treatment
■ To diagnose renal transplant rejection

PATIENT PREPARATION
■ Make sure the patient has signed an appropriate consent form.
■ Note and report all allergies.
■ Check the patient history for bleeding tendencies.
■ Restriction of food and fluids is required for 8 hours before the test.
■ A 24-hour hospital stay is usually required.
■ Preprocedure laboratory work may be ordered.
■ Explain the use of a local anesthetic.
■ Warn of a pinching pain when the needle is inserted through the back into the kidney.

Teaching points

Be sure to cover:
- the test's purpose and how it's done
- who will perform the biopsy and where
- that the test takes 15 to 30 minutes.

POSTPROCEDURE CARE

- Maintain bed rest as ordered.
- Notify the physician of gross hematuria.
- Encourage oral fluid intake as ordered.
- Resume normal diet as ordered.
- Discourage strenuous activities for several days after the procedure to prevent possible bleeding.

Monitoring

- Vital signs
- Intake and output
- Biopsy site
- Bleeding
- Infection
- Hematuria

PRECAUTIONS

- Percutaneous renal biopsy is contraindicated in:
  - hypersensitivity to contrast media
  - severe uncorrected bleeding disorder.

COMPLICATIONS

- Bleeding
- Hematoma
- Infection
- Arteriovenous fistula

Interpretation

NORMAL FINDINGS

- Kidney tissue shows Bowman's capsule, the glomerular tuft, and the capillary lumen.
- The proximal tubule is one layer of epithelial cells with microvilli that form a brush border.
- The descending loop of Henle has flat, squamous epithelial cells.
- The ascending, distal convoluted, and collecting tubules are lined with squamous epithelial cells.

ABNORMAL RESULTS

- Histologic examination of renal tissue suggests possible malignancy such as renal cell carcinoma.
- Characteristic histologic changes suggest possible renal disease, such as:
  - disseminated lupus erythematosus
  - amyloid infiltration
  - acute and chronic glomerulonephritis
  - renal vein thrombosis
  - pyelonephritis.

GENITOURINARY CARE

DISEASES

ACUTE PYELONEPHRITIS

Overview

DESCRIPTION

- One of the most common renal diseases

- Inflammation occurring mainly in the interstitial tissue and renal pelvis and occasionally in the renal tubules
- Affecting one or both kidneys
- Good prognosis; rarely extensive permanent damage occurs
- Also called acute infective tubulointerstitial nephritis

Pathophysiology
- Infection spreads from the bladder to ureters to the kidneys, commonly through vesicoureteral reflux.
- Vesicoureteral reflux may result from congenital weakness at the junction of the ureter and bladder.
- Bacteria refluxed to intrarenal tissues may create colonies of infection within 24 to 48 hours.
- Female anatomy allows for higher incidence of infection.

Causes
- Bacterial infection of the kidneys

Risk factors
- Urinary procedures that involve instrumentation such as cystoscopy
- Hematogenic infection such as septicemia
- Sexually active women
- Pregnant women
- Neurogenic bladder
- Obstructive disease
- Renal diseases

Complications
- Renal calculi
- Renal failure
- Renal abscess
- Septic shock
- Chronic pyelonephritis

Assessment

History
- Pain over one or both kidneys
- Urinary urgency and frequency
- Burning during urination
- Dysuria, nocturia, hematuria
- Anorexia, vomiting, diarrhea
- General fatigue
- Symptoms that develop rapidly over a few hours or a few days

Physical findings
- Pain on flank palpation

- Cloudy urine
- Ammonia-like or fishy odor to urine
- Fever of 102° F (38.9° C) or higher
- Shaking chills

Test results
Laboratory
- Pyuria, significant bacteriuria, low specific gravity and osmolality, slightly alkaline urine pH, or proteinuria, glycosuria, and ketonuria (less frequent) as revealed by urinalysis and culture and sensitivity testing
- Elevated white blood cell count, neutrophil count, and erythrocyte sedimentation rate

Imaging
- Kidney-ureter-bladder radiography reveals calculi, tumors, or cysts in the kidneys and urinary tract.
- Excretory urography shows asymmetrical kidneys, possibly indicating a high frequency of infection.

Treatment

General
- Identification and correction of predisposing factors to infection, such as obstruction and calculi
- Short courses of therapy for uncomplicated infections

Diet
- No restrictions
- Increased fluid intake

Activity
- No restrictions

Medication
- Antibiotics
- Urinary analgesics such as phenazopyridine

Monitoring
- Vital signs

- Intake and output
- Characteristics of urine
- Pattern of urination
- Daily weight
- Renal function studies

BENIGN PROSTATIC HYPERPLASIA

Overview

DESCRIPTION
- Prostate gland enlarges sufficiently to compress urethra, causing overt urinary obstruction
- Depending on the size of prostate, age and health of patient, and extent of obstruction, may be treated surgically or symptomatically
- Referred to as BPH

PATHOPHYSIOLOGY
- Changes occur in periurethral glandular tissue.
- Prostate enlarges; may extend into bladder.
- Compression or distortion of prostatic urethra obstructs urine outflow.
- BPH may cause a diverticulum musculature, retaining urine.

CAUSES
- Unknown
- Recent evidence suggests a link with hormonal activity

RISK FACTORS
- Age
- Intact testes

COMPLICATIONS
- Urinary stasis, urinary tract infection (UTI), or calculi
- Bladder wall trabeculation
- Detrusor muscle hypertrophy
- Bladder diverticula and saccules
- Urethral stenosis

- Hydronephrosis
- Paradoxical (overflow) incontinence
- Acute or chronic renal failure
- Acute postobstructive diuresis

Assessment

HISTORY
- Decreased urine stream caliber and force
- Interrupted urinary stream
- Urinary hesitancy and frequency
- Difficulty starting urination
- Nocturia, hematuria
- Dribbling, incontinence
- Urine retention

PHYSICAL FINDINGS
- Visible midline mass above the symphysis pubis
- Distended bladder
- Enlarged prostate

TEST RESULTS
Laboratory
- Elevated blood urea nitrogen and serum creatinine levels suggesting impaired renal function
- Bacterial count that exceeds 100,000/ml revealing hematuria, pyuria, and UTI

Imaging
- Excretory urography may indicate urinary tract obstruction.

Diagnostic procedures
- Cystourethroscopy determines the best surgical intervention and shows prostate enlargement and bladder wall changes.

Treatment

GENERAL
- Prostatic massages
- Sitz baths
- Regular sexual intercourse

GENITOURINARY CARE

Diet
■ Short-term fluid restriction (prevent bladder distention)

Activity
■ After surgery, avoiding lifting, performing strenuous exercises, and taking long automobile rides for at least 1 month
■ No sexual intercourse for several weeks after discharge

Medication
■ Antibiotics, if infection present
■ Alpha$_1$-adrenergic blockers such as terazosin
■ Finasteride (Proscar)

Surgery
■ For relief of acute urine retention, hydronephrosis, severe hematuria, and recurrent UTI or for palliative relief of intolerable symptoms
■ Suprapubic (transvesical) prostatectomy
■ Perineal prostatectomy
■ Retropubic (extravesical) prostatectomy
■ Transurethral resection
■ Balloon dilatation, ultrasound needle ablation, and use of stents

Monitoring
■ Vital signs
■ Intake and output
■ Daily weight

> *Watch for signs of postobstructive diuresis, characterized by polyuria exceeding 2 L in 8 hours and excessive electrolyte losses. Although usually self-limiting, it can result in vascular collapse and death if not promptly treated.*

After prostatic surgery
■ Pain control
■ Catheter function and drainage
■ Signs of infection

Overview

Description
■ About 90% of bladder cancers are transitional cell carcinomas, arising from the transitional epithelium of mucous membranes (they may result from malignant transformation of benign papillomas)
■ Less common bladder tumors include adenocarcinomas, epidermoid carcinomas, squamous cell carcinomas, sarcomas, tumors in bladder diverticula, and carcinoma in situ
■ Most common cancer of the urinary tract

Pathophysiology
■ Benign or malignant tumors may develop on the bladder wall surface or grow within the wall and quickly invade underlying muscles.

Causes
■ Exact cause unknown
■ Associated with chronic bladder irritation and infection in people with renal calculi, indwelling urinary catheters, chemical cystitis caused by cyclophosphamide, and pelvic irradiation

Risk factors
■ Certain environmental carcinogens, such as tobacco, nitrates, and coffee
■ Occupational exposure to other carcinogens such as 2-naphthylamine, an industrial chemical

Complications
■ Bone metastases
■ Problems resulting from tumor invasion of contiguous viscera

Assessment

HISTORY
■ Gross, painless, intermittent hematuria, often with clots
■ Suprapubic pain after voiding, which suggests invasive lesions
■ Bladder irritability, urinary frequency, nocturia, and dribbling
■ Flank pain that may indicate an obstructed ureter

PHYSICAL FINDINGS
■ Gross hematuria
■ Flank tenderness if ureteral obstruction present

TEST RESULTS
Laboratory
■ Complete blood count helping to detect anemia
■ Urinalysis detecting blood and malignant cells in the urine

Imaging
■ Excretory urography can identify a large, early-stage tumor or an infiltrating tumor.
■ Retrograde cystography evaluates bladder structure and integrity; also helps confirm a bladder cancer diagnosis.
■ Bone scan can detect metastasis.
■ Computed tomography scan can define the thickness of the involved bladder wall and disclose enlarged retroperitoneal lymph nodes.
■ Ultrasonography can find metastases in tissues beyond the bladder and can distinguish a bladder cyst from a bladder tumor.

Diagnostic procedures
■ Cystoscopy and biopsy confirm bladder cancer diagnosis.

Treatment

GENERAL
■ The cancer's stage and the patient's lifestyle, other health problems, and mental outlook will influence selection of therapy.

DIET
■ No restrictions

ACTIVITY
■ Initially postoperatively, avoid heavy lifting and contact sports
■ After recovery, no restrictions

MEDICATION
■ Intravesical chemotherapy, such as thiotepa, doxorubicin, and mitomycin
■ Attenuated bacille Calmette-Guérin vaccine live

SURGERY
■ Transurethral resection (cystoscopic approach) and fulguration (electrically)
■ Segmental bladder
■ Radical cystectomy
■ Ureterostomy, nephrostomy, continent vesicostomy (Kock pouch), ileal bladder, and ureterosigmoidostomy

MONITORING
■ Wound site
■ Postoperative complications
■ Intake and output
■ Pain control

CERVICAL CANCER

Overview

DESCRIPTION
■ Third most common cancer of the female reproductive system
■ Classified as either preinvasive or invasive

PATHOPHYSIOLOGY
Preinvasive cancer
■ Preinvasive cancer ranges from minimal cervical dysplasia, in which the lower third of the epithelium contains abnormal cells, to carcinoma in situ, in which the full thickness of epithelium contains abnormally proliferating cells.

Invasive disease
■ Cancer cells penetrate the basement membrane and can spread directly to contiguous pelvic structures or disseminate to distant sites by way of lymphatic routes.
■ Most (95%) cases are squamous cell carcinoma; 5% of cases are adenocarcinomas.

CAUSES
■ Unknown

RISK FACTORS
■ Frequent intercourse at a young age (under age 16)
■ Multiple sexual partners
■ Multiple pregnancies
■ Human papillomavirus (HPV)
■ Bacterial or viral venereal infections

COMPLICATIONS
■ Renal failure
■ Distant metastasis
■ Vaginal stenosis
■ Ureterovaginal or vesicovaginal fistula
■ Proctitis
■ Cystitis
■ Bowel obstruction

Assessment

HISTORY
■ One or more risk factors present

Preinvasive cancer
■ No symptoms or other clinical changes

Invasive cervical cancer
■ Abnormal vaginal bleeding or discharge
■ Gradually increasing flank pain

PHYSICAL FINDINGS
■ Vaginal discharge

TEST RESULTS
Imaging
■ Lymphangiography can show metastasis.
■ Cystography can show metastasis.
■ Organ and bone scans can show metastasis.

Diagnostic procedures
■ Papanicolaou (Pap) test shows abnormal cells, and colposcopy shows the source of the abnormal cells seen on the Pap test.
■ Cone biopsy is performed if endocervical curettage is positive.
■ HPV deoxyribonucleic acid testing may be performed for women who have abnormal PAP test results to detect the presence of HPV and determine the need for further evaluation.

Treatment

GENERAL
■ Accurate clinical staging used to determine type of treatment

DIET
■ Well-balanced; as tolerated

ACTIVITY
■ No restrictions

MEDICATION
■ Multidrug chemotherapy regimens

SURGERY
Preinvasive lesions
- Total excisional biopsy
- Cryosurgery
- Laser destruction
- Conization, followed by frequent Pap test follow-ups

Invasive squamous cell carcinoma
- Radical hysterectomy and radiation therapy (internal, external, or both)
- Pelvic exenteration (rare; may be performed for recurrent cervical cancer)

MONITORING
- Vital signs
- Complications
- Pain control
- Vaginal discharge
- Renal status
- Response to treatment

KIDNEY CANCER

Overview

DESCRIPTION
- 85% originate in kidneys; 15% metastasize from various primary-site carcinomas
- Also called nephrocarcinoma and renal carcinoma

PATHOPHYSIOLOGY
- Most kidney tumors are large, firm, nodular, encapsulated, unilateral, and solitary.
- Kidney cancer may affect either kidney; occasionally tumors are bilateral or multifocal.
- Renal cancers arise from the tubular epithelium.
- Tumor margins are usually clearly defined.
- Tumors can include areas of ischemia, necrosis, and focal hemorrhage.
- Tumor cells may be well differentiated to anaplastic.
- Kidney cancer can be separated histologically into clear cell, granular cell, and spindle cell types.
- The prognosis is better for patients with the clear cell type than for the other types.

CAUSES
- Unknown

RISK FACTORS
- Heavy cigarette smoking
- Regular hemodialysis treatments

COMPLICATIONS
- Hemorrhage
- Metastasis

Assessment

HISTORY
- Hematuria
- Dull, aching flank pain
- Weight loss (rare)

PHYSICAL FINDINGS
- Palpable smooth, firm, nontender abdominal mass

TEST RESULTS
Laboratory
- Increased alkaline phosphatase, bilirubin, and transaminase levels
- Prolonged prothrombin time

Imaging
- Renal ultrasonography and computed tomography scan can be used to verify renal cancer.
- Excretory urography, nephrotomography, and kidney-ureter-bladder radiography are used to aid diagnosis and help in staging.

GENITOURINARY CARE

Treatment

GENERAL
■ Because of radiation resistance, radiation used only when cancer has spread into perinephric region or lymph nodes or when primary tumor or metastatic sites can't be completely excised

DIET
■ Low-protein

ACTIVITY
■ Postoperatively, no heavy lifting or contact sports for 6 to 8 weeks

MEDICATION
■ Chemotherapy
■ Biotherapy with lymphokine-activated killer cells plus recombinant interleukin-2
■ Interferon

SURGERY
■ Radical nephrectomy, with or without regional lymph node dissection

MONITORING
■ Wound site
■ Intake and output
■ Complete blood count; serum chemistry results
■ Pain control

PROSTATIC CANCER

Overview

DESCRIPTION
■ Usually takes the form of adenocarcinoma, and typically originates in the posterior prostate gland
■ May progress to widespread bone metastases and death

PATHOPHYSIOLOGY
■ Slow-growing prostatic cancer seldom causes signs and symptoms until it's well advanced.
■ Typically, when a primary prostatic lesion spreads beyond the prostate gland, it invades the prostatic capsule and spreads along ejaculatory ducts in the space between the seminal vesicles or perivesicular fascia.
■ Endocrine factors may play a role, leading researchers to suspect that androgens speed tumor growth.
■ Malignant prostatic tumors seldom result from the benign hyperplastic enlargement that commonly develops around the prostatic urethra in older men.

CAUSES
■ Unknown

RISK FACTORS
■ Over age 40
■ Infection

COMPLICATIONS
■ Spinal cord compression
■ Deep vein thrombosis
■ Pulmonary emboli
■ Myelophthisis

Assessment

HISTORY
■ Symptoms rare in early stages
■ Later, urinary problems, such as difficulty initiating a urinary stream, dribbling, and urine retention

PHYSICAL FINDINGS
■ In early stages: nonraised, firm, nodular mass with a sharp edge
■ In advanced disease: edema of the scrotum or leg; a hard lump in the prostate region

Test results
Laboratory
■ Elevated serum prostate-specific antigen level

Imaging
■ Transrectal prostatic ultrasonography shows prostate size and presence of abnormal growths.
■ Bone scan and excretory urography can determine the extent of disease.
■ Magnetic resonance imaging and computed tomography scan can define the extent of the tumor.

Other
■ Standard screening test: digital rectal examination (recommended yearly by the American Cancer Society for men over age 40).

Treatment

General
■ Varies with cancer stage
■ Radiation therapy or internal beam radiation

Diet
■ Well-balanced, no restrictions

Activity
■ No restrictions

Medication
■ Hormonal therapy
■ Chemotherapy

Surgery
■ Prostatectomy
■ Orchiectomy
■ Radical prostatectomy
■ Transurethral resection of prostate

Monitoring
■ Pain level
■ Wound site
■ Postoperative complications
■ Medication effects

RENAL CALCULI

Overview

Description
■ Formation of calculi ("stones") anywhere in the urinary tract
■ Most common in the renal pelvis or calyces
■ Vary in size; may be solitary or multiple
■ Necessitate hospitalization in roughly 1 of every 1,000 Americans

Pathophysiology
■ Calculi form when substances normally dissolved in the urine, such as calcium oxalate and calcium phosphate, precipitate.
■ Large, rough calculi may occlude the opening to the ureteropelvic junction.

Causes
■ Unknown

Risk factors
■ Dehydration
■ Infection
■ Urine pH changes
■ Urinary tract obstruction
■ Immobilization
■ Metabolic factors

Complications
■ Renal parenchymal damage
■ Renal cell necrosis
■ Hydronephrosis
■ Complete ureteral obstruction

Assessment

History
■ Classic renal colic pain: severe pain that travels from the costovertebral angle to the flank and then to the suprapubic region and external genitalia

GENITOURINARY CARE

- With calculi in the renal pelvis and calyces: relatively constant, dull pain
- Pain of fluctuating intensity; may be excruciating at its peak
- Nausea, vomiting
- Fever, chills
- Anuria (rare)

PHYSICAL FINDINGS
- Hematuria
- Abdominal distention

TEST RESULTS
Laboratory
- 24-hour urine collection showing calcium oxalate, phosphorus, and uric acid excretion levels
- Urinalysis showing increased urine specific gravity, hematuria, crystals, casts, and pyuria

Imaging
- Kidney-ureter-bladder (KUB) radiography reveals most renal calculi.
- Excretory urography helps confirm the diagnosis and determines calculi size and location.
- Kidney ultrasonography can detect obstructive changes and radiolucent calculi not seen on KUB.

Treatment

GENERAL
- Percutaneous ultrasonic lithotripsy
- Extracorporeal shock wave lithotripsy

DIET
- Vigorous hydration (more than 3 qt [3 L]/day)
- Adequate calcium intake

ACTIVITY
- No restriction

MEDICATION
- Antibiotics
- Analgesics
- Diuretics
- Methenamine mandelate
- Allopurinol (for uric acid calculi)

SURGERY
- Parathyroidectomy for hyperparathyroidism
- Cystoscopy

MONITORING
- Intake and output
- Daily weight
- Pain control
- Catheter function and drainage
- Signs and symptoms of infection

RENAL FAILURE, ACUTE

Overview

DESCRIPTION
- Sudden interruption of renal function resulting from obstruction, reduced circulation, or renal parenchymal disease
- Classified as prerenal failure, intrarenal failure, or postrenal failure
- Usually reversible with medical treatment
- If not treated, may progress to end-stage renal disease, uremia, and death
- Normally occurs in three distinct phases: oliguric, diuretic, and recovery

Oliguric phase
- This phase may last a few days or several weeks.
- Urine output drops below 400 ml/day.
- Fluid volume excess, azotemia, and electrolyte imbalance occur.
- Local mediators are released, causing intrarenal vasoconstriction.

■ Medullary hypoxia causes cellular swelling and adherence of neutrophils to capillaries and venules.
■ Hypoperfusion occurs.
■ Cellular injury and necrosis occur.
■ Reperfusion causes reactive oxygen species to form, leading to further cellular injury.

Diuretic phase
■ Renal function is recovered.
■ Urine output gradually increases.
■ Glomerular filtration rate improves, although tubular transport systems remain abnormal.

Recovery phase
■ This phase may last 3 to 12 months, or even longer.
■ The patient gradually returns to normal or near normal renal function.

PATHOPHYSIOLOGY
Prerenal failure
■ Caused by impaired blood flow
■ Glomerular filtration rate declines because of the decrease in filtration pressure
■ Failure to restore blood volume or blood pressure that may cause acute tubular necrosis (ATN) or acute cortical necrosis

Intrarenal failure
■ A severe episode of hypotension, commonly associated with hypovolemia, that's frequently a significant contributing event
■ Ischemia generates toxic oxygen free radicals and anti-inflammatory mediators that cause cell swelling, injury, and necrosis, a form of reperfusion injury that may also be caused by nephrotoxins

Postrenal failure
■ Usually occurs with urinary tract obstruction that affects the kidneys bilaterally such as prostatic hyperplasia

CAUSES
Prerenal failure
■ Hypovolemia
■ Hemorrhagic blood loss
■ Loss of plasma volume
■ Water and electrolyte losses
■ Hypotension or hypoperfusion

Intrarenal failure
■ ATN
■ Glomerulopathies
■ Malignant hypertension
■ Coagulation defects

Postrenal failure
■ Obstructive uropathies usually bilateral
■ Ureteral destruction
■ Bladder neck obstruction

COMPLICATIONS
■ Renal shutdown
■ Electrolyte imbalance
■ Metabolic acidosis
■ Acute pulmonary edema
■ Hypertensive crisis
■ Infection
■ Death

Assessment

HISTORY
■ Predisposing disorder
■ Recent fever, chills, or central nervous system problem
■ Recent GI problem

PHYSICAL FINDINGS
■ Oliguria or anuria, depending on renal failure phase
■ Tachycardia
■ Bibasilar crackles
■ Irritability, drowsiness, or confusion

GENITOURINARY CARE

- Altered level of consciousness
- Bleeding abnormalities
- Dry, pruritic skin
- Dry mucous membranes
- Uremic breath odor

TEST RESULTS
Laboratory

- Elevated blood urea nitrogen, serum creatinine, and potassium levels
- Decreased blood pH, bicarbonate, hematocrit, and hemoglobin levels
- Urine casts, cellular debris, and decreased specific gravity
- In glomerular disease, proteinuria and urine osmolality close to serum osmolality level
- Urine sodium level below 20 mEq/L, in oliguria caused by decreased perfusion
- Urine sodium above 40 mEq/L, in oliguria from an intrarenal problem
- Urine creatinine clearance to measure glomerular filtration rate and estimate number of remaining functioning nephrons

Imaging
The following imaging tests may show the cause of renal failure:

- kidney ultrasonography
- kidney-ureter-bladder radiography
- excretory urography renal scan
- retrograde pyelography
- computed tomography scan
- nephrotomography.

Diagnostic procedures

- Electrocardiography shows tall, peaked T waves; a widening QRS complex; and disappearing P waves if hyperkalemia is present.

GENERAL

- Hemodialysis or peritoneal dialysis (if appropriate)

DIET

- High-calorie
- Low in protein, sodium, and potassium
- Fluid restriction

ACTIVITY

- Rest periods when fatigued

MEDICATION

- Supplemental vitamins
- Diuretics
- In hyperkalemia: hypertonic glucose-and-insulin infusions, sodium bicarbonate, sodium polystyrene sulfonate

SURGERY

- Creation of vascular access for hemodialysis

MONITORING

- Intake and output
- Daily weight
- Renal function studies
- Vital signs
- Effects of excess fluid volume
- Dialysis access site

RENAL FAILURE, CHRONIC

Overview

DESCRIPTION

- Usually the end result of gradually progressive loss of renal function
- Symptoms sparse until more than 75% of glomerular filtration lost; symptoms worsen as renal function declines
- Fatal unless treated; sustaining life may require maintenance dialysis or kidney transplantation

PATHOPHYSIOLOGY
■ Nephron destruction eventually causes irreversible renal damage.
■ Disease course may progress through the following stages: reduced renal reserve, renal insufficiency, renal failure, and end-stage renal disease.

CAUSES
■ Chronic glomerular disease
■ Chronic infections such as chronic pyelonephritis
■ Congenital anomalies such as polycystic kidney disease
■ Vascular diseases
■ Obstructive processes such as calculi
■ Collagen diseases such as systemic lupus erythematosus
■ Nephrotoxic agents
■ Endocrine disease

COMPLICATIONS
■ Anemia
■ Peripheral neuropathy
■ Lipid disorders
■ Platelet dysfunction
■ Pulmonary edema
■ Electrolyte imbalances
■ Sexual dysfunction

Assessment

HISTORY
■ Predisposing factor
■ Dry mouth
■ Fatigue
■ Nausea
■ Hiccups
■ Muscle cramps
■ Fasciculations, twitching
■ Infertility, decreased libido
■ Amenorrhea
■ Impotence
■ Pathologic fractures

PHYSICAL FINDINGS
■ Decreased urine output

■ Hypotension or hypertension
■ Altered level of consciousness
■ Peripheral edema
■ Cardiac arrhythmias
■ Bibasilar crackles
■ Pleural friction rub
■ Gum ulceration and bleeding
■ Uremic fetor
■ Abdominal pain on palpation
■ Poor skin turgor
■ Pale, yellowish bronze skin color
■ Thin, brittle fingernails and dry, brittle hair

TEST RESULTS
Laboratory
■ Elevated blood urea nitrogen, serum creatinine, sodium, and potassium levels
■ Arterial blood gas (ABG) values showing decreased arterial pH and bicarbonate levels
■ Low hematocrit and hemoglobin level; decreased red blood cell (RBC) survival time
■ Mild thrombocytopenia; platelet defects
■ Increased aldosterone secretion
■ Hyperglycemia, hypertriglyceridemia
■ Decreased high-density lipoprotein levels
■ ABG values showing metabolic acidosis
■ Urine specific gravity fixed at 1.010
■ Proteinuria, glycosuria; urinary RBCs, leukocytes, casts, and crystals

Imaging
■ Kidney-ureter-bladder radiography, excretory urography, nephrotomography, renal scan, and renal arteriography show reduced kidney size.

Diagnostic procedures
■ Renal biopsy allows histologic identification of the underlying pathology.

Treatment

GENERAL
■ Hemodialysis or peritoneal dialysis

DIET
■ Low-protein (with peritoneal dialysis, high-protein)
■ High-calorie
■ Low in sodium, phosphorus, and potassium
■ Fluid restriction

ACTIVITY
■ Rest periods when fatigued

MEDICATION
■ Loop diuretics
■ Cardiac glycosides
■ Antihypertensives
■ Antiemetics
■ Iron and folate supplements
■ Erythropoietin
■ Antipruritics
■ Supplementary vitamins and essential amino acids

SURGERY
■ Creation of vascular access for dialysis
■ Possible kidney transplant

MONITORING
■ Renal function studies
■ Laboratory results
■ Vital signs
■ Intake and output
■ Daily weight
■ Signs and symptoms of fluid overload
■ Signs and symptoms of bleeding

TESTICULAR CANCER

Overview

DESCRIPTION
■ Most originate from germinal cells and about 40% become seminomas.

■ Prognosis depends on cancer cell type and stage (with treatment, a more-than-5-year survival rate).

PATHOPHYSIOLOGY
■ Testicular cancer spreads through the lymphatic system to the iliac, para-aortic, and mediastinal nodes.
■ Metastases affect the lungs, liver, viscera, and bone.

CAUSES
■ Exact cause unknown

RISK FACTORS
■ Cryptorchidism
■ Mumps orchitis
■ Inguinal hernia in childhood
■ Maternal use of diethylstilbestrol (DES) or other estrogen-progestin combinations during pregnancy

COMPLICATIONS
■ Back or abdominal pain from retroperitoneal adenopathy
■ Metastasis
■ Ureteral obstruction

Assessment

HISTORY
■ Previous injuries to the scrotum
■ Viral infection (such as mumps)
■ Use of DES or other estrogen-progestin drugs by the patient's mother during pregnancy
■ Feeling of heaviness or a dragging sensation in the scrotum
■ Swollen testes or a painless lump
■ Weight loss (late sign)
■ Fatigue and weakness (late sign)

PHYSICAL FINDINGS
■ Enlarged testes
■ Gynecomastia
■ Lethargic, thin, and pallid appearance (later stages)
■ Palpable firm, smooth testicular mass

■ Enlarged lymph nodes in surrounding areas

TEST RESULTS
Laboratory
■ Levels of the proteins (tumor markers): elevated human chorionic gonadotropin (HCG) and alpha-fetoprotein (AFP) suggest testicular cancer and can differentiate a seminoma from a nonseminoma
■ Elevated HCG and AFP levels indicating a nonseminoma
■ Elevated HCG and normal AFP levels indicating a seminoma

Diagnostic procedures
■ Biopsy can be used to confirm the diagnosis and to stage the disease.

Treatment

GENERAL
■ Varies with tumor cell type and stage
■ Radiation therapy

■ Autologous bone marrow transplantation for patients nonresponsive to standard therapy

DIET
■ Well-balanced; no restrictions

ACTIVITY
■ No restrictions

MEDICATION
■ Chemotherapy
■ Hormonal therapy

SURGERY
■ Orchiectomy and retroperitoneal node dissection

MONITORING
■ Wound site
■ Vital signs
■ Hydration and nutritional status
■ Pain control
■ Effects of medication
■ Postoperative complications

TREATMENTS

GENITOURINARY CARE

BLADDER AND BOWEL RETRAINING

Overview

■ Bladder and bowel retraining may be needed to treat such elimination problems as bladder and fecal incontinence (especially in elderly patients).
■ Severe elimination problems can have serious psychosocial effects and threaten a patient's ability to live independently.

INDICATIONS
■ Loss or impairment of urinary or anal sphincter control (see *Strengthening pelvic floor muscles,* page 434)
■ Bladder or fecal incontinence
■ Age- or disease-related changes in genitourinary or GI system function or, less commonly, changes in other body systems, such as musculoskeletal and nervous systems
■ Fecal stasis and impaction

COMPLICATIONS
■ Skin breakdown
■ Infection

STRENGTHENING PELVIC FLOOR MUSCLES

Stress incontinence, the most common kind of urinary incontinence in women, usually results from weakening of the urethral sphincter. In men, it may sometimes occur after a radical prostatectomy.

You can help a patient prevent or minimize stress incontinence by teaching her pelvic floor (Kegel) exercises to strengthen the pubococcygeal muscles. Here's how.

Learning Kegel exercises

First, explain how to locate the muscles of the pelvic floor. Instruct the patient to tense the muscles around the anus, as if to retain stool.

Next, teach the patient to tighten the muscles of the pelvic floor to stop the flow of urine while urinating and then to release the muscles to restart the flow. Once learned, these exercises can be done anywhere at any time.

Establishing a regimen

Explain to the patient that contraction and relaxation exercises are essential to muscle retraining. Suggest that she start out by contracting the pelvic floor muscles for 10 seconds, then relax for 10 seconds before slowly tightening the muscles and then releasing them.

Typically, the patient starts with 15 contractions in the morning and afternoon and 20 at night. Or she may exercise for 10 minutes three times per day, working up to 25 contractions at a time as strength improves.

Advise the patient not to use stomach, leg, or buttock muscles. Also discourage leg crossing or breath holding during these exercises.

Nursing interventions

PRETREATMENT CARE

- Explain the treatment and preparation to the patient and family.
- Perform careful and continuing assessment.
- Assess for signs and symptoms of urinary tract infection.
- Provide support, and help the patient deal with feelings of shame, embarrassment, or powerlessness caused by loss of control.
- Encourage persistence, tolerance, and a positive attitude.

MONITORING

- Vital signs
- Infection
- Fluid intake after 6 p.m.
- Time voiding schedule

POSTTREATMENT CARE

- Praise the patient's successful efforts.
- Be sensitive to feelings of embarrassment and self-consciousness.
- Maximize the patient's independence level while minimizing risks to self-esteem.

PATIENT TEACHING

Be sure to cover:
- the fact that periodic incontinence doesn't mean program failure
- gradual elimination of laxative use, if necessary
- use of natural laxatives, such as prunes or prune juice
- medications, such as antibiotics for urinary tract infection, and potential adverse reactions
- signs and symptoms of infection
- complications
- when to notify the physician
- follow-up care.

Conization

Overview

- Removal of a cone of tissue; most commonly refers to excision of the entire transformation zone and endocervical canal

Indications
- Microinvasive cervical cancer
- Abnormal Papanicolaou test

Complications
- Uterine perforation
- Bleeding
- Infection
- Cervical stenosis
- Infertility
- Decreased cervical mucus
- Cervical incompetence

Nursing interventions

Pretreatment care
- Explain the treatment and preparation to the patient and family.
- Make sure the patient has signed an appropriate consent form.
- Provide emotional support.
- Obtain results of diagnostic studies, medical history, and physical examination; notify the physician of any abnormalities.
- Make sure the patient has fasted and used an enema preoperatively.
- Administer I.V. fluids as ordered.

Posttreatment care
- Administer analgesics as ordered.
- Administer fluids as ordered.
- Provide the ordered diet as tolerated.
- Institute safety precautions.

Be sure to report continuous, sharp abdominal pain that doesn't respond to analgesics, which indicates a possible symptom of uterine perforation, a potentially life-threatening complication.

Monitoring
- Vital signs
- Intake and output
- Vaginal drainage
- Infection

Patient teaching
Be sure to cover:
- medications and possible adverse reactions
- possibility of postoperative abdominal cramping and pain in the pelvis and lower back
- postoperative vaginal drainage
- abnormal bleeding
- signs and symptoms of infection
- complications
- when to notify the physician
- follow-up care
- possibility of heavier-than-normal menses for the first two or three menstrual cycles after the procedure
- avoidance of tampons, douches, or sexual intercourse until the physician approves.

Cystectomy

Overview

- Partial or total removal of the urinary bladder and surrounding structures (see *Types of Cystectomy,* page 436)
- Total cystectomy necessitates permanent urinary diversion into an ileal or colonic conduit

Indications
- Advanced bladder cancer
- Bladder disorders such as interstitial cystitis
- Frequent recurrence of widespread papillary tumors not responding to endoscopic or chemotherapeutic management

TYPES OF CYSTECTOMY

In cystectomy, surgery may be partial, simple, or radical.

■ *Partial cystectomy* involves resection of a portion of the bladder wall. Typically preserving bladder function, this surgery is most commonly indicated for a single, easily accessible bladder tumor.

■ *Simple or total cystectomy* involves resection of the entire bladder. It's indicated for benign conditions limited to the bladder. It may also be performed as a palliative measure, such as to stop bleeding, when cancer isn't curable.

■ *Radical cystectomy* is generally indicated for muscle-invasive primary bladder carcinoma. Besides removing the bladder, this procedure removes several surrounding structures. This extensive surgery typically causes impotence in men and sterility in women.

After removal of the entire bladder, the patient requires a permanent urinary diversion, such as an ileal conduit or a continent urinary pouch.

COMPLICATIONS

■ Bleeding
■ Hypotension
■ Nerve injury, such as to the genitofemoral or peroneal nerve
■ Anuria
■ Stoma stenosis
■ Urinary tract infection
■ Pouch leakage
■ Electrolyte imbalances
■ Ureteroileal junction stenosis
■ Vascular compromise
■ Loss of sexual or reproductive function
■ Psychological problems relating to changes in body image

Nursing interventions

PRETREATMENT CARE

■ Explain the treatment and preparation to the patient and family.
■ Make sure the patient has signed an appropriate consent form.
■ Arrange for a visit by a wound, ostomy, continence nurse.
■ Address the patient's concerns about inevitable loss of sexual or reproductive function.
■ Explain the equipment the patient will see immediately after surgery.
■ If possible, arrange for the patient to visit the intensive care unit.
■ Perform standard bowel preparation as ordered.
■ Administer enemas or oral polyethylene glycol-electrolyte solution as ordered.
■ Administer antibiotics as ordered.

POSTTREATMENT CARE

■ Administer medications as ordered.
■ Report urine output of less than 30 ml/hour.
■ Maintain patency of the indwelling urinary catheter or stoma as appropriate, and irrigate as ordered.
■ Test all drainage from the nasogastric tube, abdominal drains, indwelling urinary catheter, and urine collection appliance for blood; notify the physician of positive findings.
■ Change abdominal dressings, maintaining asepsis.
■ Encourage frequent position changes, coughing, deep breathing, and early ambulation.
■ Offer emotional support.

Monitoring

■ Vital signs
■ Intake and output
■ Surgical wound and dressings
■ Drainage
■ Hypovolemic shock

- Stoma (if present)
- Frank hematuria and clots
- Respiratory status
- Infection

PATIENT TEACHING

Be sure to cover:
- medications and possible adverse reactions
- signs and symptoms of infection
- abnormal bleeding, including persistent hematuria
- complications
- when to notify the physician
- urinary diversion care
- home care nursing visits if appropriate
- possibility of cancer recurrence
- follow-up care
- referral to a support group such as the United Ostomy Association if appropriate
- referral for psychological and sexual counseling as appropriate.

NEPHRECTOMY

Overview

- Surgical removal of a kidney
- May be unilateral or bilateral
- Partial nephrectomy: resection of a portion of the kidney
- Simple nephrectomy: removal of the entire kidney
- Radical nephrectomy: resection of the entire kidney and surrounding fat tissue
- Nephroureterectomy: removal of the entire kidney, entire ureter, and perinephric fat

INDICATIONS

- Renal cell carcinoma
- Harvest of a healthy kidney for transplantation
- Renal trauma or infection

- Hypertension
- Hydronephrosis
- Inoperable renal calculi

COMPLICATIONS

- Infection
- Hemorrhage
- Atelectasis
- Pneumonia
- Deep vein thrombosis
- Pulmonary embolism

Nursing interventions

PRETREATMENT CARE

- Explain the treatment and preparation to the patient and family.
- Make sure the patient has signed an appropriate consent form.
- Explain postoperative care.
- Restrict oral intake as ordered.
- Administer I.V. fluids as ordered.

POSTTREATMENT CARE

- Administer medications as ordered.
- Provide care for the I.V. line, nasogastric tube, and indwelling urinary catheter.
- Notify the physician if urine output falls below 50 ml/hour.
- Maintain drain patency.
- Change dressings as ordered.
- Resume oral feedings as ordered.
- Encourage coughing, deep breathing, incentive spirometry, and position changes.
- Encourage early and regular ambulation.
- Apply antiembolism stockings as ordered.

Monitoring

- Vital signs
- Intake and output
- Daily weight
- Complications
- Surgical wound and dressings
- Abnormal bleeding

GENITOURINARY CARE

- Drainage
- Bowel sounds
- Respiratory status
- Hemorrhage and shock
- Infection

PATIENT TEACHING

Be sure to cover:
- medications and possible adverse reactions
- coughing and deep-breathing exercises
- signs and symptoms of infection
- complications
- when to notify the physician
- intake and output monitoring
- prescribed fluid intake and dietary restrictions
- prescribed activity restrictions
- follow-up care
- importance of wearing medical identification.

PROSTATECTOMY

Overview

- Surgical removal of the prostate
- Transurethral resection of the prostate: prostate removal via insertion of a resectoscope into the urethra
- May be performed by an open surgical approach, such as suprapubic prostatectomy, retropubic prostatectomy (which allows pelvic lymph node dissection for prostate cancer staging), or perineal prostatectomy (safer for obese patients and those who have had lower abdominal or pelvic surgery)

INDICATIONS

- Prostate cancer
- Obstructive benign prostatic hyperplasia

COMPLICATIONS

- Hemorrhage

- Infection
- Urine retention and incontinence
- Impotence

Nursing interventions

PRETREATMENT CARE

- Explain the treatment and preparation to the patient and family.
- Make sure the patient has signed an appropriate consent form.
- Explain postoperative care.
- Administer an enema.
- Restrict foods and fluids as ordered.

POSTTREATMENT CARE

- Administer medications as ordered.
- Maintain urinary catheter and suprapubic tube patency as ordered.
- Keep the urinary collection container below the bladder level.
- Administer antispasmodics and analgesics as ordered.
- Offer sitz baths.
- Arrange for psychological and sexual counseling as needed.

Never administer medication rectally in a patient who has had a total prostatectomy.

Monitor for and report signs and symptoms of dilutional hyponatremia, such as altered mental status, muscle twitching, and seizures.

Monitoring

- Vital signs
- Intake and output
- Urine characteristics
- Complications
- Surgical wound and dressings
- Drainage
- Abnormal bleeding
- Infection
- Fluid and electrolyte status

Monitor for and report signs and symptoms of epididymitis, including fever, chills, groin pain, and a swollen, tender epididymis.

Patient teaching

Be sure to cover:
- medications and possible adverse reactions
- incision care
- signs and symptoms of infection and abnormal bleeding
- complications
- when to notify the physician
- importance of drinking ten 8-oz glasses of water daily
- likelihood of experiencing transient urinary frequency and dribbling after catheter removal
- how to perform Kegel exercises
- avoidance of caffeine-containing beverages
- prescribed activity restrictions
- sitz baths
- follow-up care
- annual prostate-specific antigen testing.

Instruct the patient to seek immediate medical care if he can't void or if he passes bloody urine.

URINARY DIVERSION SURGERY

Overview

- Provides an alternative route for urine excretion when disease impedes normal urine low through the bladder
- Incontinent diversion: urine flow is constant; used when the patient permanently requires an external collection device; types include ileal conduit, ureterosigmoidostomy, and nephrostomy
- Continent diversion: used when an external collection bag isn't needed; types include the Kock pouch, Indiana pouch, Mainze reservoir, and Camey procedure (see *Types of permanent urinary diversion,* page 440)

Indications

- Cystectomy
- Congenital urinary tract defect
- Severe, unmanageable urinary tract infection that threatens renal function
- Chronic cystitis
- Injury to the ureters, bladder, or urethra
- Obstructive malignancy
- Neurogenic bladder

Complications

- Skin breakdown
- Infection
- Urinary extravasation
- Ureteral obstruction
- Small-bowel obstruction
- Peritonitis
- Hydronephrosis
- Stomal stenosis
- Pyelonephritis
- Renal calculi
- Psychological problems

Nursing interventions

Pretreatment care

- Explain the treatment and preparation to the patient and family.
- Make sure the patient has signed an appropriate consent form.
- Explain postoperative care.
- Initiate referrals if the patient needs assistance with stoma management.
- Prepare the bowel as ordered (such as with a low-residue or clear liquid diet, an enema, antimicrobial drugs, total parenteral nutrition (TPN), or fluid replacement therapy).

Posttreatment care

- Administer medications as ordered.
- Provide comfort measures.
- Observe urine drainage for pus and blood; report these findings.
- Maintain patency of drainage catheters as ordered and report urine leakage from the drain or suture line.

GENITOURINARY CARE

TYPES OF PERMANENT URINARY DIVERSION

The steps involved in creating an ileal conduit or a continent urinary diversion are described here.

Ileal conduit

A short segment of the ileum is excised, and the intestine is reanastomosed. One end of the excised section is closed, and the ureters are dissected from the bladder and anastomosed to the ileal segment, as shown below. The open end of the ileal segment is brought out to the abdominal wall as a stoma. Urine will now pass through this conduit and out the opening in the abdomen.

Continent urinary diversion

A tube is formed from part of the ascending colon and ileum. One end of the tube is brought to the skin to form the stoma, as shown below. At the internal end of this tube, a nipple valve is constructed so urine won't drain out unless a catheter is inserted through the stoma into the newly formed bladder pouch. The urethral neck is sutured closed.

Another type of continent urinary diversion (not pictured here) is "hooked" back to the urethra, obviating the need for a stoma.

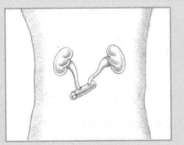
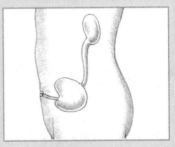

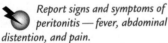
Report signs and symptoms of peritonitis — fever, abdominal distention, and pain.

■ Perform surgical wound care and dressing changes as ordered.
■ Continue I.V. replacement therapy and TPN.
■ Provide emotional support.

Monitoring

■ Vital signs
■ Intake and output
■ Surgical wound and dressings
■ Stoma and peristomal skin
■ Drainage
■ Urine characteristics
■ Abnormal bleeding
■ Complications and infection
■ Bowel sounds

PATIENT TEACHING

Be sure to cover:
■ medications and adverse reactions
■ signs and symptoms of infection
■ complications
■ when to notify the physician
■ stoma care and abnormal changes
■ with a continent internal ileal reservoir, pouch drainage tube care until it's removed (usually 3 weeks)
■ prescribed activity restrictions
■ follow-up care
■ sexual counseling as needed
■ referrals to support groups.

PROCEDURES AND EQUIPMENT

SETUP FOR CONTINUOUS BLADDER IRRIGATION

In continuous bladder irrigation, a triple-lumen catheter allows irrigating solution to flow into the bladder through one lumen and flow out through another, as shown in the inset. The third lumen is used to inflate the balloon that holds the catheter in place.

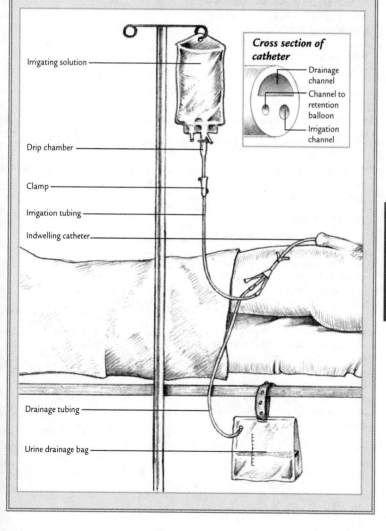

Irrigating solution

Drip chamber

Clamp

Irrigation tubing

Indwelling catheter

Drainage tubing

Urine drainage bag

Cross section of catheter

Drainage channel

Channel to retention balloon

Irrigation channel

GENITOURINARY CARE

Taping a Nephrostomy Tube

To tape a nephrostomy tube directly to the skin, cut a wide piece of hypoallergenic adhesive tape twice lengthwise to its midpoint.

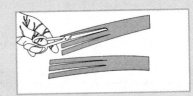

Apply the uncut end of the tape to the skin so that the midpoint meets the tube. Wrap the middle strip around the tube in a spiral fashion. Tape the other two strips to the patient's skin on both sides of the tube.

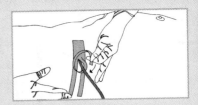

Comparing Peritoneal Dialysis Catheters

The first step in any type of peritoneal dialysis is the insertion of a catheter to allow instillation of dialyzing solution. The physician may insert one of the three different catheters described here.

Tenckhoff catheter

To implant a Tenckhoff catheter, the physician inserts the first 6¾″ (17.1 cm) of the catheter into the patient's abdomen. The next 2¾″ (7-cm) segment, which may have a Dacron cuff at one or both ends, is imbedded subcutaneously. Within a few days after insertion, the patient's tissues grow around the cuffs, forming a tight barrier against bacterial infiltration. The remaining 3⅞″ (9.8 cm) of the catheter extends outside of the abdomen and is equipped with a metal adapter at the tip that connects to dialyzer tubing.

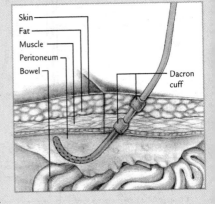

Skin — Fat — Muscle — Peritoneum — Bowel — Dacron cuff

For greater security, repeat this step with a second piece of tape, applying it in the reverse direction. You may also apply two more strips of tape perpendicular to and over the first two pieces.

Always apply another strip of tape lower down on the tube in the direction of the drainage tube to further anchor the tube. Don't put tension on sutures that prevent tube distention.

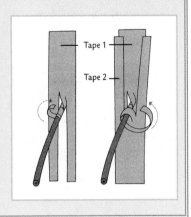

Flanged collar catheter

To insert a flanged collar catheter, the physician positions the collar just below the dermis so that the device extends through the abdominal wall. He keeps the distal end of the cuff from extending into the peritoneum, where it could cause adhesions.

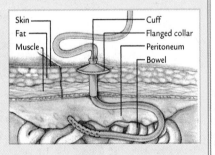

Column disk peritoneal catheter

To insert a column disk peritoneal catheter (CDPC), the physician rolls up the flexible disk section of the implant, inserts it into the peritoneal cavity, and retracts it against the abdominal wall. The implants's first cuff rests just outside the peritoneal membrane, and its second cuff rests just under the skin. Because the CDPC

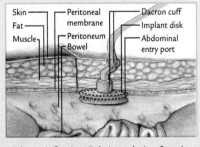

doesn't float freely in the peritoneal cavity, it keeps inflowing dialyzing solution from being directed at the sensitive organs, which increases patient comfort during dialysis.

HEMODIALYSIS ACCESS SITES

Hemodialysis requires vascular access. The site and type of access may vary, depending on the expected duration of dialysis, the surgeon's preference, and the patient's condition.

Subclavian vein catheterization

Using the Seldinger technique, the physician or surgeon inserts an introducer needle into the subclavian vein. He then inserts a guidewire through the introducer needle and removes the needle. Using the guidewire, he then threads a 5″ to 12″ (12.5 to 30.5 cm) plastic or Teflon catheter with a Y-hub into the patient's vein.

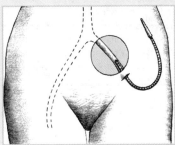

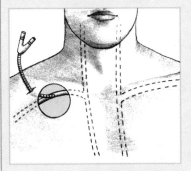

Femoral vein catheterization

Using the Seldinger technique, the physician or surgeon inserts an introducer needle into the right or left femoral vein. He then inserts a guidewire through the introducer needle and removes the needle. Using the guidewire, he then threads a 5″ to 12″ (12.5 to 30.5 cm) plastic or Teflon catheter with a Y-hub or two catheters, one for inflow and another, placed about ½″ (1.5 cm) distal to the first, for outflow.

Arteriovenous fistula

To create a fistula, the surgeon makes an incision in the patient's wrist or lower forearm, then a small incision in the side of an artery and another in a side of a vein. He then sutures the edges of the incisions together to make a common opening approximately 1″ to 3″ (2.5 to 7.5 cm) long.

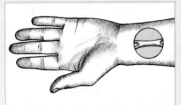

GENITOURINARY CARE

Arteriovenous shunt

To create a shunt, the surgeon makes an incision in the patient's wrist, lower forearm, or (rarely) ankle. He then inserts a 6″ to 10″ (15 to 25.5 cm) transparent Silastic cannula into an artery and another into a vein. Finally, he tunnels the cannulas out through incisions and joins them with a piece of Teflon tubing. .

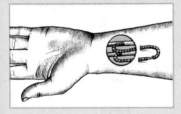

Arteriovenous graft

To create a graft, the surgeon makes an incision in the patient's forearm, upper arm, or thigh. He then tunnels a natural or synthetic graft under the skin and sutures the distal end to an artery and the proximal end to a vein.

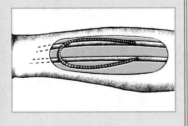

SETUP FOR PERITONEAL DIALYSIS

The illustration below shows the proper setup for peritoneal dialysis.

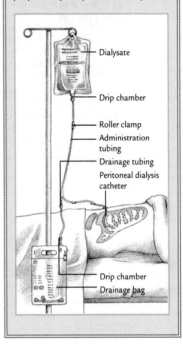

Dialysate

Drip chamber

Roller clamp

Administration tubing

Drainage tubing

Peritoneal dialysis catheter

Drip chamber

Drainage bag

COMMON SETUPS FOR CRRT

Continuous renal replacement therapy (CRRT) is used to treat patients with acute renal failure. Unlike the more traditional intermittent hemodialysis (IHD), CRRT is administered around the clock, providing patients with continuous therapy and sparing them the destabilizing hemodynamic and electrolyte changes characteristic of IHD. Illustrated here are setups for two common types of CRRT.

Continuous arteriovenous hemofiltration

In continuous arteriovenous hemofiltration (CAVH), as shown below, the physician inserts two large-bore, single-lumen catheters. One catheter is inserted into an artery — most commonly, the femoral artery. The other catheter is inserted into a vein, usually the femoral, subclavian, or internal jugular vein. During CAVH, the patient's arterial blood pressure serves as a natural pump, driving blood through the *arterial* line. A hemofilter removes water and toxic solutes (ultrafiltrate) from the blood. Replacement fluid is infused into a port on the arterial side. This same port can be used to infuse heparin. The *venous* line carries the replacement fluid and purified blood to the patient.

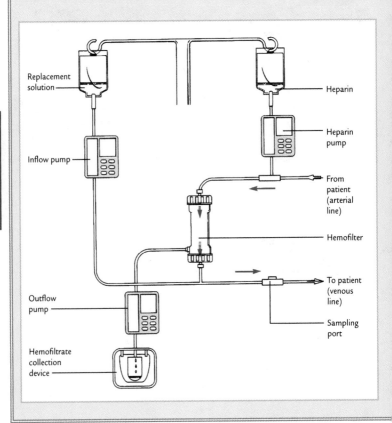

Continuous venovenous hemofiltration

With continuous venovenous hemofiltration, as shown below, the physician inserts a special double-lumen catheter into a large vein, commonly the subclavian, femoral, or internal jugular vein. Because the catheter is in a vein, an external pump is used to move blood through the system. The patient's venous blood moves through the *arterial* lumen to the pump, which pushes it through the cathe-ter to the hemofilter. Here, water and toxic solutes (ultrafiltrate) are removed and the blood drains into a collection device. Blood cells aren't removed because they are too large to pass through the filter. As the blood exits the hemofilter, it's moved through the pump's *venous* lumen back to the patient. Several pump components provide safety mechanisms. Pressure monitors maintain the flow of blood through the circuit at a constant rate. An air detector traps air bubbles before the blood returns to the patient. A venous trap collects any clots. A blood-leak detector signals when blood is found in the ultrafiltrate; a venous clamp operates if air is detected in the circuit or if there's any disconnection in the blood line.

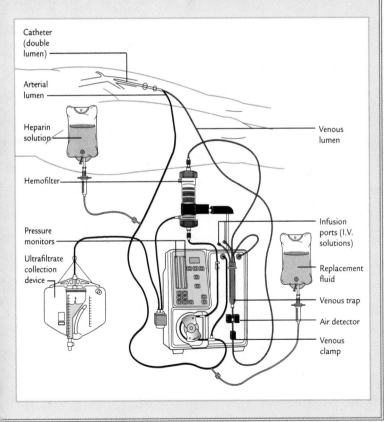

PREVENTING COMPLICATIONS OF CRRT

Measures to avoid complications during continuous renal replacement therapy (CRRT) are listed below.

Complication	Interventions
Hypotension	■ Monitor blood pressure. ■ Temporarily decrease the blood pump's speed for transient hypotension. ■ Increase the vasopressor support.
Hypothermia	■ Use an inline fluid warmer placed on the blood return line to the patient or an external warming blanket.
Fluid and electrolyte imbalances	■ Monitor the patient's fluid levels every 4 to 6 hours. ■ Monitor the patient's sodium, lactate, potassium, and calcium levels and replace as necessary.
Acid-base imbalances	■ Monitor the patient's bicarbonate and arterial blood gas levels.
Air embolism	■ Observe for air in the system. ■ Use luer-lock devices on catheter openings.
Hemorrhage	■ Check all connections and keep the dialysis line visible.
Infection	■ Perform sterile dressing changes.

DRUGS

COMMONLY USED DRUGS FOR RENAL DISORDERS

Drug	Indication	Adverse reactions	Special considerations
ADRENERGIC AGENT			
Dopamine (Intropin)	■ Low dose (less than 5 mcg/kg/min) dopamine infusions used to increase renal and mesenteric perfusion in patients with renal failure	■ Tachycardia, palpitations, angina, conduction abnormalities, ventricular arrhythmias, hypotension, hypertension, nausea and vomiting	■ Monitor cardiac rhythm ■ Correct hypovolemia before starting dopamine infusion ■ Administer I.V. infusion on infusion devise to control flow ■ Don't mix other drugs with dopamine infusion ■ Administer into a large vein to prevent the possibility of extravasations ■ If extravasation occurs, stop the infusion and infiltrate the site with phentolamine

COMMONLY USED DRUGS
FOR RENAL DISORDERS *(continued)*

Drug	Indication	Adverse reactions	Special considerations

ALKALINIZING AGENT

Drug	Indication	Adverse reactions	Special considerations
Sodium bicarbonate (Neut)	■ Treatment of metabolic acidosis in patients with renal failure	■ Metabolic alkalosis, hypernatremia, local pain and irritation at injection site	■ Use with caution in patients with heart failure or renal insufficiency, or those receiving corticosteroids ■ Assess cardiopulmonary status ■ Monitor for metabolic alkalosis and electrolyte imbalance, especially hypocalcemia and hypokalemia ■ Monitor I.V. site for irritation and infiltration (extravasation may cause tissue damage and necrosis)

LOOP DIURETICS

Drug	Indication	Adverse reactions	Special considerations
Bumetanide (Bumex); **furosemide** (Lasix); **torsemide** (Demadex)	■ Inhibit sodium reabsorption in renal tubule and promote diuresis and manage edema	■ Dizziness, muscle cramps, hypotension, headache, fluid and electrolyte imbalance (hypokalemia, hypochloremia, and hyponatremia), electrocardiogram (ECG) changes, chest pain, renal failure	■ Monitor for fluid and electrolyte imbalance ■ Monitor for cardiac arrhythmias, especially ventricular ■ Avoid in patients with sulfonamide hypersensitivity ■ Contraindicated in anuria ■ Ototoxicity may result with rapid I.V. administration of high dosages

SULFONATE CATION-EXCHANGE RESIN

Drug	Indication	Adverse reactions	Special considerations
Sodium polystyrene sulfonate (Kayexalate)	■ Treatment of hyperkalemia	■ GI irritation, anorexia, nausea, vomiting, constipation, hypokalemia, hypocalcemia, hypernatremia (due to cation exchange of sodium for potassium)	■ Monitor for electrolyte imbalance, hypokalemia, hypocalcemia ■ Monitor for ECG changes (flat, inverted T wave, prominent U wave) and ventricular arrhythmias ■ For oral administration, mix resin with water or sorbitol, never orange juice because of high potassium content ■ Monitor elderly patients for constipation and fecal impaction ■ Use cautiously in patients who require sodium restriction, such as patients with heart failure or those with hypertension, to prevent sodium overload

DRUGS AND ACUTE RENAL FAILURE

Many drugs are eliminated by the kidneys. Therefore, when your patient has acute renal failure, drug dosages may need to be adjusted to avoid overburdening the patient's already compromised kidney function. Highlighted here are some commonly used drugs that require a reduction in dosage and some examples of drugs that should be avoided for the patient with acute renal failure.

Drugs requiring reduced dosage may include:
■ angiotensin-converting enzyme inhibitors
■ cefazolin
■ ciprofloxacin
■ digoxin
■ histamine-2-receptor antagonists, such as cimetidine, famotidine, nizatidine, and ranitidine
■ magnesium-containing antacids and laxatives
■ meperidine

■ penicillins
■ phenobarbital
■ sulfonamides.

The following drugs should be avoided in patients with acute renal failure:
■ amikacin and other aminoglycosides, such as gentamicin, kanamycin, neomycin (oral form), netilmicin, tobramycin (parenteral form), because of the increased risk of nephrotoxicity
■ amiloride and other potassium-sparing diuretics such as spironolactone because of the increased risk of potassium retention, which compounds and increases the patient's risk of life-threatening hyperkalemia
■ cisplatin, because of the increased risk of nephrotoxicity
■ lithium carbonate, because of the increased risk of nephrotoxicity as well as drug toxicity. (Renal dysfunction increases the plasma half-life of the drug, predisposing the patient to possible toxic drug levels.)

10

NEUROLOGIC CARE

NEUROLOGIC SYSTEM: NORMAL FINDINGS

Inspection
- Patient can shrug his shoulders, a sign of an adequately functioning cranial nerve XI (accessory nerve).
- Pupils are equal, round, and reactive to light, a test of cranial nerves II and III.
- Eyes move freely and in a coordinated manner, a sign of adequately functioning cranial nerves III, IV, and VI.
- The lids of both eyes close when you stroke each cornea with a wisp of cotton, a test of cranial nerve V (trigeminal nerve).
- Patient can identify familiar odors, a test of cranial nerve I (olfactory nerve).
- Patient can hear a whispered voice, a test of cranial nerve VIII (acoustic nerve).
- Patient can purse his lips and puff out his cheeks, a sign of an adequately functioning cranial nerve VII (facial nerve).
- Tongue moves easily and without tremor, a sign of a properly functioning cranial nerve XII (hypoglossal nerve).

- Voice is clear and strong; uvula moves upward when the patient says "ah"; gag reflex occurs when the tongue blade touches the posterior pharynx, signs of properly functioning cranial nerves IX and X.
- No involuntary movements are detectable.
- Gait is smooth.
- Patient is oriented to himself, other people, place, and time.
- Memory and attention span are intact.
- Deep tendon reflexes are intact.

Palpation
- Strength in the facial muscles is symmetrical, a sign of adequately functioning cranial nerves V and VII (trigeminal and facial nerves).
- Muscle tone and strength are adequate.

REVIEWING CRANIAL NERVES

The cranial nerves have either sensory or motor function or both. They're assigned Roman numerals and are written: CN I, CN II, CN III, and so forth. The function of each cranial nerve is listed below.

- *CN I: Olfactory*
Smell
- *CN II: Optic*
Vision
- *CN III: Oculomotor*
Most eye movement, pupillary constriction, upper eyelid elevation

- *CN IV: Trochlear*
Downward and inward eye movement
- *CN V: Trigeminal*
Chewing, corneal reflex, face and scalp sensations
- *CN VI: Abducens*
Lateral eye movement

ASSESSING THE PUPILS

Pupillary changes can signal different conditions. Use these illustrations and lists of causes to help you detect problems.

Bilaterally equal and reactive

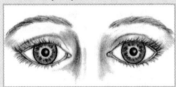

- Normal

Unilateral, dilated (4 mm), fixed, and nonreactive

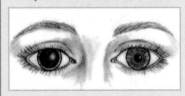

- Uncal herniation with oculomotor nerve damage
- Brain stem compression from an expanding lesion or an aneurysm

- Increased intracranial pressure
- Tentorial herniation
- Head trauma with subsequent subdural or epidural hematoma
- Normal in some people

Bilateral, dilated (4 mm), fixed, and nonreactive

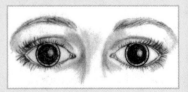

- Severe midbrain damage
- Cardiopulmonary arrest (hypoxia)
- Anticholinergic poisoning

- *CN VII: Facial*
Expressions in forehead, eye, and mouth; taste
- *CN VIII: Acoustic*
Hearing and balance
- *CN IX: Glossopharyngeal*
Swallowing, salivating, and taste
- *CN X: Vagus*

Swallowing, gag reflex, talking; sensations of throat, larynx, and abdominal viscera; activities of thoracic and abdominal viscera, such as heart rate and peristalsis
- *CN XI: Spinal accessory*
Shoulder movement and head rotation
- *CN XII: Hypoglossal*
Tongue movement

Bilateral, midsized (2 mm), fixed and nonreactive

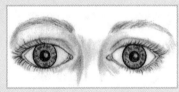

- Midbrain involvement caused by edema, hemorrhage, infarctions, lacerations, contusions

Unilateral, small (1.5 mm), and nonreactive

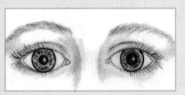

- Disruption of sympathetic nerve supply to the head caused by spinal cord lesion above T1

Bilateral, pinpoint (less than 1 mm), and usually nonreactive

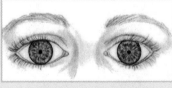

- Lesion of pons, usually after hemorrhage, leading to blocked sympathetic impulses
- Opiates, such as morphine (pupils may be reactive)

GRADING PUPIL SIZE

To ensure accurate evaluation of pupillary size, compare the patient's pupils to this scale. Keep in mind that maximum constriction may be less than 1 mm and maximum dilation greater than 9 mm.

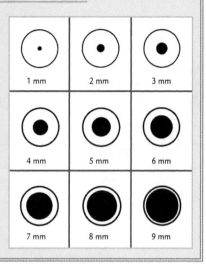

VISUAL FIELD DEFECTS

Here are some examples of visual field defects. The black areas represent visual loss.

Left	Right
A: Blindness of right eye	
B: Bitemporal hemianopsia, or loss of half the visual field	
C: Left homonymous hemianopsia	
D: Left homonymous hemianopsia, superior quadrant	

ASSESSING DEEP TENDON REFLEXES

During a neurologic examination, you assess the patient's deep tendon reflexes—that is, the biceps, triceps, brachioradialis, patellar or quadriceps, and Achilles reflexes.

Biceps reflex

Position the patient's arm so his elbow is flexed at a 45-degree angle and his arm is relaxed. Place your thumb or index finger over the biceps tendon and your remaining fingers loosely over the triceps muscle. Strike your finger with the pointed end of the reflex hammer, and watch and feel for the contraction of the biceps muscle and flexion of the forearm.

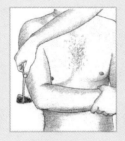

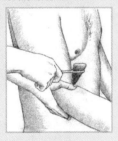

Triceps reflex

Have the patient adduct his arm and place his forearm across his chest. Strike the triceps tendon about 2″ (5 cm) above the olecranon process on the extensor surface of the upper arm. Watch for contraction of the triceps muscle and extension of the forearm.

Brachioradialis reflex

Ask the patient to rest the ulnar surface of his hand on his knee with the elbow partially flexed. Strike the radius, and watch for supination of the hand and flexion of the forearm at the elbow.

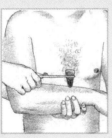

Patellar reflex

Have the patient sit with his legs dangling freely. If he can't sit up, flex his knee at a 45-degree angle, and place your nondominant hand behind it for support. Strike the

patellar tendon just below the patella, and look for contraction of the quadriceps muscle in the thigh with extension of the leg.

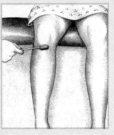

Achilles reflex

Have the patient flex his foot. Then support the plantar surface. Strike the Achilles tendon, and watch for plantar flexion of the foot at the ankle.

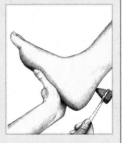

HOW TO ELICIT BABINSKI'S REFLEX

To elicit Babinski's reflex, stroke the lateral aspect of the sole of the patient's foot with your thumbnail or another moderately sharp object. Normally, this elicits flexion of all toes (a negative Babinski's reflex), as shown at right. In a positive Babinski's reflex, the great toe dorsiflexes and the other toes fan out, as shown far right.

Normal toe flexion

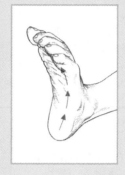

Positive Babinski's reflex

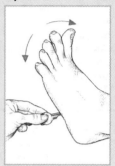

ASSESSING BRUDZINSKI'S AND KERNIG'S SIGNS

When positive, Brudzinski's and Kernig's signs indicate meningeal irritation. Follow these guidelines to test for these two signs.

Brudzinski's sign

With the patient in the supine position, place your hand under his neck and flex it forward, chin to chest. This test is positive if he flexes his ankles, knees, and hips bilaterally. In addition, the patient typically complains of pain when the neck is flexed.

Brudzinski's sign

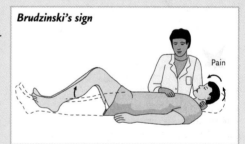

Kernig's sign

With the patient in the supine position, flex his hip and knee to form a 90-degree angle. Next, attempt to extend this leg. If he exhibits pain, resistance to extension, and spasm, the test is positive.

Kernig's sign

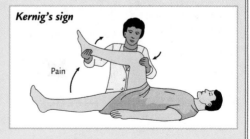

STAGES OF ALTERED AROUSAL

This chart highlights the six levels or stages of altered arousal and their manifestations..

Stage	Manifestations
Confusion	■ Loss of ability to think rapidly and clearly ■ Impaired judgment and decision making
Disorientation	■ Beginning loss of consciousness ■ Disorientation to time progressing to include disorientation to place ■ Impaired memory ■ Lack of recognition of self (last to go)
Lethargy	■ Limited spontaneous movement or speech ■ Easily aroused by normal speech or touch ■ Possible disorientation to time, place, or person
Obtundation	■ Mild to moderate reduction in arousal ■ Limited responsiveness to environment ■ Ability to fall asleep easily in absence of verbal or tactile stimulation from others ■ Minimum response to questions
Stupor	■ State of deep sleep or unresponsiveness ■ Arousable with difficulty (motor or verbal response only to vigorous and repeated stimulation) ■ Withdrawal or grabbing response to stimulation
Coma	■ Lack of motor or verbal response to external environment or any stimuli ■ No response to noxious stimuli such as deep pain ■ Can't be aroused by any stimulus

NEUROLOGIC CARE

GLASGOW COMA SCALE

The Glasgow Coma Scale provides an easy way to describe the patient's baseline neurologic status. It can also help detect neurologic changes.

A decreased score in one or more categories may signal an impending neurologic crisis. The best response is scored.

Test	Score	Patient's response
EYE OPENING		
Spontaneously	4	Opens eyes spontaneously
To speech	3	Opens eyes to verbal command
To pain	2	Opens eyes to painful stimulus
None	1	Doesn't open eyes in response to stimulus
MOTOR RESPONSE		
Obeys	6	Reacts to verbal command
Localizes	5	Identifies localized pain
Withdraws	4	Flexes and withdraws from painful stimulus
Abnormal flexion	3	Assumes a decorticate posture
Abnormal extension	2	Assumes a decerebrate posture
None	1	No response; just lies flaccid
VERBAL RESPONSE		
Oriented	5	Is oriented and converses
Confused	4	Is disoriented and confused
Inappropriate words	3	Replies randomly with incorrect words
Incomprehensible	2	Moans or screams
None	1	No response
Total score		

COMPARING DECEREBRATE AND DECORTICATE POSTURES

Decerebrate posture results from damage to the upper brain stem. In this posture, the arms are adducted and extended, with the wrists pronated and the fingers flexed. The legs are stiffly extended, with plantar flexion of the feet.

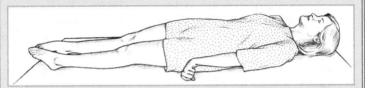

Decorticate posture results from damage to one or both corticospinal tracts. In this posture, the arms are adducted and flexed, with the wrists and fingers flexed on the chest. The legs are stiffly extended and internally rotated, with plantar flexion of the feet.

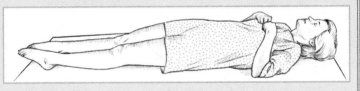

NEUROLOGIC SYSTEM: INTERPRETING YOUR FINDINGS

Your assessment will reveal a group of findings that may lead you to suspect a particular disorder. This chart shows some common groups of findings for signs and symptoms related to the neurologic system, along with their probable causes.

Sign or symptom and findings	Probable cause
APHASIA	
■ Wernicke's, Broca's, or global aphasia ■ Decreased level of consciousness (LOC) ■ Right-sided hemiparesis ■ Homonymous hemianopsia ■ Paresthesia and loss of sensation	Stroke

(continued)

NEUROLOGIC CARE

NEUROLOGIC SYSTEM:
INTERPRETING YOUR FINDINGS *(continued)*

Sign or symptom and findings	Probable cause
APHASIA *(continued)*	
■ Any type of aphasia occurring suddenly, may be transient or permanent ■ Blurred or double vision ■ Headache ■ Cerebrospinal otorrhea and rhinorrhea ■ Disorientation ■ Behavioral changes ■ Signs of increased intracranial pressure (ICP)	Head trauma
■ Any type of aphasia occurring suddenly and resolving within 24 hours ■ Transient hemiparesis ■ Hemianopsia ■ Paresthesia ■ Dizziness and confusion	Transient ischemic attack
DECREASED LOC	
■ Slowly decreasing LOC, from lethargy to coma ■ Apathy, behavior changes ■ Memory loss ■ Decreased attention span ■ Morning headache ■ Sensorimotor disturbances	Brain tumor
■ Slowly decreasing LOC, from lethargy to possible coma ■ Malaise ■ Tachycardia ■ Tachypnea ■ Orthostatic hypotension ■ Skin is hot, flushed, and diaphoretic	Heatstroke
■ Lethargy progressing to coma ■ Confusion, anxiety, and restlessness ■ Hypotension ■ Tachycardia ■ Weak pulse with narrowing pulse pressure ■ Dyspnea ■ Oliguria ■ Cool, clammy skin	Shock

NEUROLOGIC SYSTEM:
INTERPRETING YOUR FINDINGS *(continued)*

Sign or symptom and findings	Probable cause

HEADACHE

■ Excruciating headache ■ Acute eye pain ■ Blurred vision ■ Halo vision ■ Nausea and vomiting ■ Moderately dilated, fixed pupil	Acute angle-closure glaucoma
■ Slightly throbbing occipital headache on awakening that decreases in severity during the day ■ Atrial gallop ■ Restlessness ■ Blurred vision ■ Nausea and vomiting	Hypertension
■ Severe generalized or frontal headache beginning suddenly ■ Stabbing retro-orbital pain ■ Weakness, diffuse myalgia ■ Fever, chills ■ Coughing ■ Rhinorrhea	Influenza

PARALYSIS

■ Transient, unilateral, facial muscle paralysis, with sagging muscles and failure of eyelid closure ■ Increased tearing ■ Diminished or absent corneal reflex	Bell's palsy
■ Transient paralysis that gradually becomes more persistent ■ May include weak eye closure, ptosis, diplopia, lack of facial mobility, and dysphagia ■ Neck muscle weakness ■ Possible respiratory distress	Myasthenia gravis
■ Permanent spastic paralysis below the level of back injury ■ Absent reflexes may return	Spinal cord injury

NEUROLOGIC CARE

DIAGNOSTIC TESTS

CEREBRAL ANGIOGRAPHY

Overview

■ Radiographic examination of the cerebral vasculature after injection of intra-arterial contrast medium
■ Most common approach: the femoral artery; other approaches include a direct carotid or vertebral artery puncture, or the brachial, axillary, or subclavian artery
■ Indicated with suspected abnormalities of the cerebral vasculature, commonly suggested by other imaging studies

PURPOSE

■ To detect cerebrovascular abnormalities, such as aneurysm or arteriovenous malformation, thrombosis, narrowing, or occlusion
■ To evaluate vascular displacement caused by tumor, hematoma, edema, herniation, vasospasm, increased intracranial pressure, or hydrocephalus
■ To locate clips applied to blood vessels during surgery and to evaluate the postoperative status of such vessels
■ To evaluate the presence and degree of carotid artery disease

PATIENT PREPARATION

■ Make sure the patient has signed an appropriate consent form.
■ Note and report all allergies.
■ Have the patient fast for 8 to 10 hours before the test.
■ Tell the patient his head will be immobilized and he'll need to lie still.
■ A local anesthetic will be administered.

■ Warn the patient that nausea, warmth, or burning may occur with contrast injection.
■ Initiate an I.V. access and administer I.V. fluids as ordered.
■ Administer a sedative as ordered.
■ Have the patient void.
■ Document baseline vital signs and neurologic assessment data.

Teaching points

Be sure to cover:
■ the test's purpose and how it's done
■ who will perform the test and where
■ that the test takes 2 to 4 hours.

POSTPROCEDURE CARE

■ Enforce bed rest and apply an ice bag as ordered.
■ If active bleeding or expanding hematoma occurs, apply firm pressure to the puncture site and inform the physician immediately.
■ Ensure adequate hydration to assist in clearing the contrast material through the kidneys.
■ Provide analgesia as ordered.
■ Resume usual diet as ordered.

Monitoring

■ Vital signs
■ Intake and output
■ Neurovascular status of extremity distal to the access site
■ Neurologic and respiratory status
■ Puncture site for active bleeding or expanding hematoma

If the femoral approach was used, keep the involved leg straight at the hip and check pulses distal to the site as ordered. Check the temperature, color, and sensation of the affected leg because thrombosis, embolism, or hematoma can occlude distal blood flow.

If the carotid artery was used as the access site, watch for dysphagia or respiratory distress, which can result from hematoma or edema. Also watch for disorientation, weakness, or numbness in the extremities (signs of neurovascular compromise) and for arterial spasms, which produce symptoms of transient ischemic attacks (TIAs). Notify the physician immediately if abnormal signs develop.

If the brachial artery was used, keep the arm straight at the elbow and assess distal pulses (radial and ulnar) as ordered. Avoid venipuncture and blood pressures in the affected arm. Observe the extremity for changes in color, temperature, or sensation. If it becomes pale, cool, or numb, notify the physician immediately.

PRECAUTIONS
■ Check for allergy to iodine or other contrast media; notify the physician if present.
■ Cerebral angiography is contraindicated in patients with severe renal or thyroid disease, recent anticoagulation therapy, and recent thrombotic or embolic events.
■ Head movement affects the clarity of the angiographic images.

COMPLICATIONS
■ Adverse reaction to contrast media
■ Embolism
■ Bleeding
■ Infection
■ Hematoma at the puncture site
■ Vasospasm
■ Thrombosis
■ TIA or stroke

Interpretation

NORMAL FINDINGS
■ Cerebral vasculature is normal.

■ During the arterial phase of perfusion, the contrast medium fills and opacifies superficial and deep arteries and arterioles.
■ During the venous phase, the contrast medium opacifies superficial and deep veins.

ABNORMAL RESULTS
■ Changes in the caliber of vessel lumina suggest vascular disease.
■ Vessel displacement suggests a possible tumor.

COMPUTED TOMOGRAPHY, INTRACRANIAL

Overview

■ Provides a series of tomograms, translated by a computer and displayed on an oscilloscope screen; contrast enhancement commonly used
■ Provides layers of cross-sectional images of the brain
■ Reconstructs cross-sectional, horizontal, sagittal, and coronal-plane images
■ Also known as computed tomography (CT) of the brain or head

PURPOSE
■ To diagnose intracranial lesions and abnormalities
■ To monitor effects of surgery, radiotherapy, or chemotherapy in treatment of intracranial tumors
■ To guide cranial surgery
■ To assess focal neurologic abnormalities
■ To evaluate suspected head injury such as subdural hematoma

PATIENT PREPARATION
■ Make sure the patient has signed an appropriate consent form.

■ Note and report all allergies.

■ Explain restriction of food and fluids with contrast enhancement as ordered.

■ Stress the importance of remaining still during the test because movement can limit test accuracy.

■ Warn that minimal discomfort may be experienced because of lying still and immobilizing the head.

■ Warn about transient discomfort from the needle puncture and a warm or flushed feeling if an I.V. contrast medium is used.

■ Caution that clacking sounds are heard as the head of the table is moved into the scanner, which rotates around the patient's head.

Teaching points

Be sure to cover:
■ the test's purpose and how it's done
■ who will perform the test and where
■ that the test takes 15 to 30 minutes.

POSTPROCEDURE CARE

■ No specific posttest care is necessary if the test was performed without contrast enhancement.

■ If a contrast agent was used, watch for delayed adverse reactions.

■ Resume the usual diet and medications unless otherwise ordered.

PRECAUTIONS

■ Intracranial CT isn't usually recommended during pregnancy because of potential risk to the fetus.

■ Check the patient's history for hypersensitivity to shellfish, iodine, or iodinated contrast media, and document such reactions on the patient's chart.

■ Inform the physician of any sensitivities because prophylactic medications may be ordered or because contrast enhancement may not be used.

COMPLICATIONS

■ Adverse reaction to iodinated contrast media

Interpretation

NORMAL FINDINGS

■ Brain matter appears in shades of gray.

■ Ventricular and subarachnoid cerebrospinal fluid appears black.

ABNORMAL RESULTS

■ Enlarged ventricles with large sulci suggest cerebral atrophy.

In children, enlargement of the fourth ventricle usually indicates hydrocephalus.

■ Areas of marked generalized lucency suggest cerebral edema.

■ Cerebral vessels appearing with slightly increased density suggest possible arteriovenous malformation.

■ Areas of altered density or displaced vasculature or other structures may indicate:
– intracranial tumors
– intracranial hematoma
– cerebral atrophy, infarction, edema
– congenital anomalies such as hydrocephalus.

If test results are abnormal, provide psychological support to the patient. If the etiology of the abnormality indicates an emergency, the patient will likely need preparation for a surgical procedure.

ELECTROENCEPH-ALOGRAPHY

Overview

■ Involves recording a portion of the brain's electrical activity through electrodes attached to the scalp

■ Electrical impulses are transmitted to electroencephalograph, magnified, and recorded as brain waves

■ Intracranial electrodes are sometimes surgically implanted to record EEG changes for localization of seizure focus

PURPOSE

■ To determine the presence and type of epilepsy

■ To aid diagnosis of intracranial lesions

■ To evaluate brain activity in metabolic disease, head injury, meningitis, encephalitis, and psychological disorders

■ To help confirm brain death

PATIENT PREPARATION

■ Make sure the patient has signed an appropriate consent form.

■ Note and report all allergies.

■ Wash and dry the patient's hair to remove hair sprays, creams, or oils.

■ Withhold tranquilizers, barbiturates, and other sedatives for 24 to 48 hours before the test as ordered.

■ Minimize sleep (4 to 5 hours) the night before the study if ordered.

■ If a sleep EEG is ordered, administer a sedative to promote sleep during the test as ordered.

■ There's no need to restrict food and fluids before the test, but stimulants such as caffeine-containing beverages, chocolate, and smoking aren't permitted for 8 hours before the study.

■ Provide reassurance that the electrodes won't shock the patient.

■ If needle electrodes are used, warn the patient that he might feel pricking sensations during insertion.

Teaching points

Be sure to cover:

■ the test's purpose and how it's done

■ who will perform the test and where

■ that the test takes about 1 hour.

POSTPROCEDURE CARE

■ Resume medications as ordered.

■ Provide a safe environment.

■ Maintain seizure precautions.

■ Help the patient remove electrode paste from his hair.

■ If brain death is confirmed, provide emotional support for the family.

Monitoring

■ Seizure activity

■ Adverse effects of sedation if used

PRECAUTIONS

■ Skipping the meal before the test can cause hypoglycemia and alter brain wave patterns.

■ Anticonvulsants, tranquilizers, barbiturates, and other sedatives can interfere with the accuracy of test results.

COMPLICATIONS

■ Adverse effects of sedation

■ Possible seizure activity

Interpretation

NORMAL FINDINGS

■ Alpha waves:

– occur at frequencies of 8 to 13 cycles/second in a regular rhythm

– are present only in the waking state when the patient's eyes are closed but he's mentally alert

– usually disappear with visual activity or mental concentration

– are decreased by apprehension or anxiety

– are most prominent in the occipital leads.

■ Beta waves (13 to 30 cycles/second):

– indicate normal activity when the patient is alert with eyes open

– are seen most readily in the frontal and central regions of the brain.

■ Theta waves (4 to 7 cycles/second):

– are most common in children and young adults
– appear primarily in the parietal and temporal regions
– indicate drowsiness or emotional stress in adults.

■ Delta waves (less than 4 cycles/second):
– are seen in deep sleep stages and in serious brain dysfunction.

ABNORMAL RESULTS

■ Spikes and waves at a frequency of 3 cycles/second suggest absence seizures.

■ Multiple, high-voltage, spiked waves in both hemispheres suggest generalized tonic-clonic seizures.

■ Spiked waves in the affected temporal region suggest temporal lobe epilepsy.

■ Localized, spiked discharges suggest focal seizures:
– Slow waves (usually delta waves, but possibly unilateral beta waves) suggest intracranial lesions.
– Focal abnormalities in the injured area suggest vascular lesions.
– Generalized, diffuse, and slow brain waves suggest metabolic or inflammatory disorders or increased intracranial pressure.
– Absent EEG pattern or a "flat" tracing (except for artifacts) may indicate brain death.

ELECTROMYOGRAPHY

Overview

■ Records the electrical activity of selected skeletal muscle groups at rest and during voluntary contraction
■ Nerve conduction time often measured simultaneously
■ Also known as EMG

PURPOSE

■ To differentiate between primary muscle disorders, such as muscular dystrophies, and certain metabolic disorders
■ To identify diseases characterized by central neuronal degeneration such as amyotrophic lateral sclerosis (ALS)
■ To aid in diagnosis of neuromuscular disorders such as myasthenia gravis
■ To aid in diagnosis of radiculomyopathies

PATIENT PREPARATION

■ Make sure the patient has signed an appropriate consent form.
■ Note and report all allergies.
■ Check for and note medications that may interfere with test results (cholinergics, anticholinergics, anticoagulants, and skeletal muscle relaxants).
■ Foods and fluids aren't withheld before this test. Cigarettes, coffee, tea, and cola may be restricted for 2 to 3 hours before the test as ordered.
■ Warn the patient that he might experience some discomfort as a needle is inserted into selected muscles.

Teaching points

Be sure to cover:
■ the test's purpose and how it's done
■ who will perform the test and where
■ that the test takes at least 1 hour.

POSTPROCEDURE CARE

■ Apply warm compresses and administer analgesics as ordered for discomfort.
■ Resume medications or substances that were withheld before the test as ordered.

PRECAUTIONS
■ Electromyography may be contraindicated in patients with bleeding disorders.

Monitoring
■ Signs and symptoms of infection
■ Pain level and response to analgesics

COMPLICATIONS
■ Infection

Interpretation

NORMAL FINDINGS
■ At rest, a normal muscle exhibits minimal electrical activity.
■ During voluntary contraction, electrical activity increases markedly.
■ A sustained contraction, or one of increasing strength, produces a rapid "train" of motor unit potentials.

ABNORMAL RESULTS
■ Short (low amplitude) motor unit potentials, with frequent, irregular discharges suggest possible primary muscle disease such as muscular dystrophies.
■ Isolated and irregular motor unit potentials with increased amplitude and duration suggest possible disorders, such as ALS and peripheral nerve disorders.
■ Initially normal motor unit potentials, which progressively diminish in amplitude with continuing contractions, suggest possible myasthenia gravis.

LUMBAR PUNCTURE

Overview

■ Permits sampling of cerebral spinal fluid (CSF) for qualitative analysis

■ More common than cisternal or ventricular puncture
■ Also known as a spinal tap

PURPOSE
■ To measure CSF pressure
■ To aid diagnosis of viral or bacterial meningitis
■ To aid diagnosis of subarachnoid or intracranial hemorrhage
■ To aid diagnosis of tumors and brain abscesses
■ To aid diagnosis of neurosyphilis and chronic central nervous system infections

PATIENT PREPARATION
■ Make sure the patient has signed an appropriate consent form.
■ Note and report all allergies.
■ Restriction of food and fluids isn't necessary.

Teaching points
Be sure to cover:
■ the test's purpose and how it's done
■ who will perform the procedure and where
■ that the test takes at least 15 minutes
■ that headache is the most common adverse effect.

POSTPROCEDURE CARE
■ Keep the patient lying flat for 4 to 6 hours as ordered.
■ Inform him that he can turn from side to side.
■ Encourage and assist the patient to drink fluids.
■ Administer analgesics as ordered.

Monitoring
■ Vital signs
■ Intake and output
■ Neurologic status
■ Puncture site for redness, swelling, and drainage

NEUROLOGIC CARE

- Bleeding
- Infections

PRECAUTIONS

- Lumbar puncture is contraindicated in skin infections at the puncture site.

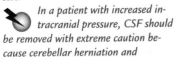 *In a patient with increased intracranial pressure, CSF should be removed with extreme caution because cerebellar herniation and medullary compression can result.*

COMPLICATIONS

- Adverse reaction to the anesthetic
- Infection
- Meningitis
- Bleeding into the spinal canal
- Leakage of CSF
- Cerebellar herniation
- Medullary compression

Interpretation

The following interpretations of CSF findings include normal findings and abnormal results.

NORMAL FINDINGS

- Pressure: 50 to 180 mm H_2O
- Appearance: clear, colorless
- Protein: 15 to 45 mg/dl
- Gamma globulin: 3% to 12% of total protein
- Glucose: 50 to 80 mg/dl
- Cell count: 0 to 5 white blood cells; no red blood cells (RBCs)
- Venereal Disease Research Laboratory (VDRL) test: nonreactive
- Chloride: 118 to 130 mEq/L
- Gram stain: no organisms

ABNORMAL RESULTS

Pressure

- Increased intracranial pressure (ICP): tumor, hemorrhage, or edema caused by trauma

- Decreased ICP: spinal subarachnoid obstruction

Appearance

- Cloudy: infection
- Xanthochromic or bloody: intracranial hemorrhage or spinal cord obstruction
- Brown, orange: increased protein levels or RBC breakdown

Protein

- Increased: tumor, trauma, diabetes mellitus, or blood in CSF
- Decreased: rapid CSF production

Gamma globulin

- Increased: demyelinating disease or Guillain-Barré syndrome

Glucose

- Increased: hyperglycemia
- Decreased: hypoglycemia, infection, or meningitis

Cell count

- Increased: meningitis, tumor, abscess, demyelinating disease
- RBCs: hemorrhage

VDRL

- Positive: neurosyphilis

Chloride

- Decreased: infected meninges

Gram stain

- Gram-positive or gram-negative organisms: bacterial meningitis

MAGNETIC RESONANCE IMAGING

Overview

■ Produces cross-sectional images of the brain and spine in multiple planes
■ Enables ability to "see through" bone and to delineate fluid-filled soft tissue
■ Magnetic resonance angiography may also be used to image the neurologic system (see *Magnetic resonance angiography: A closer look*)

PURPOSE

■ To aid diagnosis of intracranial and spinal lesions
■ To aid diagnosis of soft-tissue abnormalities
■ To detect small tumors and hemorrhages and cerebral infarction earlier than computed tomography scanning

PATIENT PREPARATION

■ Make sure the patient has signed an appropriate consent form.
■ Note and report all allergies.
■ Screen for any surgically implanted joints, pins, clips, valves, pumps, or pacemakers containing metal.
■ Remove all metallic objects from the patient.
■ Explain the need to remain still for the entire procedure.
■ Warn the patient that clicking, whirring, and thumping sounds will be heard during the procedure.
■ Advise the patient that he might receive earplugs.
■ Provide reassurance that the patient will be able to communicate at all times during the procedure.

MAGNETIC RESONANCE ANGIOGRAPHY: A CLOSER LOOK

Magnetic resonance angiography (MRA) uses magnetic resonance technology to identify and evaluate blood vessel disorders and to aid in their treatment. Although contrast material isn't necessary, a special form of I.V. contrast called gadolinium is usually given to enhance image clarity.

MRA is especially useful for evaluating intracranial arterial disease. In fact, researchers have found that when MRA is used, only patients with positive findings need a more invasive, expensive, and risky diagnostic study: cerebral arteriography.

MRA, which is a painless procedure, has no side effects and the magnetic field isn't known to cause tissue damage. Contraindications are the same as those for magnetic resonance imaging; patients with any of the following devices should avoid MRA as well: an artificial heart valve, cardiac pacemaker, implanted neurostimulator, metallic ear implant, or any metallic object within the eye socket. MRA should also be avoided if the patient has a bullet fragment or implanted vascular access device.

MRA doesn't image calcium; therefore, computed tomography angiography may be more appropriate in certain clinical situations. The image clarity of MRA is inferior to that of conventional angiography.

Teaching points

Be sure to cover:
■ the test's purpose and how it's done
■ who will perform the test and where
■ that the test takes up to 90 minutes

■ that magnetic resonance imaging (MRI) is painless and involves no exposure to radiation.

POSTPROCEDURE CARE
■ Resume normal activity as ordered.

Monitoring
■ Vital signs
■ Postural hypotension

PRECAUTIONS
■ Because of powerful magnetic fields, MRI is contraindicated in patients with pacemakers, intracranial clips, ferrous metal implants, or gunshot wounds to the head.
■ Metallic or computer-based equipment (for example, ventilators and I.V. pumps) must not enter the MRI area.
■ If the patient is claustrophobic, sedation or an open scanner may be used.

COMPLICATIONS
■ Claustrophobia
■ Postural hypotension
■ Anxiety

Interpretation

NORMAL FINDINGS
■ Brain and spinal cord structures appear distinct and sharply defined.

ABNORMAL RESULTS
■ Structural changes that increase tissue water content suggest possible cerebral edema, demyelinating disease, and pontine and cerebellar tumors.
■ Areas of demyelination (curdlike gray or gray-white areas) around the edges of ventricles suggest multiple sclerosis lesions.
■ Changes in normal anatomy suggest possible tumors.

MYELOGRAPHY

Overview

■ Combines fluoroscopy and radiography to evaluate the spinal subarachnoid space after injection of a contrast medium
■ Water-based contrast media — lighter than cerebrospinal fluid and don't need to be removed at end of study — have replaced most oil-based contrast media
■ Fluoroscopy: used to visualize flow of the contrast medium and outline of subarachnoid space

PURPOSE
■ To demonstrate lesions partially or totally blocking cerebrospinal fluid flow in the subarachnoid space (tumors and herniated intervertebral disks)
■ To detect arachnoiditis, spinal nerve root injury, or tumors in the posterior fossa of the skull

PATIENT PREPARATION
■ Make sure the patient has signed an appropriate consent form.
■ Note and report all allergies.
■ Check the patient's history for hypersensitivity to iodine and iodine-containing substances (such as shellfish) and contrast media.
■ Notify the radiologist if there's a history of epilepsy or antidepressant or phenothiazine use.

Phenothiazines in combination with metrizamide given during myelography increases the risk of toxicity.
■ Administer a sedative and anticholinergic as ordered.
■ Explain the need to restrict food and fluids before the test as ordered.

■ Warn the patient that transient burning may be felt as the contrast medium is injected and that he may experience flushing and warmth, a headache, a salty taste, or nausea and vomiting.

Teaching points

Be sure to cover:
■ the test's purpose and how it's done
■ who will perform the test and where
■ that the test takes at least 1 hour.

POSTPROCEDURE CARE
■ Determine the type of contrast medium used for the test.
■ If an oil-based contrast agent was used, keep the patient flat in bed for 8 to 12 hours.
■ If a water-based contrast agent was used, elevate the head of the bed for 6 to 8 hours.
■ Maintain bed rest as ordered.
■ Encourage oral fluid intake to assist the kidneys in eliminating the contrast media.
■ Notify the physician if the patient fails to void within 8 hours.
■ Resume a usual diet and activities the day after the test as ordered.

If a water-based contrast is used, care must be taken that the large dye load doesn't reach the surface of the brain; to prevent this, the patient's head is kept elevated for 30 to 45 minutes after the procedure.

MONITORING
■ Vital signs
■ Intake and output
■ Neurologic status
■ Puncture site
■ Bleeding
■ Infection
■ Seizure activity

If radicular pain, fever, back pain, or signs and symptoms of meningeal irritation (headache, irritability, or neck stiffness) develop, inform the physician immediately. Keep the room quiet and dark, and provide an analgesic or an antipyretic as ordered.

PRECAUTIONS
■ Myelography is contraindicated in:
– increased intracranial pressure
– hypersensitivity to contrast media
– infection at the puncture site.
■ Improper positioning after the test may affect recovery.

COMPLICATIONS
■ Bleeding
■ Infection
■ Meningeal irritation
■ Seizures
■ Dehydration

Interpretation

NORMAL FINDINGS
■ Contrast medium flows freely through the subarachnoid space.
■ No obstruction or structural abnormality is found.

ABNORMAL RESULTS
■ Extradural lesions suggest possible herniated intervertebral disks or metastatic tumors.
■ Lesions within the subarachnoid space suggest possible neurofibromas or meningiomas.
■ Lesions within the spinal cord suggest possible ependymomas or astrocytomas.
■ Fluid-filled cavities in the spinal cord and widening of the cord itself suggest possible syringomyelia.

NEUROLOGIC CARE

DISEASES

ALZHEIMER'S DISEASE

Overview

DESCRIPTION
- Degenerative disorder of the cerebral cortex (especially the frontal lobe) accounts for more than half of all cases
- Poor prognosis
- No cure or definitive treatment

PATHOPHYSIOLOGY
- Genetic abnormality on chromosome 21
- Brain damage caused by genetic substance (amyloid)
- Three distinguishing features of brain tissue: neurofibrillary tangles, neuritic plaques, and granulovacuolar degeneration

CAUSES
- Unknown

RISK FACTORS
Neurochemical
- Deficiencies of the neurotransmitters

Environmental
- Aluminum and manganese
- Trauma
- Genetic abnormality on chromosome 21
- Slow-growing central nervous system viruses

COMPLICATIONS
- Injury from violent behavior, wandering, or unsupervised activity
- Pneumonia and other infections
- Malnutrition and dehydration

Assessment

HISTORY
- History obtained from a family member or caregiver
- Insidious onset
- Initial changes almost imperceptible
- Forgetfulness and subtle memory loss
- Recent memory loss
- Difficulty learning and remembering new information
- General deterioration in personal hygiene
- Inability to concentrate
- Tendency to perform repetitive actions and experience restlessness
- Negative personality changes (irritability, depression, paranoia, hostility)
- Nocturnal awakening
- Disorientation
- Suspicious and fearful of imaginary people and situations
- Misperceives own environment
- Misidentifies objects and people
- Complains of stolen or misplaced objects
- Emotions may be described as labile
- Mood swings, sudden angry outbursts, and sleep disturbances

PHYSICAL FINDINGS
- Impaired sense of smell (usually an early symptom)
- Impaired stereognosis
- Gait disorders
- Tremors
- Loss of recent memory
- Positive snout reflex
- Organic brain disease in adults
- Urinary or fecal incontinence
- Seizures

TEST RESULTS

- Diagnosed by exclusion; tests performed to rule out other diseases.
- Positive diagnosis is made on autopsy.

Imaging

- Position emission tomography reveals metabolic activity of the cerebral cortex.
- Computed tomography scan shows excessive and progressive brain atrophy.
- Magnetic resonance imaging rules out intracranial lesions.
- Cerebral blood flow studies reveal abnormalities in blood flow to the brain.

Diagnostic procedures

- Cerebrospinal fluid analysis shows chronic neurologic infection.

Other

- EEG evaluates the brain's electrical activity and may show slowing of the brain waves in late stages of the disease.
- Neuropsychologic tests may show impaired cognitive ability and reasoning.

Treatment

GENERAL

- Hyperbaric oxygen

DIET

- Avoidance of coffee, tea, cola, and chocolate

ACTIVITY

- No restrictions; as tolerated

MEDICATION

- Cerebral vasodilators
- Psychostimulators
- Antidepressants
- Anticholinesterase agents

MONITORING

- Response to medication
- Fluid intake and nutrition status

AMYOTROPHIC LATERAL SCLEROSIS

Overview

DESCRIPTION

- Most common motor neuron disease of muscular atrophy
- Chronic, progressive, and debilitating disease that's invariably fatal
- No cure
- Also known as Lou Gehrig disease

PATHOPHYSIOLOGY

- An excitatory neurotransmitter that accumulates to toxic levels
- Motor units that no longer innervate
- Progressive degeneration of axons that cause loss of myelin
- Progressive degeneration of upper and lower motor neurons
- Progressive degenerations of motor nuclei in the cerebral cortex and corticospinal tracts

CAUSES

- Exact cause unknown
- 10% of patients with amyotrophic lateral sclerosis (ALS) inherit the disease as an autosomal dominant trait
- Virus that creates metabolic disturbances in motor neurons
- Immune complexes such as those formed in autoimmune disorders

Precipitating factors that cause acute deterioration

- Severe stress such as myocardial infarction
- Traumatic injury
- Viral infections
- Physical exhaustion

COMPLICATIONS
- Respiratory tract infections
- Complications of physical immobility

Assessment

HISTORY
- Mental function intact
- Family history of ALS
- Asymmetrical weakness first noticed in one limb
- Easy fatigue and easy cramping in the affected muscles

PHYSICAL FINDINGS
- Location of the affected motor neurons
- Severity of the disease
- Fasciculations in the affected muscles
- Progressive weakness in muscles of the arms, legs, and trunk
- Brisk and overactive stretch reflexes
- Difficulty talking, chewing, swallowing, and breathing
- Shortness of breath and occasional drooling

TEST RESULTS
Laboratory
- Increased protein in cerebrospinal fluid

Imaging
- Computed tomography scan rules out other disorders.

Diagnostic procedures
- Muscle biopsy discloses atrophic fibers.

Other
- EEG rules out other disorders.
- Electromyography shows the electrical abnormalities of involved muscles.
- Nerve conduction studies appear normal.

Treatment

GENERAL
- Rehabilitative measures

DIET
- May need tube feedings

ACTIVITY
- No restrictions; as tolerated

MEDICATION
- Muscle relaxants
- Dantrolene
- Baclofen
- I.V. or intrathecal administration of thyrotropin-releasing hormone

MONITORING
- Muscle weakness
- Respiratory status
- Speech
- Swallowing ability
- Skin integrity
- Nutritional status
- Response to treatment
- Complications
- Signs and symptoms of infection

BRAIN TUMOR, MALIGNANT

Overview

DESCRIPTION
- Growths within the intracranial space; tumors of the brain tissue, meninges, pituitary gland, and blood vessels
- In adults, the most common tumor types are gliomas and meningiomas, which usually occur above the covering of the cerebellum, or supratentorial tumors
- In children, most common tumor types are astrocytomas, medulloblastomas, ependymomas, and brain stem gliomas

■ The most common cause of cancer death in children

PATHOPHYSIOLOGY
■ Classified based on histology or grade of cell malignancy
■ Central nervous system changes by invading and destroying tissues and by secondary effect — mainly compression of the brain, cranial nerves, and cerebral vessels; cerebral edema; and increased intracranial pressure (ICP)

CAUSES
■ Cause unknown

RISK FACTORS
■ Preexisting cancer

COMPLICATIONS
■ Radiation encephalopathy

Life-threatening complications from increased ICP
■ Coma
■ Respiratory or cardiac arrest
■ Brain herniation

Assessment

HISTORY
■ Insidious onset
■ Headache
■ Nausea and vomiting

PHYSICAL FINDINGS
Signs and symptoms of increased ICP
■ Vision disturbances
■ Weakness, paralysis
■ Aphasia, dysphagia
■ Ataxia, incoordination
■ Seizure

TEST RESULTS
Imaging
■ Skull X-rays confirming presence of tumor

■ Brain scan confirming presence of tumor
■ Computed tomography scan confirming presence of tumor
■ Magnetic resonance imaging confirming presence of tumor
■ Cerebral angiography confirming presence of tumor

Diagnostic procedures
■ Tissue biopsy confirms presence of tumor.

Other
■ Lumbar puncture shows increased cerebrospinal fluid (CSF) pressure, which reflects ICP, increased protein levels, decreased glucose levels and, occasionally, tumor cells in CSF.

Treatment

GENERAL
■ Treatments vary with tumor histologic type, radiosensitivity, and location.

DIET
■ No restrictions unless swallowing impaired

ACTIVITY
■ Ability may be altered based on neurologic status

MEDICATION
■ Chemotherapy such as nitrosoureas
■ Steroids
■ Antacids and histamine-receptor antagonists
■ Anticonvulsants

SURGERY
For glioma
■ Resection by craniotomy
■ Radiation therapy and chemotherapy follow resection

For low-grade cystic cerebellar astrocytoma
■ Surgical resection

For astrocytoma
■ Repeated surgeries, radiation therapy, and shunting of fluid from obstructed CSF pathways

For oligodendroglioma and ependymoma
■ Surgical resection and radiation therapy

For medulloblastoma
■ Surgical resection
■ Possibly, intrathecal infusion and methotrexate or another antineoplastic drug

For meningioma
■ Surgical resection, including dura mater and bone

For schwannoma
■ Microsurgical technique

MONITORING
■ Neurologic status
■ Vital signs
■ Wound site
■ Postoperative complications

CONCUSSION

Overview

DESCRIPTION
■ Acceleration-deceleration injury
■ Blow to the head forceful enough to jostle the brain and make it strike the skull (see *Types of head injury,* pages 478 to 481)
■ Causes temporary (less than 48 hours) neural dysfunction

PATHOPHYSIOLOGY
■ Concussion causes diffuse soft tissue damage.
■ Inflammation occurs.
■ Structural damage is usually minimal.

CAUSES
■ Trauma to the head

COMPLICATIONS
■ Seizures
■ Persistent vomiting
■ Intracranial hemorrhage (rare)

Assessment

HISTORY
■ Trauma to head
■ Short-term loss of consciousness
■ Vomiting
■ Antegrade and retrograde amnesia
■ Change in level of consciousness
■ Dizziness
■ Nausea
■ Severe headache

PHYSICAL FINDINGS
■ Tenderness or hematomas on skull palpation

TEST RESULTS
Imaging
■ Computed tomography scan and magnetic resonance imaging help to rule out fractures and more serious injuries.

Treatment

GENERAL
■ Observation for changes in mental status

DIET
■ No restriction
■ Clear liquids if vomiting occurs

ACTIVITY
■ Bed rest initially
■ Avoidance of contact sports until fully recovered

MEDICATION
■ Nonopioid analgesics

MONITORING
■ Vital signs
■ Neurologic status
■ Pain

CREUTZFELDT-JAKOB DISEASE

Overview

DESCRIPTION
■ Rapidly progressive prion disease that attacks the central nervous system (CNS)
■ Always fatal
■ Not transmitted by normal casual contact (although iatrogenic transmission can occur)
■ Typical duration of Creutzfeldt-Jakob disease (CJD) is 4 months
■ New variant of CJD (nvCJD) emerged in Europe in 1996
■ No cure and its progress can't be slowed

PATHOPHYSIOLOGY
■ CJD is caused by the abnormal accumulation or metabolism of prion proteins.
■ These modified proteins are resistant to proteolytic digestion and aggregate in the brain to produce rod-like particles.
■ The accumulation of these modified cellular proteins results in neuronal degeneration and spongiform changes in brain tissue.

CAUSES
■ Familial or genetically inherited form
■ Sporadic form of unknown etiology
■ Iatrogenic or acquired form due to inadvertent exposure to CJD-contaminated equipment or material as a result of brain surgery, corneal grafts, or use of human pituitary-derived growth hormones or gonadotropin

COMPLICATIONS
■ Severe, progressive dementia
■ CNS abnormalities
■ Death

Assessment

HISTORY
■ Mood changes
■ Emotional lability
■ Poor concentration
■ Lethargy
■ Impaired judgment
■ Memory loss
■ Involuntary muscle movements
■ Vision disturbances or other types of hallucinations
■ Gait disturbances

PHYSICAL FINDINGS
■ Dementia
■ Myoclonus
■ Spasticity
■ Agitation
■ Tremor
■ Clumsiness
■ Ataxia
■ Hypokinesis and rigidity
■ Hyperreflexia

TEST RESULTS
Laboratory
■ Cerebral spinal fluid (CSF) immunoassay possibly showing abnormal protein species

(Text continues on page 482.)

NEUROLOGIC CARE

TYPES OF HEAD INJURY

Type	Description
Concussion (closed head injury)	■ A blow to the head hard enough to make the brain hit the skull but not hard enough to cause a cerebral contusion causes temporary neural dysfunction. ■ Recovery is usually complete within 24 to 48 hours. ■ Repeated injuries exact a cumulative toll on the brain.
Contusion (bruising of brain tissue; more serious than concussion)	■ Most common in people ages 20 to 40. ■ Most result from arterial bleeding. ■ Blood commonly accumulates between the skull and dura. Injury to the middle meningeal artery in the parietotemporal area is most common and is frequently accompanied by linear skull fractures in the temporal region over the middle meningeal artery. ■ Less commonly arises from dural venous sinuses.
Epidural hematoma	■ Acceleration-deceleration or coup-contrecoup injuries disrupt normal nerve functions in the bruised area. ■ Injury is directly beneath the site of impact when the brain rebounds against the skull from the force of a blow (a beating with a blunt instrument, for example), when the force of the blow drives the brain against the opposite side of the skull, or when the head is hurled forward and stopped abruptly (as in an automobile accident when the driver's head strikes the windshield). ■ The brain continues moving and slaps against the skull (acceleration), then rebounds (deceleration). The brain may strike bony prominences inside the skull (especially the sphenoidal ridges), causing intracranial hemorrhage or hematoma that may result in tentorial herniation.

Signs and symptoms	Diagnostic test findings
■ Short-term loss of consciousness secondary to disruption of reticular activating system (RAS), possibly due to abrupt pressure changes in the areas responsible for consciousness, changes in polarity of the neurons, ischemia, or structural distortion of neurons ■ Vomiting from localized injury and compression ■ Anterograde and retrograde amnesia (patient can't recall events immediately after the injury or events that led up to the traumatic incident) correlating with severity of injury; all related to disruption of RAS ■ Irritability or lethargy from localized injury and compression ■ Behavior out of character due to focal injury ■ Complaints of dizziness, nausea, or severe headache due to focal injury and compression	■ Computed tomography (CT) scan reveals no sign of fracture, bleeding, or other nervous system lesion.
■ Severe scalp wounds from direct injury ■ Labored respiration and loss of consciousness secondary to increased pressure from bruising ■ Drowsiness, confusion, disorientation, agitation, or violence from increased intracranial pressure (ICP) associated with trauma ■ Hemiparesis related to interrupted blood flow to the site of injury ■ Decorticate or decerebrate posturing from cortical damage or hemispheric dysfunction ■ Unequal pupillary response from brain stem involvement	■ CT scan shows changes in tissue density, possible displacement of the surrounding structures, and evidence of ischemic tissue, hematomas, and fractures. ■ Lumbar puncture with cerebrospinal fluid (CSF) analysis reveals increased pressure and blood (not performed if hemorrhage is suspected). ■ EEG recordings directly over area of contusion reveal progressive abnormalities by appearance of high-amplitude theta and delta waves
■ Brief period of unconsciousness after injury due to concussive effects of head trauma, then a lucid interval of 10 minutes to hours or, rarely, days ■ Severe headache ■ Progressive loss of consciousness and deterioration in neurologic signs resulting from expanding lesion and extrusion of medial portion of temporal lobe through tentorial opening ■ Compression of brainstem by temporal lobe causing clinical manifestations of intracranial hypertension ■ Deterioration in level of consciousness resulting from compression of brainstem reticular formation as temporal lobe herniates on its upper portion ■ Respirations, initially deep and labored, becoming shallow and irregular as brainstem is impacted ■ Contralateral motor deficits reflecting compression of corticospinal tracts that pass through the brainstem	■ CT scan or magnetic resonance imaging (MRI) identifies abnormal masses or structural shifts within the cranium.

NEUROLOGIC CARE

(continued)

TYPES OF HEAD INJURY *(continued)*

Type	Description
Epidural hematoma *(continued)*	
Subdural hematoma	■ Meningeal hemorrhages, resulting from accumulation of blood in subdural space (between dura mater and the arachnoid), are most common. ■ May be acute, subacute, and chronic: unilateral or bilateral. ■ Usually associated with torn connecting veins in cerebral cortex; rarely from arteries. ■ Acute hematomas are a surgical emergency.
Intracerebral hematoma	■ Subacute hematomas have better prognosis because venous bleeding tends to be slower. ■ Traumatic or spontaneous disruption of cerebral vessels in brain parenchyma cause neurologic deficits, depending on the site and amount of bleeding. ■ Shear forces from brain movement frequently cause vessel laceration and hemorrhage into the parenchyma. ■ Frontal and temporal lobes are common sites. Trauma is associated with few intracerebral hematomas; most caused by result of hypertension.
Skull fracture	■ There are four types of skull fractures: linear, comminuted, depressed, basilar. ■ Fractures of anterior and middle fossae are associated with severe head trauma and are more common than those of posterior fossa. ■ Blows to the head cause one or more types of skull fractures. May not be problematic unless the brain is exposed or bone fragments are driven into neural tissue.

Signs and symptoms	Diagnostic test findings
■ Ipsilateral (same-side) pupillary dilation due to compression of third cranial nerve ■ Seizures possible from high ICP ■ Continued bleeding leading to progressive neurologic degeneration, evidenced by bilateral pupillary dilation, bilateral decerebrate response, increased systemic blood pressure, decreased pulse, and profound coma with irregular respiratory patterns	
■ Similar to epidural hematoma but significantly slower in onset because bleeding is typically of venous origin	■ CT scan, X-rays, and arteriography reveal mass and altered blood flow in the area, confirming hematoma. ■ CT scan or MRI reveals evidence of masses and tissue shifting. ■ CSF is yellow and has relatively low protein (chronic subdural hematoma).
■ Unresponsive immediately or experiencing a lucid period before lapsing into a coma from increasing ICP and mass effect of hemorrhage ■ Possible motor deficits and decorticate or decerebrate responses from compression of corticospinal tracts and brain stem	■ CT scan or cerebral arteriography identifies bleeding site. CSF pressure elevated; fluid may appear bloody or xanthochromic (yellow or straw-colored) from hemoglobin breakdown.
■ Possibly asymptomatic, depending on underlying brain trauma ■ Discontinuity and displacement of bone structure with severe fracture ■ Motor sensory and cranial nerve dysfunction with associated facial fractures ■ People with anterior fossa basilar skull fractures may have periorbital ecchymosis (raccoon eyes), anosmia (loss of smell due to first cranial nerve involvement) and pupil abnormalities (second and third cranial nerve involvement) ■ CSF rhinorrhea (leakage through nose), CSF otorrhea (leakage from the ear), hemotympanum (blood accumulation at the tympanic membrane), ecchymosis over the mastoid bone (Battle's sign), and facial paralysis (seventh cranial nerve injury) accompany middle fossa basilar skull fractures ■ Signs of medullary dysfunction, such as cardiovascular and respiratory failure, accompany posterior fossa basilar skull fracture	■ CT scan and MRI reveal intracranial hemorrhage from ruptured blood vessels and swelling. ■ Skull X-ray may reveal fracture. ■ Lumbar puncture contraindicated by expanding lesions.

NEUROLOGIC CARE

■ CSF analysis possibly showing mildly elevated protein level

Imaging
■ Computed tomography scan and magnetic resonance imaging of the brain may show evidence of generalized cortical atrophy.

Diagnostic procedures
■ EEG may show typical changes in brain wave activity.
■ Brain biopsy may show spongiform changes.

Other
■ Autopsy of brain tissue allows definitive diagnosis.

Treatment

GENERAL
■ Palliative care to make the patient comfortable and to ease symptoms

DIET
■ Well-balanced
■ Adequate fluid intake

ACTIVITY
■ As tolerated

MEDICATION
■ No specific drug therapy

SURGERY
■ Possible brain biopsy for diagnosis

MONITORING
■ Vital signs
■ Intake and output
■ Neurologic status
■ Mental status

EPILEPSY

Overview

DESCRIPTION
■ Susceptibility to recurrent seizures
■ Doesn't affect intelligence
■ About 80% of patients have good seizure control with strict adherence to prescribed treatment
■ Also known as seizure disorder

PATHOPHYSIOLOGY
■ Seizures are paroxysmal events involving abnormal electrical discharges of neurons in the brain and cell membrane potential that's less negative than usual. (See *Seizure types,* pages 484 and 485.)
■ On stimulation, the neuron fires, the discharge spreads to surrounding cells, and stimulation continues to one side or both sides of the brain.

CAUSES
■ Half of cases are idiopathic

Nonidiopathic epilepsy
■ Birth trauma
■ Anoxia
■ Perinatal infection
■ Genetic abnormalities (tuberous sclerosis and phenylketonuria)
■ Perinatal injuries
■ Metabolic abnormalities (hypoglycemia, pyridoxine deficiency, hypoparathyroidism)
■ Brain tumors or other space-occupying lesions
■ Meningitis, encephalitis, or brain abscess
■ Traumatic injury
■ Ingestion of toxins, such as mercury, lead, or carbon monoxide
■ Stroke
■ Apparent familial incidence in some seizure disorders

COMPLICATIONS
- Anoxia
- Traumatic injury

Assessment

HISTORY
- Seizure occurrence unpredictable and unrelated to activities
- Precipitating factors or events possibly reported
- Headache
- Mood changes
- Lethargy
- Myoclonic jerking
- Description of an aura
- Pungent smell
- GI distress
- Rising or sinking feeling in the stomach
- Dreamy feeling
- Unusual taste in the mouth
- Visual disturbance

PHYSICAL FINDINGS
- Findings possibly normal while patient isn't having a seizure and when the cause is idiopathic
- Findings related to underlying cause of the seizure
- The hallmark of epilepsy is recurring seizures, which can be classified as partial, generalized, status epilepticus, or unclassified. Some patients may be affected by more than one type.

TEST RESULTS
Laboratory
- Serum glucose and calcium study results ruling out other diagnoses

Imaging
- Computed tomography scan and magnetic resonance imaging may indicate abnormalities in internal structures.
- Skull radiography may show certain neoplasms within the brain substance or skull fractures.
- Brain scan may show malignant lesions when X-ray findings are normal or questionable.
- Cerebral angiography may show cerebrovascular abnormalities, such as aneurysm or tumor.

Treatment

GENERAL
- Vagal nerve stimulation by pacemaker
- A detailed presurgical evaluation to characterize seizure type, frequency, site of onset, psychological functioning, and degree of disability to select candidates for surgery in medically intractable patients

DIET
- No restrictions
- Regular meals

ACTIVITY
- As tolerated

MEDICATION
- Anticonvulsants

SURGERY
- Removal of a demonstrated focal lesion
- Correction of the underlying problem

MONITORING
- Response to anticonvulsants
- Vital signs
- Seizure activity
- Respiratory status
- Adverse drug reactions
- Associated injuries

NEUROLOGIC CARE

SEIZURE TYPES

The various types of seizures — partial, generalized, status epilepticus, and unclassified — have distinct signs and symptoms.

Partial seizures

Arising from a localized area of the brain, partial seizures cause focal symptoms. These seizures are classified by their effect on consciousness and whether they spread throughout the motor pathway, causing a generalized seizure.

- A *simple partial seizure* begins locally and generally doesn't cause an alteration in consciousness. It may present with sensory symptoms (lights flashing, smells, hearing hallucinations), autonomic symptoms (sweating, flushing, pupil dilation), and psychic symptoms (dream states, anger, fear). The seizure lasts for a few seconds and occurs without preceding or provoking events. This type can be motor or sensory.
- A *complex partial seizure* alters consciousness. Amnesia for events that occur during and immediately after the seizure is a differentiating characteristic. During the seizure, the patient may follow simple commands. This seizure usually lasts for 1 to 3 minutes.

Generalized seizures

As the term suggests, generalized seizures cause a generalized electrical abnormality within the brain. They can be convulsive or nonconvulsive and include several types:

- *Absence seizures* occur most commonly in children, although they may affect adults. They usually begin with a brief change in level of consciousness, indicated by a blinking or rolling of the eyes, a blank stare, and slight mouth movements. The patient retains his posture and continues preseizure activity without difficulty. Typically, each seizure lasts from 1 to 10 seconds. If not properly treated, seizures can recur as often as 100 times per day. An absence seizure is a nonconvulsive seizure, but it may progress to a generalized tonic-clonic seizure.
- *Myoclonic seizures* are brief, involuntary muscular jerks of the body or extremities, often occurring in early morning.
- *Clonic seizures* are characterized by bilateral rhythmic movements.

GUILLAIN-BARRÉ SYNDROME

Overview

DESCRIPTION

- A form of polyneuritis
- Acute, rapidly progressive, and potentially fatal
- Three phases:
- Acute: lasting from first symptom, ending in 1 to 3 weeks
- Plateau: lasting several days to 2 weeks

- Recovery: coincides with remyelination and axonal process regrowth; extends over 4 to 6 months and may take up to 2 to 3 years; recovery possibly not complete

PATHOPHYSIOLOGY

- Segmented demyelination of peripheral nerves occurs, preventing normal transmission of electrical impulses.
- Sensorimotor nerve roots are affected; autonomic nerve transmission may also be affected.

■ *Tonic seizures* are characterized by a sudden stiffening of muscle tone, usually of the arms, but possibly including the legs.

■ *Generalized tonic-clonic seizures* typically begin with a loud cry, precipitated by air rushing from the lungs through the vocal cords. The patient then loses consciousness and falls to the ground. The body stiffens (tonic phase) and then alternates between episodes of muscle spasm and relaxation (clonic phase). Tongue biting, incontinence, labored breathing, apnea, and subsequent cyanosis may occur. The seizure stops in 2 to 5 minutes, when abnormal electrical conduction ceases. When the patient regains consciousness, he's confused and may have difficulty talking. If he can talk, he may complain of drowsiness, fatigue, headache, muscle soreness, and arm or leg weakness. He may fall into a deep sleep after the seizure.

■ *Atonic seizures* are characterized by a general loss of postural tone and a temporary loss of consciousness. They occur in young children and are sometimes called "drop attacks" because they cause the child to fall.

Status epilepticus

Status epilepticus is a continuous seizure state that can occur in all seizure types. The most life-threatening example is generalized tonic-clonic status epilepticus, a continuous generalized tonic-clonic seizure. Status epilepticus is accompanied by respiratory distress leading to hypoxia or anoxia. It can result from abrupt withdrawal of anticonvulsant medications, hypoxic encephalopathy, acute head trauma, metabolic encephalopathy, or septicemia secondary to encephalitis or meningitis.

Unclassified seizures

This category is reserved for seizures that don't fit the characteristics of partial or generalized seizures or status epilepticus. Included as unclassified are events that lack the data to make a more definitive diagnosis.

CAUSES

■ Unknown
■ Virus can cause cell-mediated immunologic attack on peripheral nerves

RISK FACTORS

■ Surgery
■ Rabies or swine influenza vaccination
■ Viral illness
■ Hodgkin's or some other malignant disease
■ Lupus erythematosus

COMPLICATIONS

■ Thrombophlebitis
■ Pressure ulcers
■ Contractures
■ Muscle wasting
■ Aspiration
■ Respiratory tract infections
■ Life-threatening respiratory and cardiac compromise

Assessment

HISTORY

■ Minor febrile illness 1 to 4 weeks before current symptoms

- Tingling and numbness in the legs
- Progression of symptoms to arms, trunk and, finally, the face
- Stiffness and pain in the calves

PHYSICAL FINDINGS
- Muscle weakness (the major neurologic sign)
- Sensory loss, usually in the legs (spreads to arms)
- Difficulty talking, chewing, and swallowing
- Paralysis of the ocular, facial, and oropharyngeal muscles
- Loss of position sense
- Diminished or absent deep tendon reflexes

TEST RESULTS
Diagnostic procedures
- Cerebrospinal fluid (CSF) analysis may show a normal white blood cell count, an elevated protein count and, in severe disease, increased CSF pressure.

Other
- Electromyography may demonstrate repeated firing of the same motor unit instead of widespread sectional stimulation.
- Nerve conduction studies show marked slowing of nerve conduction velocities.

Treatment

GENERAL
- Primarily supportive
- Possible endotracheal intubation or tracheotomy
- Volume replacement
- Plasmapheresis

DIET
- Possible tube feedings with endotracheal intubation
- Adequate caloric intake

ACTIVITY
- Exercise program to prevent contractures

MEDICATION
- I.V. beta-adrenergic blockers
- Parasympatholytics
- I.V. immune globulin

SURGERY
- Possible tracheostomy
- Possible gastrostomy or jejunotomy feeding tube insertion

MONITORING
- Vital signs
- Breath sounds
- Arterial blood gas measurements
- Level of consciousness
- Continual respiratory function
- Pulse oximetry
- Signs of thrombophlebitis
- Signs of urine retention
- Response to medications

MENINGITIS

Overview

DESCRIPTION
- Inflammation of brain and spinal cord meninges
- May affect all three meningeal membranes (dura mater, arachnoid membrane, and pia mater)
- Usually follows onset of respiratory symptoms
- Sudden onset, causing serious illness within 24 hours
- Prognosis is good; complications are rare

PATHOPHYSIOLOGY
- Inflammation of pia-arachnoid progresses to congestion of adjacent tissues.
- Nerve cells are destroyed.

■ Intracranial pressure (ICP) increases because of exudates.

■ Results can include:
– engorged blood vessels
– disrupted blood supply
– thrombosis
– rupture.

CAUSES

■ Bacterial infection, usually from *Neisseria meningitidis* and *Streptococcus pneumoniae* (Before the 1990s, *Haemophilus influenzae* type b [Hib] was the leading cause of bacterial meningitis. However, new vaccines have reduced its occurrence in children.)

■ Viruses

■ Protozoa

■ Fungi

■ Secondary to another bacterial infection such as pneumonia

■ May follow skull fracture, penetrating head wound, lumbar puncture, or ventricular shunting procedures

COMPLICATIONS

■ Visual impairment; optic neuritis

■ Cranial nerve palsies; deafness

■ Paresis or paralysis

■ Endocarditis

■ Coma

■ Vasculitis

■ Cerebral infarction

Assessment

HISTORY

■ Headache

■ Fever

■ Nausea, vomiting

■ Weakness

■ Myalgia

■ Photophobia

■ Confusion, delirium

■ Seizures

PHYSICAL FINDINGS

■ Meningismus

■ Rigors

■ Profuse sweating

■ Kernig's and Brudzinski's signs elicited in only 50% of adults

■ Declining level of consciousness (LOC)

■ Cranial nerve palsies

■ Focal neurologic deficits such as visual field defects

■ Signs of increased ICP (in later stages)

Elderly patients may exhibit an insidious onset, exhibiting lethargy and variable signs of meningismus and no fever.

TEST RESULTS
Laboratory

■ White blood cell count showing leukocytosis

■ Positive blood cultures in bacterial meningitis, depending on the pathogen

Imaging

■ Chest X-rays may reveal a coexisting pneumonia.

■ Neuroimaging techniques, such as computed tomography scan and magnetic resonance imaging, may detect complications and a parameningeal source of infection.

Diagnostic procedures

■ Lumbar puncture and cerebrospinal fluid analysis shows:
– increased opening pressure
– neutrophilic pleocytosis
– elevated protein
– hypoglycorrhachia
– positive Gram stain
– positive culture.

Treatment

GENERAL

■ Hypothermia

■ Fluid therapy

DIET
■ Generally no restrictions

ACTIVITY
■ Bed rest (in acute phase)

MEDICATION
■ I.V. antibiotics
■ Oral antibiotics
■ Antiarrhythmics
■ Osmotic diuretics
■ Anticonvulsants
■ Aspirin or acetaminophen

MONITORING
■ Neurologic status
■ Vital signs
■ Signs and symptoms of cranial nerve involvement
■ Signs and symptoms of increased ICP
■ LOC
■ Seizures
■ Respiratory status
■ Arterial blood gas results
■ Fluid balance
■ Response to medications
■ Complications

MULTIPLE SCLEROSIS

Overview

DESCRIPTION
■ Progressive demyelination of white matter of brain and spinal cord
■ Characterized by exacerbations and remissions
■ May progress rapidly, causing death within months
■ Prognosis varies (70% lead active lives with prolonged remissions)

PATHOPHYSIOLOGY
■ Sporadic patches of demyelination occur in the central nervous system, resulting in widespread and varied neurologic dysfunction.

CAUSES
■ Exact cause unknown
■ Slowly acting viral infection
■ An autoimmune response of the nervous system
■ Allergic response
■ Events that precede the onset:
– Emotional stress
– Overwork
– Fatigue
– Pregnancy
– Acute respiratory tract infections
■ Genetic factors possibly involved

RISK FACTORS
■ Trauma
■ Toxins
■ Nutritional deficiencies

COMPLICATIONS
■ Injuries from falls
■ Urinary tract infections
■ Constipation
■ Contractures
■ Pressure ulcers
■ Pneumonia

Assessment

HISTORY
■ Symptoms related to extent and site of myelin destruction, extent of re-myelination, and adequacy of subsequent restored synaptic transmission
■ Symptoms possibly transient or last for hours or weeks
■ Symptoms unpredictable and difficult to describe
■ Visual problems and sensory impairment (the first signs)
■ Blurred vision or diplopia
■ Urinary problems
■ Emotional lability
■ Dysphagia
■ Bowel disturbances (involuntary evacuation or constipation)
■ Fatigue (typically the most disabling symptom)

Physical findings
- Poor articulation
- Muscle weakness of the involved area
- Spasticity; hyperreflexia
- Intention tremor
- Gait ataxia
- Paralysis, ranging from monoplegia to quadriplegia
- Nystagmus; scotoma
- Optic neuritis
- Ophthalmoplegia

Test results
- Years of testing and observation may be required for diagnosis.

Laboratory
- Cerebrospinal fluid analysis showing mononuclear cell pleocytosis, an elevation in the level of total immunoglobulin (Ig) G, and presence of oligoclonal Ig

Imaging
- Magnetic resonance imaging is the most sensitive method of detecting multiple sclerosis focal lesions.

Other
- EEG abnormalities occur in one-third of patients.

Treatment

General
- For acute exacerbations
- For the disease process
- For related signs and symptoms

Diet
- High fluid and fiber intake in case of constipation

Activity
- Frequent rest periods

Medication
- I.V. steroids followed by oral steroids
- Immunosuppressants
- Antimetabolites
- Alkylating drugs
- Biological response modifiers

Monitoring
- Response to medications
- Adverse drug reactions
- Sensory impairment
- Muscle dysfunction
- Energy level
- Signs and symptoms of infection
- Speech
- Elimination patterns
- Vision changes
- Laboratory results

Parkinson's disease

Overview

Description
- Brain disorder causing progressive deterioration, with muscle rigidity, akinesia, and involuntary tremors
- Usual cause of death: aspiration pneumonia
- One of the most common crippling diseases in the United States

Pathophysiology
- Dopaminergic neurons degenerate, causing loss of available dopamine.
- Dopamine deficiency prevents affected brain cells from performing their normal inhibitory function.
- Excess excitatory acetylcholine occurs at synapses.
- Nondopaminergic receptors are also involved.
- Motor neurons are depressed.

Causes
- Usually unknown
- Exposure to such toxins as manganese dust and carbon monoxide

COMPLICATIONS
- Injury from falls
- Food aspiration
- Urinary tract infections
- Skin breakdown

Assessment

HISTORY
- Muscle rigidity
- Akinesia
- Insidious (unilateral pill-roll) tremor, which increases during stress or anxiety and decreases with purposeful movement and sleep
- Dysphagia
- Fatigue with activities of daily living
- Muscle cramps of legs, neck, and trunk
- Oily skin
- Increased perspiration
- Insomnia
- Mood changes
- Dysarthria

PHYSICAL FINDINGS
- High-pitched, monotonous voice
- Drooling
- Masklike facial expression
- Difficulty walking
- Lack of parallel motion in gait
- Loss of posture control with walking
- Oculogyric crises (eyes fixed upward, with involuntary tonic movements)
- Muscle rigidity causing resistance to passive muscle stretching
- Difficulty pivoting
- Loss of balance

TEST RESULTS
Imaging
- Computed tomography scan or magnetic resonance can rule out other disorders such as intracranial tumors.

Treatment

DIET
- Small, frequent meals
- High-bulk foods

ACTIVITY
- Physical therapy
- Assistive devices to aid ambulation

MEDICATION
- Dopamine replacement drugs
- Anticholinergics
- Antihistamines
- Antiviral agents
- Enzyme-inhibiting agents
- Tricyclic antidepressants

SURGERY
- Used when drug therapy fails
- Stereotaxic neurosurgery
- Destruction of ventrolateral nucleus of thalamus

MONITORING
- Vital signs
- Intake and output
- Drug therapy
- Adverse reactions to medications
- Postoperatively: signs of hemorrhage and increased intracranial pressure

STROKE

Overview

DESCRIPTION
- Most common cause of neurologic disability
- Sudden impairment of cerebral circulation in blood vessels to the brain
- About 50% of stroke survivors permanently disabled
- Recurrences possible within weeks, months, or years

■ Also known as *cerebrovascular accident* or *brain attack*

PATHOPHYSIOLOGY
■ The oxygen supply to the brain is interrupted or diminished.
■ In thrombotic or embolic stroke, neurons die from lack of oxygen.
■ In hemorrhagic stroke, impaired cerebral perfusion causes infarction.

CAUSES
Cerebral thrombosis
■ Most common cause of stroke
■ Obstruction of a blood vessel in the extracerebral vessels
■ Site possibly intracerebral

Cerebral embolism
■ Second most common cause of stroke
■ Develops rapidly, in 10 to 20 seconds, and without warning
■ Left middle cerebral artery most commonly involved

Cerebral hemorrhage
■ Third most common cause of stroke

RISK FACTORS
■ History of transient ischemic attack (see *Understanding transient ischemic attacks*)
■ Heart disease
■ Obesity
■ Alcohol
■ High red blood cell count
■ Arrhythmias
■ Diabetes mellitus
■ Gout
■ High serum triglyceride levels
■ Use of hormonal contraceptives in conjunction with smoking and hypertension
■ Smoking
■ Family history of cerebrovascular disease

> ## UNDERSTANDING TRANSIENT ISCHEMIC ATTACKS
>
> A transient ischemic attack (TIA) is an episode of neurologic deficit resulting from cerebral ischemia. The recurrent attacks may last from seconds to hours and clear within 12 to 24 hours. TIAs are commonly considered a warning sign for stroke and have been reported in more than one-half of the patients who later developed a stroke, usually within 2 to 5 years.
>
> In a TIA, microemboli released from a thrombus may temporarily interrupt blood flow, especially in the small, distal branches of the brain's arterial tree. Small spasms in those arterioles may impair blood flow and also precede a TIA.
>
> The most distinctive features of TIAs are transient focal deficits with complete return of function. The deficits usually involve some degree of motor or sensory dysfunction. They may progress to loss of consciousness and loss of motor or sensory function for a brief period. The patient typically experiences weakness in the lower part of the face and arms, hands, fingers, and legs on the side opposite the affected region. Other manifestations may include transient dysphagia, numbness or tingling of the face and lips, double vision, slurred speech, and vertigo.

COMPLICATIONS
■ Unstable blood pressure from loss of vasomotor control
■ Fluid and electrolyte imbalances
■ Malnutrition
■ Infections
■ Sensory impairment
■ Altered level of consciousness

- Aspiration
- Contractures
- Skin breakdown
- Deep vein thrombosis
- Pulmonary emboli
- Depression

Assessment

HISTORY
- Varying clinical features, depending on:
  - Artery affected
  - Severity of damage
  - Extent of collateral circulation
- One or more risk factors present
- Sudden onset of hemiparesis or hemiplegia
- Gradual onset of dizziness, mental disturbances, or seizures
- Loss of consciousness or sudden aphasia

PHYSICAL FINDINGS
- With stroke in left hemisphere, signs and symptoms seen on right side
- With stroke in right hemisphere, signs and symptoms seen on left side
- With stroke that causes cranial nerve damage, signs and symptoms seen on same side
- Unconsciousness or changes in LOC
- With conscious patient, anxiety along with communication and mobility difficulties (see *Cincinnati prehospital stroke scale*)
- Urinary incontinence
- Loss of voluntary muscle control
- Hemiparesis or hemiplegia on one side of the body
- Decreased deep tendon reflexes
- Hemianopsia on the affected side of the body
- With left-sided hemiplegia, problems with visuospatial relations
- Sensory losses

TEST RESULTS
Laboratory
- Laboratory tests — including anticardiolipin antibodies, antiphospholipid, factor V (Leiden) mutation, antithrombin III, protein S, and protein C — possibly showing increased thrombotic risk

Imaging
- Magnetic resonance imaging and magnetic resonance angiography allow evaluation of the lesion's location and size.
- Cerebral angiography details the disruption of cerebral circulation and is the test of choice for examining the entire cerebral blood flow.
- Computed tomography scan is used to detect structural abnormalities.
- Positron emission tomography provides data on cerebral metabolism and on cerebral blood flow changes.

Other
- Transcranial Doppler studies are used to evaluate the velocity of blood flow.
- Carotid Doppler is used to measure flow through the carotid arteries.
- Two-dimensional echocardiogram is used to evaluate the heart for dysfunction.
- Cerebral blood flow studies are used to measure blood flow to the brain.
- EEG shows reduced electrical activity in an area of cortical infarction.

Treatment

GENERAL
- Careful blood pressure management
- Varies, depending on cause and clinical manifestations (see *Treating suspected stroke*, pages 494 and 495)

CINCINNATI PREHOSPITAL STROKE SCALE

If any one of the three signs described here is abnormal, the probability of a stroke is 72%.

Facial droop

Tell the patient to show his teeth or smile. If he hasn't had a stroke, both sides of his face will move equally. If he has had a stroke, one side of his face won't move as well as the other side.

Other findings, such as pronator grip, may be helpful.

If the patient has had a stroke, one arm won't move or one arm will drift down compared with the other arm.

Normal

Normal response

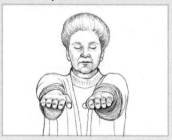

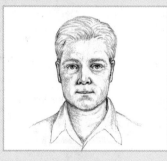

Stroke patient with facial droop on right side of face

One-sided motor weakness (right arm)

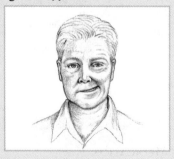

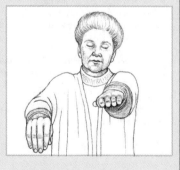

Arm drift

Tell the patient to close her eyes and hold both arms straight out in front of her for 20 seconds. If she hasn't had a stroke, her arms won't move or, if they do move, they'll move the same amount.

Abnormal speech

Have the patient say "You can't teach an old dog new tricks." If he hasn't had a stroke, he'll use correct words and his speech won't be slurred. If he has had a stroke, his words will be slurred, he may use the wrong words, or he may be unable to speak at all.

Adapted with permission from Kothari, R., et al. "Early Stroke Recognition: Developing an Out-of-Hospital NIH Stroke Scale," *Academy of Emergency Medicine* 4(10):986-90, October 1997.

NEUROLOGIC CARE

TREATING SUSPECTED STROKE

This algorithm is used for suspected stroke. The patient's survival depends on prompt recognition of symptoms and treatment.

Detection, Dispatch, Delivery to Door

Immediate general assessment: first 10 minutes after arrival
- Assess ABCs and vital signs.
- Provide oxygen by nasal cannula.
- Obtain I.V. access; obtain blood samples (complete blood count, electrolyte levels, coagulation studies).
- Check blood glucose levels; treat if indicated.
- Obtain 12-lead electrocardiogram; check for arrhythmias.
- Perform general neurologic screening assessment.
- Alert stroke team, neurologist, radiologist, computed tomography (CT) technician.

Immediate neurologic assessment: first 25 minutes after arrival
- Review patient history.
- Establish onset (< 3 hours required for fibrinolytics).
- Perform physical examination.
- Perform neurologic examination: Determine level of consciousness (Glasgow Coma Scale) and level of stroke severity (NIH Stroke Scale or Hunt and Hess Scale).
- Order urgent noncontrast CT scan (door-to-CT scan performed: goal < 25 minutes from arrival).
- Read CT scan (door-to-CT scan read: goal < 45 minutes from arrival).
- Perform lateral cervical spine X-ray (if patient is comatose or has a history of trauma).

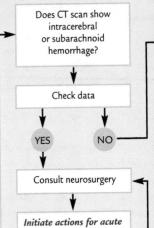

Does CT scan show intracerebral or subarachnoid hemorrhage?

Check data

YES   NO

Consult neurosurgery

Initiate actions for acute hemorrhage
- Reverse any anticoagulants.
- Reverse any bleeding disorder.
- Monitor neurologic condition.
- Treat hypertension in acute patients.

DIET
- Pureed dysphagia diet or tube feedings if indicated

ACTIVITY
- Physical, speech, and occupational rehabilitation
- Care measures to help the patient adapt to specific deficits

MEDICATION
- Fibrinolytic therapy
- Anticonvulsants
- Stool softeners
- Anticoagulants
- Analgesics
- Antidepressants
- Antiplatelets
- Lipid-lowering agents
- Antihypertensives

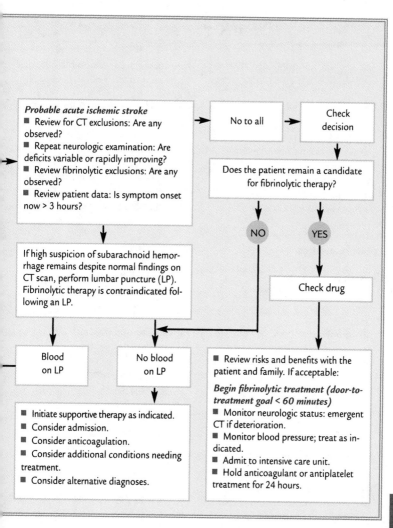

Probable acute ischemic stroke
- Review for CT exclusions: Are any observed?
- Repeat neurologic examination: Are deficits variable or rapidly improving?
- Review fibrinolytic exclusions: Are any observed?
- Review patient data: Is symptom onset now > 3 hours?

No to all → Check decision

Does the patient remain a candidate for fibrinolytic therapy?

NO   YES

If high suspicion of subarachnoid hemorrhage remains despite normal findings on CT scan, perform lumbar puncture (LP). Fibrinolytic therapy is contraindicated following an LP.

Check drug

Blood on LP

No blood on LP

- Initiate supportive therapy as indicated.
- Consider admission.
- Consider anticoagulation.
- Consider additional conditions needing treatment.
- Consider alternative diagnoses.

- Review risks and benefits with the patient and family. If acceptable:

Begin fibrinolytic treatment (door-to-treatment goal < 60 minutes)
- Monitor neurologic status: emergent CT if deterioration.
- Monitor blood pressure; treat as indicated.
- Admit to intensive care unit.
- Hold anticoagulant or antiplatelet treatment for 24 hours.

SURGERY
- Craniotomy
- Endarterectomy
- Extracranial-intracranial bypass
- Ventricular shunts

MONITORING
- Continuous neurologic assessment
- Continuous respiratory support
- Continuous monitoring of vital signs
- Continuous monitoring of GI problems
- Fluid, electrolyte, and nutritional intake
- Development of deep vein thrombosis and pulmonary embolus
- Response to medication

NEUROLOGIC CARE

TREATMENTS

CRANIOTOMY

Overview

■ A surgical opening into the skull, exposing the brain for treatment

INDICATIONS
■ Ventricular shunt
■ Tumor excision
■ Abscess drainage
■ Hematoma aspiration
■ Aneurysm clipping

COMPLICATIONS
■ Infection
■ Vasospasm
■ Hemorrhage
■ Air embolism
■ Respiratory compromise
■ Increased intracranial pressure (ICP)
■ Diabetes insipidus
■ Syndrome of inappropriate antidiuretic hormone secretion
■ Seizures
■ Cranial nerve damage

Nursing interventions

PRETREATMENT CARE
■ Explain the treatment and preparation to the patient and family.
■ Make sure the patient has signed an appropriate consent form.
■ Tell the patient that his head will be shaved in the operating room.
■ Explain the intensive care unit and equipment the patient will see postoperatively.
■ Perform a complete neurologic assessment.

POSTTREATMENT CARE
■ Administer medications as ordered.

■ Position the patient on his side with the head of the bed elevated 15 to 30 degrees.
■ Turn the patient carefully every 2 hours.
■ Encourage careful deep breathing and coughing.
■ Suction gently as needed.
■ Make sure the dressings stay clean, dry, and intact.
■ Ensure a quiet, calm environment.
■ Maintain seizure precautions.

Monitoring
■ Vital signs
■ Intake and output
■ Level of consciousness
■ Respiratory status
■ ICP
■ Heart rate and rhythm
■ Hemodynamic values
■ Fluid and electrolyte balance
■ Urine specific gravity
■ Daily weight
■ Drain patency
■ Surgical wound, dressings, drainage
■ Complications

Notify the physician immediately if you detect a worsening mental status, pupillary changes, or focal signs, such as increasing weakness in an arm or leg. These findings may indicate increased ICP.

PATIENT TEACHING
Be sure to cover:
■ medications and possible adverse reactions
■ surgical wound care
■ probability of headache and facial swelling for 2 to 3 days after surgery
■ postoperative leg exercises and deep breathing
■ use of antiembolism stockings or a pneumatic compression device

- signs and symptoms of infection
- complications
- when to notify the physician
- use of a wig, hat, or scarf until hair grows back
- avoidance of alcohol and smoking
- follow-up care.

HYPOPHYSECTOMY

Overview

- Excision of the hypophysis cerebri
- Transfrontal approach: entry into the sella turcica through the cranium
- Transsphenoidal approach: entry into the sella turcica from the inner aspect of the upper lip through the sphenoid sinus
- Alternative approach: laser surgery

INDICATIONS

- Pituitary tumor
- Palliative measure for metastatic breast or prostate cancer

COMPLICATIONS

- Diabetes insipidus
- Transient syndrome of inappropriate antidiuretic hormone
- Infection
- Cerebrospinal fluid leakage
- Hemorrhage
- Vision defects
- Loss of smell and taste

Nursing interventions

PRETREATMENT CARE

- Explain the treatment and preparation to the patient and family.
- Make sure the patient has signed an appropriate consent form.
- Explain postoperative care, including presence of a nasal catheter and packing for 1 to 2 days after surgery.

- Arrange for baseline visual field tests and other appropriate tests and examinations as ordered.

POSTTREATMENT CARE

- Administer medications as ordered.
- Maintain bed rest for 24 hours, then encourage ambulation.
- Elevate the head of the bed.
- For diabetes insipidus, administer fluids, aqueous vasopressin, or sublingual desmopressin acetate as ordered.
- Arrange for visual field testing.
- Evaluate the need for hormone replacement.

Monitoring

- Vital signs
- Intake and output
- Complications
- Surgical wound and dressings
- Drainage
- Diabetes insipidus
- Pituitary hormone levels

PATIENT TEACHING

Be sure to cover:
- medications and possible adverse reactions
- signs and symptoms of diabetes insipidus
- fluid restrictions if indicated
- avoidance of sneezing, coughing, blowing the nose, or bending over for several days postoperatively
- avoidance of brushing the teeth for 2 weeks if ordered (suggest the use of mouthwash instead)
- signs and symptoms of excessive or insufficient cortisol or thyroid hormone replacement (if ordered)
- complications
- when to notify the physician
- importance of wearing medical identification
- follow-up care.

NEUROLOGIC CARE

PROCEDURES AND EQUIPMENT

BISPECTRAL INDEX MONITORING

Bispectral index monitoring consists of a monitor and cable connected to a sensor applied to the patient's forehead (as shown below).

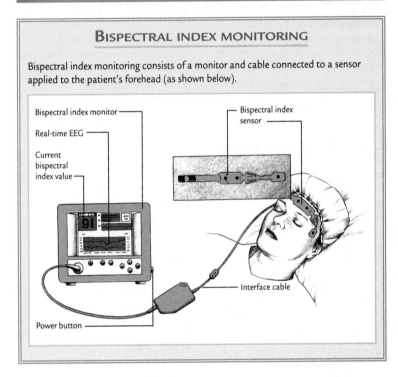

Bispectral index monitor

Real-time EEG

Current bispectral index value

Bispectral index sensor

Interface cable

Power button

TROUBLESHOOTING SENSOR PROBLEMS

When initiating bispectral index monitoring, be aware that the monitor may display messages that indicate a problem. This chart highlights these messages and offers possible solutions.

Message	Possible solutions
High impedance message	Check sensor adhesion; reapply firm pressure to each of the numbered circles on the sensor for 5 seconds each; if message continues, check the connection between the sensor and the monitor; if necessary, apply a new sensor.
Noise message	Remove possible pressure on the sensor; investigate possible large stimulus such as electrocautery.
Lead-off message	Check sensor for electrode displacement or lifting; reapply with firm pressure or, if necessary, apply a new sensor.

NEUROLOGIC CARE

INTERPRETING BISPECTRAL INDEX VALUES

Use the following guidelines to interpret patient's bispectral index value:

Bispectral index		
100	Awake	
	Light to moderate sedation	⎫ Light hypnotic
70	Deep sedation (low probability of explicit recall)	⎬ state
60	General anesthesia (low probability of consciousness)	⎫ Moderate
40	Deep hypnotic state	⎬ hypnotic state
0	Flat-line EEG	

NEUROLOGIC PARAMETERS

Parameter	Potential causes of high values	Potential causes of low values
Mixed venous oxygen saturation ($S\overline{v}o_2$) Normal: 60% to 80% Formula: (CO x Cao_2 x 10) – Vo_2	■ Increased oxygen supply ■ Decreased oxygen demand ■ Decreased use of oxygen by tissues ■ Hypertension	■ Decreased oxygen supply ■ Increased oxygen demand ■ Hypovolemic shock ■ Myocardial infarction (MI) ■ Pericardial tamponade ■ Pulmonary embolism
Cerebral perfusion pressure Normal: 70 to 80 mm Hg Formula: MAP – (ICP)	■ Hypertension	■ Acute hydrocephalus ■ Intracranial hematoma ■ Cerebral edema ■ Arrhythmias ■ MI ■ Dehydration ■ Osmotic drugs ■ Diabetes insipidus ■ Blood pressure medications (antihypertensives)
Intracranial pressure Normal: 0 to 10 mm Hg Formula: N/A	■ Cerebral edema ■ Acute hydrocephalus ■ Intracranial hematoma ■ Ischemia	

NEUROLOGIC CARE

Types of ICP monitoring

Intracranial pressure (ICP) can be monitored by using one of four systems.

Intraventricular catheter monitoring

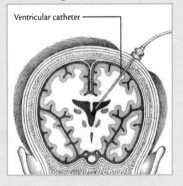

Subarachnoid bolt monitoring

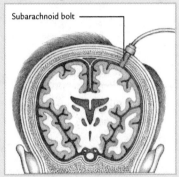

In intraventricular catheter monitoring, which monitors ICP directly, the physician inserts a small polyethylene or silicone catheter into the lateral ventricle through a burr hole.

This is the only type of ICP monitoring that allows evaluation of brain compliance and drainage of significant amounts of cerebrospinal fluid (CSF). Although this method measures ICP most accurately, it also carries the greatest risk of infection.

Contraindications usually include stenotic cerebral ventricles, cerebral aneurysms in the path of catheter placement, and suspected vascular lesions.

Subarachnoid bolt monitoring involves the insertion of a special bolt into the subarachnoid space through a twist-drill hole that's positioned in the front of the skull behind the hairline.

Placing the bolt is easier than placing an intraventricular catheter, especially if a computed tomography scan reveals that the cerebrum has shifted or the ventricles have collapsed. This type of ICP monitoring also carries less risk of infection and parenchymal damage because the bolt doesn't penetrate the cerebrum.

Epidural or subdural sensor monitoring

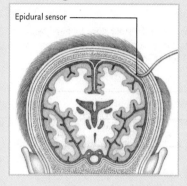

Epidural sensor

Intraparenchymal monitoring

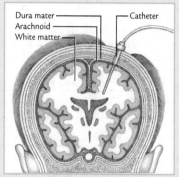

Dura mater — Catheter
Arachnoid
White matter

ICP can also be monitored from the epidural or subdural space. For epidural monitoring, a fiberoptic sensor is inserted into the epidural space through a burr hole. This system's main drawback is its questionable accuracy because ICP isn't being measured directly from a CSF-filled space.

For subdural monitoring, a fiber-optic transducer–tipped catheter is tunneled through a burr hole and its tip is placed on brain tissue under the dura mater. The main drawback to this method is its inability to drain CSF.

,,..,.In intraparenchymal monitoring, the physician inserts a catheter through a small subarachnoid bolt and, after puncturing the dura, advances the catheter a few centimeters into the brain's white matter. There's no need to balance or calibrate the equipment after insertion.

Although this method doesn't provide direct access to CSF, measurements are accurate because brain tissue pressure correlates well with ventricular pressures. Intraparenchymal monitoring may be used to obtain ICP measurements in patients with compressed or dislocated ventricles.

INTERPRETING ICP WAVEFORMS

Three waveforms — A, B, and C — are used to monitor intracranial pressure (ICP). A waves are an ominous sign of intracranial decompensation and poor compliance. B waves correlate with changes in respiration, and C waves correlate with changes in arterial pressure.

Normal waveform

A normal ICP waveform typically shows a steep upward systolic slope followed by a downward diastolic slope with a dicrotic notch. In most cases, this waveform occurs continuously and indicates an ICP between 0 and 15 mm Hg — normal pressure.

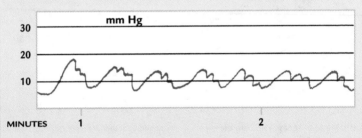

A waves

The most clinically significant ICP waveforms are A waves (shown below), which may reach elevations of 50 to 100 mm Hg, persist for 5 to 20 minutes, then drop sharply — signaling exhaustion of the brain's compliance mechanisms. A waves may come and go, spiking from temporary rises in thoracic pressure or from any condition that increases ICP beyond the brain's compliance limits. Activities, such as sustained coughing or straining during defecation, can cause temporary elevations in thoracic pressure.

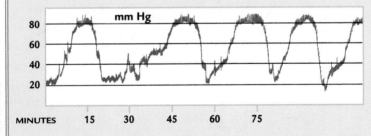

B waves

B waves, which appear sharp and rhythmic with a sawtooth pattern, occur every 1½ to 2 minutes and may reach elevations of 50 mm Hg. The clinical significance of B waves isn't clear, but the waves correlate with respiratory changes and may occur more frequently with decreasing compensation. Because B waves sometimes precede A waves, notify the physician if B waves occur frequently.

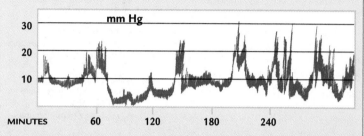

C waves

Like B waves, C waves are rapid and rhythmic, but they aren't as sharp. Clinically insignificant, they may fluctuate with respirations or systemic blood pressure changes.

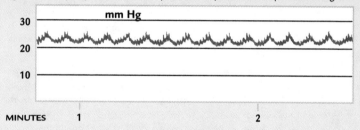

Waveform showing equipment problem

A waveform that looks like the one shown below signals a problem with the transducer or monitor. Check for line obstruction, and determine if the transducer needs rebalancing.

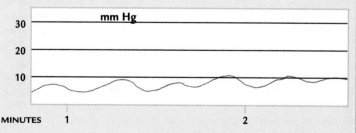

TROUBLESHOOTING
INTRACRANIAL PRESSURE MONITORS

Problem	Possible causes	Interventions
Damped or absent waveform	■ Transducer needs recalibration	■ Turn stopcock off to the patient. ■ Open transducer's stopcock to air and balance transducer. ■ Recalibrate transducer and monitor.
	■ Air in line	■ Turn stopcock off to the patient. ■ Flush air out through an open stopcock port with a syringe and sterile normal saline solution. ■ Don't use heparin to flush because some of the drug could inadvertently be injected into the patient and cause bleeding. ■ Rebalance and recalibrate transducer and monitor.
	■ Loose connection	■ Check tubing and stopcocks for possible moisture, which may indicate a loose connection. ■ Turn stopcock off to the patient, and then tighten all connections. ■ Make sure tubing is long enough to allow the patient to turn head without pulling on the tubing.
	■ Disconnection in the line	■ Turn stopcock off to the patient immediately. ■ Keep in mind that with a ventricular catheter, rapid cerebrospinal fluid loss may allow intracranial pressure to drop precipitously, causing brain herniation. ■ Replace equipment to reduce the risk of infection.
	■ Change in the patient's position	■ Reposition transducer's balancing port level with the foramen of Monro. ■ Rebalance and recalibrate transducer and monitor. ■ Remember to rebalance and recalibrate at least once every 4 hours and whenever the patient is repositioned.
	■ Tubing, catheter, or screw occluded with blood or brain tissue	■ Notify the physician, because he may want to irrigate the screw or catheter with a small amount of sterile normal saline. ■ Never irrigate the screw or catheter by yourself.

TROUBLESHOOTING
INTRACRANIAL PRESSURE MONITORS *(continued)*

Problem	Possible causes	Interventions
False pressure readings, high or low	■ Air in line	■ Turn stopcock off to the patient. ■ Flush air out through an open stopcock port with a syringe and sterile normal saline solution. ■ Rebalance and recalibrate transducer and monitor.
	■ Transducer placed too low (causing high pressure reading) or too high (causing low pressure reading)	■ Reposition transducer's balancing port level with the foramen of Monro. ■ Rebalance and recalibrate transducer and monitor.

CSF DRAINAGE USING A VENTRICULAR DRAIN

Cerebrospinal fluid (CSF) drainage aims to control intracranial pressure (ICP) during treatment for traumatic injury or other conditions that cause an increase in ICP. A commonly used procedure is described below.

Ventricular drain
For a ventricular drain, the physician makes a burr hole in the patient's skull and inserts the catheter into the ventricle. The distal end of the catheter is connected to a closed drainage system.

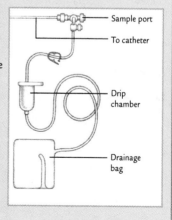

Sample port

To catheter

Drip chamber

Drainage bag

NEUROLOGIC CARE

DRUGS

COMMON NEUROLOGIC DRUGS

Use this table to find out about common neurologic drugs, their indications and adverse effects, and related special considerations.

Drug	Indications	Adverse reactions	Special considerations
NONOPIOID ANALGESICS			
Acetaminophen (Tylenol)	■ Mild pain, headache	■ Severe liver damage, neutropenia, thrombocytopenia	■ Monitor total daily intake of acetaminophen because of risk for liver toxicity. Use cautiously in elderly patients and those with liver disease.
OPIOID ANALGESICS			
Morphine	■ Severe pain	■ Respiratory depression, apnea, bradycardia, seizures, sedation	■ Monitor for respiratory depression. Use cautiously in elderly patients and those with head injury, seizures, or increased intracranial pressure (ICP). Contraindicated in patients with acute bronchial asthma.
Codeine	■ Mild to moderate pain	■ Respiratory depression, bradycardia, sedation, constipation	■ Monitor for respiratory depression. Use cautiously in elderly patients and those with head injury, seizures, or increased ICP.
ANTICONVULSANTS			
Carbamazepine (Tegretol)	■ Generalized tonic-clonic seizures, complex partial seizures, mixed seizures	■ Heart failure, worsening of seizure, atrioventricular block, hepatitis, thrombocytopenia, Stevens-Johnson syndrome	■ Use cautiously in patients with mixed seizure disorders because it can increase their risk of seizure. Use cautiously in patients with hepatic dysfunction. Obtain baseline liver function, complete blood count, and blood urea nitrogen level. Monitor blood levels of the drug; therapeutic level is 4 to 12 mcg/ml.

COMMON NEUROLOGIC DRUGS *(continued)*

Drug	Indications	Adverse reactions	Special considerations
ANTICONVULSANTS *(continued)*			
Fosphenytoin (Cerebyx)	■ Status epilepticus, seizures during neurosurgery	■ Increased intracranial pressure, cerebral edema, somnolence, bradycardia, QT prolongation, heart block	■ Stop administration of the drug in patients who develop acute hepatotoxicity. May cause hyperglycemia; monitor blood glucose levels in patients who are diabetic. Fosphenytoin should be prescribed and dispensed in phenytoin sodium equivalent units. Monitor for cardiac arrhythmias and QT prolongation.
Phenytoin (Dilantin)	■ Generalized tonic-clonic seizures, status epilepticus, nonepileptic seizures after head trauma	■ Agranulocytosis, thrombocytopenia, toxic hepatitis, slurred speech, Stevens-Johnson syndrome	■ Abrupt withdrawal can trigger status epilepticus. Contraindicated in patients with heart block. Use cautiously in patients with hepatic disease and myocardial insufficiency. Monitor blood levels of drug; therapeutic range is 10 to 20 mcg/ml. If rash appears, stop administration.
Primidone (Mysoline)	■ Generalized tonic-clonic seizures, focal seizures, complex partial seizures	■ Thrombocytopenia, drowsiness, ataxia	■ Abrupt withdrawal can cause status epilepticus. Reduce dosage in elderly patients.
Valproic acid (Depakene)	■ Complex partial seizures, simple and complex absence seizures	■ Thrombocytopenia, pancreatitis, toxic hepatitis, sedation, ataxia	■ Obtain baseline liver function tests. Avoid use in patients with a high risk for hepatotoxicity. Abrupt withdrawal may worsen seizures. Monitor blood levels of drug; therapeutic range is 50 to 100 mcg/ml.

NEUROLOGIC CARE

(continued)

COMMON NEUROLOGIC DRUGS *(continued)*

Drug	Indications	Adverse reactions	Special considerations
ANTICOAGULANTS			
Heparin	■ Embolism prophylaxis after cerebral thrombosis in evolving stroke	■ Hemorrhage, thrombocytopenia	■ Monitor for bleeding. Obtain baseline international normalized ratio (INR), prothrombin time (PT), and partial thromboplastin time (PTT). Monitor PTT at regular intervals. Protamine reverses the effects of heparin.
ANTIPLATELETS			
Aspirin (A.S.A.)	■ Transient ischemic attacks, thromboembolic disorders	■ GI bleeding, acute renal insufficiency, thrombocytopenia, liver dysfunction	■ Monitor for bleeding. Avoid using in patients with a peptic ulcer and GI inflammation.
Sulfinpyrazone (Anturane)	■ Thrombotic stroke prophylaxis	■ Blood dyscrasia, thrombocytopenia, bronchoconstriction	■ Monitor for bleeding. Avoid using in patients with a peptic ulcer and GI inflammation.
Ticlopidine (Ticlid)	■ Thrombotic stroke prophylaxis	■ Thrombocytopenia, agranulocytosis	■ Monitor for bleeding. Avoid using in patients with hepatic impairment and a peptic ulcer.
BARBITURATES			
Phenobarbital (Barbita)	■ All types of seizures except absence seizures and febrile seizures in children; also used for status epilepticus, sedation, and drug withdrawal	■ Respiratory depression, apnea, bradycardia, angioedema, Stevens-Johnson syndrome	■ Monitor for respiratory depression and bradycardia. Keep resuscitation equipment on hand when administering I.V.; monitor respirations.

COMMON NEUROLOGIC DRUGS *(continued)*

Drug	Indications	Adverse reactions	Special considerations
BENZODIAZEPINES			
Clonazepam (Klonopin)	■ Absence and atypical seizures, generalized tonic-clonic seizures, status epilepticus, panic disorder	■ Respiratory depression, thrombocytopenia, leukopenia, drowsiness, ataxia	■ Abrupt withdrawal may precipitate status epilepticus. Elderly patients are at a greater risk for central nervous system (CNS) depression and may require a lower dose.
Diazepam (Valium)	■ Status epilepticus, anxiety, acute alcohol withdrawal, muscle spasm	■ Respiratory depression, bradycardia, cardiovascular collapse, drowsiness, acute withdrawal syndrome	■ Monitor for respiratory depression and cardiac arrhythmia. Don't stop administration abruptly; can cause acute withdrawal in persons who are physically dependent.
Lorazepam (Ativan)	■ Status epilepticus, anxiety and agitation	■ Drowsiness, acute withdrawal syndrome	■ Don't stop administration abruptly; can cause acute withdrawal in persons who are physically dependent. Monitor for CNS depressant effects in elderly patients.
CALCIUM CHANNEL BLOCKERS			
Nimodipine (Nimotop)	■ Neurologic deficits caused by cerebral vasospasm after congenital aneurysm rupture	■ Decreased blood pressure, tachycardia, edema	■ Use cautiously in patients with hepatic failure. Monitor for hypotension and tachycardia.
CORTICOSTEROIDS			
Dexamethasone (Decadron); **methylprednisolone** (Solu-Medrol)	■ Cerebral edema, severe inflammation	■ Heart failure, cardiac arrhythmias, edema, circulatory collapse, thromboembolism, pancreatitis, peptic ulceration	■ Use cautiously in patients with recent myocardial infarction (MI), hypertension, renal disease, and GI ulcer. Monitor blood pressure and blood glucose levels.

(continued)

NEUROLOGIC CARE

COMMON NEUROLOGIC DRUGS *(continued)*

Drug	Indications	Adverse reactions	Special considerations
DIURETICS			
Loop diuretic: furosemide (Lasix)	■ Edema, hypertension	■ Renal failure, thrombocytopenia, agranulocytosis, volume depletion, dehydration	■ Monitor blood pressure, pulse, and intake and output. Monitor serum electrolytes, especially potassium levels. Monitor for cardiac arrhythmias.
Osmotic diuretic: mannitol (Osmitrol)	■ Cerebral edema, increased intracranial pressure	■ Heart failure, seizures, fluid and electrolyte imbalance	■ Contraindicated in patients with severe pulmonary congestion and heart failure. Monitor blood pressure, heart rate, and intake and output. Monitor serum electrolytes. Use with caution in patients with renal dysfunction.
THROMBOLYTICS			
Alteplase (recombinant alteplase, tissue-type plasminogen) (Activase); **streptokinase** (Streptase)	■ Acute ischemic stroke	■ Cerebral hemorrhage, spontaneous bleeding, allergic reaction	■ Contraindicated in patients with intracranial or subarachnoid hemorrhage. The patient must meet criteria for thrombolytic therapy prior to initiation of therapy. Monitor baseline laboratory values: hemoglobin, hematocrit, PTT, PT, and INR. Monitor vital signs. Monitor for signs of bleeding.

11

MUSCULOSKELETAL CARE

ASSESSMENT

MUSCULOSKELETAL SYSTEM: NORMAL FINDINGS

Inspection
- No gross deformities are apparent.
- Body parts are symmetrical.
- Body alignment is good.
- No involuntary movements are detectable.
- Gait is smooth.
- All muscles and joints have active range of motion with no pain.
- No swelling or inflammation is visible in the joints or muscles.
- Bilateral limb length is equal and muscle mass is symmetrical.

Palpation
- Shape is normal, with no swelling or tenderness.
- Bilateral muscle tone, texture, and strength are equal.
- No involuntary contractions or twitching is detectable.
- Bilateral pulses are equally strong.

GRADING MUSCLE STRENGTH

Grade muscle strength on a scale of 0 to 5, as follows:
- 5/5: normal; patient moves joint through full range of motion (ROM) and against gravity with full resistance
- 4/5: good; patient completes ROM against gravity with moderate resistance
- 3/5: fair; patient completes ROM against gravity only
- 2/5: poor; patient completes full ROM with gravity eliminated (passive motion)
- 1/5: trace; patient's attempt at muscle contraction is palpable but without joint movement
- 0/5: zero; no evidence of muscle contraction.

TESTING MUSCLE STRENGTH

To test the muscle strength of your patient's arm and ankle muscles, use the techniques shown here.

Biceps strength

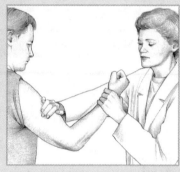

Triceps strength

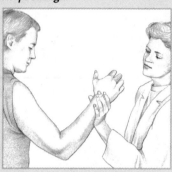

THE 5 P'S OF MUSCULOSKELETAL INJURY

To swiftly assess a musculoskeletal injury, remember the 5 P's—pain, paresthesia, paralysis, pallor, and pulse.

Pain

Ask the patient whether he feels pain. If he does, assess the location, severity, and quality of the pain.

Paresthesia

Assess the patient for loss of sensation by touching the injured area with the tip of an open safety pin. Abnormal sensation or loss of sensation indicates neurovascular involvement.

Paralysis

Assess whether the patient can move the affected area. If he can't, he might have nerve or tendon damage.

Pallor

Paleness, discoloration, and coolness on the injured side may indicate neurovascular compromise.

Pulse

Check all pulses distal to the injury site. If a pulse is decreased or absent, blood supply to the area is reduced.

Ankle strength: Plantar flexion

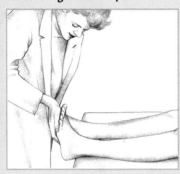

Ankle strength: Dorsiflexion

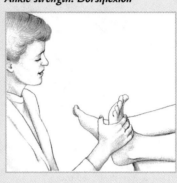

BULGE SIGN

The bulge sign indicates excess fluid in the joint. To assess the patient for this sign, ask him to lie down so that you can palpate his knee. Then give the medial side of his knee two to four firm strokes, as shown, to displace excess fluid.

Lateral check
Next, tap the lateral aspect of the knee while checking for a fluid wave on the medial aspect, as shown.

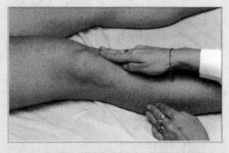

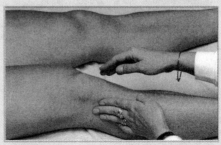

MUSCULOSKELETAL SYSTEM: INTERPRETING YOUR FINDINGS

After you assess the patient, a group of findings may lead you to suspect a particular disorder. This chart shows some common groups of findings for signs and symptoms of the musculoskeletal system, along with their probable causes.

Sign or symptom and findings	Probable cause
ARM PAIN	
■ Pain radiating through the arm ■ Pain worsens with movement ■ Crepitus, felt and heard ■ Deformity (if bones are misaligned) ■ Local ecchymosis and edema ■ Impaired distal circulation ■ Paresthesia	Fracture
■ Left arm pain ■ Deep and crushing chest pain ■ Weakness ■ Pallor ■ Dyspnea ■ Diaphoresis ■ Apprehension	Myocardial infarction
■ Severe arm pain with passive muscle stretching ■ Impaired distal circulation ■ Muscle weakness ■ Decreased reflex response ■ Paresthesia ■ Edema ■ Ominous signs: paralysis and absent pulse	Compartment syndrome
LEG PAIN	
■ Severe, acute leg pain, particularly with movement ■ Ecchymosis and edema ■ Leg unable to bear weight ■ Impaired neurovascular status distal to injury ■ Deformity, crepitus, and muscle spasms	Fracture
■ Shooting, aching, or tingling pain that radiates down the leg ■ Pain exacerbated by activity and relieved by rest ■ Limping ■ Difficulty moving from a sitting to a standing position	Sciatica
■ Discomfort ranging from calf tenderness to severe pain ■ Edema and a feeling of heaviness in the affected leg ■ Warmth ■ Fever, chills, malaise, muscle cramps ■ Positive Homans' sign	Thrombophlebitis

MUSCULOSKELETAL SYSTEM:
INTERPRETING YOUR FINDINGS *(continued)*

Sign or symptom and findings	Probable cause

MUSCLE SPASM

■ Spasms and intermittent claudication ■ Loss of peripheral pulses ■ Pallor or cyanosis ■ Decreased sensation ■ Hair loss ■ Dry or scaling skin ■ Edema ■ Ulcerations	Arterial occlusive disease
■ Localized spasms and pain ■ Swelling ■ Limited mobility ■ Bony crepitation	Fracture
■ Tetany (muscle cramps and twitching, carpopedal and facial muscle spasms, and seizures) ■ Positive Chvostek's and Trousseau's signs ■ Paresthesia of the lips, fingers, and toes ■ Choreiform movements ■ Hyperactive deep tendon reflexes ■ Fatigue ■ Palpitations ■ Cardiac arrhythmias	Hypocalcemia

MUSCLE WEAKNESS

■ Unilateral or bilateral weakness of the arms, legs, face, or tongue ■ Dysarthria ■ Aphasia ■ Paresthesia or sensory loss ■ Vision disturbances ■ Bowel and bladder dysfunction	Stroke
■ Muscle weakness, disuse, and possible atrophy ■ Altered level of consciousness ■ Personality changes ■ Severe lower back pain, possibly radiating to the buttocks, legs, and feet (usually unilateral) ■ Diminished reflexes ■ Sensory changes	Herniated disk

(continued)

MUSCULOSKELETAL SYSTEM: INTERPRETING YOUR FINDINGS (continued)

Sign or symptom and findings	Probable cause
MUSCLE WEAKNESS (continued)	
■ Muscle weakness in one or more limbs which may lead to atrophy, spasticity, and contractures ■ Diplopia, blurred vision, or vision loss ■ Hyperactive deep tendon reflexes ■ Paresthesia or sensory loss ■ Incoordination ■ Intention tremors	Multiple sclerosis

DIAGNOSTIC TESTS

ARTHROSCOPY

Overview

■ Visual examination of the interior of a joint using a fiber-optic endoscope
■ Most commonly used to examine the knee joint
■ Permits concurrent surgery or biopsy using triangulation, in which instruments are passed through a separate cannula
■ Usually an outpatient procedure

PURPOSE

■ To evaluate suspected or confirmed joint disease
■ To provide a safe, convenient alternative to open surgery (arthrotomy) and separate biopsy
■ To detect and diagnose meniscal, patellar, condylar, extrasynovial, and synovial diseases
■ To monitor progression of disease
■ To monitor effectiveness of therapy

PATIENT PREPARATION

■ Make sure the patient has signed an appropriate consent form.
■ Note and report all allergies.
■ Instruct the patient that fasting is required after midnight before the procedure.
■ Warn the patient that transient discomfort may be felt from injection of the local anesthetic and pressure of the tourniquet on the leg.
■ Explain that a thumping sensation may be felt as the cannula is inserted into the joint capsule.

TEACHING POINTS

Be sure to cover:
■ the test's purpose and how it's done
■ who will perform the study and where
■ that the study takes about 1 hour
■ the need to avoid tub baths until after the postoperative visit. (Showers are permitted 48 hours after the study.)

POSTPROCEDURE CARE

- Administer analgesics as ordered.
- Elevate the leg and apply ice for the first 24 hours.
- Report any fever, bleeding, drainage, or increased swelling or pain in the joint.
- Limit weight bearing by using a walker, cane, or crutches for 48 hours.
- Apply an immobilizer if ordered.
- Resume the patient's usual diet.

Monitoring

- Fever
- Swelling
- Increased pain
- Localized inflammation
- Neurovascular status of the extremity

PRECAUTIONS

- Check the patient's history for hypersensitivity to the anesthetic or sedation.
- Contraindications include:
- fibrous ankylosis with flexion of less than 50 degrees
- local skin or wound infections.

COMPLICATIONS

- Infection
- Hematoma
- Thrombophlebitis
- Joint injury

Interpretation

NORMAL FINDINGS

- The knee is a diarthrodial joint surrounded by muscles, ligaments, cartilage, and tendons and lined with synovial membrane.
- Articular cartilage appears smooth and white.
- Ligaments and tendons appear cablelike and silvery.
- The synovium is smooth and marked by a fine vascular network.
- Degenerative changes begin during adolescence.

ABNORMAL RESULTS

- Meniscal abnormalities may suggest torn medial or lateral meniscus.
- Patellar abnormalities may suggest chondromalacia, dislocation, subluxation, fracture, or parapatellar synovitis.
- Condylar abnormalities may suggest degenerative articular cartilage, osteochondritis dissecans, or loose bodies.
- Extrasynovial abnormalities may suggest torn anterior cruciate or tibial collateral ligaments, Baker's cyst, and ganglion cyst.
- Synovial abnormalities may suggest synovitis and rheumatoid and degenerative arthritis.
- Foreign bodies may suggest gout, pseudogout, and osteochondromatosis.

BONE BIOPSY

Overview

- Removal of a piece or a core of bone for histologic examination
- Performed using a special drill needle under local anesthesia, or by surgical excision under general anesthesia
- Indicated in patients with bone pain and tenderness after a bone scan, a computed tomography scan, radiographs, or arteriography reveals a mass or deformity
- Excision provides larger specimen than drill biopsy and permits immediate surgical treatment if rapid histologic analysis of the specimen reveals malignant tumor

PURPOSE

■ To distinguish between benign and malignant bone tumors

PATIENT PREPARATION

■ Make sure the patient has signed an appropriate consent form.
■ Note and report all allergies.
■ Fasting overnight before the test is necessary with open biopsy. Food and fluids restriction isn't generally necessary with drill biopsy.
■ A local anesthetic is administered before drill biopsy.
■ Warn the patient that some discomfort and pressure will be experienced when the biopsy needle enters the bone in drill biopsy.

Teaching points

Be sure to cover:
■ the test's purpose and how it's done
■ who will perform the biopsy and where

POSTPROCEDURE CARE

■ Notify the physician of excessive drainage or bleeding at the biopsy site.
■ Administer analgesics as ordered.
■ Resume the patient's usual diet after full recovery from anesthesia.

Monitoring

■ Vital signs
■ Biopsy site
■ Signs and symptoms of infection

For several days after the biopsy, watch for indications of bone infection, including fever, headache, pain on movement, and tissue redness or abscess at or near the biopsy site. Notify the physician if these symptoms develop.

PRECAUTIONS

■ Check the patient's history for hypersensitivity to the anesthetic.

■ Bone biopsy is performed cautiously in patients with uncorrected coagulopathy.
■ Send the specimen to the laboratory immediately.
■ Failure to obtain a representative bone specimen or to use the proper fixative may alter test results.

COMPLICATIONS

■ Bone fracture
■ Damage to surrounding tissue
■ Infection (osteomyelitis)

Interpretation

NORMAL FINDINGS

■ Bone tissue is classified as one of two histologic types: compact or cancellous.
■ Compact bone has dense, concentric layers of mineral deposits, or lamellae.
■ Cancellous bone has widely spaced lamellae with osteocytes and red and yellow marrow between them.

ABNORMAL RESULTS

■ Well circumscribed and nonmetastasizing lesions suggest benign tumors, such as osteoid osteoma, osteoblastoma, osteochondroma, unicameral bone cyst, benign giant cell tumor, and fibroma.
■ Irregularly and rapidly spreading lesions suggest malignant tumors, such as multiple myeloma and osteosarcoma.

BONE DENSITOMETRY

Overview

■ A noninvasive means to measure bone mass

■ Uses a radiography tube and computer-analyzed images to measure bone mineral density
■ Performed in the radiology department, a physician's office, or a clinic
■ Exposes the patient to minimal radiation
■ Also known as dual energy X-ray absorptiometry or DEXA

PURPOSE

■ To determine bone mineral density
■ To identify people at risk for osteoporosis
■ To evaluate clinical response to therapy aimed at reducing the rate of bone loss

PATIENT PREPARATION

■ Remove all metal objects from the area to be scanned.

Teaching points

Be sure to cover:
■ the test's purpose and how it's done
■ who will perform the test and where
■ that the test is painless and exposure to radiation is minimal
■ that the test takes from 10 minutes to 1 hour, depending on the areas scanned.

POSTPROCEDURE CARE

■ No specific postprocedure care is required.

PRECAUTIONS

■ Bone densitometry is contraindicated during pregnancy.
■ The accuracy of test results may be influenced by:
– osteoarthritis
– fractures
– size of the region to be scanned
– fat tissue distribution.

COMPLICATIONS

■ None known

Interpretation

NORMAL FINDINGS

■ T-score is above –1.

ABNORMAL RESULTS

■ A T-score between –1 and –2.5 may suggest osteopenia.
■ A T-score at or below –2.5 may suggest osteoporosis.

BONE SCAN

Overview

■ Permits imaging of the skeleton by a scanning camera after I.V. injection of a radioactive tracer compound
■ Tracer of choice is radioactive technetium diphosphonate
■ Increased concentrations of tracer collect in bone tissue at sites of abnormal metabolism; when scanned, these sites appear as hot spots (commonly detectable months before radiography reveals lesion)
■ May be performed with gallium scan to promote early detection of lesions
■ Primary indications:
– Symptoms of metastatic bone disease
– Bone trauma
– Known degenerative disorders that require monitoring for signs of progression

PURPOSE

■ To detect malignant bone lesions when radiographic findings are normal but cancer is confirmed or suspected
■ To rule out suspected bone lesions
■ To detect occult bone trauma associated with pathologic fractures
■ To monitor degenerative bone disorders

- To detect infection
- To evaluate unexplained bone pain
- To assist in staging cancer

PATIENT PREPARATION

- Make sure the patient has signed an appropriate consent form, if required.
- Note all allergies.
- There are no dietary restrictions.
- Instruct the patient to drink fluids to maintain hydration and to reduce the radiation dose to the bladder after tracer injection and before scanning.
- Explain the importance of holding still during scanning.

Teaching points

Be sure to cover:
- the purpose of the study and how it's done
- who will perform the test and where
- that the scan is painless and takes about 1 hour
- that the radioactive isotope emits less radiation than a standard radiograph machine
- that analgesics will be given as ordered for positional discomfort.

POSTPROCEDURE CARE

- Instruct the patient to drink additional fluids and to empty his bladder frequently for the next 24 to 48 hours.

Monitoring

- Signs and symptoms of infection at injection site
- Intake and output

PRECAUTIONS

- A bone scan is contraindicated during pregnancy or lactation.
- Avoid exposing infants to radiation.
- Allergic reactions to the radionuclide are rare.
- A bone scan doesn't distinguish between normal and abnormal bone formation.

- Antihypertensives may affect test results.
- A distended bladder may obscure pelvic detail.
- Improper injection technique allows the tracer to seep into muscle tissue, producing erroneous hot spots.
- Avoid scheduling additional radionuclide tests for the next 24 to 48 hours.

COMPLICATIONS

- Infection at the injection site
- Allergic reactions to radionuclide (rare)

Interpretation

NORMAL FINDINGS

- Uptake of the tracer is symmetrical and uniform.
- The tracer concentrates at sites of new bone formation or increased metabolism.
- The epiphyses of growing bone are normal sites of high concentration or hot spots.

ABNORMAL RESULTS

- Increased uptake of tracer where bone formation is occurring faster than in surrounding bone may suggest:
  - all types of bone cancer
  - infection
  - fracture
  - additional disorders when used in conjunction with the patient's medical and surgical history, radiographic findings, and laboratory test results.

MAGNETIC RESONANCE IMAGING OF BONE AND SOFT TISSUE

Overview

■ Noninvasive technique producing clear and sensitive tomographic images of bone and soft tissue
■ Provides superior contrast of body tissues and allows imaging of multiple planes, including direct sagittal and coronal views
■ Eliminates the risks associated with exposure to radiation from X-rays and causes no known harm to cells

PURPOSE

■ To evaluate bony and soft-tissue tumors
■ To identify changes in the bone marrow cavity
■ To identify spinal disorders

PATIENT PREPARATION

■ Make sure the patient has signed an appropriate consent form.
■ Note and report all allergies.
■ Make sure the scanner can accommodate the patient's weight and abdominal girth.
■ Screen for surgically implanted joints, pins, clips, valves, pumps, or pacemakers containing metal.
■ Discontinue I.V. infusion pumps, feeding tubes with metal tips, pulmonary artery catheters, and similar devices before the test as ordered.
■ Explain to the patient that he'll the scanner clicking, whirring, and thumping, so he may use earplugs.
■ Provide reassurance to the patient that he'll be able to communicate with the technician at all times.

■ An I.V. line may be started for injection of a contrast agent for certain types of magnetic resonance imaging (MRI).
■ If the patient is claustrophobic, sedation or an open scanner may be used.
■ Stress the importance of removing all metallic objects, such as jewelry, hairpins, and a watch.

Teaching points
Be sure to cover:
■ the test's purpose and how it's done
■ who will perform the test and where
■ that the test takes 30 to 90 minutes
■ that MRI is painless and involves no exposure to radiation.

POSTPROCEDURE CARE

■ Provide comfort measures as needed.
■ Resume normal activities as ordered.

Monitoring

■ Vital signs
■ Postural hypotension

PRECAUTIONS

■ Monitor for claustrophobia and anxiety.
■ MRI involves using a powerful magnetic field, so don't allow any metal objects, such as I.V. pumps, ventilators, and other metallic equipment, or computer-based equipment to enter the MRI area.

If the patient is unstable, make sure an I.V. line without metal components is in place and that all equipment is compatible with MRI imaging; monitor oxygen saturation, cardiac rhythm, and respiratory status during the test. An anesthesiologist may be needed to monitor a heavily sedated patient.

COMPLICATIONS
- Claustrophobia
- Anxiety
- Postural hypotension

Interpretation

NORMAL FINDINGS
- There's no evidence of pathology in bone, muscles, and joints.

ABNORMAL RESULTS
- Structural abnormalities suggest possible primary and metastatic tumors and various disorders of the bone, muscles, and joints.

DISEASES

ACCELERATION-DECELERATION INJURIES

Overview

DESCRIPTION
- Injury resulting from sharp hyperextension and flexion of the neck that damages muscles, ligaments, disks, and nerve tissue
- Excellent prognosis; symptoms usually subside with symptomatic treatment
- Also called whiplash

PATHOPHYSIOLOGY
- Unexpected force causes the head to jerk back and then forward.
- The bones of the neck snap out of position, causing injury.
- Irritated nerves can interfere with blood flow and transmission of nerve impulses.
- Pinched nerves can affect certain body part functions.

CAUSES
- Motor vehicle accidents
- Sports accidents
- Falls

Risks
- Absence of head restraint in automobile
- Osteoporosis
- Driving under the influence of alcohol or drugs

COMPLICATIONS
- Temporomandibular disorder

Assessment

HISTORY
- Moderate to severe pain in the anterior and posterior neck
- Dizziness
- Headache
- Back pain

PHYSICAL FINDINGS
- Neck muscle asymmetry
- Gait disturbances
- Rigidity or numbness in the arms
- Pain at the exact location of the injury

TEST RESULTS
Imaging
- Full cervical spine X-rays rule out cervical fracture.

Treatment

GENERAL
■ Protect the cervical spine with a soft cervical collar
■ Ice packs
■ Physical therapy

DIET
■ No restrictions

ACTIVITY
■ Limit activity during the first 72 hours after the injury
■ Limit neck movement
■ Avoid strenuous activities, such as lifting and contact sports

MEDICATION
■ Oral analgesics (acetaminophen, nonsteroidal anti-inflammatory drugs, Percocet)

SURGERY
■ Surgical stabilization may be necessary in severe cervical acceleration-deceleration injuries

MONITORING
■ Level of pain
■ Response to medications
■ Complications
■ Neurologic status

CARPAL TUNNEL SYNDROME

Overview

DESCRIPTION
■ Compression of the median nerve in the wrist
■ Most common nerve entrapment syndrome
■ May pose a serious occupational health problem

PATHOPHYSIOLOGY
■ The median nerve controls motions in the forearm, wrist, and hand and supplies sensation to the index, middle, and ring fingers.
■ Compression of the median nerve interrupts normal function.

CAUSES
■ Exact cause unknown
■ Repetitive wrist motions involving excessive flexion or extension
■ Dislocation
■ Acute sprain that may damage the median nerve

RISK FACTORS
■ Amyloidosis
■ Edema-producing conditions

COMPLICATIONS
■ Tendon inflammation
■ Compression
■ Neural ischemia
■ Permanent nerve damage with loss of movement and sensation

Assessment

HISTORY
■ Occupation or hobby requiring strenuous or repetitive use of the hands
■ Condition that causes swelling in carpal tunnel structures
■ Weakness, pain, burning, numbness, or tingling that occurs in one or both hands
■ Paresthesia that worsens at night and in the morning
■ Pain that spreads to the forearm and, in severe cases, as far as the shoulder
■ Pain can be relieved by:
– shaking hands vigorously
– dangling the arms at sides

ELICITING SIGNS OF CARPAL TUNNEL SYNDROME

Two simple tests — for Tinel's sign and Phalen's sign — may confirm carpal tunnel syndrome. The tests prove that certain wrist movements compress the median nerve, causing pain, burning, numbness, or tingling in the hand and fingers.

Tinel's sign

Lightly percuss the transverse carpal ligament over the median nerve where the patient's palm and wrist meet. If this action produces discomfort, such as numbness or tingling that shoots into the palm and fingers, the patient has Tinel's sign.

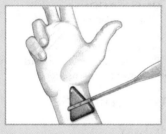

Phalen's sign

If flexing the patient's wrist for about 30 seconds causes the patient to feel subsequent pain or numbness in her hand or fingers, the patient has Phalen's sign. The more severe the carpal tunnel syndrome, the more rapidly the symptoms develop.

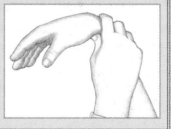

PHYSICAL FINDINGS

■ Inability to make a fist (see *Eliciting signs of carpal tunnel syndrome*)
■ Fingernails may be atrophied, with surrounding dry, shiny skin

TEST RESULTS
Imaging

■ Electromyography shows a median nerve motor conduction delay of more than 5 msec.
■ Digital electrical stimulation shows median nerve compression by measuring the length and intensity of stimulation from the fingers to the median nerve in the wrist.

Other

■ Compression test result supports the diagnosis.

Treatment

GENERAL

■ Conservative initially:
– Splinting the wrist for 1 to 2 weeks
– Possible occupational changes
– Correction of any underlying disorder

DIET

■ No restrictions

ACTIVITY

■ As tolerated

MEDICATION

■ Nonsteroidal anti-inflammatory drugs
■ Corticosteroids
■ Vitamin B complex

SURGERY

■ Decompression of the nerve
■ Neurolysis

MONITORING

■ Response to analgesia

■ After surgery, vital signs
■ Color, sensation, and motion of the affected hand

DISLOCATIONS AND SUBLUXATIONS

Overview

DESCRIPTION
■ Dislocation — displacement of joint bones so that articulating surfaces totally lose contact
■ Subluxation — partial displacement of articulating surfaces
■ May accompany fractures of joints

PATHOPHYSIOLOGY
■ Trauma causes displacement of the joint.
■ Joint structures (blood vessels, ligaments, tendons and nerves) are damaged.
■ Injuries may result in deposition of fracture fragments between joint surfaces, damaging surrounding structures.
■ Joint function is impaired.

CAUSES
■ Congenital
■ Trauma
■ Paget's disease of surrounding joint tissues

RISK FACTORS
■ Participation in contact sports

COMPLICATIONS
■ Avascular necrosis
■ Bone necrosis

Assessment

HISTORY
■ Trauma or fall
■ Extreme pain at injury site

PHYSICAL FINDINGS
■ Joint surface fractures
■ Deformity around the joint
■ Change in the length of the involved extremity
■ Impaired joint mobility
■ Point tenderness

TEST RESULTS
Imaging
■ X-rays are used to confirm the diagnosis and show any associated fractures.

Treatment

GENERAL
■ Immediate reduction and immobilization that can prevent additional tissue damage and vascular impairment
■ Closed reduction

DIET
■ Nothing by mouth if surgery scheduled
■ No restriction

ACTIVITY
■ Limitations based on injury
■ Active range-of-motion exercises for adjacent joints that aren't immobilized

MEDICATIONS
■ Sedation
■ Analgesics
■ Muscle relaxants

SURGERY
■ Open reduction
■ Skeletal traction
■ Ligament repair

MONITORING
■ Respiratory status when I.V. sedatives used

■ Neurovascular status of extremity involved
■ Integrity of skin

HERNIATED INTERVERTEBRAL DISK

Overview

DESCRIPTION
■ Protrusion of part of the nucleus pulposus, an intervertebral disk's gelatinous center, through a tear in the posterior rim of the outer ring or annulus fibrosus
■ Resultant pressure on spinal nerve roots or spinal cord causes back pain and other symptoms of nerve root irritation
■ Most common site for herniation is L4–L5 disk space; other sites include L5–S1, L2–L3, L3–L4, C6–C7, and C5–C6
■ Clinical manifestations determined by:
– Location and size of the herniation into the spinal canal
– Amount of space that exists inside the spinal canal
■ Also known as herniated nucleus pulposus or "slipped disk"

PATHOPHYSIOLOGY
■ The ligament and posterior capsule of the disk are usually torn, allowing the nucleus pulposus to extrude, compressing the nerve root.
■ Occasionally, the injury tears the entire disk loose, causing protrusion onto the nerve root or compression of the spinal cord.
■ Large amounts of extruded nucleus pulposus or complete disk herniation of the capsule and nucleus pulposus may compress the spinal cord.

CAUSES
■ Trauma or strain
■ Degenerative disk disease

RISK FACTORS
■ Advanced age
■ Congenitally small lumbar spinal canal
■ Osteophytes along the vertebrae

COMPLICATIONS
■ Neurologic deficits
■ Bowel and bladder dysfunction

Assessment

HISTORY
■ Previous traumatic injury or back strain
■ Unilateral, low back pain
■ Pain that may radiate to the buttocks, legs, and feet
■ Pain that may begin suddenly, subside in a few days, and then recur at shorter intervals with progressive intensity
■ Sciatic pain beginning as a dull ache in the buttocks, worsening with Valsalva's maneuver, coughing, sneezing, or bending
■ Pain that may subside with rest
■ Muscle spasms

PHYSICAL FINDINGS
■ Limited ability to bend forward
■ A posture favoring the affected side
■ Muscle atrophy, in later stages
■ Tenderness over the affected region
■ Radicular pain with straight leg raising in lumbar herniation
■ Increased pain with neck movement in cervical herniation

TEST RESULTS
Imaging
■ X-ray studies of the spine show degenerative changes.

■ Myelography shows the level of the herniation.

■ Computed tomography scan shows bone and soft-tissue abnormalities; can also show spinal canal compression.

■ Magnetic resonance imaging shows soft-tissue abnormalities.

Other

■ Nerve conduction studies show sensory and motor loss.

Treatment

GENERAL

■ Unless neurologic impairment progresses rapidly, initial treatment is conservative

■ Possible traction

■ Supportive devices such as a brace

■ Heat or ice applications

■ Transcutaneous electrical nerve stimulation

■ Chemonucleolysis

DIET

■ As tolerated

ACTIVITY

■ Bed rest, initially

■ Prescribed exercise program

MEDICATION

■ Nonsteroidal anti-inflammatory agents

■ Steroids

■ Muscle relaxants

SURGERY

■ Laminectomy

■ Spinal fusion

■ Microdiskectomy

MONITORING

■ Vital signs

■ Intake and output

■ Pain

■ Range of motion

■ Mobility

■ Motor strength

■ Deep vein thrombosis

■ Bowel and bladder function

After surgery

■ Blood drainage system

■ Drainage

■ Incisions

■ Dressings

■ Neurovascular status

■ Bowel sounds and abdominal distention

HIP FRACTURE

Overview

DESCRIPTION

■ Break in the head or neck of the femur

■ Most common fall-related injury resulting in hospitalization

■ Leading cause of disability among older adults

■ May permanently change level of functioning and independence

■ Almost one-fourth of patients die within 1 year following hip fracture

PATHOPHYSIOLOGY

■ With bone fracture, the periosteum and blood vessels in the marrow, cortex, and surrounding soft tissues are disrupted.

■ This results in bleeding from the damaged ends of the bone and from the neighboring soft tissue.

■ Clot formation occurs within the medullary canal, between the fractured bone ends, and beneath the periosteum.

■ Bone tissue immediately adjacent to the fracture dies, and the necrotic tissue causes an intense inflammatory response.

■ Vascular tissue invades the fracture area from surrounding soft tissue and marrow cavity within 48 hours, increasing blood flow to the entire bone.
■ Bone-forming cells in the periosteum, endosteum, and marrow are activated to produce subperiosteal procallus along the outer surface of the shaft and over the fractured ends of the bone.
■ Collagen and matrix, which become mineralized to form callus, are synthesized by osteoblasts within the procallus.

CAUSES
■ Falls
■ Trauma
■ Cancer metastasis
■ Osteoporosis
■ Skeletal disease

COMPLICATIONS
■ Pneumonia
■ Venous thrombosis
■ Pressure ulcers
■ Social isolation
■ Depression
■ Bladder dysfunction
■ Deep vein thrombosis
■ Pulmonary embolus

Assessment

HISTORY
■ Falls or trauma to the bones
■ Pain in the affected hip and leg
■ Movement exacerbates pain

PHYSICAL FINDINGS
■ Outward rotation of affected extremity
■ Affected extremity may appear shorter
■ Limited or abnormal range of motion (ROM)
■ Edema and discoloration of the surrounding tissue

■ In an open fracture, bone protruding through the skin

TEST RESULTS
Imaging
■ X-rays showing the location of the fracture
■ Computed tomography scan showing abnormalities in complicated fractures

Treatment

GENERAL
■ Depends on age, comorbidities, cognitive functioning, support systems, and functional ability
■ Possible skin traction
■ Physical therapy
■ Non–weight-bearing transfers

DIET
■ Well-balanced
■ Foods rich in vitamin C and A, calcium, and protein
■ Adequate vitamin D

ACTIVITY
■ Bed rest initially
■ Ambulation as soon as possible after surgery

MEDICATION
■ Analgesics

SURGERY
■ Total hip arthroplasty
■ Hemiarthroplasty
■ Percutaneous pinning
■ Internal fixation using a compression screw and plate

MONITORING
■ Vital signs
■ Intake and output
■ Pain
■ Mobility and ROM
■ Incision and dressings

- Complications
- Coagulation study results
- Signs of bleeding
- Neurovascular status
- Skin integrity
- Signs and symptoms of infection

Following surgery, assess the patient for complications, such as deep vein thrombosis, pulmonary embolus, and hip dislocation.

OSTEOARTHRITIS

Overview

DESCRIPTION
- Most common form of arthritis
- Disability from minor limitation to near immobility
- Varying progression rates

PATHOPHYSIOLOGY
- Deterioration of the joint cartilage occurs.
- Reactive new bone forms at the margins and subchondral areas.
- Breakdown of chondrocytes occurs in the hips and knees.
- Cartilage flakes irritate synovial lining.
- The cartilage lining becomes fibrotic.
- Joint movement is limited.

CAUSES
- Advancing age
- Hereditary, possibly
- Secondary osteoarthritis
- Traumatic injury
- Congenital abnormality
- Endocrine disorders such as diabetes mellitus
- Metabolic disorders such as chondrocalcinosis

COMPLICATIONS
- Flexion contractures
- Subluxation
- Deformity
- Ankylosis
- Bony cysts
- Gross bony overgrowth
- Central cord syndrome
- Nerve root compression
- Cauda equina syndrome

Assessment

HISTORY
- Predisposing traumatic injury
- Deep, aching joint pain
- Pain after exercise or weight bearing
- Pain possibly relieved by rest
- Stiffness in morning and after exercise
- Aching during changes in weather
- "Grating" feeling when the joint moves
- Limited movement

PHYSICAL FINDINGS
- Contractures
- Joint swelling
- Muscle atrophy
- Deformity of the involved areas
- Gait abnormalities
- Hard nodes that may be red, swollen, and tender on the distal and proximal interphalangeal joints (see *Signs of osteoarthritis*, page 530)
- Loss of finger dexterity
- Muscle spasms, limited movement, and joint instability

TEST RESULTS
Laboratory
- Synovial fluid analysis ruling out inflammatory arthritis

Imaging
- X-rays of the affected joint may show a narrowing of the joint space or margin, cystlike bony deposits in the joint space and margins, sclerosis of the subchondral space, joint deformi-

SIGNS OF OSTEOARTHRITIS

Heberden's nodes appear on the dorsolateral aspect of the distal interphalangeal joints. These bony and cartilaginous enlargements are usually hard and painless. They typically occur in middle-aged and elderly patients with osteoarthritis. Bouchard's nodes are similar to Heberden's nodes but are less common and appear on the proximal interphalangeal joints.

Heberden's nodes

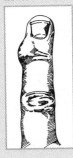

Bouchard's nodes

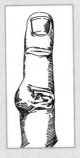

ty or articular damage, bony growths at weight-bearing areas, and possible joint fusion.
■ Radionuclide bone scan may be used to rule out inflammatory arthritis by showing normal uptake of the radionuclide.
■ Magnetic resonance imaging shows affected joint, adjacent bones, and disease progression.

Diagnostic procedures
■ Neuromuscular tests may show reduced muscle strength.

Treatment

GENERAL
■ To relieve pain
■ To improve mobility
■ To minimize disability

DIET
■ No restrictions

ACTIVITY
■ As tolerated
■ Physical therapy
■ Assistive mobility devices

MEDICATION
■ Analgesics

SURGERY
■ Arthroplasty (partial or total)
■ Arthrodesis
■ Osteoplasty
■ Osteotomy

MONITORING
■ Pain pattern
■ Response to analgesics
■ ROM

OSTEOMYELITIS

Overview

DESCRIPTION
■ Pyogenic bone infection
■ Chronic or acute
■ Prognosis for acute form good with prompt treatment
■ Prognosis for chronic form poor

PATHOPHYSIOLOGY
■ Organisms settle in a hematoma or weakened area and spread directly to bone.
■ Pus is produced and pressure builds within the rigid medullary cavity.

- Pus is forced through the haversian canals.
- Subperiosteal abscess forms.
- Bone is deprived of its blood supply.
- Necrosis results and new bone formation is stimulated.
- Dead bone detaches and exits through an abscess or the sinuses.
- Osteomyelitis becomes chronic.

CAUSES
- Minor traumatic injury
- Acute infection originating elsewhere in the body
- *Staphylococcus aureus*
- *Streptococcus pyogenes*
- *Pseudomonas aeruginosa*
- *Escherichia coli*
- *Proteus vulgaris*
- Fungi or viruses

COMPLICATIONS
- Chronic infection
- Skeletal deformities
- Joint deformities
- Disturbed bone growth in children
- Differing leg lengths
- Impaired mobility

Assessment

HISTORY
- Previous injury, surgery, or primary infection
- Sudden, severe pain in the affected bone
- Pain unrelieved by rest and worse with motion
- Related chills, nausea, and malaise
- Refusal to use the affected area

PHYSICAL FINDINGS
- Tachycardia and fever
- Swelling and restricted movement over the infection site
- Tenderness and warmth over the infection site

- Persistent pus drainage from an old pocket in a sinus tract

TEST RESULTS
Laboratory
- White blood cell count showing leukocytosis
- Increased erythrocyte sedimentation rate
- Blood culture identifying pathogen

Imaging
- X-rays may show bone involvement.
- Bone scans may detect early infection.
- Computed tomography scan and magnetic resonance imaging can show extent of infection.

Treatment

GENERAL
- To decrease internal bone pressure
- To prevent bone necrosis
- Hyperbaric oxygen therapy
- Free tissue transfers
- I.V. fluids as needed

DIET
- High-protein, rich in vitamin C

ACTIVITY
- Bed rest
- Immobilization of involved bone and joint with a cast or traction

MEDICATION
- I.V. antibiotics
- Analgesics
- Intracavitary instillation of antibiotics for open wounds

SURGERY
- Surgical drainage
- Local muscle flaps
- Sequestrectomy
- Amputation for chronic and unrelieved symptoms

MONITORING

- Vital signs
- Wound appearance
- New pain
- Drainage and suctioning equipment
- Sudden malpositioning of the limb
- Response to analgesics

OSTEOPOROSIS

Overview

DESCRIPTION

- Loss of calcium and phosphate from bones
- Bone abnormally vulnerable to fractures
- Primary or secondary to underlying disease
- Types of primary osteoporosis: postmenopausal osteoporosis (type I) and age-associated osteoporosis (type II)
- Secondary osteoporosis: caused by an identifiable agent or disease

PATHOPHYSIOLOGY

- The rate of bone resorption accelerates as the rate of bone formation decelerates.
- Decreased bone mass results and bones become porous and brittle.

CAUSES

- Exact cause unknown
- Prolonged therapy with steroids or heparin
- Bone immobilization
- Alcoholism
- Malnutrition
- Rheumatoid arthritis
- Liver disease
- Malabsorption
- Scurvy
- Lactose intolerance
- Hyperthyroidism
- Osteogenesis imperfecta
- Sudeck's atrophy (localized in hands and feet, with recurring attacks)

RISK FACTORS

- Mild, prolonged negative calcium balance
- Declining gonadal adrenal function
- Faulty protein metabolism (caused by estrogen deficiency)
- Sedentary lifestyle

COMPLICATIONS

- Bone fractures (vertebrae, femoral neck, and distal radius)

Assessment

HISTORY

- Postmenopausal patient
- Condition known to cause secondary osteoporosis
- Snapping sound or sudden pain in lower back when bending down to lift something
- Possible slow development of pain (over several years)
- With vertebral collapse, backache and pain radiating around the trunk
- Pain aggravated by movement or jarring

PHYSICAL FINDINGS

- Humped back
- Markedly aged appearance
- Loss of height
- Muscle spasm
- Decreased spinal movement with flexion more limited than extension

Laboratory

- Normal serum calcium, phosphorus, and alkaline levels
- Elevated parathyroid hormone level

Imaging

■ X-ray studies show characteristic degeneration in the lower thoracolumbar vertebrae.
■ Computed tomography scan accurately assesses spinal bone loss.
■ Bone scans show injured or diseased areas.

Diagnostic procedures

■ Bone biopsy shows thin, porous, but otherwise normal bone.

Other

■ Dual or single photon absorptiometry (measurement of bone mass) shows loss of bone mass.

Treatment

GENERAL

■ To control bone loss
■ To prevent additional fractures
■ To control pain
■ Reduction and immobilization of Colles' fracture

DIET

■ Rich in vitamin D, calcium, and protein

ACTIVITY

■ Physical therapy program of gentle exercise and activity
■ Supportive devices

MEDICATION

■ Bisphosphonate (Alendronate)
■ Hormone replacement therapy at lowest effective dose (controversial therapy; research is on-going)
■ Calcium and vitamin D supplements
■ Calcitonin

SURGERY

■ Open reduction and internal fixation for femur fractures

MONITORING

■ Skin for redness, warmth, and new pain sites
■ Response to analgesia
■ Nutritional status
■ Height
■ Exercise tolerance
■ Joint mobility

RHEUMATOID ARTHRITIS

Overview

DESCRIPTION

■ Chronic, systemic, symmetrical inflammatory disease
■ Primarily attacks peripheral joints and surrounding muscles, tendons, ligaments, and blood vessels
■ Marked by spontaneous remissions and unpredictable exacerbations
■ Potentially crippling

PATHOPHYSIOLOGY

■ Cartilage damage resulting from inflammation triggers further immune responses, including complement activation.
■ Complement, in turn, attracts polymorphonuclear leukocytes and stimulates release of inflammatory mediators, which exacerbates joint destruction.

CAUSES

■ Unknown
■ Possible influence of infection (viral or bacterial), hormonal factors, and lifestyle

COMPLICATIONS

■ Fibrous or bony ankylosis
■ Soft-tissue contractures
■ Joint deformities
■ Sjögren's syndrome
■ Spinal cord compression

- Carpal tunnel syndrome
- Osteoporosis
- Recurrent infections
- Hip joint necrosis

Assessment

HISTORY

- Insidious onset of nonspecific symptoms, including fatigue, malaise, anorexia, persistent low-grade fever, weight loss, and vague articular symptoms
- Later, more specific localized articular symptoms, commonly in the fingers
- Bilateral and symmetrical symptoms, which may extend to the wrists, elbows, knees, and ankles
- Painful, red, swollen arms
- Stiff joints
- Stiff, weak, or painful muscles
- Numbness or tingling in the feet or weakness or loss of sensation in the fingers
- Pain on inspiration
- Shortness of breath

PHYSICAL FINDINGS

- Joint deformities and contractures
- Foreshortened hands
- Boggy wrists
- Rheumatoid nodules
- Leg ulcers
- Eye redness
- Joints that are warm to the touch
- Pericardial friction rub
- Positive Babinski's sign

TEST RESULTS
Laboratory

- Positive rheumatoid factor test (in 75% to 80% of patients), as indicated by titer of 1:160 or higher (see *Classifying rheumatoid arthritis*)
- Synovial fluid analysis showing increased volume and turbidity but decreased viscosity and complement (C3 and C4) levels, with white blood cell count possible exceeding 10,000/µl
- Elevated serum globulin levels
- Elevated erythrocyte sedimentation rate
- Complete blood count showing moderate anemia and slight leukocytosis

Imaging

- In early stages, X-rays show bone demineralization and soft-tissue swelling. Later, they help determine the extent of cartilage and bone destruction, erosion, subluxations, and deformities and show the characteristic pattern of these abnormalities.
- Magnetic resonance imaging and computed tomography scan may provide information about the extent of damage.

Treatment

GENERAL

- Increased sleep (8 to 10 hours every night)
- Splinting
- Range-of-motion exercises and carefully individualized therapeutic exercises
- Moist heat application

DIET

- No restrictions

ACTIVITY

- Frequent rest periods between activities

MEDICATION

- Salicylates
- Nonsteroidal anti-inflammatory drugs
- Antimalarials (hydroxychloroquine)
- Gold salts

CLASSIFYING RHEUMATOID ARTHRITIS

The criteria of the American College of Rheumatology allow the classification of rheumatoid arthritis.

Guidelines

A patient who meets four of seven criteria is classified as having rheumatoid arthritis. She must experience the first four criteria for at least 6 weeks, and a physician must observe the second through fifth criteria.

A patient with two or more other clinical diagnoses can also be diagnosed with rheumatoid arthritis.

Criteria

■ Morning stiffness in and around the joints that lasts for 1 hour before full improvement

■ Arthritis in three or more joint areas, with at least three joint areas (as observed by a physician) exhibiting soft-tissue swelling or joint effusions, not just bony overgrowth (the 14 possible areas involved include the right and left proximal interphalangeal, metacarpophalangeal, wrist, elbow, knee, ankle, and metatarsophalangeal joints)

■ Arthritis of hand joints, including the wrist, the metacarpophalangeal joint, or the proximal interphalangeal joint

■ Arthritis that involves the same joint areas on both sides of the body

■ Subcutaneous rheumatoid nodules over bony prominences

■ Demonstration of abnormal amounts of serum rheumatoid factor by any method that produces a positive result in less than 5% of patients without rheumatoid arthritis

■ Radiographic changes, usually on posteroanterior hand and wrist radiographs; these changes must show erosions or unequivocal bony decalcification localized in or most noticeable adjacent to the involved joints

---

■ Penicillamine
■ Corticosteroids

SURGERY

■ Metatarsal head and distal ulnar resectional arthroplasty and insertion of silastic prosthesis between the metacarpophalangeal and proximal interphalangeal joints
■ Arthrodesis (joint fusion)
■ Synovectomy
■ Osteotomy
■ Repair of ruptured tendon
■ In advanced disease: joint reconstruction or total joint arthroplasty

MONITORING

■ Joint stiffness
■ Skin integrity
■ Vital signs
■ Daily weight
■ Sensory disturbances
■ Pain level
■ Serum electrolyte, hemoglobin and hematocrit levels
■ Complications of corticosteroid therapy

TREATMENTS

AMPUTATION

Overview

- Surgical removal of an extremity
- Closed technique: skin flaps are used to cover the bone stump
- Open (guillotine) amputation: tissue and bone are cut flush, and the wound is left open to be repaired in a second operation

INDICATIONS

- To preserve function in a remaining part
- To prevent death
- Severe trauma
- Gangrene
- Cancer
- Vascular disease
- Congenital deformity
- Thermal injury

COMPLICATIONS

- Infection
- Contractures
- Skin breakdown
- Phantom pain

Nursing interventions

PRETREATMENT CARE

- Explain the treatment and preparation to the patient and family.
- Make sure the patient has signed an appropriate consent form.
- Provide emotional support.
- Arrange for the patient to meet with a well-adjusted amputee if possible.
- Demonstrate prescribed exercises.
- Administer broad-spectrum antibiotics as ordered.

POSTTREATMENT CARE

- Elevate the affected limb as ordered.
- Provide analgesics as ordered.
- Keep the stump wrapped properly with elastic compression bandages or a stump shrinker as ordered.
- Provide cast care if a rigid plaster dressing has been applied.
- Maintain the patient in proper body alignment.
- Provide regular physical therapy.
- Encourage frequent ambulation.
- Encourage active or passive range-of-motion exercises.
- Help the patient with turning and positioning without propping the limb on a pillow.

Monitoring

- Vital signs
- Intake and output
- Surgical wound and dressings
- Bleeding
- Drain patency and drainage
- Pain

PATIENT TEACHING

Be sure to cover:
- medications and possible adverse reactions
- postoperative care and rehabilitation
- prosthesis and its care
- phantom limb sensation
- daily examination of the distal limb
- daily limb care and dressings
- signs and symptoms of infection
- complications
- when to notify the physician
- use of elastic bandages or a stump shrinker
- proper crutch use as appropriate
- activities to toughen the residual limb
- follow-up care

- referral for psychological counseling or social services as indicated
- referral to a local support group.

CARPAL TUNNEL RELEASE

Overview

- Surgery to decompress the median nerve
- Relieves pain and restores function in the wrist and hand

INDICATIONS

- Carpal tunnel syndrome unrelieved by splinting or medication

COMPLICATIONS

- Hematoma
- Infection
- Painful scar formation
- Tenosynovitis

Nursing interventions

PRETREATMENT CARE

- Explain the treatment and preparation to the patient and family.
- Make sure the patient has signed an appropriate consent form.
- Explain that the patient will have a dressing wrapped around the hand and lower arm after surgery and that this will remain in place for 1 to 2 days.
- Tell the patient that pain may occur once the anesthetic wears off but that analgesics will be available.
- Demonstrate rehabilitative exercises, and have the patient perform a return demonstration.

POSTTREATMENT CARE

- Keep the affected hand elevated to reduce swelling and discomfort.
- Administer analgesics as ordered.

- Report severe, persistent pain or tenderness.
- Encourage the patient to perform wrist and finger exercises.
- Assess the need for home care.

Monitoring

- Vital signs
- Circulation in the affected arm and hand
- Sensory and motor function in the affected arm and hand
- Surgical dressings
- Drainage or bleeding
- Pain
- Complications
- Response to treatment

PATIENT TEACHING

Be sure to cover:
- medications and possible adverse reactions
- surgical incision care
- dressing changes
- daily wrist and finger exercises
- avoidance of overusing the affected wrist or lifting objects heavier than a thin magazine
- signs and symptoms of infection
- complications
- when to notify the physician
- follow-up care
- referral to occupational therapy, especially if the disorder is work related.

HIP REPLACEMENT

Overview

- Total or partial replacement of the hip joint with a synthetic prosthesis
- Results in improved, pain-free mobility and an increased sense of independence

INDICATIONS

- Primary degenerative arthritis

- Severe chronic arthritis
- Extensive joint trauma
- Hip fracture
- Protruding acetabulum associated with rheumatoid arthritis
- Osteomalacia
- Paget's disease

COMPLICATIONS
- Hip fracture or dislocation
- Stroke
- Myocardial infarction
- Fat embolism
- Infection
- Hypovolemic shock
- Pulmonary edema
- Arterial thrombosis
- Pseudoaneurysm
- Hematoma
- Fracture of the joint cement
- Displaced prosthetic head

Nursing interventions

PRETREATMENT CARE
- Explain the treatment and preparation to the patient and family.
- Make sure the patient has signed an appropriate consent form.
- Explain postoperative care.
- Make sure the patient's medical history and physical, laboratory studies, and diagnostic tests are completed; report abnormal results.
- Check for a history of allergies.
- Make sure blood typing and crossmatching is completed; verify if blood is to be kept on hold for the patient.

POSTTREATMENT CARE
- Administer medications as ordered.
- Administer I.V. fluids as ordered.
- Transfuse blood products as ordered.
- Maintain bed rest for the prescribed period.

- Maintain the hip in proper alignment, using a triangular abduction pillow.
- Provide surgical wound care.
- Reposition the patient frequently.
- Encourage frequent coughing and deep breathing.
- Assist the patient in exercising the affected leg.

Monitoring
- Vital signs
- Intake and output
- Complications
- Infection
- Neurovascular status distal to the operative site
- Surgical wound and dressings
- Drainage
- Abnormal bleeding
- Heart rate and rhythm

Watch for and immediately report early clinical changes that may indicate fat embolism syndrome (FES), including: altered level of consciousness, tachypnea, dyspnea, elevated temperature without other cause, and tachycardia. An arterial oxygen tension of less than 60 mm Hg indicates possible FES.

Stay alert for and report signs and symptoms of dislocation. These include sudden, severe pain; shortening of the involved leg; and external leg rotation.

PATIENT TEACHING
Be sure to cover:
- medications and possible adverse reactions
- proper use of an abductor pillow, splints, and assistive devices
- transfer and pivoting techniques
- prescribed exercise program
- prescribed activity restrictions
- signs and symptoms of infection
- complications
- when to notify the physician

- incision care
- referrals for home physical therapy and assistive devices as indicated
- follow-up care.

JOINT REPLACEMENT

Overview

- Total or partial replacement of a joint with a synthetic prosthesis; also called arthroplasty
- Restores joint mobility and stability and relieves pain
- May involve any joint except a spinal joint
- Most commonly involves the hip and knee

INDICATIONS
- Severe chronic arthritis
- Degenerative joint disorders
- Extensive joint trauma

COMPLICATIONS
- Infection
- Hypovolemic shock
- Fat embolism
- Thromboembolism
- Pulmonary embolism (PE)
- Nerve compromise
- Prosthesis dislocation or loosening
- Heterotrophic ossification
- Avascular necrosis
- Atelectasis
- Pneumonia
- Deep vein thrombosis (DVT)

Nursing interventions

PRETREATMENT CARE
- Explain the treatment and patient preparation.
- Make sure the patient has signed an appropriate consent form.
- Explain postoperative care.

- Reassure the patient that analgesics will be available as needed.
- Provide emotional support.

POSTTREATMENT CARE
- Administer medications as ordered.
- Maintain bed rest for the prescribed period.
- Maintain the affected joint in proper alignment.
- Assess the patient's pain level and provide analgesics as ordered.
- Change dressings as ordered.
- Reposition the patient frequently.
- Encourage frequent coughing and deep breathing.
- Encourage adequate fluid intake.
- Exercise the affected joint as ordered.
- If joint displacement occurs, notify the physician.
- If traction is used to correct joint displacement, periodically check weights and other equipment.

Monitoring
- Vital signs
- Intake and output
- Complications
- Surgical wound and dressings
- Drainage
- Abnormal bleeding
- Respiratory status
- Neurovascular status of the affected extremity
- Infection

PATIENT TEACHING
Be sure to cover:
- medications and possible adverse reactions
- signs and symptoms of infection
- signs and symptoms of joint dislodgment
- complications
- when to notify the physician
- incision care
- follow-up care
- signs and symptoms of DVT and PE

- prescribed exercise regimen
- prescribed activity restrictions
- physical therapy
- range-of-motion exercises and use of a continuous passive motion device as appropriate
- infective endocarditis prophylaxis.

After hip replacement

Be sure to cover:
- importance of maintaining hip abduction
- avoidance of crossing his legs when sitting
- avoidance of flexing his hips more than 90 degrees when rising from a bed or chair
- using a chair with high arms and a firm seat
- importance of sleeping on a firm mattress
- proper use of crutches or a cane.

After shoulder joint replacement

Be sure to cover:
- importance of keeping the affected arm in a sling until postoperative swelling subsides.

LAMINECTOMY AND SPINAL FUSION

Overview

- Laminectomy: removal of one or more of the bony laminae that cover the vertebrae; typically done to relieve pressure on the spinal cord or spinal nerve roots
- Spinal fusion: grafting of bone chips between the vertebral spaces to stabilize the spine; it follows laminectomy
- Spinal fusion used when more conservative treatments (wuch as prolonged bed rest, traction, and use of a back brace) prove ineffective

- Percutaneous (endoscopic) discectomy: alternative to laminectomy for decompressing and repairing damaged lumbar disks (see *Laminectomy alternative*)

INDICATIONS
- Herniated disk
- Compression fracture
- Vertebral dislocation
- Spinal cord tumor
- Vertebrae seriously weakened by trauma or disease

COMPLICATIONS
- Herniation relapse
- Arachnoiditis
- Chronic neuritis
- Immobility
- Nerve or muscle damage

Nursing interventions

PRETREATMENT CARE
- Explain the treatment and preparation to the patient and family.
- Make sure the patient has signed an appropriate consent form.
- Explain postoperative care; reassure the patient that analgesics and muscle relaxants will be available.
- Inform the patient that relief will come after chronic nerve irritation and swelling subside.
- Perform a baseline assessment of motor function and sensation.
- Show the patient how to perform the logrolling method of turning, and explain that he'll use this technique later to get in and out of bed by himself.

POSTTREATMENT CARE
- Administer medications as ordered.
- Keep the head of the bed flat or elevated no more than 45 degrees for at least 24 hours after surgery.

■ Urge the patient to remain in a supine position for the prescribed period.

■ When the patient can lie on his side, make sure the spine is straight, with his knees flexed and drawn up toward his chest.

■ Insert a pillow between the patient's knees.

■ Assist the surgeon with the initial dressing change.

■ If the patient doesn't void within 8 to 12 hours after surgery, notify the physician, and prepare to insert a urinary catheter (or assist with insertion).

■ If the patient can void normally, provide assistance in getting on and off the bedpan while maintaining proper body alignment.

Monitoring
■ Vital signs
■ Intake and output
■ Surgical wound and dressings
■ Drainage
■ Abnormal bleeding
■ Cerebrospinal fluid leakage
■ Motor and neurologic function
■ Peripheral vascular status
■ Bowel sounds
■ Respiratory status

PATIENT TEACHING

Be sure to cover:
■ medications and possible adverse reactions
■ incision care
■ signs and symptoms of infection
■ complications
■ when to notify the physician
■ showering with his back facing away from the stream of water
■ prescribed activity restrictions
■ prescribed exercises
■ proper body mechanics
■ avoidance of lying on his stomach or on his back with legs flat

---

LAMINECTOMY ALTERNATIVE

Percutaneous (endoscopic) diskectomy is an alternative to traditional surgery for a herniated disk. In this technique, the physician uses suction and X-ray visualization to remove only the disk portion that's causing pain. Typically used for smaller, less severe disk abnormalities, percutaneous automated diskectomy has only a 50% success rate, perhaps because the operative site isn't visualized directly. One report indicates a high incidence of postoperative diskitis.

Nursing care after diskectomy resembles post-laminectomy care. Typically, the patient is allowed out of bed in 24 to 48 hours and is encouraged to ambulate without assistance as soon as possible.

■ sitting up straight with his feet on a low stool
■ using a firm, straight-backed chair
■ alternating placing each foot on a low stool
■ sleeping only on a firm mattress or inserting a bed board between the mattress and box spring
■ follow-up care.

TRACTION

Overview

■ Treatment that exerts a pulling force on a part of the body, usually the spine, pelvis, or a long bone of the arm or leg
■ The type of mechanical traction used (skin or skeletal) determined by the physician, based on the patient's condition, age, weight, and skin con-

dition as well as the purpose and expected duration of traction
■ Skin traction: applied directly to the skin (indirectly to the bone); used when a light, temporary, or noncontinuous pulling force is required
■ Skeletal traction: device inserted through the bone and attached to traction equipment to exert a direct, constant, longitudinal pulling force; applied by an orthopedist

INDICATIONS
■ Fracture
■ Dislocation
■ Deformity
■ Contracture
■ Muscle spasm

COMPLICATIONS
■ Pressure ulcers
■ Muscle atrophy
■ Weakness
■ Contractures
■ Osteoporosis
■ Urinary stasis and calculi
■ Pneumonia
■ Thrombophlebitis
■ Osteomyelitis
■ Nonunion or delayed union of bone
■ Complications of immobility
■ Feelings of depression

Nursing interventions

PRETREATMENT CARE
■ Explain the treatment and preparation to the patient and family.
■ Make sure the patient has signed an appropriate consent form.
■ Set up appropriate traction equipment and a frame according to established facility policy.

POSTTREATMENT CARE
■ Administer medications as ordered.
■ Show the patient how much movement is permitted.

■ Provide comfort measures.
■ Unwrap skin traction every shift and assess the skin for redness, warmth, blisters, and other signs of breakdown.
■ Maintain the patient in proper body alignment; reposition as necessary.
■ Provide meticulous skin care.
■ Administer pin care as ordered.
■ Encourage coughing and deep-breathing exercises.
■ Assist with ordered range-of-motion exercises for unaffected extremities.
■ Apply elastic support stockings as ordered.
■ Provide dietary fiber and sufficient fluids.
■ Administer stool softeners, laxatives, or enemas as needed and ordered.
■ Inspect traction equipment for kinks, knots, or frays in ropes; make sure the weights hang freely and don't touch the floor.

Monitoring
■ Vital signs
■ Intake and output
■ Skin condition
■ Infection
■ Complications of immobility
■ Neurovascular status of extremities

PATIENT TEACHING
Be sure to cover:
■ medications and possible adverse reactions
■ set-up and care of traction equipment
■ use of an overhead trapeze
■ pin care
■ signs and symptoms of infection
■ complications
■ when to notify the physician
■ preventing and managing complications of immobility
■ dietary recommendations
■ follow-up care.

PROCEDURES AND EQUIPMENT

USING AN AIR SPLINT

In an emergency, an air splint can be applied to immobilize a fracture or control bleeding, especially from a forearm or lower leg. This compact, comfortable splint is made 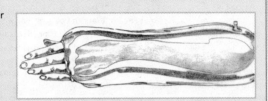 of double-walled plastic and provides gentle, diffuse pressure over an injured area. The appropriate splint is chosen, wrapped around the affected extremity, secured with Velcro or other strips, and then inflated. The fit should be snug enough to immobilize the extremity without impairing circulation.

An air splint may actually control bleeding better than a local pressure bandage. The device's clear plastic construction simplifies inspection of the affected site for bleeding, pallor, or cyanosis. An air splint also allows the patient to be moved without further damage to the injured limb.

HOW TO PETAL A CAST

Rough cast edges can be cushioned by petaling them with adhesive tape or moleskin. To do this, first cut several 4″ × 2″ (10 × 5 cm) strips. Round off one end of each strip to keep it from curling. Make sure the rounded end of the strip is on the outside of the cast, then tuck the straight end just inside the cast edge.

Smooth the moleskin with your finger until you're sure it's secured inside and out. Repeat the procedure, overlapping the moleskin pieces until you've gone all the way around the cast edge.

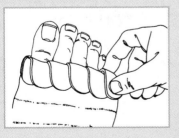
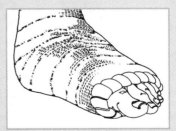

REMOVING A CAST

Typically, a cast is removed when a fracture heals or requires further manipulation. Less common indications include cast damage, a pressure ulcer under the cast, excessive drainage or bleeding, and a constrictive cast.

Explain the procedure to the patient. Tell him he'll feel some heat and vibration as the cast is split with the cast saw. If the patient is a child, tell him that the saw is very noisy but won't cut the skin beneath. Warn the patient that when the padding is cut, he'll see discolored skin and signs of poor muscle tone. Reassure him that you'll stay with him. The illustrations here show how a plaster cast is removed.

The physician cuts one side of the cast, then the other. As he does so, closely monitor the patient's anxiety level.

Next, the physician opens the cast pieces with a spreader.

Finally, using cast scissors, the physician cuts through the cast padding.

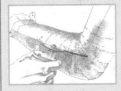
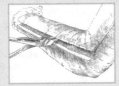
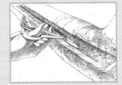

When the cast is removed, provide skin care to remove accumulated dead skin and to begin restoring the extremity's normal appearance.

FITTING A PATIENT FOR A CRUTCH

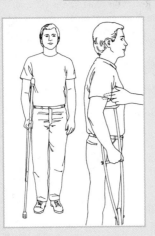

Position the crutch so that it extends from a point 4″ to 6″ (10 to 15 cm) to the side and 4″ to 6″ in front of the patient's feet to 1½″ to 2″ (4 to 5 cm) below the axillae (about the width of two fingers). Then adjust the handgrips so that the patient's elbows are flexed at a 15-degree angle when he's standing with the crutches in the resting position.

IMMOBILIZING A SHOULDER DISLOCATION

When a shoulder disloca-
tion has been reduced, an
external immobilization
device, such as the elastic
shoulder immobilizer or
the stockinette Velpeau
splint, can maintain the
position until healing
takes place. The device
should remain on for
about 3 weeks.

Elastic shoulder immobilizer

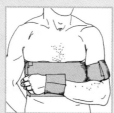

Stockinette Velpeau splint

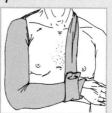

WRAPPING A STUMP

Proper stump care protects the limb, reduces swelling, and prepares the limb for a
prosthesis. As you perform the procedure, teach the patient.

Start by obtaining two 4″
elastic bandages. Center
the end of the first 4″
bandage at the top of the
patient's thigh. Unroll the
bandage downward over
the stump and to the
back of the leg (as shown
below).

Make three figure-eight
turns to adequately cover
the ends of the stump. As
you wrap, include the roll
of flesh in the groin area.
Use enough pressure to
ensure that the stump
narrows toward the end
so that it fits comfortably
into the prosthesis.

Use the second 4″ ban-
dage to anchor the first
bandage around the
waist. For a below-the-
knee amputation, use the
knee to anchor the ban-
dage in place. Secure the
bandage with clips, safety
pins, or adhesive tape.
Check the stump bandage
regularly and rewrap it if
it bunches at the end.

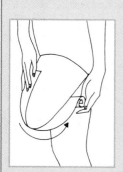

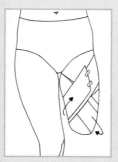

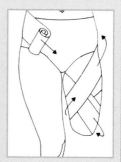

DRUGS

COMMON DRUGS FOR MUSCULOSKELETAL PAIN

Drug	Indications	Adverse reactions
ASPIRIN		
Aspirin (A.S.A.)	■ Mild pain ■ Rheumatoid arthritis and osteoarthritis ■ Fever	■ Abdominal pain GI bleeding, acute renal insufficiency, tinnitus ■ Other reactions: heartburn, indigestion, thrombocytopenia
NONOPIOID ANALGESIC		
Acetaminophen (Tylenol)	■ Mild pain ■ Osteoarthritis ■ Fever	■ Servere liver damage, neutropenia, thrombocytopenia ■ Other reactions: headache, hematuria, rash
NONSTEROIDAL ANTI-INFLAMMATORY DRUGS		
Diflunisal (Dolobid); **ibuprofen** (Motrin); **indomethacin** (Indocin); **naproxen** (Naprosyn)	■ Mild to moderate pain ■ Rheumatoid arthritis ■ Osteoarthritis	■ Bleeding, bloody or tarry stools, bruises, rash, wheezing, acute renal failure, Stevens-Johnson syndrome ■ Other reactions: diarrhea, dizziness, drowsiness, heartburn, indigestion, nausea, vomiting, peripheral edema
SKELETAL MUSCLE RELAXANTS		
Carisoprodol (Soma)	■ Relief of discomfort in acute, painful musculoskeletal conditions	■ Drowsiness, dizziness, itching, rash, shortness of breath, angioedema, tachycardia, wheezing ■ Other reactions: hiccups, nausea, vomiting
Cyclobenzaprine (Flexeril)	■ Adjunct in acute, painful musculoskeletal conditions	■ Confusion, severe drowsiness, dizziness, tachycardia, arrhythmias, hypotension ■ Other reactions: dry mouth, rash, urticaria, urine retention, blurred vision

Special considerations

- Use cautiously in patients with a history of GI disease, especially peptic ulcer disease.
- Assess for signs and symptoms of bleeding, such as petechiae, bruising, coffee ground emesis, and black, tarry stools.
- Give with food or after meals.
- Advise the patient to avoid aspirin and other salicylates for 5 days before any surgery or dental work to avoid increased bleeding.

- Monitor the patient's total daily intake of acetaminophen because of potential liver toxicity.
- Use cautiously in elderly patients and those with liver disease.
- Advise the patient on high-dose or long-term therapy that regular visits to his health care provider are essential.

- Monitor the patient's cardiopulmonary status closely. Observe for fluid retention and monitor for bleeding.
- Give with food or after meals.
- If the drug makes the patient drowsy, advise him not to perform activities that require alertness, such as driving or operating heavy machinery.

- Use cautiously with other central nervous system depressants; effects may be cumulative.
- Withdrawal symptoms may occur with abrupt termination of the drug.
- Cautioun the patient not to perform tasks requiring mental or physical alertness, such as driving or operating heavy machinery, if he feeks dizzy or drowsy.

- Use with caution in elderly patients and those with a history of urine retention.
- Because this drug may cause dizziness or drowsiness, caution the patient to get out of bed and change positions slowly. Warn
against driving or operating machinery when he feels dizzy.
- Contraindicated in patients with hyperthyroidism, heart block, and conduction disturbances.

12

ENDOCRINE CARE

ASSESSMENT

PALPATING THE THYROID

To palpate the thyroid *from the front*, stand in front of the patient and place your index and middle fingers below the cricoid cartilage on both sides of the trachea. Palpate for the thyroid isthmus as he swallows. Next, ask the patient to flex his neck toward the side being examined as you gently palpate each lobe. In most cases, you'll feel only the isthmus connecting the two lobes. However, if the patient has a thin neck, you may feel the whole gland. If he has a short, stocky neck, you may have trouble palpating even an enlarged thyroid.

To locate the right lobe, use your right hand to displace the thyroid cartilage slightly to your left. Hook your left

Palpating the right lobe, from the front

Sternocleidomastoid muscles

Thyroid gland

Thyroid cartilage

Isthmus

Trachea

index and middle fingers around the sternocleidomastoid muscle to palpate for thyroid enlargement. Then examine the left lobe, using your left hand to displace the thyroid cartilage and your right hand to palpate the lobe.

ASSESSING ENDOCRINE DYSFUNCTION: SOME COMMON SIGNS AND SYMPTOMS

Sign or symptom	Possible cause
Abdominal pain	Diabetic ketoacidosis (DKA), myxedema, addisonian crisis, thyroid storm
Anemia	Hypothyroidism, panhypopituitarism, adrenal insufficiency, Cushing's disease, hyperparathyroidism
Anorexia	Hyperparathyroidism, Addison's disease, DKA, hypothyroidism
Body temperature change	*Increase:* Thyrotoxicosis, thyroid storm, primary hypothalamic disease (after pituitary surgery) *Decrease:* Addison's disease, hypoglycemia, myxedema coma, DKA
Hypertension	Primary aldosteronism, pheochromocytoma, Cushing's syndrome
Libido changes, sexual dysfunction	Thyroid or adrenocortical hypofunction or hyperfunction, diabetes mellitus, hypopituitarism, gonadal failure
Skin changes	*Hyperpigmentation:* Addison's disease (after bilateral adrenalectomy for Cushing's syndrome), corticotropin-secreting pituitary tumor *Hirsutism:* Cushing's syndrome, adrenal hyperplasia, adrenal tumor, acromegaly *Coarse, dry skin:* Myxedema, hypoparathyroidism, acromegaly *Excessive sweating:* Thyrotoxicosis, acromegaly, pheochromocytoma, hypoglycemia
Tachycardia	Hyperthyroidism, pheochromocytoma, hypoglycemia, DKA
Weakness, fatigue	Addison's disease, Cushing's syndrome, hypothyroidism, hyperparathyroidism, hyperglycemia or hypoglycemia, pheochromocytoma
Weight gain	Cushing's syndrome, hypothyroidism, pituitary tumor
Weight loss	Hyperthyroidism, pheochromocytoma, Addison's disease, hyperparathyroidism, diabetes mellitus, diabetes insipidus

ENDOCRINE CARE

DIAGNOSTIC TESTS

RADIOACTIVE IODINE UPTAKE

Overview

- Used to evaluate thyroid function by measuring the amount of orally ingested radioactive isotopes of iodine, ^{123}I or ^{131}I, that accumulate in the thyroid gland after 2, 6, and 24 hours
- Used to accurately diagnose hyperthyroidism (about 90%), but less accurate for hypothyroidism; also used to distinguish between permanent causes of hyperthyroidism (Grave's disease) and temporary causes such as thyroiditis
- Also known as RAIU test
- Perchlorate suppression test possibly used in addition to RAIU in patient with suspected Hashimoto's disease

PURPOSE

- To evaluate thyroid function
- To aid diagnosis of hyperthyroidism or hypothyroidism
- To distinguish between primary and secondary thyroid disorders
- To differentiate Graves' disease from hyperfunctioning toxic adenoma, when performed concurrently with radionuclide thyroid imaging and the triiodothyronine resin uptake test

PATIENT PREPARATION

- Make sure the patient has signed an appropriate consent form.
- Note and report all allergies.
- Check the patient history for past or present iodine exposure, including use of iodine preparations or thyroid medication, which may interfere with test results.
- Check for previous radiologic tests using contrast media or nuclear medicine procedures.
- Instruct the patient to fast from midnight before the test
- Provide reassurance that the study is painless.

Teaching points

Be sure to cover:
- the purpose of the study and how it's done
- who will perform the study and where
- that scan takes 1 to 1½ hours
- that radiation exposure is minimal and harmless.

POSTPROCEDURE CARE

- Resume a light diet 2 hours after taking the oral dose of ^{123}I or ^{131}I as ordered.

PRECAUTIONS

- An iodine-deficient diet or ingestion of phenothiazines can increase iodine uptake, affecting the accuracy of test results.
- Contraindications include:
  - pregnancy
  - iodine or shellfish allergy.

COMPLICATIONS

- None known

Interpretation

NORMAL FINDINGS

- After 2 hours, 4% to 12% of the radioactive iodine should accumulate in the thyroid; after 6 hours, 5% to 20%; after 24 hours, 8% to 29%.

■ Local variations in the normal range of iodine uptake may stem from regional differences in dietary iodine intake or procedural differences among individual laboratories.

Abnormal results

■ Below-normal percentages of iodine uptake may suggest:
- hypothyroidism
- subacute thyroiditis
- iodine overload.

■ Above-normal percentages may suggest:
- hyperthyroidism
- early Hashimoto's disease
- hypoalbuminemia
- ingestion of lithium
- iodine-deficient goiter.

Thyroid imaging, radionuclide

Overview

■ Allows visualization of the thyroid gland by a gamma camera after administration of a radioisotope (usually ^{131}I, ^{131}I, or technetium-99m [^{99m}Tc] pertechnetate); ^{131}I and ^{131}I used most often because of their short half-lives (which limit exposure to radiation) and to enable measurement of thyroid function

■ Usually recommended after discovery of a palpable mass, enlarged gland, or asymmetrical goiter

■ Usually performed concurrently with measurement of serum triiodothyronine (T_3) and serum thyroxine levels and thyroid uptake tests

Purpose

■ To assess size, structure, and position of the thyroid gland
■ To evaluate thyroid function in conjunction with other thyroid tests

Patient preparation

■ Make sure the patient has signed an appropriate consent form.
■ Note and report all allergies.
■ Determine if the patient has undergone tests that used radiographic contrast media within the past 60 days; note such tests or the use of drugs that may interfere with iodine uptake on the radiograph request.
■ Two to three weeks before the test, discontinue administration of thyroid hormones, thyroid hormone antagonists, and iodine preparations (Lugol's solution, some multivitamins, and cough syrups), phenothiazines, corticosteroids, salicylates, anticoagulants, and antihistamines as ordered.
■ Instruct the patient to avoid iodized salt, iodinated salt substitutes, and seafood for 14 to 21 days as ordered.
■ Discontinue liothyronine, propylthiouracil, and methimazole 3 days before the test as ordered.
■ Discontinue thyroxine 10 days before the test as ordered.
■ Tell the patient to fast after midnight the night before the test (if scheduled to receive an oral dose of ^{123}I or ^{131}I); fasting is necessary for another 2 hours after it's administered.
■ There's no need to fast if the patient will receive an I.V. injection of ^{99m}Tc pertechnetate.

Teaching points

Be sure to cover:
■ the purpose of the study and how it's done
■ who will perform the study and where
■ that imaging takes only 30 minutes and that radiation exposure is minimal.

Postprocedure care

■ Resume medications as ordered.
■ Resume a normal diet as ordered.

PRECAUTIONS

■ Contraindications include:
– pregnancy
– lactation
– previous allergy to iodine, shellfish, or radioactive tracers.

COMPLICATIONS

■ Adverse reaction to the radioactive tracer (rare)

Interpretation

NORMAL FINDINGS

■ Thyroid gland should be about 2″ (5 cm) long and 1″ (2.5 cm) wide, with uniform uptake of the radioisotope and without tumors.
■ The gland should be butterfly-shaped, with the isthmus located at the midline.
■ Occasionally, a third lobe called the pyramidal lobe may be present; this is a normal variant.

ABNORMAL RESULTS

■ Areas of excessive iodine uptake, appearing as black regions called hot spots, suggest hyperfunctioning nodules.
■ White or light gray regions, appearing as areas of little or no iodine uptake called cold spots, suggest hypofunctioning nodules.

ULTRASONOGRAPHY OF THE PANCREAS

Overview

■ Cross-sectional images of the pancreas produced by channeling high-frequency sound waves into the epigastric region, converting the resultant echoes to electrical impulses, and displaying them as real-time images on a monitor; pattern varies with tissue density and represents the size, shape, and position of the pancreas and surrounding viscera
■ Can't provide a sensitive measure of pancreatic function, but useful in detecting anatomic abnormalities, such as pancreatic carcinoma and pseudocysts, and to guide the insertion of biopsy needles
■ Doesn't expose the patient to radiation, so this procedure has largely replaced hypotonic duodenography, endoscopic retrograde cholangiopancreatography, radioisotope studies, and arteriography

PURPOSE

■ To aid diagnosis of pancreatitis, pseudocysts, and pancreatic carcinoma

PATIENT PREPARATION

■ Make sure the patient has signed an appropriate consent form.
■ Note and report all allergies.
■ Fasting is required for 8 to 12 hours before the test to reduce bowel gas, which hinders transmission of ultrasound.

Teaching points

Be sure to cover:
■ the purpose of the study and how it's done
■ that the test takes 30 minutes.

POSTPROCEDURE CARE

■ Remove the lubricating jelly from the patient's skin.
■ Resume the patient's usual diet as ordered.

PRECAUTIONS

■ Factors that may affect test results include:
– failure to fast
– bowel gas
– dehydration

– barium from previous diagnostic tests

– obesity.

COMPLICATIONS
■ None known

Interpretation

NORMAL FINDINGS
■ The pancreas demonstrates a coarse, uniform echo pattern (reflecting tissue density) and usually appears more echogenic than the adjacent liver.

ABNORMAL RESULTS
■ Alterations in the size, contour, and parenchymal texture of the pancreas suggest possible pancreatic disease.
■ An enlarged pancreas with decreased echogenicity and distinct borders suggests pancreatitis.
■ A well-defined mass with an essentially echo-free interior suggests pseudocyst.
■ An ill-defined mass with scattered internal echoes, or a mass in the head of the pancreas (obstructing the common bile duct) and a large noncontracting gallbladder suggests pancreatic carcinoma.

ULTRASONOGRAPHY OF THE THYROID

Overview

■ Pulses emitted from a piezoelectric crystal in a transducer, directed at the thyroid gland, and reflected back to the transducer; pulses are converted electronically to produce structural visualization on oscilloscope screen
■ Used to differentiate between a cyst and a tumor larger than 1 cm with about 85% accuracy when mass is located by palpation or by thyroid imaging
■ Especially useful in evaluating thyroid nodules during pregnancy because it doesn't expose the fetus to radioactive iodine used in other diagnostic procedures
■ Can also be performed on parathyroid glands

PURPOSE
■ To evaluate thyroid structure
■ To differentiate between a cyst and a solid tumor
■ To monitor the size of the thyroid gland during suppressive therapy
■ To allow accurate measurement of a nodule's size
■ To aid in performance of thyroid needle biopsy

PATIENT PREPARATION
■ Make sure the patient has signed an appropriate consent form.
■ Note and report all allergies.
■ Restriction of food and fluids before the test isn't necessary.

Teaching points
Be sure to cover:
■ the purpose of the study and how it's done
■ that the test takes approximately 10 minutes and the results are almost immediately available
■ that the study is painless and safe.

POSTPROCEDURE CARE
■ Thoroughly clean the patient's neck to remove the contact solution.

PRECAUTIONS
■ No precautions are necessary.

COMPLICATIONS
■ None known

Interpretation

NORMAL FINDINGS
- A uniform echo pattern is found throughout the gland.
- No anatomical abnormalities are present.

ABNORMAL RESULTS
- Smooth-bordered, echo-free areas with enhanced sound transmission suggest cysts.
- Solid and well-demarcated areas with identical echo patterns may suggest adenomas and carcinomas.

DISEASES

DIABETES MELLITUS

Overview

DESCRIPTION
- Chronic disease of absolute or relative insulin deficiency or resistance
- Characterized by disturbances in carbohydrate, protein, and fat metabolism
- Two primary forms:
- Type 1, characterized by absolute insufficiency
- Type 2, characterized by insulin resistance with varying degrees of insulin secretory defects

PATHOPHYSIOLOGY
- The effects of diabetes mellitus result from insulin deficiency or resistance to endogenous insulin.
- Insulin allows glucose transport into the cells for use as energy or storage as glycogen.
- Insulin also stimulates protein synthesis and free fatty acid storage in the adipose tissues.
- Insulin deficiency compromises the body tissues' access to essential nutrients for fuel and storage.

CAUSES
- Genetic factors
- Autoimmune disease (type 1)

RISK FACTORS
- Viral infections (type 1)
- Obesity (type 2)
- Physiologic or emotional stress
- Sedentary lifestyle (type 2)
- Pregnancy

COMPLICATIONS
- Ketoacidosis (occurs most often in patients with type 1 diabetes mellitus)
- Hyperosmolar, hyperglycemic non-ketotic syndrome (more common in older patients with type 2 diabetes mellitus; see *Understanding the difference between HHNS and DKA*)
- Cardiovascular disease
- Peripheral vascular disease
- Retinopathy, blindness
- Nephropathy, renal failure
- Diabetic dermopathy
- Peripheral neuropathy
- Autonomic neuropathy
- Amputations
- Impaired resistance to infection
- Cognitive depression

Assessment

HISTORY
- Polyuria, nocturia
- Dehydration
- Polydipsia
- Dry mucous membranes
- Poor skin turgor
- Weight loss and hunger

UNDERSTANDING THE DIFFERENCE BETWEEN HHNS AND DKA

Hyperosmolar hyperglycemic nonketotic syndrome (HHNS) and diabetic ketoacidosis (DKA), both acute complications associated with diabetes, share some similarities, but they're two distinct conditions. Use the flowchart below to help determine which condition your patient is experiencing.

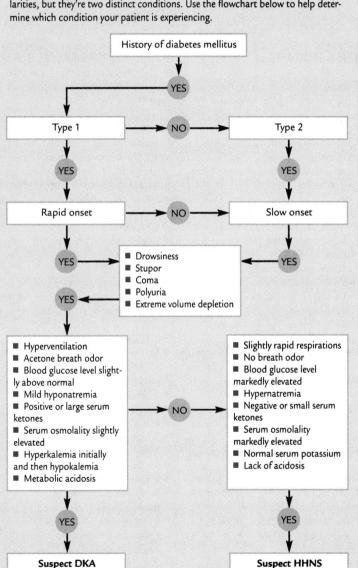

- Weakness; fatigue
- Vision changes
- Frequent skin and urinary tract infections
- Dry, itchy skin
- Sexual problems
- Numbness or pain in the hands or feet
- Postprandial feeling of nausea or fullness
- Nocturnal diarrhea

Type 1
- Rapidly developing symptoms

Type 2
- Vague, long-standing symptoms that develop gradually
- Family history of diabetes mellitus
- Gestational diabetes

PHYSICAL FINDINGS
- Retinopathy or cataract formation
- Skin changes, especially on the legs and feet
- Muscle wasting and loss of subcutaneous fat (type 1)
- Obesity, particularly in the abdominal area (type 2)
- Characteristic "fruity" breath odor in ketoacidosis
- Possible hypovolemia and shock in ketoacidosis and hyperosmolar hyperglycemic state

TEST RESULTS

Laboratory
- Fasting plasma glucose level greater than or equal to 126 mg/dl on at least two occasions
- Random blood glucose level greater than or equal to 200 mg/dl
- Two-hour postprandial blood glucose level greater than or equal to 200 mg/dl
- Glycosylated hemoglobin (Hb A_{1C}) increased

- Urinalysis possibly showing acetone or glucose

Diagnostic procedures
- Ophthalmologic examination may show diabetic retinopathy.

Treatment

GENERAL
- Exercise and diet for type 2 diabetes
- Tight glycemic control for prevention of complications in type 1 and type 2

DIET
- Modest caloric restriction for weight loss or maintenance
- American Diabetes Association recommendations to reach target glucose, Hb A_{1c} lipid, and blood pressure levels

ACTIVITY
- Regular aerobic exercise

MEDICATION
- Exogenous insulin (type 1)
- Oral antihyperglycemic drugs (type 2); insulin may be required

SURGERY
- Pancreas transplantation

MONITORING
- Vital signs
- Intake and output
- Daily weights
- Serum glucose
- Urine acetone
- Renal status
- Cardiovascular status
- Signs and symptoms of:
  – hypoglycemia
  – hyperglycemia
  – hyperosmolar coma
  – urinary tract and vaginal infections
  – diabetic neuropathy

HYPOTHYROIDISM

Overview

DESCRIPTION
- Clinical condition characterized by either decreased circulating levels of or resistance to free thyroid hormone
- Classified as primary or secondary
- Severe hypothyroidism known as myxedema

PATHOPHYSIOLOGY
- In primary hypothyroidism, a decrease in thyroid hormone production is a result of the loss of thyroid tissue.
- This results in an increased secretion of thyroid-stimulating hormone (TSH) that leads to a goiter.
- In secondary hypothyroidism, typically the pituitary fails to synthesize or secrete adequate amounts of TSH, or target tissues fail to respond to normal blood levels of thyroid hormone.
- Either type may progress to myxedema, which is clinically more severe and considered a medical emergency.

CAUSES
- Thyroid gland surgery
- Radioactive iodine therapy
- Inflammatory conditions
- Autoimmune thyroiditis
- Endemic iodine deficiency
- Antithyroid drugs
- Congenital defects
- Amyloidosis
- Sarcoidosis (rare)
- External radiation to the neck
- Pituitary failure to produce TSH
- Pituitary tumor
- Idiopathic

COMPLICATIONS
Cardiovascular complications
- Cardiomegaly
- Heart failure
- Pleural and pericardial effusion

GI complications
- Megacolon

Other complications
- Conductive or sensorineural deafness
- Psychiatric disturbances
- Carpal tunnel syndrome
- Impaired fertility
- Myxedema coma

Assessment

HISTORY
- Vague and varied symptoms that developed slowly over time
- Energy loss, fatigue
- Forgetfulness
- Sensitivity to cold
- Unexplained weight gain
- Constipation
- Anorexia
- Decreased libido
- Menorrhagia
- Paresthesia
- Joint stiffness
- Muscle cramping

PHYSICAL FINDINGS
- Slight mental slowing to severe obtundation
- Thick, dry tongue
- Hoarseness; slow, slurred speech
- Dry, flaky, inelastic skin
- Puffy face, hands, and feet
- Periorbital edema; drooping upper eyelids
- Dry, sparse hair with patchy hair loss
- Loss of the outer third of the eyebrow
- Thick and brittle nails with transverse and longitudinal grooves
- Ataxia, intention tremor; nystagmus

- Weak pulse and bradycardia
- Muscle weakness
- Sacral or peripheral edema
- Delayed reflex relaxation time
- Possible goiter
- Absent or decreased bowel sounds
- Hypotension
- A gallop or distant heart sounds
- Adventitious breath sounds
- Abdominal distention or ascites

TEST RESULTS
Laboratory
- Radioimmunoassay showing decreased serum levels of T_3 and T_4
- Serum TSH level increased with thyroid insufficiency; decreased with hypothalamic or pituitary insufficiency
- Serum cholesterol, alkaline phosphatase, and triglycerides levels elevated
- Serum electrolytes showing low serum sodium levels in myxedema coma

Imaging
- Skull X-ray, computed tomography scan, and magnetic resonance imaging may show pituitary or hypothalamic lesions.

Treatment

GENERAL
- To restore and maintain a normal thyroid state
- Need for long-term thyroid replacement

DIET
- Low-fat, low-cholesterol
- High-fiber
- Low-sodium
- Possible fluid restriction

ACTIVITY
- As tolerated

MEDICATION
- Synthetic hormone levothyroxine
- Synthetic liothyronine

SURGERY
- For underlying cause such as pituitary tumor

MONITORING
- Vital signs
- Intake and output
- Daily weight
- Cardiovascular status
- Pulmonary status
- Edema
- Bowel sounds, abdominal distention, frequency of bowel movements
- Mental and neurologic status
- Signs and symptoms of hyperthyroidism

THYROID CANCER

Overview

DESCRIPTION
- The most common endocrine malignancy
- Papillary carcinomas: 50% of all cases
- Medullary cancer: may be associated with pheochromocytoma; curable when detected before it causes symptoms

PATHOPHYSIOLOGY
- Papillary cancer is usually multifocal and bilateral. It metastasizes slowly into regional nodes of the neck, mediastinum, lungs, and other distant organs.
- Follicular cancer is less common but is more likely to recur and metastasize to the regional lymph nodes and spread through blood vessels into the bones, liver, and lungs.

■ Medullary (solid) carcinoma originates in the parafollicular cells derived from the last branchial pouch and contains amyloid and calcium deposits.

Causes
■ Previous exposure to radiation treatment in the neck area
■ Prolonged secretion of thyroid-stimulating hormone (radiation or heredity)

Risk factors
■ Familial predisposition
■ Chronic goiter

Complications
■ Dysphagia
■ Stridor
■ Hormone alterations
■ Distant metastasis

Assessment

History
■ Sensitivity to cold and mental apathy (hypothyroidism)
■ Sensitivity to heat, restlessness, and overactivity (hyperthyroidism)
■ Diarrhea
■ Dysphagia
■ Anorexia
■ Irritability
■ Ear pain

Physical findings
■ Hard, painless nodule in an enlarged thyroid gland or palpable lymph nodes with thyroid enlargement
■ Hoarseness and vocal stridor
■ Disfiguring thyroid mass
■ Bruits

Test results
Laboratory
■ Calcitonin assay identifies silent medullary carcinoma; calcitonin level measuring during a resting state and during a calcium infusion, that shows an elevated fasting calcitonin level and an abnormal response to calcium stimulation—a high release of calcitonin from the node in comparison with the rest of the gland—indicating medullary cancer

Imaging
■ Thyroid scan is used to differentiate functional nodes, which are rarely malignant, from hypofunctional nodes, which are commonly malignant.
■ Ultrasonography shows changes in the size of thyroid nodules after thyroxine suppression therapy and is used to guide fine-needle aspiration and to detect recurrent disease.
■ Magnetic resonance imaging and computed tomography scans provide a basis for treatment planning because they establish the extent of the disease within the thyroid and in surrounding structures.

Diagnostic procedures
■ Fine-needle aspiration biopsy is used to differentiate benign from malignant thyroid nodules.
■ Histologic analysis is used to stage the disease and thereby guide treatment plans.

Treatment

General
■ Radioisotope (^{131}I) therapy with external radiation (sometimes postoperatively in lieu of radical neck excision) or alone (for metastasis)

DIET
■ Soft diet with small frequent meals if dysphagia occurs

ACTIVITY
■ No limitations

MEDICATION
■ Suppressive thyroid hormone therapy
■ Chemotherapy

SURGERY
■ Total or subtotal thyroidectomy with modified node dissection
■ Total thyroidectomy and radical neck excision

MONITORING
■ Vital signs
■ Wound site
■ Pain control
■ Serum calcium levels (if the parathyroid glands were removed)
■ Postoperative complications
■ Hydration and nutritional status

THYROTOXICOSIS

Overview

DESCRIPTION
■ An alteration in thyroid function in which thyroid hormones exert greater than normal responses
■ Management determined by cause
■ Hyperthyroidism: a form of thyrotoxicosis in which excess thyroid hormones are secreted by the thyroid gland
■ Thyrotoxicoses not associated with hyperthyroidism: subacute thyroiditis, ectopic thyroid tissue, and ingestion of excessive thyroid hormone
■ Graves' disease (also known as toxic diffuse goiter): an autoimmune disease, the most common form of thyrotoxicosis
■ Also known as hyperthyroidism

PATHOPHYSIOLOGY
■ In Graves' disease, thyroid-stimulating antibodies bind to and stimulate the thyroid-stimulating hormone (TSH) receptors of the thyroid gland.
■ The trigger for this autoimmune disease is unclear.
■ It's associated with the production of autoantibodies possibly caused by a defect in suppressor-T-lymphocyte function that allows the formation of these autoantibodies.

CAUSES
■ Diseases that can cause hyperthyroidism:
– Graves' disease
– Toxic multinodular goiter
– Thyroid cancer
– Increased TSH secretion
– Genetic and immunologic factors
■ Precipitating factors:
– Excessive intake of iodine
– Stress
– Surgery
– Infection
– Toxemia of pregnancy
– Diabetic ketoacidosis

COMPLICATIONS
■ Arrhythmias
■ Left ventricular hypertrophy
■ Heart failure
■ Muscle weakness and atrophy
■ Osteoporosis
■ Thyrotoxic crisis or thyroid storm

Assessment

HISTORY
Graves' disease
■ Nervousness, tremor
■ Heat intolerance

- Weight loss despite increased appetite
- Sweating
- Frequent bowel movements
- Palpitations
- Poor concentration
- Shaky handwriting
- Clumsiness
- Emotional instability and mood swings
- Thin, brittle nails
- Hair loss
- Nausea and vomiting
- Weakness and fatigue
- Oligomenorrhea or amenorrhea
- Fertility problems
- Diminished libido
- Diplopia

PHYSICAL FINDINGS
Graves' disease
- Enlarged thyroid (goiter)
- Exophthalmos
- Tremor
- Smooth, warm, flushed skin
- Fine, soft hair
- Premature graying and increased hair loss
- Friable nails and onycholysis
- Pretibial myxedema
- Thickened skin
- Accentuated hair follicles
- Tachycardia at rest
- Full, bounding pulses
- Arrhythmias, especially atrial fibrillation
- Wide pulse pressure
- Possible systolic murmur
- Dyspnea
- Hepatomegaly
- Hyperactive bowel sounds

When thyrotoxicosis escalates to thyroid storm, these signs and symptoms can be accompanied by extreme irritability, hypertension, tachycardia, vomiting, temperature up to 106° F (41.1° C), delirium, and coma.

TEST RESULTS
Laboratory
- Radioimmunoassay showing increased serum triiodothyronine and thyroxine concentrations
- Increased serum protein-bound iodine
- Decreased serum cholesterol and total lipid levels
- Decreased TSH

Imaging
- Thyroid scan shows increased uptake of radioactive iodine (^{131}I).
- Ultrasonography shows subclinical ophthalmopathy.

Treatment

GENERAL
- In hyperthyroidism, drugs, radioiodine, and surgery
- Treatment with ^{131}I: a single oral dose; treatment of choice for women past reproductive age or men and women not planning to have children

DIET
- Adequate caloric intake

ACTIVITY
- As tolerated

MEDICATION
- Thyroid hormone antagonists
- Beta-adrenergic antagonists
- Corticosteroids
- Sedatives

SURGERY
- Subtotal (partial) thyroidectomy
- Surgical decompression

MONITORING
- Vital signs
- Daily weight
- Intake and output
- Daily neck circumference

ENDOCRINE CARE

- Serum electrolyte results
- Hyperglycemia and glycosuria
- Electrocardiogram for arrhythmias and ST-segment changes
- Complete blood count results
- Signs and symptoms of heart failure
- Frequency and characteristics of stools

After thyroidectomy
- Dressings
- Signs and symptoms of hemorrhage into the neck
- Surgical incision
- Dysphagia or hoarseness
- Signs and symptoms of hypocalcemia

TREATMENTS

ADRENALECTOMY

Overview

- Surgical resection or removal of one or both of the adrenal glands

INDICATIONS
- Adrenal hyperfunction
- Hyperaldosteronism
- Benign or malignant adrenal tumor
- Secondary treatment of neoplasms
- Secondary treatment of corticotropin oversecretion

COMPLICATIONS
- Acute life-threatening adrenal crisis (see *Understanding acute adrenal crisis*)
- Hemorrhage
- Poor wound healing
- Hypoglycemia
- Electrolyte disturbances
- Pancreatic injury
- Hypotension (with gland removal)
- Hypertension (with gland manipulation)

Nursing interventions

PRETREATMENT CARE
- Explain the treatment and preparation to the patient and his family.

- Make sure the patient has signed an appropriate consent form.
- Administer medications to control hypertension, edema, diabetes, cardiovascular symptoms, and increased infection risk as needed and ordered.
- Administer aldosterone antagonists for blood pressure control as ordered.
- Give glucocorticoids on the morning of surgery as ordered.
- Draw blood samples for laboratory test as ordered.
- Administer potassium supplements as ordered.
- Provide a low-sodium, high-potassium diet as ordered.

Monitoring
- Arrhythmias
- Palpitations
- Severe headache
- Hypertension
- Hyperglycemia
- Nausea, vomiting
- Diaphoresis
- Vision disturbances

POSTTREATMENT CARE
- Administer I.V. vasopressors; titrate the dosage to the patient's blood pressure response as ordered.
- Increase the I.V. fluid rate as ordered.

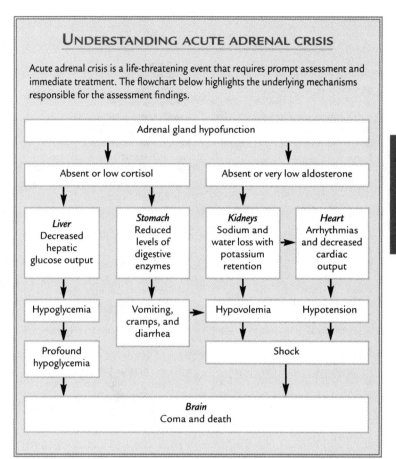

UNDERSTANDING ACUTE ADRENAL CRISIS

Acute adrenal crisis is a life-threatening event that requires prompt assessment and immediate treatment. The flowchart below highlights the underlying mechanisms responsible for the assessment findings.

Adrenal gland hypofunction

Absent or low cortisol — Absent or very low aldosterone

Liver Decreased hepatic glucose output

Stomach Reduced levels of digestive enzymes

Kidneys Sodium and water loss with potassium retention

Heart Arrhythmias and decreased cardiac output

Hypoglycemia

Vomiting, cramps, and diarrhea → Hypovolemia — Hypotension

Profound hypoglycemia

Shock

Brain Coma and death

- Administer glucocorticoids I.V. as ordered.
- Administer analgesics as ordered.

Monitoring
- Vital signs
- Intake and output
- Hemorrhage and shock
- Invasive arterial pressure
- Adrenal hypofunction
- Acute adrenal crisis
- Hypoglycemia
- Serum electrolyte levels
- Surgical wound and dressings

- Abdominal distention and return of bowel sounds

PATIENT TEACHING
Be sure to cover:
- medications and possible adverse reactions
- avoidance of sudden steroid withdrawal
- complications
- when to notify the physician
- follow-up medical care

PANCREAS TRANSPLANTATION

Pancreas transplantation involves the replacement of a person's pancreas with a donor pancreas. It's indicated for patients with end-stage pancreatic disease, primarily type 1 diabetes mellitus. These patients generally have serious complications of the disease, including neuropathies, macrovascular and microvascular disease. Thus, the risks associated with transplantation surgery and immunosuppressive therapy are less than those associated with the disease complications. The goal of pancreas transplantation is to restore blood glucose levels to normal and limit the progression of complications.

Contraindications for pancreas transplantation include:
■ heart disease that can't be controlled
■ active infection
■ positive serology for human immunodeficiency virus or hepatitis B surface antigen
■ malignancy within the past 3 years
■ current and active substance abuse
■ history of noncompliance or serious psychiatric illness
■ active untreated peptic ulcer disease
■ irreversible liver or lung dysfunction

■ other systemic illnesses that would delay or prevent recovery

Most commonly, pancreas transplantation occurs simultaneously with renal transplantation, referred to as simultaneous pancreas-kidney (SPK) transplant. Pancreas transplantation can also be done after renal transplantation, termed pancreas-after-kidney transplant, or as a single transplant procedure, referred to as pancreas-transplant alone. Surgical complications include graft thrombosis, infection, pancreatitis, intrapancreatic abscess, leakage at the anastomosis site, and organ rejection.

When caring for a patient undergoing a pancreas transplant, major nursing responsibilities include preprocedure patient preparation, patient education, and monitoring the patient postprocedure for complications and organ rejection.

SPK transplantation

The illustration below depicts SPK transplant, in which the donor pancreas is anastomosed using the systemic bladder technique.

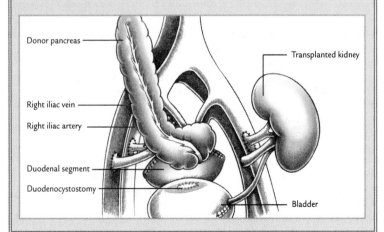

Donor pancreas

Right iliac vein

Right iliac artery

Duodenal segment

Duodenocystostomy

Transplanted kidney

Bladder

THYROIDECTOMY

Overview

■ Surgical removal of all or part of the thyroid gland

INDICATIONS
■ Hyperthyroidism
■ Respiratory obstruction caused by goiter
■ Thyroid cancer

COMPLICATIONS
■ Hemorrhage
■ Parathyroid damage
■ Hypocalcemia
■ Tetany
■ Laryngeal nerve damage
■ Vocal cord paralysis
■ Thyroid storm

Nursing interventions

PRETREATMENT CARE
■ Explain the treatment and preparation to the patient and his family.
■ Make sure the patient has signed an appropriate consent form.
■ Explain postoperative care.
■ Inform the patient that some hoarseness and a sore throat will occur after surgery.
■ Make sure the patient has followed the preoperative drug regimen as ordered.
■ Collect blood samples for serum thyroid hormone measurement.
■ Obtain a 12-lead electrocardiogram.

POSTTREATMENT CARE
■ Administer medications as ordered.
■ Keep the patient in high-Fowler's position.
■ Evaluate the patient's speech for signs of laryngeal nerve damage.
■ Keep a tracheotomy tray at the bedside for 24 hours after surgery.
■ Provide surgical wound care and dressing changes as ordered.
■ Provide comfort measures.
■ Maintain patency of drains.

Monitoring
■ Vital signs
■ Intake and output
■ Surgical wound and dressings
■ Drainage
■ Abnormal bleeding
■ Respiratory status
■ Hypocalcemia (Chvostek's and Trousseau's signs)
■ Thyroid storm

PATIENT TEACHING
Be sure to cover:
■ medications and possible adverse reactions
■ signs and symptoms of respiratory distress
■ signs and symptoms of hypothyroidism and hyperthyroidism
■ signs and symptoms of infection
■ signs and symptoms of hypocalcemia
■ abnormal bleeding
■ complications
■ when to notify the physician
■ prescribed thyroid hormone replacement therapy
■ calcium supplements as indicated
■ incision care and dressing changes
■ follow-up care.

PROCEDURES AND EQUIPMENT

BEDSIDE BLOOD GLUCOSE MONITORING

Nurses frequently use blood glucose monitoring at the bedside for patients who are at risk for hypoglycemia and hyperglycemia, and to monitor the effectiveness of insulin administration. The fast, accurate results obtained allow for immediate interventions, as needed. Numerous testing systems are available and most meters use a drop of capillary blood obtained by fingerstick or heel stick; newer blood glucose meters require smaller amounts of blood and the puncture may also be performed on the forearm.

Before using the blood glucose meter, calibrate it and run it with a control sample to ensure accurate test results. Follow the manufacturer's instructions for calibration. Assess the skin area that will be used for the puncture and avoid sites with bruising, open lesions, or areas that are cold, swollen or cyanotic.

Blood glucose meters are convenient for the patient's home use, and the nurse plays a vital role in providing initial patient education for self-monitoring of blood glucose.

Types of insulin infusion pumps

A subcutaneous insulin infusion pump provides continuous, long-term insulin therapy for patients with type I diabetes mellitus. Complications include infection at the injection site, catheter clogging, and insulin loss from loose reservoir-catheter connections. Insulin pumps work on either an open-loop or a closed-loop system.

Open-loop system
The open-loop pump is used most commonly. It infuses insulin but can't respond to changes in serum glucose levels. These portable, self-contained, programmable insulin pumps are smaller and less obtrusive than ever — about the size of a credit card — and have fewer buttons.

The pump delivers insulin in small (basal) doses every few minutes and large (bolus) doses that the patient sets manually. The system consists of a reservoir containing the insulin syringe, a small pump, an infusion-rate selector that allows insulin release adjustments, a battery, and a plastic catheter with an attached needle leading from the syringe to the subcutaneous injection site. The needle is typically held in place with waterproof tape. The patient can wear the pump on his belt or in his pocket — practically anywhere as long as the infusion line has a clear path to the injection site.

The infusion-rate selector automatically releases about one-half the total daily insulin requirement. The patient re-leases the remainder in bolus doses before meals and snacks. The patient must change the syringe daily; he must change the needle, catheter, and injection site every other day.

Closed-loop system
The self-contained closed-loop system detects and responds to changing serum glucose levels. The typical closed-loop system includes a glucose sensor, a programmable computer, a power supply, a pump, and an insulin reservoir. The computer triggers continuous insulin delivery in appropriate amounts from the reservoir.

Nonneedle catheter system
In the nonneedle delivery system, a tiny plastic catheter is inserted into the skin over a needle using a special insertion device (shown below). The needle is then withdrawn, leaving the catheter in place (shown in inset). This catheter can be placed in the abdomen, thigh, or flank and should be changed every 2 to 3 days.

ENDOCRINE CARE

COMMONLY USED MEDICATIONS FOR ENDOCRINE DISORDERS

Drug	Indications	Adverse reactions	Special considerations
ORAL ANTIDIABETICS			
Sulfonylureas **Glipizide** (Glucotrol); **glyburide** (DiaBeta)	■ Type 2 diabetes management	■ Hypoglycemia ■ Weight gain ■ Nervousness ■ Dizziness ■ Nausea ■ Leukopenia	■ Check for signs and symptoms of hypoglycemia and hyperglycemia. ■ Monitor blood glucose. ■ Risk of hypoglycemia increases when drug is given in combination with insulin.
Biguanides **Metformin** (Glucophage)	■ Type 2 diabetes management	■ Nausea or vomiting ■ Flatulence ■ Diarrhea ■ Headache ■ Hypoglycemia (rare if used as a single agent) ■ Lactic acidosis	■ Give drug with meals. ■ Assess renal function. ■ Monitor for lactic acidosis, especially patients with renal insufficiency ■ Monitor for lactic acidosis after administration of contrast dye.
Thiazolidinediones **Pioglitazone** (Actos); **rosiglitazone** (Avandia)	■ Type 2 diabetes management	■ Weight gain ■ Upper respiratory infection ■ Edema ■ Headache ■ Hypoglycemia (rare if used as a single agent)	■ Monitor liver function studies. ■ Avoid in patients with active liver disease. ■ Use with caution in patients with edema or heart failure.
INSULINS			
(long-, intermediate-, fast-, and rapid-acting)	■ All types of diabetes ■ Diabetic ketoacidosis ■ Hyperosmolar hyperglycemic nonketotic syndrome	■ Hypoglycemia ■ Weight gain	■ Monitor for hypoglycemia. ■ Monitor blood glucose levels. ■ Teach patient the symptoms and treatment of hypoglycemia and hyperglycemia.

COMMONLY USED MEDICATIONS
FOR ENDOCRINE DISORDERS *(continued)*

Drug	Indications	Adverse reactions	Special considerations
ANTITHYROID MEDICATIONS			
Propylthioura-cil (Propyl-Thyracil)	■ Hyper-thyroidism	■ Lethargy ■ Weakness ■ Intolerance to cold ■ Weight gain ■ Edema ■ Drowsiness ■ Headache ■ Vertigo ■ Loss of taste perception ■ Constipation ■ Arthralgia ■ Systemic lupus erythematosus-like syndrome ■ Myxedema coma	■ Use with caution with anticoagulants (bleeding risk increased). ■ Monitor for signs of bleeding. ■ Monitor effects of cardiac medications after hyperthyroidism corrected (cardiac medication dosages may need to be decreased). ■ Monitor thyroid tests frequently to adjust dosing. ■ Teach patient the symptoms of hypothyroidism (myxedema coma).
THYROID REPLACEMENT MEDICATIONS			
Levothyroxine (Synthroid)	■ Hypo-thyroidism	■ Irritability ■ Restlessness ■ Intolerance to heat ■ Weight loss ■ Hypertension ■ Tachycardia ■ Nervousness ■ Menstrual irregularities ■ Insomnia ■ Sleep disturbances ■ Thyrotoxicosis	■ Instruct patient to take medications in the early morning on an empty stomach. ■ Monitor thyroid tests. ■ Monitor for cardiac arrhythmias, such as tachycardia and drug toxicity. ■ Teach patient the symptoms of toxicity (thyrotoxicosis symptoms). ■ Use with caution in elderly patients and in patients with renal impairment or cardiovascular disorders.

13

HEMATOLOGIC AND IMMUNE CARE

ASSESSMENT

PALPATING THE LYMPH NODES

When assessing a patient for signs of an immune disorder, you need to palpate the superficial lymph nodes of the head, neck and axillary, epitrochlear inguinal, and popliteal areas, using the pads of the index and middle fingers. Always palpate gently; begin with light pressure and gradually increase the pressure.

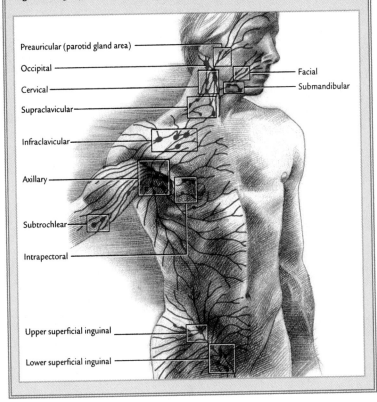

Preauricular (parotid gland area)
Occipital
Facial
Cervical
Submandibular
Supraclavicular
Infraclavicular
Axillary
Subtrochlear
Intrapectoral
Upper superficial inguinal
Lower superficial inguinal

PERCUSSING AND PALPATING THE SPLEEN

To assess the spleen, use percussion to estimate its size and palpation to detect tenderness and enlargement.

Percussion

To percuss the spleen, follow these steps.
1. Percuss the lowest intercostal space in the left anterior axillary line; percussion notes should be tympanic.

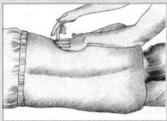

2. Ask the patient to take a deep breath, and then percuss this area again. If the spleen is normal in size, the area will remain tympanic. If the tympanic percussion note changes on inspiration to dullness, the spleen is probably enlarged.
3. To estimate spleen size, outline the spleen's edges by percussing in several directions from areas of tympany to areas of dullness.

Palpation

To palpate the spleen, follow these steps.
1. With the patient in a supine position and you at his right side, reach across him to support the posterior lower left rib cage with your left hand. Place your right hand below the left costal margin and press inward.

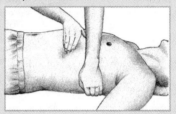

2. Instruct him to take a deep breath. The spleen normally shouldn't descend on deep inspiration below the ninth or tenth intercostal space in the posterior midaxillary line. If the spleen is enlarged, you'll feel its rigid border. Don't overpalpate the spleen; an enlarged spleen can rupture easily.

INTERPRETING IMMUNOLOGIC ASSESSMENT FINDINGS

After completing your assessment, you're ready to put together a nursing care plan. You're also in a position to form a diagnostic impression of the patient's condition. This chart will help you form such an impression by showing groups of signs and symptoms, related assessment findings you may discover during the health history and physical assessment, and the possible cause of these findings.

Key signs and symptoms	Related findings	Possible causes
■ Fatigue and weakness ■ Lymphadenopathy ■ Cough ■ Weight loss	■ Infection with unusual pathogen ■ Recurrent infections ■ Homosexual or bisexual preference ■ I.V. drug use ■ History of hemophilia with blood transfusions before 1985 ■ Unsafe sexual practices ■ Weight loss greater than 10% of body weight	Acquired immunodeficiency syndrome
■ Fatigue, fever, and weakness ■ Painless lymphadenopathy ■ Occasional abnormal bleeding ■ Joint pain at multiple sites ■ Anorexia, malaise, and weight loss ■ Muscle pain ■ Cough ■ Photosensitivity	■ Female gender ■ Butterfly rash on cheeks and bridge of nose ■ Pigmentation changes ■ Alopecia ■ Raynaud's phenomenon ■ Myocarditis, nephritis, pericarditis, pleural effusion ■ Hepatomegaly, splenomegaly ■ Mental status alterations ■ Seizures	Systemic lupus erythematosus

DIAGNOSTIC TESTS

BONE MARROW ASPIRATION AND BIOPSY

Overview

■ Involves collection of a specimen of the soft tissue in the medullary canals of long bone and interstices of cancellous bone for histologic and hematologic examination
■ Performed by aspiration or needle biopsy under local anesthesia
■ Aspiration biopsy: involves removal of a fluid specimen from the bone marrow
■ Needle biopsy: involves removal of a core of marrow cells, not fluid

■ Both methods commonly used concurrently to obtain the best possible marrow specimens

■ Minimal complications associated with sampling of the iliac crest, the preferred site

PURPOSE

■ To diagnose thrombocytopenia, leukemias, granulomas, and anemias

■ To diagnose primary and metastatic tumors

■ To determine causes of infection

■ To aid in disease staging, such as with Hodgkin's disease

■ To evaluate chemotherapy

■ To monitor myelosuppression

PATIENT PREPARATION

■ Make sure the patient has signed an appropriate consent form.

■ Note all allergies.

■ Explain that a blood sample will be collected before the biopsy for laboratory testing.

■ Explain that pressure on insertion of the biopsy needle and a brief, pulling pain on removal of the marrow will be felt.

■ Administer a mild sedative 1 hour before the test as ordered.

Teaching points

Be sure to cover:

■ the purpose of the study and how it's done

■ that it usually takes only 5 to 10 minutes

■ which bone site (sternum, anterior or posterior iliac crest, vertebral spinous process, rib, or tibia) will be used.

POSTPROCEDURE CARE
Monitoring

■ Vital signs

■ Biopsy site for bleeding

■ Signs and symptoms of hemorrhage

■ Signs and symptoms of infection

PRECAUTIONS

■ Bone marrow biopsy is contraindicated in patients with bleeding disorders.

■ Check the patient's history for hypersensitivity to the local anesthetic.

COMPLICATIONS

■ Bleeding

■ Infection

■ Puncture of the heart and major vessels (sternum)

■ Hemorrhage

■ Puncture of the mediastinum (sternum)

Interpretation

NORMAL FINDINGS

■ Yellow marrow contains fat cells and connective tissue.

■ Red marrow contains hematopoietic cells, fat cells, and connective tissue.

■ The iron stain, which measures hemosiderin (storage iron), has a +2 level.

■ The Sudan black B stain, which shows granulocytes, is negative.

■ The periodic acid–Schiff stain, which detects glycogen reactions, is negative.

ABNORMAL RESULTS

■ Decreased hemosiderin levels in an iron stain may indicate a true iron deficiency.

■ Increased hemosiderin levels may suggest other types of anemias or blood disorders.

■ A positive Sudan black B stain can differentiate acute myelogenous leukemia from acute lymphoblastic leukemia (negative Sudan black B stain).

■ A positive periodic acid–Schiff stain may suggest acute or chronic lymphocytic leukemia, amyloidosis, thalassemia, lymphoma, infectious mononucleosis, iron-deficiency anemia, or sideroblastic anemia.

DISEASES

ACQUIRED IMMUNODEFICIENCY SYNDROME AND HUMAN IMMUNODEFICIENCY VIRUS

Overview

DESCRIPTION
■ Marked by progressive failure of the immune system
■ Patients becoming susceptible to opportunistic infections, unusual cancers, and other abnormalities that define acquired immunodeficiency syndrome (AIDS)
■ The human immunodeficiency virus (HIV) type I, a retrovirus, primarily causing AIDS
■ Transmission of HIV occurring by contact with infected blood or body fluids and associated with identifiable high-risk behaviors

PATHOPHYSIOLOGY
■ HIV strikes helper T cells bearing the CD4+ antigen.
■ The antigen serves as a receptor for the retrovirus and lets it enter the cell.
■ After invading a cell, HIV replicates, leading to cell death, or becomes latent.
■ HIV infection leads to profound pathology, either directly, through destruction of CD4+ cells, other immune cells, and neuroglial cells, or indirectly, through the secondary effects of CD4+ T cell dysfunction and resultant immunosuppression.

CAUSES
■ Infection with HIV, a retrovirus

COMPLICATIONS
■ Repeated opportunistic infections
■ Neoplasms
■ Premalignant diseases
■ Organ-specific syndrome

Assessment

HISTORY
■ After a high-risk exposure and inoculation, a mononucleosis-like syndrome usually develops; then may remain asymptomatic for years.
■ In the latent stage, the only sign of HIV infection is laboratory evidence of seroconversion.

PHYSICAL FINDINGS
■ Persistent generalized adenopathy
■ Nonspecific symptoms (weight loss, fatigue, night sweats, fevers)
■ Neurologic symptoms resulting from HIV encephalopathy
■ Opportunistic infection or cancer

TEST RESULTS
Laboratory
■ A CD4+ T cell count of at least 200 cells/ml confirms HIV infection
■ Presence of HIV antibodies that indicate HIV infection

Treatment

GENERAL
■ Variety of therapeutic options for opportunistic infections (the leading cause of morbidity and mortality in patients infected with HIV)
■ Disease-specific therapy for a variety of neoplastic and premalignant diseases
■ For organ-specific syndromes

Diet
■ Balanced, nutritious

Activity
■ Regular exercise, as tolerated
■ Adequate rest periods

Medication
■ Immunomodulatory agents
■ Anti-infective agents
■ Antineoplastic agents

Primary therapy
■ Protease inhibitors
■ Nucleoside reverse transcriptase inhibitors
■ Nonnucleoside reverse transcriptase inhibitors

Monitoring
■ Fever, noting any pattern, and for signs of skin breakdown, cough, sore throat, and diarrhea
■ Swollen, tender lymph nodes
■ Laboratory values
■ Calorie intake
■ Progression of lesions in Kaposi's sarcoma
■ Opportunistic infections or signs of disease progression

ANAPHYLAXIS

Overview

Description
■ Dramatic, acute atopic reaction
■ Marked by sudden onset of rapidly progressive urticaria and respiratory distress
■ Severe reactions may initiate vascular collapse, leading to systemic shock and, possibly, death

Pathophysiology
■ After initial exposure to an antigen, the immune system produces specific immunoglobulin (Ig) antibodies in the lymph nodes. Helper T cells enhance the process.
■ The antibodies (IgE) then bind to membrane receptors located on mast cells and basophils.
■ After the body reencounters the antigen, the IgE antibodies, or cross-linked IgE receptors, recognize the antigen as foreign; this activates the release of power chemical mediators.
■ IgG or IgM enters into the reaction and activates the release of complement factors.

Causes
■ Systemic exposure to sensitizing drugs, foods, insect venom, latex, or other specific antigens

Complications
■ Respiratory obstruction
■ Systemic vascular collapse
■ Death

Assessment

History
■ Immediately after exposure, complaints of a feeling of impending doom or fright and exhibiting apprehension, restlessness, cyanosis, cool and clammy skin, erythema, edema, tachypnea, weakness, sweating, sneezing, dyspnea, nasal pruritus, and urticaria
■ Angioedema may cause a "lump" in the patient's throat
■ Dyspnea and complaints of chest tightness

Physical findings
■ Hives
■ Hoarseness or stridor, wheezing
■ Severe abdominal cramps, nausea, diarrhea

- Dizziness, drowsiness, headache, restlessness, and seizures
- Hypotension, shock; sometimes, angina and cardiac arrhythmias

TEST RESULTS
- No tests are required to identify anaphylaxis. The patient's history and signs and symptoms establish the diagnosis.

Laboratory
- Skin testing may help to identify a specific allergen.

Treatment

GENERAL
- Patent airway must be established and maintained
- Cardiopulmonary resuscitation, if cardiac arrest occurs

DIET
- Nothing by mouth, until stable

ACTIVITY
- Bed rest, until stable

MEDICATION
- *Immediate* injection of epinephrine 1:1,000 aqueous solution for mild signs and symptoms
- Corticosteroids
- Diphenhydramine I.V.
- Volume expander infusions, as needed
- Vasopressors
- Norepinephrine
- Dopamine

MONITORING
- Vital signs
- Adverse reactions from radiographic contrast media
- Respiratory status
- Serious allergic response after skin or scratch testing

- Neurologic status
- Response to treatment
- Complications

ANEMIA, APLASTIC

Overview

DESCRIPTION
- Can be potentially fatal; results from injury to or destruction of stem cells in bone marrow or the bone marrow matrix

PATHOPHYSIOLOGY
- Usually develops when damaged or destroyed stem cells inhibit red blood cell (RBC) production.
- Less commonly, develops when damaged bone marrow microvasculature creates an unfavorable environment for cell growth and maturation.

CAUSES
- Result of adverse drug reactions
- Immunologic factors; severe disease, especially hepatitis; viral infection, especially in children; and preleukemic and neoplastic infiltration of bone marrow
- Congenital hypoplastic anemia
- May also be idiopathic

COMPLICATIONS
- Hemorrhage
- Infection
- Heart failure

Assessment

HISTORY
- Signs and symptoms of anemia, or signs of thrombocytopenia

PHYSICAL FINDINGS
- Pallor, ecchymosis, petechiae, or retinal hemorrhage

- Alterations in level of consciousness, weakness, fatigue
- Bibasilar crackles, tachycardia, and a gallop murmur
- Fever, oral and rectal ulcers, and sore throat
- Nausea
- Decreased hair and skin quality

TEST RESULTS
Laboratory
- RBC count of count of 1 million/μl or less, usually with normochromic and normocytic cells (although macrocytosis [larger-than-normal erythrocytes] and anisocytosis [excessive variation in erythrocyte size] may exist); very low absolute reticulocyte count
- Elevated serum iron levels (unless bleeding occurs), but normal or slightly reduced total iron-binding capacity
- Decreased serum platelet and white blood cell counts

Diagnostic procedures
- Bone marrow biopsies performed at several sites may yield a dry tap or show severely hypocellular or aplastic marrow

Treatment

GENERAL
- Effective treatment must eliminate any identifiable cause
- Vigorous supportive measures, such as packed RBCs, platelets, and experimental histocompatibility antigen-matched leukocyte transfusions
- Respiratory support with oxygen in addition to blood transfusions
- Bone marrow transplantation (for severe aplasia and patients who need constant RBC transfusions)
- Prevention of infection

DIET
- No restrictions
- Foods high in nutritional value

ACTIVITY
- Isolation procedures may be necessary if neutropenic

MEDICATION
- Antibiotics
- Corticosteroids
- Marrow-stimulating agents, such as androgens; antilymphocyte globulin (experimental); and immunosuppressant agents

MONITORING
- Blood studies in patients receiving anemia-inducing drugs
- Early detection of bleeding

ANEMIA, IRON DEFICIENCY

Overview

DESCRIPTION
- Stems from an inadequate supply of iron for optimal formation of red blood cells (RBCs)
- Produces smaller (microcytic) cells with less color on staining (hypochromia)

PATHOPHYSIOLOGY
- Body stores of iron, including plasma iron, decrease.
- Transferrin, which binds with and transports iron, also decreases.
- Insufficient body stores of iron lead to a depleted RBC mass and to a decreased hemoglobin concentration.
- Results in decreased oxygen-carrying capacity of the blood.

CAUSES
- Inadequate dietary intake of iron

- Iron malabsorption
- Blood loss secondary to drug-induced GI bleeding or due to heavy menses, hemorrhage from trauma, GI ulcers, malignant tumors, and varices
- Pregnancy
- Intravascular hemolysis-induced hemoglobinuria or paroxysmal nocturnal hemoglobinuria
- Mechanical erythrocyte trauma caused by a prosthetic heart valve or vena cava filter

COMPLICATIONS
- Infection
- Pneumonia

Assessment

HISTORY
- Can persist for years without signs and symptoms
- Fatigue, inability to concentrate, headache, and shortness of breath (especially on exertion) that may not develop until long after iron stores and circulating iron become low
- May report increased frequency of infections and pica, an uncontrollable urge to eat strange things, such as clay, starch, ice and, in children, lead
- Menorrhagia
- Dysphagia
- Vasomotor disturbances, numbness and tingling of the extremities, and neuralgic pain

PHYSICAL FINDINGS
- Red, swollen, smooth, shiny, and tender tongue (glossitis)
- Corners of the mouth may be eroded, tender, and swollen (angular stomatitis)
- Spoon-shaped, brittle nails
- Tachycardia

TEST RESULTS
Laboratory
- Low serum hemoglobin (males, less than 12 g/dl; females, less than 10 g/dl) or decreased mean corpuscular hemoglobin in severe anemia
- Low serum hematocrit (males, less than 47 ml/dl; females, less than 42 ml/dl)
- Low serum iron levels with high binding capacity
- Low serum ferritin levels
- Low serum RBC count with microcytic and hypochromic cells (in early stages, RBC count may be normal, except in infants and children)

Diagnostic procedures
- Bone marrow studies reveal depleted or absent iron stores.
- GI studies, such as guaiac stool tests, barium swallow and enema, endoscopy, and sigmoidoscopy, rule out or confirm the diagnosis of bleeding causing the iron deficiency.

Treatment

GENERAL
- Underlying cause of anemia must first be determined

DIET
- Nutritious, nonirritating foods

ACTIVITY
- No restrictions
- Planned rest periods

MEDICATION
- Oral preparation of iron or a combination of iron and ascorbic acid
- I.M. iron in rare cases
- Total-dose I.V. infusions of supplemental iron for pregnant and elderly patients with severe disease

Monitoring
- Vital signs
- Compliance with prescribed iron supplement therapy
- Iron replacement overdose

Anemia, pernicious

Overview

Description
- Characterized by decreased gastric production of hydrochloric acid and deficiency of intrinsic factor, essential for vitamin B_{12} absorption
- Deficiency of vitamin B_{12} that causes serious neurologic, psychological, gastric, and intestinal abnormalities
- Also known as Addison's anemia

Pathophysiology
- An inherited autoimmune response may cause gastric mucosal atrophy and resultant decreased hydrochloric acid and intrinsic factor production, a substance normally secreted by the parietal cells of the gastric mucosa.
- Intrinsic factor deficiency impairs vitamin B_{12} absorption.
- Vitamin B_{12} deficiency inhibits the growth of all cells, particularly red blood cells (RBCs), leading to insufficient and deformed RBCs with poor oxygen-carrying capacity.

Causes
- Genetic predisposition
- Secondary pernicious anemia results from partial removal of the stomach
- Chronic gastric inflammation

Complications
- Heart failure with severe anemia
- Myocardial ischemia

Assessment

History
- Characteristic triad of symptoms: weakness; a beefy red, sore tongue; and numbness and tingling in the extremities
- May also complain of nausea, vomiting, anorexia, weight loss, flatulence, diarrhea, and constipation
- Peripheral numbness and paresthesia
- Light-headedness
- Headache
- Diplopia and blurred vision
- Taste
- Tinnitus

Physical findings
- Lips, gums, and tongue that appear markedly bloodless
- Slightly jaundiced sclera and pale to bright yellow skin
- Tachycardia
- Systolic murmur
- Enlarged liver and spleen
- Weakness in the extremities
- Disturbed position sense
- Lack of coordination
- Impaired fine finger movement

Test results
Laboratory
- Complete blood count: decreased hemoglobin levels (4 to 5 g/dl) and decreased RBC count, increased mean corpuscular volume; because larger-than-normal RBCs each contain increased amounts of hemoglobin, mean corpuscular hemoglobin concentration is also increased; possibly low white blood cell and platelet counts and large, malformed platelets; serum vitamin B_{12} tests may show levels less than 0.1 µg/ml; serum lactate dehydrogenase tests may show elevated serum lactate dehydrogenase levels

DIAGNOSTIC PROCEDURES
■ Bone marrow studies reveal erythroid hyperplasia with increased numbers of megaloblasts but few normally developing RBCs.
■ Gastric analysis shows an absence of free hydrochloric acid after histamine or pentagastrin injection.
■ The Schilling test may reveal a urinary excretion of less than 3% in the first 24 hours in patients with pernicious anemia; may reveal normal excretion of vitamin B_{12} when repeated with intrinsic factor added.

Treatment

GENERAL
■ Based on underlying cause

DIET
■ Well-balanced, including foods high in vitamin B_{12}
■ Sodium and fluid restriction for heart failure

ACTIVITY
■ If anemia causes extreme fatigue, bed rest until hemoglobin increases

MEDICATION
■ Early I.M. vitamin B_{12} replacement
■ Maintenance levels (monthly) of vitamin B_{12} doses, after the patient's condition improves

MONITORING
■ Vital signs
■ Mental and neurologic status

ANEMIA, SICKLE CELL

Overview

DESCRIPTION
■ Congenital hemolytic disease that results from a defective hemoglobin (Hb) molecule (HbS) that causes red blood cells (RBCs) to become sickle shaped
■ Sickle-shaped cells impair circulation, resulting in chronic ill health (fatigue, dyspnea on exertion, swollen joints), periodic crises, long-term complications, and premature death
■ No cure

PATHOPHYSIOLOGY
■ The abnormal HbS found in the patient's RBCs becomes insoluble whenever hypoxia occurs.
■ The RBCs become rigid, rough, and elongated, forming a crescent or sickle shape.
■ Sickling can produce hemolysis (cell destruction).
■ The altered cells accumulate in capillaries and smaller blood vessels, making the blood more viscous.
■ Normal circulation is impaired, causing pain, tissue infarctions, and swelling.

CAUSES
■ Homozygous inheritance of the HbS-producing gene (defective Hb gene from each parent)

COMPLICATIONS
■ Chronic obstructive pulmonary disease
■ Heart failure
■ Retinopathy
■ Nephropathy

Assessment

HISTORY
■ Signs and symptoms usually don't develop until after age 6 months
■ Chronic fatigue
■ Unexplained dyspnea or dyspnea on exertion
■ Joint swelling
■ Aching bones

- Chest pain
- Ischemic leg ulcers
- Increased susceptibility to infection
- Pulmonary infarctions and cardiomegaly

PHYSICAL FINDINGS

- Jaundice or pallor
- May appear small in stature for age
- Delayed growth and puberty
- Spiderlike body build (narrow shoulders and hips, long extremities, curved spine, and barrel chest) in adult
- Tachycardia
- Hepatomegaly and, in children, splenomegaly
- Systolic and diastolic murmurs
- Sleepiness with difficulty awakening
- Hematuria
- Pale lips, tongue, palms, and nail beds
- Body temperature over 104° F (40° C) or a temperature of 100° F (37.8° C) that persists for 2 or more days

TEST RESULTS
Laboratory

- Stained blood smear that shows sickle cells and Hb electrophoresis showing HbS (Electrophoresis should be done on umbilical cord blood samples at birth to provide sickle cell disease screening for all neonates at risk.)
- Low RBC counts, elevated white blood cell and platelet counts, decreased erythrocyte sedimentation rate, increased serum iron levels
- Complete blood count (CBC) that reveals decreased RBC survival and reticulocytosis; normal or low Hb levels

Imaging

- A lateral chest X-ray detects the characteristic "Lincoln log" deformity. (This spinal abnormality develops in many adults and some adolescents with sickle cell anemia, leaving the vertebrae resembling logs that form the corner of a cabin.)

Diagnostic procedures

- Corkscrew or comma-shaped vessels in the conjunctivae are detected by an ophthalmoscopic examination.

Treatment

GENERAL

- Avoidance of extreme temperatures
- Avoidance of stress

DIET

- Well-balanced
- Adequate amounts of folic acid-rich foods
- Adequate fluid intake

ACTIVITY

- Bed rest with crises
- As tolerated

MEDICATION

- Anti-infectives and vaccines to prevent illness
- Analgesics
- Iron supplements
- Transfusion of packed RBCs, if Hb level decreases suddenly or if condition deteriorates rapidly
- Sedation and administration of analgesics, blood transfusion, oxygen therapy, and large amounts of oral or I.V. fluids, in an acute sequestration crisis

MONITORING

- Vital signs
- Intake and output
- CBC and other laboratory study results

HEMATOLOGIC AND
IMMUNE CARE

DISSEMINATED INTRAVASCULAR COAGULATION

Overview

DESCRIPTION

- Complicates diseases and conditions that accelerate clotting, causing occlusion of small blood vessels, organ necrosis, depletion of circulating clotting factors and platelets, and activation of the fibrinolytic system
- Also known as DIC, consumption coagulopathy, and defibrination syndrome

PATHOPHYSIOLOGY

- Typical accelerated clotting results in generalized activation of prothrombin and a consequent excess of thrombin.
- Excess thrombin converts fibrinogen to fibrin, producing fibrin clots in the microcirculation.
- This process consumes exorbitant amounts of coagulation factors (especially platelets, factor V, prothrombin, fibrinogen, and factor VIII), causing thrombocytopenia, deficiencies in factors V and VIII, hypoprothrombinemia, and hypofibrinogenemia.
- Circulating thrombin activates the fibrinolytic system, which lyses fibrin clots into fibrin degradation products.
- The hemorrhage that occurs may be due largely to the anticoagulant activity of fibrin degradation products and depletion of plasma coagulation factors.

CAUSES

- Infection, sepsis
- Obstetric complications
- Neoplastic disease
- Disorders that produce necrosis, such as extensive burns and trauma
- Other disorders, such as heatstroke, shock, incompatible blood transfusion, drug reactions, cardiac arrest, surgery necessitating cardiopulmonary bypass, adult respiratory distress syndrome, diabetic ketoacidosis, pulmonary embolism

COMPLICATIONS

- Renal failure
- Hepatic damage
- Stroke
- Ischemic bowel
- Respiratory distress
- Death (mortality is greater than 50%)

Assessment

HISTORY

- Abnormal bleeding *without* a history of a serious hemorrhagic disorder; bleeding may occur at all bodily orifices
- Possible presence of one of the causes of DIC
- Possible signs of bleeding into the skin, such as cutaneous oozing, petechiae, ecchymoses, and hematomas
- Possible bleeding from surgical or invasive procedure sites, such as incisions or venipuncture sites
- Possible nausea and vomiting; severe muscle, back, and abdominal pain; chest pain; hemoptysis; epistaxis; seizures; and oliguria
- Possible GI bleeding, hematuria

PHYSICAL FINDINGS

- Petechiae
- Acrocyanosis
- Dyspnea, tachypnea
- Mental status changes, including confusion

TEST RESULTS
Laboratory

- Decreased serum platelet count (less than 100,00/µl)

- Decreased serum fibrinogen level (less than 150 mg/dl)
- Prolonged prothrombin time (more than 15 seconds)
- Prolonged partial thromboplastin time (more than 60 seconds)
- Increased fibrin degradation products (commonly greater than 45 mcg/ml)
- Positive D-dimer test (specific fibrinogen test for DIC) at less than 1:8 dilution
- Prolonged thrombin time
- Diminished blood clotting factors V and VIII
- Complete blood count showing decreased hemoglobin levels (less than 10 g/dl)
- Elevated blood urea nitrogen (greater than 25 mg/dl) and elevated serum creatinine levels (greater than 1.3 mg/dl)

Treatment

GENERAL
- Possibly supportive care alone if the patient isn't actively bleeding

DIET
- No restrictions

ACTIVITY
- As tolerated

MEDICATION
If the patient is actively bleeding
- Administration of blood, fresh frozen plasma, platelets, or packed red blood cells
- Heparin therapy
- Antithrombin III
- Fluid replacement

MONITORING
- Vital signs
- Results of serial blood studies
- Venipuncture sites and injection sites (apply pressure to injection sites for at least 15 minutes)
- Abdominal girth
- Signs of shock
- Intake and output, especially when administering blood products
- Test stool and urine for occult blood

SYSTEMIC LUPUS ERYTHEMATOSUS

Overview

DESCRIPTION
- A chronic inflammatory autoimmune disorder that affects connective tissues
- Two forms: discoid lupus erythematosus (DLE) and systemic lupus erythematosus (SLE)
- Only the skin affected by DLE

PATHOPHYSIOLOGY
- The body produces antibodies, such as antinuclear antibodies (ANAs), against its own cells.
- The formed antigen-antibody complexes suppress the body's normal immunity and damage tissues.

CAUSES
- Unknown
- Predisposing factors: stress, streptococcal or viral infections, exposure to sunlight or ultraviolet light, injury, surgery, exhaustion, emotional upsets, immunization, pregnancy, and abnormal estrogen metabolism

COMPLICATIONS
- Pleurisy
- Pleural effusions
- Pericarditis, myocarditis, endocarditis
- Coronary atherosclerosis
- Renal failure

Assessment

HISTORY
- Onset acute or insidious; no characteristic clinical pattern
- Possible fever, anorexia, weight loss, malaise, fatigue, abdominal pain, nausea, vomiting, diarrhea, constipation, rash, and polyarthralgia
- Possible drug history with one of 25 drugs that can cause SLE-like reaction
- Irregular menstruation
- Chest pain and dyspnea
- Emotional instability, headaches, irritability, and depression
- Oliguria, urinary frequency, dysuria

PHYSICAL FINDINGS
- Joint involvement that resembles rheumatoid arthritis
- Raynaud's phenomenon
- Skin eruptions provoked or aggravated by sunlight or ultraviolet light
- Tachycardia, central cyanosis, and hypotension
- Altered level of consciousness, weakness of the extremities, and speech disturbances
- Skin lesions
- Butterfly rash over nose and cheeks
- Patchy alopecia (common)
- Vasculitis
- Lymph node enlargement (diffuse or local and nontender)
- Pericardial friction rub

TEST RESULTS
Laboratory
- Complete blood count with differential showing anemia and a reduced white blood cell (WBC) count; decreased platelet count; elevated erythrocyte sedimentation rate; and serum electrophoresis showing hypergammaglobulinemia
- Positive ANA, anti-DNA, and lupus erythematosus cell test findings in most patients with active SLE, but only slightly useful in diagnosing the disease (the ANA test is sensitive but not specific for SLE)
- Urine studies showing red blood cells, WBCs, urine casts and sediment, and significant protein loss
- Blood studies demonstrating decreased serum complement (C3 and C4) levels, indicating active disease
- Increased C-reactive protein during flare-ups
- Positive rheumatoid factor in 30% to 40% of patients

Imaging
- Chest X-rays may disclose pleurisy.

Diagnostic procedures
- Central nervous system (CNS) involvement may account for abnormal EEG. But brain and magnetic resonance imaging scans may be normal in patients with SLE despite CNS disease.
- Electrocardiography may show a conduction defect with cardiac involvement or pericarditis.
- Renal biopsy shows progression of SLE and the extent of renal involvement.

Treatment

GENERAL
- Use of sunscreen agents with sun protection factor of at least 15

DIET
- No restrictions unless renal failure

ACTIVITY
- Regular exercise program

MEDICATION
- Nonsteroidal anti-inflammatory drugs
- Topical corticosteroid creams
- Fluorinated steroids

- Antimalarials
- Corticosteroids
- Cytotoxic drugs
- Antihypertensives

SURGERY
- Possible joint replacement

MONITORING
- Signs and symptoms of organ involvement
- Urine, stools, and GI secretions for blood
- Scalp for hair loss and skin and mucous membranes for petechiae, bleeding, ulceration, pallor, and bruising
- Response to treatment
- Complications
- Nutritional status
- Joint mobility
- Seizure activity

THALASSEMIA

Overview

DESCRIPTION
- A group of genetic disorders
- Characterized by defective synthesis in one or more of the polypeptide chains necessary for hemoglobin (Hb) production
- Most commonly occurring as a result of reduced or absent production of alpha or beta chains
- Affects Hb production and impairs red blood cell (RBC) synthesis

PATHOPHYSIOLOGY
In beta-thalassemia
- The fundamental defect is the uncoupling of alpha- and beta-chain synthesis.
- Beta-chain production is depressed—moderately in beta-thalassemia minor and severely in beta-thalassemia major (also called Cooley's anemia).
- Depression of beta-chain synthesis results in erythrocytes with reduced hemoglobin and accumulations of free-alpha chains.
- The free-alpha chains are unstable and easily precipitate in the cell; most erythroblasts that contain precipitates are destroyed by mononuclear phagocytes in the marrow, resulting in ineffective erythropoiesis and anemia.
- Some precipitate-carrying cells mature and enter the bloodstream but are destroyed prematurely in the spleen, resulting in mild hemolytic anemia.

In alpha-thalassemia
- Four forms exist:
  – alpha trait (the carrier trait): a single alpha-chain-forming gene is defective
  – alpha-thalassemia minor: two genes are defective
  – hemoglobin H disease: three genes are defective
  – alpha-thalassemia major: all four alpha-chain-forming genes are defective; death is inevitable because alpha chains are absent and oxygen can't be released to the tissues.

CAUSES
- Inherited autosomal recessive disorder

COMPLICATIONS
- Iron overload from RBC transfusions
- Pathologic fractures
- Cardiac arrhythmias
- Liver failure
- Heart failure
- Death

Assessment

HISTORY
■ Severity of anemia and symptoms range from mild to severe, including:
– fatigue
– shortness of breath
– headache
– angina.

PHYSICAL FINDINGS
■ Pallor or bronze appearance
■ Dyspnea on exertion
■ Splenomegaly
■ Hepatomegaly
■ Tachycardia
■ Systolic murmur (in moderate or severe anemia)

TEST RESULTS
Laboratory
■ Complete blood count showing decreased Hb, hematocrit, and mean corpuscular volume
■ Normal or increased serum iron
■ Normal or increased serum ferritin
■ Normal total iron-binding capacity
■ Normal or increased reticulocyte count
■ Hb electrophoresis showing decreased alpha- or beta-hemoglobulin chains

Imaging
■ In thalassemia major, X-rays of the skull and long bones show thinning and widening of the marrow space because of overactive bone marrow.

Long bones may show areas of osteoporosis. The phalanges may also be deformed (rectangular or biconvex). The bones of the skull and vertebrae may appear granular.

Treatment

GENERAL
■ No treatment for mild or moderate forms
■ Iron supplements contraindicated in all forms

DIET
■ Avoidance of iron-rich foods

ACTIVITY
■ Avoidance of strenuous activities

MEDICATION
■ Transfusions of packed RBCs
■ Desferal (chelation therapy)

SURGERY
■ Splenectomy
■ Bone marrow transplantation

MONITORING
■ Transfusion reaction
■ Signs and symptoms of iron overload
■ Complications
■ Cardiac arrhythmias
■ Anemia symptom severity
■ Response to treatment

TREATMENTS

BONE MARROW TRANSPLANTATION

Overview

- Infusion of fresh or stored bone marrow
- Autologous donation: bone marrow harvested from the patient (before chemotherapy or radiation, or during remission) and frozen for later use
- Syngeneic donation: bone marrow donated by the patient's identical twin
- Allogeneic donation: bone marrow donated by a histocompatible individual
- Peripheral stem cell transplantation: peripheral stem cells collected from the patient (usually after chemotherapy or growth factor treatment) and stored for later reinfusion

INDICATIONS

- Aplastic anemia
- Severe combined immunodeficiency disease
- Acute leukemia
- Chronic leukemia
- Lymphoma
- Multiple myeloma
- Certain solid tumors
- Sickle cell anemia

COMPLICATIONS
During infusion

- Fluid volume overload
- Anaphylaxis
- Pulmonary fat embolism

After infusion

- Infection
- Abnormal bleeding
- Renal insufficiency
- Venous occlusive disease

- With allogeneic donation: graft-versus-host disease (GVHD)

Nursing interventions

PRETREATMENT CARE

- Explain the treatment and patient preparation.
- Make sure the patient has signed an appropriate consent form.
- Keep diphenhydramine and epinephrine readily available to manage transfusion reactions.
- Start an I.V. line.
- Administer I.V. fluids as ordered.
- Obtain an administration set without a filter for bone marrow infusion.
- Administer medications such as prophylactic antiemetics as ordered.

Monitoring

- During pretransplantation regimen: adverse reactions
- During transfusion: vital signs
- Bronchospasm
- Urticaria
- Erythema
- Chest pain
- Back pain

POSTTREATMENT CARE

- Maintain asepsis.
- Institute safety measures.
- Administer ordered transfusions.
- Obtain blood samples for laboratory analysis as ordered.

Monitoring

- Vital signs
- Infection
- Hemorrhage
- Laboratory results
- GVHD

PATIENT TEACHING

Be sure to cover:
- medications and possible adverse reactions
- infection control measures
- bleeding precautions
- central venous catheter care
- signs and symptoms of transplant failure
- complications
- when to notify the physician
- emergency telephone numbers
- follow-up care.

SPLENECTOMY

Overview

- Surgical removal of the spleen

INDICATIONS

- Hematologic disorders
- Traumatic splenic rupture
- Hypersplenism
- Hereditary spherocytosis
- Chronic idiopathic thrombocytopenic purpura
- Hodgkin's disease

COMPLICATIONS

- Bleeding
- Infection
- Pneumonia
- Atelectasis

Nursing interventions

PRETREATMENT CARE

- Explain the treatment and preparation to the patient and his family.
- Make sure the patient has signed an appropriate consent form.
- Report abnormal results of blood studies.
- Administer blood products, vitamin K, or fresh frozen plasma as ordered.

- Obtain vital signs, and perform a baseline respiratory assessment.
- Notify the physician if you suspect respiratory infection; surgery may be delayed.
- Explain postoperative care.

POSTTREATMENT CARE

- Administer medications and I.V. fluids as ordered.
- Assist with early ambulation.
- Encourage coughing, deep breathing, and incentive spirometry use.
- Administer analgesics as needed and ordered.
- Provide comfort measures.
- Provide incision care as ordered.
- Change dressings as ordered.
- Maintain patency of drains.

Monitoring

- Vital signs
- Intake and output
- Complications
- Surgical wound and dressings
- Drainage
- Abnormal bleeding
- Hematologic studies
- Infection

PATIENT TEACHING

Be sure to cover:
- medications and potential adverse reactions
- coughing and deep-breathing techniques
- signs and symptoms of infection
- complications
- when to notify the physician
- ways to prevent infection
- incision care
- follow-up care.

PROCEDURES
AND EQUIPMENT

BLOOD TRANSFUSIONS:
CHECK, VERIFY, AND INSPECT

The most common cause of a severe transfusion reaction is receiving the wrong blood. Before administering any blood or blood product, take the steps described here.

Check
Check to make sure an informed consent form was signed. Then double-check the patient's name, medical record number, ABO blood group, Rh status (and other compatibility factors), and blood bank identification number against the label on the blood bag. Also check the expiration date on the bag.

Verify
Ask another nurse or physician to verify all information, according to your facility's policy. (Some facilities routinely require double identification.) Make sure

that you and the nurse or physician who checked the blood or blood product have signed the blood confirmation slip. If even a slight discrepancy exists, don't administer the blood or blood product. Instead, immediately notify the blood bank.

Inspect
Inspect the blood or blood product to detect abnormalities. Then confirm the patient's identity by checking the name, room number, and bed number on his wristband.

TRANSFUSION DON'TS

A blood transfusion requires extreme care. Here are some tips on what not to do when administering a transfusion:

■ Don't add any medications to the blood bag.
■ Never give blood products without checking the order against the blood bag label — the only way to tell if the request form has been stamped with the wrong name. Most life-threatening reactions occur when this step is omitted.
■ Don't transfuse the blood product if you discover a discrepancy in the blood number, blood slip type, or patient identification number.
■ Don't piggyback blood into the port of an existing infusion set. Most solu-

tions, including dextrose in water, are incompatible with blood. Administer blood only with normal saline solution.
■ Don't hesitate to stop the transfusion if your patient shows changes in vital signs, is dyspneic or restless, or develops chills, hematuria, or pain in the flank, chest, or back. Your patient could go into shock, so don't remove the I.V. device that's in place. Keep it open with a slow infusion of normal saline solution; call the physician and the laboratory.

MONITORING A BLOOD TRANSFUSION

To help avoid transfusion reactions and safeguard your patient, follow these guidelines:

■ Record vital signs before the transfusion, 15 minutes after the start of the transfusion, and just after the transfusion is complete, and more frequently if warranted by the patient's condition and transfusion history or the facility's policy. Most acute hemolytic reactions occur during the first 30 minutes of the transfusion, so watch your patient extra carefully during the first 30 minutes.

■ Always have sterile normal saline solution — an isotonic solution — set up as a primary line along with the transfusion.

■ Act promptly if your patient develops wheezing and bronchospasm. These signs may indicate an allergic reaction or anaphylaxis. If, after a few milliliters of blood are transfused, the patient becomes dyspneic and shows generalized flushing and chest pain (with or without vomiting and diarrhea), he could be having an anaphylactic reaction. Stop the blood transfusion immediately, start the normal saline solution, check and document vital signs, and call the physician and initiate anaphylaxis procedure.

■ If the patient develops a transfusion reaction, return the remaining blood together with a posttransfusion blood sample and any other required specimens to the blood bank.

TRANSFUSING PLASMA OR PLASMA FRACTIONS

To transfuse plasma or plasma fractions, follow these steps:

■ Obtain baseline vital signs.

■ Flush the patient's venous access device with normal saline solution.

■ Attach the plasma, fresh frozen plasma, albumin, factor VIII concentrate, prothrombin complex, platelets, or cryoprecipitate to the patient's venous access device.

■ Begin the transfusion, and adjust the flow rate as ordered.

■ Take the patient's vital signs, and assess him frequently for signs or symptoms of a transfusion reaction, such as fever, chills, or nausea.

■ After the infusion, flush the line with 20 to 30 ml of normal saline solution. Then disconnect the I.V. line. If therapy is to continue, resume the prescribed infusate and adjust the flow rate, as ordered.

■ Record the type and amount of plasma or plasma fraction administered, duration of transfusion, baseline vital signs, and any adverse reactions.

DRUGS

A LOOK AT COMMON HEMATOLOGIC MEDICATIONS

Drug	Indications	Adverse reactions	Special considerations
ANTICOAGULANTS			
Heparin (Heparin Sodium Injection	■ Prevention of pulmonary embolism and deep vein thrombosis (DVT) after hip or knee replacement surgery ■ Continuous I.V. or S.C. therapy for DVT, myocardial infarction (MI), pulmonary embolism	■ Hemorrhage, thrombocytopenia, chills, fever, pruritus, urticaria, anaphylactoid reactions	■ Never administer I.M. ■ Don't massage site after S.C. injection and rotate sites, keep record of sites. ■ Monitor platelet count and for signs of bleeding. ■ Check I.V. infusions regularly for under- and overdosing. Measure partial thromboplastin time (PTT) regularly. PTT values 1½ to 2 times the control values indicate anticoagulation. ■ Never piggyback other drugs into an infusion line while heparin infusion is running.
Warfarin (Coumadin)	■ Treatment of pulmonary embolism; prevention and treatment of DVT, MI, rheumatic heart disease with heart valve damage, atrial arrhythmias	■ Anorexia, nausea, vomiting, hematuria, hemorrhage, jaundice, urticaria, fever, headache	■ Prothrombin time (PT) determinations essential for proper controls; maintain PT at 1½ to 2 times normal. ■ Give drug at same time daily. ■ Regularly inspect for bleeding gums, bruises, petechiae, nosebleeds, melena, hematuria, and hematemesis. ■ Tell the patient to use electric razor, avoid scratching skin, and use soft toothbrush.

HEMATOLOGIC AND IMMUNE CARE

(continued)

A LOOK AT COMMON HEMATOLOGIC MEDICATIONS *(continued)*

Drug	Indications	Adverse reactions	Special considerations
BLOOD DERIVATIVES			
Normal serum albumin 5% (Albuminar-5); **normal serum albumin 25%** Albuminar-25)	■ Shock, hypoproteinemia	Headache, vascular overload after rapid infusion, hypotension, tachycardia, nausea, vomiting, dyspnea, pulmonary edema, chills, fever	■ Don't give more than 250 g in 48 hours. ■ Watch for hemorrhage or shock if used after surgery or injury ■ Watch for signs of vascular overload (heart failure or pulmonary edema). ■ Don't use cloudy solutions or those with sediment.
Plasma protein fractions (Plasmanate)	■ Shock, hypoproteinemia	■ Headache, hypotension or vascular overload after rapid infusion, tachycardia, nausea, vomiting, dyspnea, pulmonary edema, rash, fever, chills, back pain	■ Monitor blood pressure; slow infusion if hypotension occurs. ■ Watch for signs of vascular overload (heart failure or pulmonary edema). ■ Monitor intake and output; watch for decreased urine output. ■ Don't give more than 250 g in 48 hours.
HEMATINICS			
Ferrous sulfate (Feosol)	■ Iron deficiency	■ Nausea, epigastric pain, vomiting, constipation, black stools, diarrhea, anorexia	■ Dilute liquid preparations in orange juice or water, not milk or antacids. Give tablets with orange juice to promote absorption. ■ Give elixir with straw to avoid staining teeth. ■ May give between meals to avoid GI upset related to dose.

A LOOK AT COMMON HEMATOLOGIC MEDICATIONS *(continued)*

Drug	Indications	Adverse reactions	Special considerations
HEMOSTATICS			
Aminocaproic acid (Amicar)	■ Excessive bleeding resulting from hyperfibrinolysis	■ Dizziness, malaise, headache, seizures, arrhythmias, tinnitus, nausea, cramps, diarrhea, generalized thrombosis, elevated liver function tests, rash	■ Monitor coagulation studies, heart rhythm, and blood pressure; notify physician of changes. ■ Dilute solution with sterile water for injection, normal saline solution, D_5W, or Ringer's injection.
HEPARIN ANTAGONIST			
Protamine	■ Heparin overdose	■ Bradycardia, circulatory collapse, nausea, vomiting, pulmonary edema, acute pulmonary hypertension, anaphylaxis	■ Use cautiously after cardiac surgery. ■ Give slowly to reduce adverse reactions. ■ Watch for spontaneous bleeding.

DRUGS FOR IMMUNE DISORDERS

Drug	Indications	Adverse reactions	Special considerations
ANTIVIRALS			
Lamivudine (Epivir)	■ Treatment of human immunodeficiency virus (HIV) infection in combination with AZT	■ Headache, fatigue, dizziness, insomnia, neutropenia, anemia, thrombocytopenia, cough, fever, chills	■ Monitor serum amylase levels. Stop drug if clinical signs and symptoms suggest pancreatitis ■ Give with AZT. Not indicated for use alone.

(continued)

	DRUGS FOR IMMUNE DISORDERS *(continued)*		
Drug	**Indications**	**Adverse reactions**	**Special considerations**
ANTIVIRALS *(continued)*			
Stavudine (Zerit)	■ Treatment of HIV-infected patients who have received prolonged AZT therapy	■ Peripheral neuropathy, headache, malaise, insomnia, anxiety, dizziness, chest pain, abdominal pain, diarrhea, nausea, anorexia, weight loss, neutropenia, thrombocytopenia, anemia, rash, hepatotoxicity, chills, fever	■ May be taken with or without food. ■ Teach patient signs and symptoms of peripheral neuropathy, which is the major dose-limiting effect. It may not resolve after drug is discontinued.
Zalcitabine (Hivid)	■ Treatment of patients with advanced HIV infection who have demonstrated significant clinical or immunology deterioration	■ Peripheral neuropathy; headache; fatigue; confusion; seizures; heart failure; chest pain; cough; nausea; vomiting; diarrhea; constipation; esophageal ulcer; neutropenia; leukopenia thrombocytopenia; increased aspartate aminotransferase, alanine aminotransferase, and alkaline phosphate; pruritus; night sweats; arthralgia	■ Monitor liver function studies and pancreatic enzymes. ■ Use with extreme caution in patients with peripheral neuropathy. ■ Use cautiously in patients with a history of pancreatitis.
Zidovudine AZT (Retrovir)	■ Symptomatic HIV infection; including acquired immunodeficiency syndrome (AIDS)	■ Headache; seizures; paresthesia; somnolence; anorexia; nausea; vomiting; diarrhea; constipation; severe bone marrow suppression (resulting in anemia); rash; myalgia; fever; increased liver enzymes	■ Can cause a low red blood cell count. ■ Monitor blood studies every 2 weeks to detect anemia or granulocytopenia. ■ For I.V. use, dilute before administration. Remove the calculated dose from the vial; add to D_5W injection to achieve a concentration not exceeding 4 mg/ml. Infuse over 1 hour at a constant rate. Avoid rapid infusion or bolus injection

DRUGS FOR IMMUNE DISORDERS *(continued)*

Drug	Indications	Adverse reactions	Special considerations
IMMUNE SERUMS			
Hepatitis B immune globulin (HBIG, Bayhep)	■ Hepatitis B exposure	■ Urticaria; pain and tenderness at injection site; anaphylaxis; angioedema	■ Obtain history of allergies and reaction to immunizations. ■ Anterolateral aspect of thigh or deltoid areas are the preferred adult injection sites. ■ Requires immunization for exposure to hepatitis B.
Immune globulin, I.V. (Gamimune)	■ Bone marrow transplant, hepatitis exposure	■ Headache, faintness, nausea, vomiting, hip pain, chest pain, chest tightness, dyspnea, urticaria, muscle stiffness (at injection site), anaphylaxis, fever, chills, malaise	■ Inject into different sites, preferably anterolateral aspect of thigh or deltoid muscle for adults. ■ Use cautiously in patients with a history of cardiovascular disease or thrombotic episodes. ■ Have epinephrine available for anaphylactic reaction.
IMMUNOSUPPRESSANTS			
Cyclosporine (Sandimmune)	■ Prophylaxis of organ rejection in kidney, liver, bone marrow, and heart transplants	■ Tremor, headache, seizures, confusion, hypertension, nephrotoxicity, leukopenia, thrombocytopenia, hepatotoxicity, flushing, acne, infections, increased low-density lipoproteins, anaphylaxis	■ Measure oral doses carefully in an oral syringe. To increase palatability, mix with whole milk, chocolate milk, or fruit juice. Use a glass container to minimize adherence to container walls. ■ Dosage should be given once daily in the morning at the same time each day. ■ Patient may take with meals if drug causes nausea.

14

Eye, ear, nose, and throat care

ASSESSMENT

Eyes and ears: Normal findings

Inspection

■ No edema, scaling, or lesions on eyelids are apparent.

■ Eyelids completely cover the corneas when closed.

■ Eyelid color is the same as surrounding skin color.

■ Palpebral fissures are of equal height.

■ Margin of the upper lid falls between superior pupil margin and superior limbus.

■ Upper eyelids are symmetrical and lesion free, and don't sag or droop when the patient opens his eyes.

■ Eyelashes are evenly distributed and curve outward.

■ Globe of the eye neither protrudes from nor is sunken into the orbit.

■ Eyebrows are of equal size, color, and distribution.

■ Nystagmus isn't present.

■ Conjunctiva is clear with visible small blood vessels and no signs of drainage.

■ White sclera is visible through conjunctiva.

■ Anterior chamber is transparent and contains no visible material when you shine a penlight into the side of the eye.

■ Cornea is transparent, smooth, and bright, with no visible irregularities or lesions.

■ Lids of both eyes close when you stroke each cornea with a wisp of cotton, a test of cranial nerve V, the trigeminal nerve.

■ Pupils are round and equal sized, and they react normally to light and accommodation.

■ Both pupils constrict when you shine a light on one.

■ Lacrimal structures are free from exudate, swelling, and excessive tearing.

■ Eyes are properly aligned.

■ Eye movement in each of the six cardinal fields of gaze is parallel.

■ Auricles are bilaterally symmetrical and proportionately sized, with a vertical measurement of 1½″ to 4″ (3.5 to 10 cm).

■ Tip of the ear crosses the eye-occiput line, an imaginary line extending from the lateral aspect of the eye to the occipital protuberance.

■ Long axis of the ear is perpendicular to — or no more than 10 degrees from perpendicular to — the eye-occiput line.

Eyes and ears: Normal findings *(continued)*

- Ears and facial skin are the same color.
- No inflammation, lesions, or nodules are apparent.
- No cracking, thickening, scaling, or lesions are detectable behind the ear when you bend the auricle forward.
- There's no visible discharge from the auditory canal.
- External meatus is patent.
- Skin color on the mastoid process matches the skin color of the surrounding area.
- No redness or swelling is apparent.
- Otoscopic examination reveals normal drum landmarks and bright reflex, with no canal inflammation or drainage.

Palpation
- Eyelids show no evidence of swelling or tenderness.
- Globes feel equally firm, not overly hard or spongy.
- Lacrimal sacs don't regurgitate fluid.
- No masses or tenderness on the auricle or tragus is detectable during manipulation.
- Either there are small, nonpalpable lymph nodes behind the auricle or discrete, mobile lymph nodes with no signs of tenderness.
- Mastoid process has well-defined, bony edges, with no signs of tenderness.

NOSE AND THROAT: NORMAL FINDINGS

Inspection
Nose
■ Nose is symmetrical and lesion free, with no deviation of the septum or discharge.
■ Little or no nasal flaring is apparent.
■ Frontal and maxillary sinuses are nonedematous.
■ Patient can identify familiar odors.
■ Nasal mucosa is pinkish red, with no visible lesions and no purulent drainage.
■ There's no evidence of foreign bodies or dried blood in the nose.

Mouth
■ Lips are pink, with no dryness, cracking, lesions, or cyanosis.
■ Facial structures are symmetrical.
■ Patient can purse his lips and puff out his cheeks, a sign of an adequately functioning cranial nerve VII (facial nerve).
■ Patient can easily open and close his mouth.
■ Oral mucosa is light pink and moist, with no ulcers or lesions.
■ Palate is white and hard, or pink and soft.
■ Gums are pink, with no tartar, inflammation, or hemorrhage.
■ Teeth are intact, with no signs of occlusion, caries, or breakage.
■ Tongue is pink, with no swelling, coating, ulcers, or lesions.
■ Tongue moves easily and without tremor, a sign of a properly functioning cranial nerve XII (hypoglossal nerve).
■ Anterior and posterior arches are free from swelling and inflammation.
■ Posterior pharynx is free from lesions and inflammation.
■ Tonsils are lesion free and the right size for the patient's age.

■ The uvula moves upward when the patient says "ah," and the gag reflex occurs when a tongue blade touches the posterior pharynx, both of which are signs of properly functioning cranial nerves IX and X.

Throat
■ Neck is symmetrical with intact skin and no visible pulsations, masses, swelling, venous distention, or thyroid or lymph node enlargement.
■ There's normal rising of the larynx, trachea, and thyroid as the patient swallows.

Palpation
Nose
■ External nose is free from structural deviation, tenderness, and swelling.
■ Frontal and maxillary sinuses are free from tenderness and edema.

Mouth
■ Lips are free from pain and induration.
■ No lesions, unusual color, tenderness, or swelling is apparent on the tongue's posterior and lateral surfaces.
■ Floor of the mouth is free from tenderness, nodules, and swelling.

Throat
■ Lymph nodes are nonpalpable or feel soft, mobile, and nontender.
■ Thyroid isthmus rises when the patient swallows.

Auscultation
Throat
■ No bruits are heard over the carotid arteries or over the thyroid gland.

Eyes and ears: Interpreting your findings

After you assess the patient, a group of findings may lead you to suspect a particular disorder. The chart below shows common groups of findings for the signs and symptoms of the eyes and ears, along with their probable causes.

Sign or symptom and findings	Probable cause
Earache	
■ Sensation of blockage or fullness in the ear ■ Itching ■ Partial hearing loss ■ Possibly dizziness	Cerumen impaction
■ Mild to moderate ear pain that occurs with tragus manipulation ■ Low-grade fever ■ Sticky yellow or purulent ear discharge ■ Partial hearing loss ■ Feeling of blockage in the ear ■ Swelling of the tragus, external meatus, and external canal ■ Lymphadenopathy	Otitis externa, acute
■ Severe, deep, throbbing ear pain ■ Hearing loss ■ High fever ■ Bulging, fiery red eardrum	Otitis media, acute suppurative
Eye discharge	
■ Purulent or mucopurulent, greenish white discharge that occurs unilaterally ■ Sticky crusts that form on the eyelids during sleep ■ Itching and burning ■ Excessive tearing ■ Sensation of a foreign body in the eye	Bacterial conjunctivitis
■ Scant but continuous purulent discharge that's easily expressed from the tear sac ■ Excessive tearing ■ Pain and tenderness near the tear sac ■ Eyelid inflammation and edema noticeable around the lacrimal punctum	Dacryocystitis
■ Continuous frothy discharge ■ Chronically red eyes with inflamed lid margins ■ Soft, foul-smelling, cheesy yellow discharge elicited by pressure on the meibomian glands	Meibomianitis

(continued)

EYES AND EARS: INTERPRETING YOUR FINDINGS *(continued)*

Sign or symptom and findings	Probable cause
HEARING LOSS	
■ Conductive hearing loss ■ Ear pain or a feeling of fullness ■ Nasal congestion ■ Conjunctivitis	Allergies
■ Sudden or intermittent conductive hearing loss ■ Bony projections visible in the ear canal ■ Normal tympanic membrane	Osteoma
■ Abrupt hearing loss ■ Ear pain ■ Tinnitus ■ Vertigo ■ Sense of fullness in the ear	Tympanic membrane perforation
VISUAL BLURRING	
■ Gradual visual blurring ■ Halo vision ■ Visual glare in bright light ■ Progressive vision loss ■ Gray pupil that later turns milky white	Cataract
■ Constant morning headache that decreases in severity during the day ■ Possible severe, throbbing headache ■ Restlessness ■ Confusion ■ Nausea and vomiting ■ Seizures ■ Decreased level of consciousness	Hypertension
■ Paroxysmal attacks of severe, throbbing, unilateral or bilateral headache ■ Nausea and vomiting ■ Sensitivity to light and noise ■ Sensory or visual auras	Migraine headache

NOSE AND THROAT: INTERPRETING YOUR FINDINGS

After you assess the patient, a group of findings may lead you to suspect a particular disorder. The chart below shows common groups of findings for the signs and symptoms of the nose and throat, along with their probable causes.

Sign or symptom and findings	Probable cause
DYSPHAGIA	
■ Signs of respiratory distress, such as crowing and stridor ■ Phase 2 dysphagia with gagging and dysphonia	Airway obstruction
■ Phase 2 and 3 dysphagia ■ Rapid weight loss ■ Steady chest pain ■ Cough with hemoptysis ■ Hoarseness ■ Sore throat ■ Hiccups	Esophageal cancer
■ Painless, progressive dysphagia ■ Lead line on the gums ■ Metallic taste ■ Papilledema ■ Ocular palsy ■ Footdrop or wristdrop ■ Mental impairment or seizures	Lead poisoning
EPISTAXIS	
■ Ecchymoses ■ Petechiae ■ Bleeding from the gums, mouth, and I.V. puncture sites ■ Menorrhagia ■ Signs of GI bleeding, such as melena and hematemesis	Coagulation disorders
■ Unilateral or bilateral epistaxis ■ Nasal swelling ■ Periorbital ecchymoses and edema ■ Pain ■ Nasal deformity ■ Crepitation of the nasal bones	Nasal fracture
■ Oozing epistaxis ■ Dry cough ■ Abrupt onset of chills and high fever ■ "Rose-spot" rash ■ Vomiting ■ Profound fatigue ■ Anorexia	Typhoid fever

(continued)

EYES AND EARS: INTERPRETING YOUR FINDINGS *(continued)*

Sign or symptom and findings	Probable cause

NASAL OBSTRUCTION

- Watery nasal discharge
- Sneezing
- Temporary loss of smell and taste
- Sore throat
- Malaise
- Arthralgia
- Mild headache

Common cold

- Anosmia
- Clear, watery nasal discharge
- History of allergies, chronic sinusitis, trauma, cystic fibrosis, or asthma
- Translucent, pear-shaped polyps that are unilateral or bilateral

Nasal polyps

- Thick, purulent drainage
- Severe pain over the sinuses
- Fever
- Inflamed nasal mucosa with purulent mucus

Sinusitis

THROAT PAIN

- Throat pain that occurs seasonally or year-round
- Nasal congestion with a thin nasal discharge and postnasal drip
- Paroxysmal sneezing
- Decreased sense of smell
- Frontal or temporal headache
- Pale and glistening nasal mucosa with edematous nasal turbinates
- Watery eyes

Allergic rhinitis

- Mild to severe hoarseness
- Temporary loss of voice
- Malaise
- Low-grade fever
- Dysphagia
- Dry cough
- Tender, enlarged cervical lymph nodes

Laryngitis

- Mild to severe sore throat
- Pain may radiate to the ears
- Dysphagia
- Headache
- Malaise
- Fever with chills
- Tender cervical lymphadenopathy

Tonsillitis, acute

PROCEDURES

LARYNGOSCOPY, DIRECT

Overview

■ Visualization of the larynx using a fiber-optic endoscope, or laryngoscope, passed through the mouth or nose and pharynx to the larynx
■ Usually follows indirect laryngoscopy, a more common procedure

PURPOSE

■ To detect lesions, strictures, or foreign bodies in the larynx
■ To aid diagnosis of laryngeal cancer or vocal cord impairment
■ To remove benign lesions or foreign bodies from the larynx
■ To examine the larynx when the view provided by indirect laryngoscopy is inadequate
■ To evaluate symptoms of pharyngeal or laryngeal disease (stridor or hemoptysis)

PATIENT PREPARATION

■ Make sure the patient has signed an appropriate consent form.
■ Note and report all allergies.
■ Check the patient's history for hypersensitivity to the anesthetic.
■ Fasting is required for 6 to 8 hours before the test.
■ Sedation is administered to help the patient relax.
■ Medication is administered to reduce secretions.
■ A general or local anesthetic is administered to numb the gag reflex.

Teaching points
Be sure to cover:

■ the purpose of the study and how it's done.

POSTPROCEDURE CARE
■ Place the patient on his side with his head slightly elevated to prevent aspiration.
■ Restrict food and fluids until the gag reflex returns (usually in 2 hours).
■ Reassure that voice loss, hoarseness, and sore throat are most likely temporary.
■ Provide throat lozenges or a soothing liquid gargle after gag reflex returns.
■ Immediately report adverse reaction to the anesthetic or sedative.
■ Apply an ice collar to prevent or minimize laryngeal edema.
■ Observe sputum for blood and notify the physician immediately if excessive bleeding or respiratory compromise occurs.
■ After biopsy, instruct the patient to refrain from clearing the throat and coughing, and to avoid smoking as ordered.

Immediately report subcutaneous crepitus around the patient's face and neck — a sign of tracheal perforation.

Observe the patient with epiglottiditis for signs of airway obstruction. Immediately report signs of respiratory difficulty, such as laryngeal stridor or dyspnea. Keep emergency resuscitation equipment and a tracheotomy tray readily available for 24 hours.

Monitoring
■ Vital signs
■ Respiratory status
■ Voice quality
■ Adverse reaction to medications
■ Edema
■ Sputum

■ Subcutaneous emphysema
■ Bleeding

PRECAUTIONS
■ Direct laryngoscopy is contraindicated in patients with epiglottiditis unless performed in the operating room with resuscitative equipment immediately available.

COMPLICATIONS
■ Tracheal perforation
■ Adverse reaction to medications
■ Respiratory distress
■ Bleeding

Interpretation

NORMAL FINDINGS
■ There's no evidence of inflammation, lesions, strictures, or foreign bodies.

ABNORMAL RESULTS
■ Combined with results of biopsy, abnormal lesions suggest possible laryngeal cancer or benign lesions.
■ Narrowing suggests stricture.
■ Inflammation suggests possible laryngeal edema secondary to radiation or tumor.
■ Asynchronous vocal cords suggests possible vocal cord dysfunction.

OPHTHALMOSCOPY, HANDHELD

Overview

■ Magnified examination of living vascular and nerve tissue of the fundus, including the optic disk, retinal vessels, macula, and retina
■ Ophthalmoscope: used directly or indirectly; direct model is easier to use than indirect model

PURPOSE
■ To detect and evaluate eye disorders
■ To detect and evaluate ocular manifestations of systemic disease, such as diabetes mellitus and hypertension
■ To identify opacities of the cornea, lens, and vitreous as well as lesions of the retina and optic nerve

PATIENT PREPARATION
■ Make sure the patient has signed an appropriate consent form.
■ Note and report all allergies.
■ Check the patient's history for previous use of dilating eyedrops.
■ Check the patient's history for angle-closure glaucoma.
■ Advise the patient that eyedrops may be instilled to dilate the pupils.

Teaching points
Be sure to cover:
■ the purpose of the study and how it's done
■ who will perform the test and where.

POSTPROCEDURE CARE
■ If the eyes are dilated, protect the eyes from bright lights and explain the need to avoid driving or operating machinery until vision returns to normal.

PRECAUTIONS
Don't administer dilating eyedrops to a patient who has angle-closure glaucoma or a history of hypersensitivity reactions to the drops. Don't dilate the patient's pupils if head trauma or acute disease of the central nervous system is suspected.

COMPLICATIONS
■ Adverse reaction to mydriatics, if used, including photophobia and increased intraocular pressure

Interpretation

NORMAL FINDINGS

■ A visible red reflex is found.

■ A slightly oval optic disk, measuring 5 mm vertically lies to the nasal side of the fundus center. It's usually pink with darker edges at its nasal border.

■ The physiologic cup varies in size and tends to be larger in myopia and smaller in hyperopia; appears as a central depression in the surface of the disc.

■ A semitransparent retina surrounds the optic disk.

■ Retinal vessels, including venules and the slightly smaller arterioles, branch out from the disk.

■ Vessel diameter progressively decreases with distance from the optic disk.

■ Retinal arterioles are medium red in color; venules appear dark red or blue.

■ The macula, a small avascular area, appears darker than the surrounding retina.

■ In the macula's center lies a small, even darker spot, the fovea.

■ A tiny light reflex can be seen at the center of the fovea.

ABNORMAL RESULTS

■ Absent or diminished red reflex suggests possible gross corneal lesions, dense opacities of the aqueous or vitreous humor, cataracts, or detached retina.

■ Cloudy vitreous humor suggests possible inflammatory disease of the optic disk, retina, or uvea.

■ An elevated, increased vascular optic disk suggests possible optic neuritis.

■ A white-appearing disk suggests possible optic nerve atrophy.

■ Abnormal elevation of the disk, blurring of disk margins, engorged vessels, and hemorrhages suggest papilledema.

■ An enlarged physiologic cup appearing gray, with white edges suggests glaucoma.

■ A milky-white retina suggests the acute phase of central retinal artery occlusion.

■ Gray, elevated areas suggest retinal detachment.

■ A dark lesion suggests possible a choroidal tumor.

■ Retinal fibroses, patches of white exudate, and microaneurysms suggest complications of diabetes mellitus.

OTOSCOPY

Overview

■ Direct visualization of the external auditory canal and tympanic membrane (TM) through use of an otoscope

■ Indirectly provides information about the eustachian tube and middle ear cavity

PURPOSE

■ To detect foreign bodies, cerumen, or stenosis in the external canal

■ To detect external or middle ear pathology (infection or perforation)

■ To evaluate integrity and appearance of the TM

PATIENT PREPARATION

■ Make sure the patient has signed an appropriate consent form, if indicated.

Teaching points

Be sure to cover:

■ the purpose of the study and how it's done.

POSTPROCEDURE CARE

■ No specific postprocedure care is necessary.

Precautions

■ The otoscope should be held securely in the dominant hand.
■ The otoscope should be advanced slowly and gently.
■ Obstruction of the ear canal by cerumen or foreign matter obscures the TM.

Continuing to insert an otoscope against resistance can cause a perforation or other injury.

Complications
■ Perforation of TM

Interpretation

Normal findings
■ The TM is thin, translucent, shiny, and slightly concave. It appears pearl gray or pale pink, and reflects light in its inferior portion (cone of light) with clearly defined landmarks.
■ The short process of the malleus, manubrium, and umbo are visible but not prominent.
■ Blood vessels should be visible only in the periphery.

Abnormal results
■ Scarring, discoloration, retraction or bulging of the TM as well as the presence of drainage and scaly surface areas suggest pathology.
■ Movement of the TM in tandem with respiration suggests abnormal patency of the eustachian tube.
■ A dry, flaky auditory canal lining may suggest eczema.
■ An inflamed, swollen, and narrowed auditory canal, possibly with discharge, suggests otitis externa.

Diseases

Cataract

Overview

Description
■ Opacity of the lens or lens capsule of the eye
■ Common cause of gradual vision loss
■ Commonly affects both eyes
■ Traumatic cataracts usually unilateral

Pathophysiology
■ The clouded lens blocks light shining through the cornea.
■ Images cast onto the retina are blurred.
■ The brain interprets a hazy image.

Causes
■ Classified according to cause

Senile cataracts
■ Chemical changes in lens proteins in elderly patients

Congenital cataracts
■ Inborn errors of metabolism
■ Maternal rubella infection during the first trimester
■ Congenital anomaly
■ Genetic causes
■ Recessive cataracts may be sex-linked

Traumatic cataracts
■ Foreign bodies causing aqueous or vitreous humor to enter lens capsule

Complicated cataracts
■ Uveitis
■ Glaucoma
■ Retinitis pigmentosa
■ Retinal detachment
■ Diabetes

- Hypoparathyroidism
- Atopic dermatitis
- Ionizing radiation or infrared rays

Toxic cataracts
- Drug or chemical toxicity

COMPLICATIONS
- Complete vision loss

Possible complications of surgery
- Loss of vitreous
- Wound dehiscence
- Pupillary block glaucoma
- Retinal detachment
- Infection

Assessment

HISTORY
- Painless, gradual vision loss
- Blinding glare from headlights with night driving
- Poor reading vision
- Annoying glare
- Poor vision in bright sunlight
- Better vision in dim light than in bright light (central opacity)

PHYSICAL FINDINGS
- Milky white pupil on inspection with a penlight
- Grayish white area behind the pupil (advanced cataract)
- Red reflex is lost (mature cataract)

TEST RESULTS
Diagnostic procedures
- Indirect ophthalmoscopy reveals a dark area in the normally homogeneous red reflex.
- Slit-lamp examination confirms lens opacity.
- Visual acuity test result establishes the degree of vision loss.

Treatment

GENERAL
- Prior to surgery, eyeglasses and contact lenses that may help to improve vision
- Sunglasses in bright light and lamps that provide reflected lighting rather than direct lighting decreasing glare and aid vision

DIET
- No restrictions

ACTIVITY
- Restricted according to vision loss

MEDICATION
For cataract removal
- Nonsteroidal anti-inflammatory drugs
- Short-acting local anesthetic

SURGERY
- Lens extraction and implantation of intraocular lens
- Extracapsular cataract extraction
- Intracapsular cataract extraction
- Phacoemulsification

MONITORING
- Vital signs
- Visual acuity
- Complications of surgery

EYE, EAR, NOSE AND THROAT CARE

GLAUCOMA

Overview

DESCRIPTION
- Group of disorders characterized by high intraocular pressure (IOP) and optic nerve damage
- Two forms:
  - Open-angle (also known as chronic, simple, or wide-angle) glaucoma, which begins insidiously and progresses slowly

– Angle-closure (also known as acute or narrow-angle) glaucoma, which occurs suddenly and can cause permanent vision loss in 48 to 72 hours

PATHOPHYSIOLOGY

Open-angle glaucoma
■ Degenerative changes in the trabecular meshwork block the flow of aqueous humor from the eye, increasing IOP and resulting in optic nerve damage.

Angle-closure glaucoma
■ Obstruction to the outflow of aqueous humor is caused by an anatomically narrow angle between the iris and the cornea.
■ IOP increases suddenly.

CAUSES
Open-angle glaucoma
■ Degenerative changes

Angle-closure glaucoma
■ Anatomically narrow angle between the iris and the cornea
■ Attacks triggered by trauma, pupillary dilation, stress, or ocular changes that push the iris forward

RISK FACTORS
Open-angle glaucoma
■ Family history
■ Myopia
■ Ethnic origin

Angle-closure glaucoma
■ Family history
■ Cataracts
■ Hyperopia

COMPLICATIONS
■ Varying degrees of vision loss
■ Total blindness

Assessment

HISTORY
Open-angle glaucoma
■ Possibly no symptoms
■ Dull, morning headache
■ Mild aching in the eyes
■ Loss of peripheral vision
■ Halos around lights
■ Reduced visual acuity (especially at night) not corrected by glasses

Angle-closure glaucoma
 Angle-closure glaucoma typically has a rapid onset and is an emergency.
■ Pain and pressure over the eye
■ Blurred vision
■ Decreased visual acuity
■ Halos around lights
■ Nausea and vomiting (from increased IOP)

PHYSICAL FINDINGS
■ Unilateral eye inflammation
■ Cloudy cornea
■ Moderately dilated pupil, nonreactive to light
■ With gentle fingertip pressure to the closed eyelids, one eye feels harder than the other (in angle-closure glaucoma)

TEST RESULTS
Diagnostic procedures
■ Tonometry measurement shows increased IOP.
■ Slit-lamp examination shows effects of glaucoma on the anterior eye structures.
■ Gonioscopy shows angle of the eye's anterior chamber.
■ Ophthalmoscopy aids visualization of the fundus.
■ Perimetry or visual field tests show extent of peripheral vision loss.
■ Fundus photography shows optic disk changes.

Treatment

GENERAL
■ Reduction of IOP by decreasing aqueous humor production with medications

DIET
■ No restrictions

ACTIVITY
■ Bed rest (with acute angle-closure glaucoma)

MEDICATION
■ Topical adrenergic agonists
■ Cholinergic agonists
■ Beta-adrenergic blockers
■ Topical or oral carbonic anhydrase inhibitors

Occasionally, systemic absorption of a beta-adrenergic blocker from eyedrops can be sufficient to cause bradycardia, hypotension, heart block, bronchospasm, impotence, or depression.

SURGERY
■ For patients who don't respond to drug therapy:
– Argon laser trabeculoplasty
– Trabeculectomy

Angle-closure glaucoma
■ Laser iridectomy
■ Surgical peripheral iridectomy
■ In end-stage glaucoma, tube shunt or valve

LARYNGEAL CANCER

Overview

DESCRIPTION
■ Cancer of the larynx or voice box in which malignant cells are found in the tissues of the larynx

■ Squamous cell carcinoma most common form (95% of cases)
■ Adenocarcinoma and sarcoma are rare (5% of cases)
■ Tumor intrinsic (located on the true vocal cords; tends not to spread because underlying connective tissues lack lymph nodes) or extrinsic (located on another part of the larynx; tends to spread easily)

PATHOPHYSIOLOGY
■ Laryngeal cancer is classified by its location:
– supraglottic (on the false vocal cords)
– glottic (on the true vocal cords)
– subglottic (rare downward extension from the vocal cords).
■ Malignant cells that proliferate can cause swallowing and breathing impairment.
■ A tumor can decrease mobility of the vocal cords.

CAUSES
■ Unknown

RISK FACTORS
■ Smoking
■ Alcoholism
■ Chronic inhalation of noxious fumes
■ Familial disposition
■ History of gastroesophageal reflux disease

COMPLICATIONS
■ Increased swallowing difficulty and pain
■ Metastasis

Assessment

HISTORY
Stage I
■ Complaints of local throat irritation
■ 2-week history of hoarseness

Stages II and III
- Hoarseness
- Sore throat
- Voice volume reduced to whisper

Stage IV
- Pain radiating to ears
- Dysphagia
- Dyspnea

PHYSICAL FINDINGS
Stage I
- None

Stage II
- Possible abnormal movement of vocal cords

Stage III
- Abnormal movement of vocal cords; possible lymphadenopathy

Stage IV
- Neck mass or enlarged cervical nodes

TEST RESULTS
Imaging
- Xeroradiography, laryngeal tomography, computed tomography scan, and laryngography confirm the presence of a mass
- Chest X-ray result rules out metastasis

Diagnostic procedures
- Laryngoscopy allows definitive staging by obtaining multiple biopsy specimens to establish a primary diagnosis, to determine the extent of the disease, and to identify additional premalignant lesions or second primaries.

Other
- Biopsy identifies cancer cells.

Treatment

GENERAL
- Precancerous lesions — laser surgery
- Early lesions — laser surgery or radiation therapy
- Advanced lesions — radiation therapy and chemotherapy
- Speech preservation
- Speech rehabilitation (when speech preservation impossible) — esophageal speech, prosthetic devices, or experimental surgical reconstruction of the voice box

DIET
- Based on treatment options
- May require enteral feeding

ACTIVITY
- Frequent rest periods
- No restrictions

MEDICATION
- Chemotherapeutic agents
- Analgesics

SURGERY
- Cordectomy
- Partial or total laryngectomy
- Supraglottic laryngectomy or total laryngectomy with laryngoplasty

MONITORING
After partial laryngectomy
- Hydration and nutritional status
- Tracheostomy tube care
- Use of voice

After total laryngectomy
- Laryngectomy tube care
- Vital signs
- Postoperative complications
- Pain control
- Nasogastric tube placement and function

Otitis media

Overview

Description
- Inflammation of the middle ear associated with fluid accumulation
- Acute, chronic, suppurative, or secretory

Pathophysiology
- Differs with otitis media type.

Suppurative form
- Nasopharyngeal flora reflux through the eustachian tube and colonize the middle ear.
- Respiratory tract infections, allergic reactions, and position changes allow reflux of nasopharyngeal flora through the eustachian tube and colonization in the middle ear.

Secretory form
- Obstruction of the eustachian tube promotes transudation of sterile serous fluid from blood vessels in the middle ear membrane.

Causes
- Suppurative otitis media: bacterial infection with pneumococci, group A beta-hemolytic streptococci, staphylococci, and gram-negative bacteria
- Chronic suppurative otitis media: inadequate treatment of acute otitis episodes or infection by resistant strains of bacteria
- Secretory otitis media: viral infection, allergy, or barotrauma
- Chronic secretory otitis media: adenoidal tissue overgrowth, edema, chronic sinus infection, or inadequate treatment of acute suppurative otitis media

Complications
- Spontaneous rupture of the tympanic membrane
- Persistent perforation
- Chronic otitis media
- Mastoiditis
- Meningitis
- Cholesteatomas
- Abscesses, septicemia
- Lymphadenopathy, leukocytosis
- Permanent hearing loss and tympanosclerosis
- Vertigo

Assessment

History
- Upper respiratory tract infection
- Allergies
- Severe, deep, throbbing ear pain
- Dizziness
- Nausea, vomiting

Acute secretory otitis media
- Sensation of fullness in the ear
- Popping, crackling, or clicking sounds on swallowing or moving the jaw
- Describes hearing an echo when speaking

Tympanic membrane rupture
- Pain that suddenly stops
- Recent air travel or scuba diving

Physical findings
- Sneezing and coughing with upper respiratory tract infection
- Mild to high fever
- Painless, purulent discharge in chronic suppurative otitis media
- Obscured or distorted bony landmarks of the tympanic membrane in acute suppurative otitis media
- Tympanic membrane retraction in acute secretory otitis media
- Clear or amber fluid behind the tympanic membrane

■ Blue-black tympanic membrane with hemorrhage into the middle ear
■ Pulsating discharge with tympanic perforation
■ Conductive hearing loss

Chronic otitis media

■ Thickening and scarring of tympanic membrane
■ Decreased or absent tympanic membrane mobility
■ Cholesteatoma

TEST RESULTS
Laboratory

■ Culture and sensitivity tests of exudate showing the causative organism
■ Complete blood count showing leukocytosis

Imaging

■ Radiographic studies demonstrate mastoid involvement.

Diagnostic procedures

■ Pneumatoscopy shows decreased tympanic membrane mobility.
■ Tympanometry detects hearing loss and evaluates the condition of the middle ear.
■ Audiometry shows degree of hearing loss.
■ Pneumatic otoscopy may show decreased tympanic membrane mobility.

In adults, unilateral serous otitis media should always be evaluated for a nasopharyngeal-obstructing lesion such as carcinoma.

Treatment

GENERAL

■ In acute secretory otitis media, Valsalva's maneuver several times per day (may be the only treatment required)
■ Concomitant treatment of the underlying cause
■ Elimination of eustachian tube obstruction

DIET

■ No restrictions

ACTIVITY

■ No restrictions

MEDICATION

■ Antibiotic therapy
■ Aspirin or acetaminophen
■ Analgesics
■ Sedatives (small children)
■ Nasopharyngeal decongestant therapy

SURGERY

■ Myringotomy and aspiration of middle ear fluid, followed by insertion of a polyethylene tube into the tympanic membrane
■ Myringoplasty
■ Tympanoplasty
■ Mastoidectomy
■ Cholesteatoma excision
■ Stapedectomy for otosclerosis

MONITORING

■ Pain level
■ Excessive bleeding or discharge
■ Auditory acuity
■ Response to treatment
■ Complications

Watch for and immediately report pain and fever due to acute secretory otitis media.

RETINAL DETACHMENT

Overview

DESCRIPTION

■ Separation of the sensory retina from the underlying pigment epithelium
■ May be primary or secondary
■ Usually involves only one eye; may occur in the contralateral eye later

■ Rarely heals spontaneously; usually can be reattached successfully with surgery

■ Carries varying prognosis depending on the retinal area affected

PATHOPHYSIOLOGY

■ A hole or tear in the retina allows the liquid vitreous to seep between the retinal layers.

■ Liquid separates the sensory retinal layer from its choroidal blood supply.

CAUSES

■ Intraocular inflammation

■ Trauma

■ Age-related degenerative changes

■ Tumors

■ Systemic disease

■ Traction placed on the retina by vitreous bands or membranes

■ Hereditary factors, usually in association with myopia

RISK FACTORS

■ Myopia

■ Cataract surgery

■ Trauma

COMPLICATIONS

■ Severe vision impairment

■ Blindness

Assessment

HISTORY

■ Sensation of seeing floaters and flashes

■ Painless vision loss, described as sensation of looking through a veil, curtain, or cobweb

PHYSICAL FINDINGS

■ Visual field loss

TEST RESULTS
Imaging

■ Ocular ultrasonography may be used to examine the retina if the lens is opaque and shows intraocular and intraorbital pathology. It also commonly detects retinal detachments, characteristically producing a dense, sheetlike echo or a B-mode scan.

Diagnostic procedures

■ Direct ophthalmoscopy shows folds or discoloration in the usually transparent retina.

■ Indirect ophthalmoscopy shows retinal tears.

Treatment

GENERAL

■ Varies with location and severity of detachment

DIET

■ Nothing by mouth before surgery

ACTIVITY

■ Bed rest before surgery

■ Restriction of eye movements before surgery

■ Positioning of the patient's head to allow gravity to pull the detached retina closer to the choroid

MEDICATION

■ Antiemetics

■ Analgesics

■ Cycloplegics

■ Steroidal eyedrops

■ Antibiotic eyedrops

SURGERY

■ Cryothermy

■ Laser therapy

■ Scleral buckling

MONITORING

■ Localized corneal edema and perilimbal congestion after laser therapy

■ Persistent pain

■ Vital signs

■ Visual acuity

■ Response to treatment

TREATMENTS

CATARACT REMOVAL

Overview

- Removal of a cataract, or lens opacity
- May involve intracapsular or extracapsular cataract extraction
- May be followed by immediate placement of an intraocular lens implant

INDICATIONS

- Congenital cataract
- Traumatic cataract

COMPLICATIONS

- Pupillary block
- Corneal decompensation
- Vitreous loss
- Hemorrhage
- Cystoid macular edema
- Lens dislocation
- Secondary membrane opacification
- Retinal detachment

Nursing interventions

PRETREATMENT CARE

- Explain the treatment and preparation to the patient.
- Make sure the patient has signed an appropriate consent form.
- Explain that the patient will wear an eye patch temporarily after surgery.
- Perform an antiseptic facial scrub as ordered.

POSTTREATMENT CARE

- Institute safety precautions.
- Assist the patient with ambulation.
- Have the patient wear an eye shield, especially when sleeping.
- Maintain the eye patch.
- Approach the patient from the unaffected side.

Monitoring

- Vital signs
- Pain
- Bleeding
- Drainage
- Intraocular pressure
- Complications

PATIENT TEACHING

Be sure to cover:

- medications and possible adverse reactions
- importance of sleeping on the unaffected side
- temporary loss of depth perception and decrease in peripheral vision on the operative side
- avoidance of activities that increase intraocular pressure
- avoidance of strenuous exercise for 6 to 10 weeks postoperatively
- when to change the eye patch
- use of eye shield, especially during sleep
- importance of wearing dark glasses to relieve glare
- contact lens care if applicable
- likelihood of visual instability for several weeks after surgery
- increase in visual acuity as the affected eye heals
- follow-up care
- complications
- when to notify the physician (especially for sudden eye pain, red or watery eyes, photophobia, or sudden vision changes).

COCHLEAR IMPLANT

Overview

- Auditory prosthetic device that improves auditory awareness

■ Works by directly stimulating the auditory nerve that transmits impulses to the brain's hearing center

INDICATIONS
■ Deafness secondary to sensorineural hearing loss

COMPLICATIONS
■ Infection
■ Feelings of depression

Nursing interventions

PRETREATMENT CARE
■ Explain the treatment and preparation to the patient and his family.
■ Make sure the patient has signed an appropriate consent form.
■ When addressing the patient, speak slowly in a clear, loud voice. Give the patient time to process the information and respond.
■ Develop alternative communication methods if the patient can't hear.

POSTTREATMENT CARE
■ Report incisional redness, swelling, or drainage.
■ Administer analgesics as ordered.

Monitoring
■ Vital signs
■ Incision site
■ Drainage
■ Infection

PATIENT TEACHING
Be sure to cover:
■ medications and possible adverse reactions
■ sensorineural hearing loss
■ the fact that hearing won't return to preloss level
■ importance of learning how to interpret sounds produced by the device
■ complications
■ when to notify the physician
■ follow-up care.

CORNEAL TRANSPLANTATION

Overview

■ Replacement of a damaged part of the cornea with healthy corneal tissue from a human donor
■ May involve the full thickness or partial thickness of the cornea
■ Vision not completely functional until healing is complete; healing may take up to 1 year, during which time the sutures remain in place
■ Also called keratoplasty

INDICATIONS
■ Altered corneal clarity secondary to injury, inflammation, ulceration, or a chemical burn
■ Corneal dystrophy

COMPLICATIONS
■ Graft rejection
■ Wound leakage
■ Loosening of sutures
■ Dehiscence
■ Infection

Nursing interventions

PRETREATMENT CARE
■ Explain the treatment and preparation to the patient and his family.
■ Make sure the patient has signed an appropriate consent form.
■ Explain that a bandage and protective shield will be placed over the eye postoperatively.
■ Administer a sedative or an osmotic agent as ordered, to reduce intraocular pressure.

POSTTREATMENT CARE
■ Instill corticosteroid eyedrops or topical antibiotics as ordered.
■ Administer analgesics as ordered.

- Assist the patient to lie on the back or the unaffected side.
- Keep the head of the bed flat or slightly elevated as ordered.
- Assist the patient with ambulation.
- Keep all personal items within the patient's field of vision.

Monitoring

- Vital signs
- Dressings
- Drainage
- Pain

Immediately report sudden, sharp, or excessive pain; bloody, purulent, or clear viscous drainage; and fever.

PATIENT TEACHING

Be sure to cover:

- medications and possible adverse reactions
- signs and symptoms of graft rejection
- importance of assessing the graft *daily* for the rest of the patient's life
- the fact that healing will be slow and vision may not be completely restored until sutures are removed
- follow-up care
- avoidance of activities that increase intraocular pressure
- photophobia precautions
- importance of using an eye shield when sleeping
- avoidance of driving or participating in physical activities until the physician approves
- complications
- when to notify the physician.

PROCEDURES AND EQUIPMENT

HOW TO IRRIGATE THE EAR CANAL

Follow these guidelines for irrigating the ear canal.

- Gently pull the auricle up and back to straighten the ear canal. (For a child, pull the ear down and back.)
- Have the patient hold an emesis basin beneath the ear to catch returning irrigant. Position the tip of the irrigating syringe at the meatus of the auditory canal. Don't block the meatus because you'll impede backflow and raise pressure in the canal.

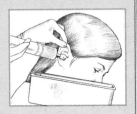

- Tilt the patient's head toward the opposite ear, and point the syringe tip upward and toward the posterior ear canal. This angle prevents damage to the tympanic membrane and guards against pushing debris farther into the canal.
- Direct a steady stream of irrigant against the upper wall of the ear canal, and inspect return fluid for cloudiness, cerumen, blood, or foreign matter.

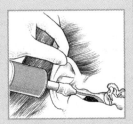

THREE DEVICES FOR EYE IRRIGATION

Depending on the type and extent of injury, the patient's eye may need to be irrigated using different devices.

Squeeze bottle

For moderate-volume irrigation — to remove eye secretions, for example — apply sterile ophthalmic irrigant to the eye directly from the squeeze bottle container. Direct the stream at the inner canthus, and position the patient so the stream washes across the cornea and exits at the outer canthus.

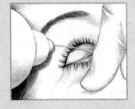

I.V. tube

For copious irrigation — to treat chemical burns, for example — set up an I.V. bag and tubing without a needle. Use the procedure described for moderate irrigation to flush the eye for at least 15 minutes. Alkali burns may require irrigation for several hours.

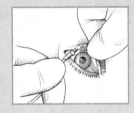

Morgan lens

Connected to irrigation tubing, a Morgan lens permits continuous lavage and delivers medication to the eye. Use an adapter to connect the lens to the I.V. tubing and the solution container. Begin the irrigation at the prescribed flow rate. To insert the device, ask the patient to look down as you insert the lens under the upper eyelid. Then have her look up as you retract and release the lower eyelid over the lens.

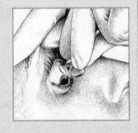

DRUGS

DRUG THERAPY FOR GLAUCOMA

Drug	Indications	Adverse reactions	Special considerations
ADRENERGICS			
Brimonidine (Alphagan); **dipivefrin** (Propine)	■ Intraocular pressure; reduction in open-angle glaucoma or ocular hypertension	■ Palpations and tachycardia ■ Blurred vision, headache, ocular stinging and burning ■ Photophobia, dry mouth	■ Explain that blurred vision may occur for a few minutes after application. Advise the patient not to drive until his vision clears. ■ Tell the patient that stinging and burning should diminish with continued therapy. If they don't, tell him to report it. ■ Tell him to discard the solution if it changes color. Also tell him to keep it refrigerated, protected from light, and tightly closed when not in use.
BETA-ADRENERGIC BLOCKERS			
Betaxolol (Betoptic); **carteolol** (Cartrol); **timolol** (Timoptic)	■ Chronic open-angle glaucoma and ocular hypertension	■ Insomnia, dizziness, headache ■ Hypertension, bradycardia, heart failure ■ Photophobia, eye stinging	■ Monitor vital signs and cardiac status. ■ Advise the patient to wash his hands before and after instilling and to apply light finger pressure on lacrimal sac for 1 minute after instilling. Advise him not to touch tip of dropper to eye. ■ Use cautiously in patients with chronic obstructive pulmonary disease, diabetes mellitus.

DRUG THERAPY FOR GLAUCOMA *(continued)*

Drug	Indications	Adverse reactions	Special considerations
CARBONIC ANHYDRASE INHIBITORS			
Acetazolamide (Diamox)	■ Chronic open-angle glaucoma ■ Preoperative management of acute angle-closure glaucoma	■ Confusion, drowsiness ■ Tinnitus, transient myopia ■ Anorexia, altered taste, hematuria	■ Monitor intake and output, weight, serum electrolyte levels. ■ Instruct the patient to consume fluids and foods high in potassium, such as orange juice and bananas. ■ If the patient is taking a single dose, advise him to take it in the morning after breakfast. If he's taking more than one dose a day, tell him not to take the last dose after 6 p.m. ■ Advise the patient to take the drug with meals if he has gastric upset. Tell him to drink plenty of fluids to prevent calculi formation.
DIRECT-ACTING CHOLINERGICS			
Carbachol (Carboptic); **pilocarpine hydrochloride** (Isopto Carpine)	■ Open-angle glaucoma ■ Emergency treatment of acute angle-closure glaucoma	■ Myopia, blurred vision, brow pain ■ Hypertension, tachycardia, bronchoconstriction	■ Tell the patient that blurred vision usually disappears in 10 to 14 days of therapy. Avoid operating machinery or driving until it subsides. ■ Use cautiously in the patient with acute cardiac failure, bronchial asthma, hyperthyroidism, GI spasm.

COMMON DRUGS FOR ALLERGIC RHINITIS

Drug	Indications	Adverse reactions	Special considerations
ANTIHISTAMINES			
Cetirizine (Zyrtec); **fexofenadine** (Allegra); **loratadine** Claritin)	■ Seasonal allergic rhinitis ■ Perennial allergies, rhinitis	■ Dizziness, gastric distress, hallucinations, drowsiness, dry mouth or throat ■ Cough, bronchospasm ■ Nausea, headache	■ Tell the patient that he can relieve a dry mouth by using warm water rinses, artificial saliva, ice chips, or sugarless gum or candy. ■ Warn him to avoid activities that require alertness, such as driving a car or operating machinery, until he knows how the drug affects his central nervous system (CNS). ■ Tell him that he can reduce GI distress by taking the drug with food or milk. ■ Caution him to consult his health care provider before using alcoholic beverages, tranquilizers, sedatives, pain relievers, sleeping medications, or other CNS depressants because these agents may increase sedation. ■ If he's taking an antihistamine, warn him to stop taking it 3 to 4 days before diagnostic skin (allergy) tests to ensure the validity of his test response.

COMMON DRUGS FOR ALLERGIC RHINITIS *(continued)*

Drug	Indications	Adverse reactions	Special considerations
CORTICOSTEROIDS (NASAL INHALANT)			
Beclomethasone (Vancenase); **budesonide** (Rhinocort); **flunisolide** (Nasalide)	■ Perennial or seasonal allergic rhinitis	■ Headache, dry mouth ■ Mild transient nasal burning and stinging ■ Nasal congestion ■ Epistaxis ■ Nasopharyngeal fungal infection	■ Instruct the patient to use the drug only as directed. ■ Use nasal inhalant cautiously in patients with tuberculosis, untreated fungal, bacterial, or systemic viral or ocular herpes simplex infections, or septal ulcers or nasal trauma. ■ Instruct the patient to shake container before use, to blow his nose to clear nasal passages, and to tilt his head slightly forward and insert the nozzle into nostril, pointing away from septum. Tell him to hold other nostril closed and inhale gently while spraying. Repeat in other nostril. Tell him to clean the nosepiece according to the manufacturer's instructions.

(continued)

COMMON DRUGS FOR ALLERGIC RHINITIS *(continued)*

Drug	Indications	Adverse reactions	Special considerations
DECONGESTANTS (NASAL)			
Naphazoline (Privine); **oxymetazoline** (Afrin); **phenylephrine hydrochloride** (Neo-Synephrine)	■ Nasal congestion	■ Restlessness, anxiety, headache ■ Rebound nasal congestion, sneezing, dryness of mucosa	■ Instruct the patient to rinse the tip of the spray bottle or nose dropper with hot water and dry it with a clean tissue. ■ Direct him to blow his nose gently to clear nasal passages before using medication. ■ For nasal drops, instruct the patient to tilt his head back as far as possible, instill drops, lean forward while inhaling, and then repeat the procedure for other nostril. ■ For nose drops, instruct the patient to tilt his head back as far as possible, instill the drops, then lean forward while inhaling. Repeat the procedure for the other nostril. ■ Emphasize that only one person should use a particular nose dropper or nasal spray device. ■ Advise him not to exceed the recommended dosage and to use the drug only when needed because rebound congestion may result from overuse. ■ Caution the patient with hypertension to use this drug only as directed.

COMMON DRUGS FOR ALLERGIC RHINITIS *(continued)*

Drug	Indications	Adverse reactions	Special considerations
DECONGESTANTS (NASAL) *(continued)*			
Pseudoephedrine hydrochloride (Sudafed)	■ Nasal and eustachian tube decongestion	■ Anxiety, tremor, dizziness, insomnia, nervousness ■ Cardiac arrhythmias, tachycardia, palpitations, hypertension ■ Nausea, vomiting, difficulty urinating	■ Use cautiously in patients with hypertension, cardiac disease, diabetes, glaucoma, hyperthyroidism, and prostatic hyperplasia. ■ Contraindicated in patients with severe hypertension and severe coronary artery disease.
MISCELLANEOUS			
Cromolyn sodium (Nasalcrom)	■ Prevention and treatment of allergic rhinitis	■ Monitor for anaphylaxis (angioedema, chest tightness, urticaria, increased wheezing), nausea, nosebleeds, painful urination, severe headache, and vomiting. ■ Bad taste in the mouth, cough, dizziness, joint pain and swelling, mild headache, nasal burning, nasal congestion, and sneezing	■ Instruct the patient to administer the drug at regular intervals to ensure effectiveness. ■ Direct him to clear his nasal passages by blowing his nose before administering the drug. ■ Mention that therapeutic effects may not occur for 2 to 4 weeks after initiating therapy. ■ If the patient is taking an adrenocorticoid, tell him to continue taking it during cromolyn therapy, unless his health care provider instructs him to do otherwise. ■ If the patient also uses a prescribed nasal decongestant, advise him to take a dose about 5 minutes before he takes cromolyn (unless otherwise indicated). This helps to distribute cromolyn in the airway.

INDEX